MEDICAL RADIOLOGY

Diagnostic Imaging and Radiation Oncology

Springer
Berlin
Heidelberg
New York
Barcelona
Hong Kong
London
Milan
Paris
Singapore
Tokyo

C. T. W. Moonen · P. A. Bandettini (Eds.)

Functional MRI

With Contributions by

G. K. Aguirre · D. C. Alsop · H. J. Aronen · J. Ashburner · P. A. Bandettini · V. Belle
K. F. Berman · J. R. Binder · B. B. Biswal · A. S. Bloom · T. S. Braver · R. L. Buckner
K. Bushara · R. B. Buxton · J. H. Callicott · B. J. Casey · W. Chen · E. R. Cohen · M. S. Cohen
R. J. Davidson · M. Décorps · C. Delon-Martin · M. D'Esposito · J. A. Detre · J. H. Duyn
G. F. Eden · J. A. Frank · L. R. Frank · K. J. Friston · J. S. Gati · G. H. Glover · R. Gollub
B. Goodyear · E. M. Haacke · M. Hallett · T. A. Hammeke · M. P. Harms · J. Hennig
M. Honda · X. Hu · W. Huang · J. S. Hyde · R. J. Ilmoniemi · W. Irwin · K. Ishii · C. R. Jack
C. Janz · P. Jezzard · A. Kastrup · R. P. Kennan · S.-G. Kim · W. Kuschinsky · S. Lai
L. Lamalle · N. Lange · T. H. Le · C. C. Lee · S. P. Lee · T. Q. Li · P. J. Magistretti · R. Massarelli
V. S. Mattay · B. Mazoyer · A. C. McLaughlin · J. R. Melcher · R. S. Menon · C. T. W. Moonen
M. E. Moseley · D. C. Noll · S. Ogawa · I. Pályka · C. S. Patlak · L. Pellerin · S. J. Peltier
N. F. Ramsey · M. E. Ravicz · S. J. Riederer · R. Risinger · M. Roth · B. K. Rutt · N. Sadato
R. Savoy · C. Segebarth · A. C. Silva · C. S. Springer, Jr. · E. A. Stein · V. A. Stenger
T. M. Talavage · K. R. Thulborn · K. M. Thomas · K. Ugurbil · P. Van Gelderen
A. L. Vazquez · A. Villringer · D. Waldvogel · H. A. Ward · D. R. Weinberger · R. M. Weisskoff
E. C. Wong · E. Yacoub · F. Q. Ye · T. A. Zeffiro

Series Editor's Foreword by
A. L. Baert

With 250 Figures in 398 Separate Illustrations, 110 in Color

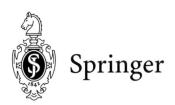 Springer

CHRIT MOONEN, PhD
Résonance Magnétique des Sytèmes Biologiques (RMSB)
UMR 5536 CNRS/Université Victor Segalen Bordeaux 2
146 rue Léo-Saignat, Case 93
F-33076 Bordeaux Cedex
France

PETER A. BANDETTINI, PhD
Assistant Professor
Biophysics Research Institute
Medical Colege of Wisconsin
8701 W. Watertown Plank Rd.
Milwaukee, WI 53226
USA

MEDICAL RADIOLOGY · Diagnostic Imaging and Radiation Oncology

Continuation of
Handbuch der medizinischen Radiologie
Encyclopedia of Medical Radiology

ISBN 3-540-64263-3 Springer-Verlag Berlin Heidelberg New York

Library of Congress Cataloging-in-Publication Data. Functional MRI / C. T. W. Moonen, P. A. Bandettini, eds.   p.   cm. -- (Medical radiology) Includes bibliographical references and index.   ISBN 3-540-64263-3 (alk. paper)   1. Brain-- Magnetic resonance imaging.   I. Moonen, C. T. W. (Chrit T. W.), 1955– . II Bandettini, P. A. (Peter A.)   III. Series. RC386.6.M34F86   1999   612.8'2--dc21   98-45190   CIP

Printed in Germany

Typesetting: Verlagsservice Teichmann, Mauer

SPIN: 10656324   21/3135 – 5 4 3 2 1 0 – Printed on acid-free paper

Foreword

With the advent of the new cross-sectional modalities: sonography, computed tomography, and magnetic resonance imaging, radiologic scientists have been able to achieve unprecedented precision in visualizing human morphology, including an amazingly exact display of normal anatomy of the living person as well as of the gross pathology of organs and diseases.

There cannot be any doubt that due to the revolutionary and innovative data provided by these new radiologic modalities, substantial progress has been achieved in delivering clinical care more appropriately and more rapidly and in better managing numerous illnesses in all organ areas and systems of the human body. It is now universally recognized that these diagnostic techniques, by virtue of their revolutionary morphological capabilities, have made a decisive impact on daily clinical practice in almost all disciplines of modern medicine.

However, during the last decade it has become increasingly more evident that, in addition to their morphologic dimension, the new cross-sectional modalities also possess a great potential for providing dynamic and functional information on physiologic and physiopathologic processes of the human body. The functional capabilities of sonography are receiving ever more attention due to the interesting possibilities provided by Doppler, color Doppler and power Doppler imaging. Functional applications of computed tomography have been proposed for several organs and are now routinely used in clinical practice in many institutions.

Exciting results have also been produced by research on the applications of functional magnetic resonance imaging (fMRI) to the cardiovascular system and the brain. More particularly, our ability to visualize active processes occurring in the human mind has ignited a great deal of enthusiasm among scientists and set off an explosive surge in research activity in the field of fMRI.

I am very grateful that C.T.W. Moonen and P.A. Bandettini, both leading specialists in the field of fMRI, accepted the challenging task of compiling and presenting a structured view of the numerous facts and data that have become available during the last few years in this emerging and rapidly evolving discipline. The editors have proven to be gifted and very successful in their selection of an impressive group of international experts in the field of fMRI. It is my great pleasure and privilege to congratulate the editors and the contributing authors on the excellent and up-to-date material that they have brought together in this latest volume of our series in Medical Radiology. Their impressive, combined efforts have resulted in an excellent work that will provide a solid learning base and efficient guidelines for clinical and research professionals engaged in this fascinating new discipline. I am convinced that this book will be well received by all of the latter and will enjoy great success. I would appreciate any constructive criticism that might be offered.

Leuven   ALBERT L. BAERT

Preface

The first papers on functional magnetic resonance imaging (fMRI) were published in 1991 and 1992, and in the short time since then, fMRI has already assumed a major role in mapping human brain activation. This explosive worldwide growth of fMRI is due to several of its distinctly advantageous characteristics. These include noninvasiveness, relatively high spatial and temporal resolution, and the ease in imaging underlying anatomy. In addition, fMRI can be performed on most conventional MRI scanners and has enough sensitivity to allow for the creation of high-quality functional maps within minutes. These advantages allow fMRI to be used for intra- and intersubject comparisons, which open up unique avenues of study and utility, including the study of mental disorders, brain plasticity, and learning-related changes.

The rapid feedback provided by fMRI data increases its clinical utility. Clinical uses include or will include presurgical mapping, evaluation of recovery from trauma, diagnostic aid for mental disorders, and baseline quantitative perfusion and blood volume maps for evaluation of vascular reserve, risk of stroke, or regions of chronically compromised blood perfusion.

Increased neuronal firing triggers local changes to many aspects of brain metabolism and brain physiology, changes that fMRI can often detect. BOLD (blood oxygen level dependent) contrast, for example, is sensitive to the regional level of deoxyhemoglobin. Other methods are sensitive to arterial, capillary, and venous flow. Interpretation of the fMRI signal in terms of such classic physiological parameters as perfusion, oxygen consumption, blood volume, and metabolic rate is, however, not straightforward and requires careful pulse sequence design, physiologic model construction, and MRI measurement techniques. In addition, fMRI signal changes are generally small, and attention must be paid to very rapid imaging methods, elimination of imaging artifacts, proper data processing, and statistical methods.

The purpose of this book is to provide a detailed, yet comprehensive overview of fMRI contrast mechanisms, implementation methods, temporal and spatial limits, and both basic and clinical applications. The intended audience includes all disciplines involved in fMRI: neuroscience, physics, statistics and mathematics, physiology, biochemistry, radiology, neurology, neurosurgery, psychology, pharmacology, and psychiatry. This book addresses both cutting edge topics such as event-related fMRI and basic issues such as the field strength dependence of BOLD contrast. Readers at all levels of fMRI knowledge and experience will find this book to be at once an in-depth and broad source of information on fMRI.

Experts from all fields of fMRI have participated in writing this book. In mid-1997 an outline of the book was our starting point. Our method was to approach several world experts in each field that was to be covered, and to provide them with this outline. The authors were asked to cover their specific subject within the field, but excursions into related fields were tolerated. We are very grateful to the overwhelmingly positive and timely responses of the authors, and for the many suggestions we received. We would like to thank all authors for their excellent and up-to-date chapters. Some overlap was unavoidable, and we did not make strict attempts to avoid it in the review process. Finally, we would like to extend our thanks to Prof. Albert Baert for giving us this wonderful opportunity to bring together all of the aspects of the current state of the art of fMRI and to Ursula Davis for advice and continuous guidance.

Bordeaux   C. T. W. Moonen

Milwaukee   P. A. Bandettini

Contents

General Physiology

1 Physiological Changes During Brain Activation

A. Villringer

CONTENTS

1.1
Introduction

The goal of functional neuroimaging is to map the activity of the living brain in space and time. The gold standard for measuring brain cell activity is direct and invasive electrical recording of membrane potential of individual neurons; however, such measurements are limited to certain experimental conditions. For studies on human subjects, noninvasive methods have to be applied and these methods have inherent limitations. There are two main approaches for noninvasive functional neuroimaging: (1) electrophysiological methods and (2) metabolic/vascular methods.

Electrophysiological methods, such as electroencephalography (EEG) and magnetoencephalography (MEG) (YANG et al. 1993), measure signals which arise as summations of electrical events in individual cells. The main advantage of these methods

is their excellent temporal resolution; the main disadvantage stems from the fact that only weighted averages (centers of gravity) of electrical brain activity can be recorded. It can be difficult to relate these signals to a defined anatomical structure and it is currently not possible to clearly define the spatial extent of an activated area.

Another group of functional neuroimaging methods measures metabolic or vascular parameters (for an overview see Table 1.1). The most important of these are positron emission tomography (PET) and functional magnetic resonance imaging (fMRI). Although these approaches are more indirect, they offer significant advantages, in particular very good spatial resolution, good delineation of the spatial extent of an activated area and precise matching to anatomical structures. The physiological basis of these methods is the fact that brain cell activity is associated with local changes in metabolism, in particular with glucose and oxygen consumption and via the so-called neurovascular coupling in cerebral blood flow (CBF) and oxygenation. In a way, nature performs a functional convolution of brain cell activity, f(x,t) at a given location x and time t with the function "g" which produces a certain change in metabolism and with the function "i" which produces a certain change in CBF (neurovascular coupling). The results are maps of metabolic [g(f(x,t)] and vascular [i(f(x,t)] events associated with changes in brain activity (Fig. 1.1). These maps can be measured by noninvasive imaging tools. The process of producing functional images by these imaging devices again can be regarded as a functional convolution. In order to understand the functional images obtained with these methods, it is therefore important to understand: (1) the relationship between local brain activity and the physiological parameters which are measured, and (2) the relationship between these physiological parameters and the obtained functional image (Fig. 1.1). In this chapter, both of these issues are discussed in detail.

A. Villringer, MD, Professor, Department of Neurology, Humboldt University, Schumannstrasse 20-21, 10117 Berlin, Germany

Table 1.1. Functional neuroimaging and physiological parameters

Physiological parameter	Method
Glucose consumption	FDG-PET, FDG-SPET
Oxygen consumption	O_2-PET
Cytochrome-C oxidase redox state	NIRS
Cerebral blood flow	H_2O-PET; xenon-, ECD-, HMPAO-SPET; fMRI (bolus track, flow-dependent); xenon-CCT; NIRS+contrast agent; TCD
Cerebral blood oxygenation (deoxy-Hb, oxy-Hb concentration)	fMRI (BOLD); NIRS, intrinsic optical signals

FDG, fluoro-deoxy glucose; PET, positron emission tomography; SPET, single photon emission tomography; NIRS, near-infrared spectroscopy; fMRI, functional magnetic resonance imaging; TCD, transcranial Doppler sonography; BOLD, blood oxygenation level-dependent contrast; ECD, ethyl cysteinate dimer; HMPAO, hexamethylpropyleneamineoxime; CCT, cranial computerized tomography.

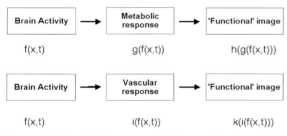

Fig. 1.1. Relationship between an ideal map of brain activity and metabolic and vascular maps, respectively, and generation of functional images

1.2
Translation of Maps of Brain Activity into Maps of Metabolism and Blood Flow

The replacement of the ideal map of brain activity at a level of individual cells by a map of the associated metabolic or vascular events is associated with a loss of information. This information loss occurs on at least three levels: (1) a qualitative reduction of many different types of brain cell activity into just one dimension of more or less brain activity; (2) a loss of spatial resolution; and (3) a loss of temporal resolution.

1.2.1
Reduction of Different Types of Brain Cell Activity into One Dimension of "Brain Activity"

The many different facets of brain activity such as synaptic excitation, synaptic inhibition, action potential of the neuron soma, and subthreshold depolarization are not reflected one by one in the metabolic or vascular response, rather they are all translated into just one dimension of metabolism/blood flow according to the respective energy need (JUEPTNER and WEILLER 1995). The metabolic change is probably not induced by the neuronal activity such as synaptic activity or the action potential itself but rather their consequences require energy and induce a metabolic response. A study on energy consuming processes in axonal terminals found that uptake of glucose correlated with the activity of the ouabain-sensitive sodium pump and it was concluded that this represented the critical event coupling energy consumption and neuronal activity (MATA et al. 1980). It seems it is in particular synaptic activity, rather than action potentials, in neuronal somata which is associated with changes in energy consumption. These conclusions are based on high-resolution autoradiography studies at a cellular level in rats (DUNCAN and STUMPF 1991, DUNCAN et al. 1987). These studies showed that most uptake of deoxy-glucose occurred in the neuropil and not in the cell bodies or in the glial cells. These results were confirmed by others (CLARKE and SOKOLOFF 1994, WREE and SCHLEICHER 1988). Regarding glial cells, however, the deoxy-glucose method may be misleading as an indicator of metabolic activity, since data by Magistretti's group (MAGISTRETTI and PELLERIN 1996) indicate that lactate, which stems from nonoxidative metabolism of glucose, in neurons is transported to glial cells which in turn produce energy from oxidative metabolism of lactate (see Chap. 3, this volume).

A number of studies have concluded that it is mainly presynaptic rather than postsynaptic activity which induces an increase in glucose utilization (SCHWARTZ et al. 1979; KADEKARO et al. 1985). A close coupling between synaptic activity induced by the major excitatory amino acid glutamate and oxidative glucose consumption has been reported recently (SIBSON et al. 1998). In this magnetic resonance spectroscopy study a stoichiometry of approximately 1:1 was found between oxidative glucose metabolism and glutamate-neurotransmitter cycling (between neurons and astrocytes). The authors concluded that (at least in their model of forepaw stimulation of the rat) a map of cortical oxidative glucose metabolism could provide a quantitative measure of synaptic glutamate release (SIBSON et al. 1998).

However, there are also other types of synaptic activity, in particular there is also inhibitory synaptic activity, and if presynaptic activity is the major determinant of related brain cell energy demand it seems questionable whether there should be a difference between excitatory vs inhibitory synaptic activity. Indeed, it has been shown that inhibitory as well as excitatory events may both induce increased energy need. In the context of functional activation, this has been demonstrated very nicely in a study on deoxy-glucose uptake in the lateral superior olive (LSO) within the brain stem auditory system during acoustic stimulation (NUDO and MASTERON 1986). It is known that the afferents from the ipsilateral ear are excitatory while the afferents from the contralateral ear are inhibitory. Stimulation, however, led to increased deoxy-glucose uptake in both, in the ipsilateral as well as in the contralateral auditory system (NUDO and MASTERTON 1986). Since there is a very close relationship between glucose consumption and blood flow it seems likely that these inhibitory and excitatory synaptic events also produce a blood flow change in the same direction.

Thus, with excitation and inhibition inducing the same type of changes, maps of metabolism and blood flow are principally ambiguous with respect to the underlying neurophysiological event. The phrase "increased brain activity," as it is used subsequently and (frequently unreflected) in most of the literature concerning brain metabolism and blood flow, therefore means a certain state of a certain volume of brain tissue which, through the summation of neuronal (and non-neuronal) events, is associated with increased energy need and blood flow. This underlying physiological event could be excitation or inhibition or any other energy consuming process.

However, to emphasize these principal shortcoming of metabolic/vascular neuroimaging does not mean that there are not ways to overcome them, at least partially. In many circumstances, previous knowledge of events in certain brain regions may help to constrain the possible types of neuronal events. For example, during the performance of saccades it has been shown, in invasive studies on monkeys, that the spontaneous neuronal activity in certain occipital neurons decreases (DUFFY and BURCHFIEL 1975). Based on this finding, a drop in metabolism/blood flow would be expected in the occipital cortex. Indeed, in human subjects, during performance of saccades, this has been found in a PET study (PAUS et al. 1995) as well as in fMRI (WENZEL et al. 1997). In this case, it therefore seems a plausible interpretation that the observed drop in CBF is related to the electrophysiological finding in monkeys of a decreased spontaneous brain cell activity in occipital neurons.

1.2.2
Loss of Spatial Resolution

Beside the qualitative reduction of several types of brain cell activity into just one dimension of more or less brain activity, there may also be a blurring of spatial information with regard to the underlying brain cell activity. For the metabolic response as measured, e.g., by glucose consumption, the spatial error is probably very small, whereas for the vascular response, it may be quite significant.

For the vascular response the spatial relationship to brain activity is given by the smallest vascular unit which adapts independently to brain activity. This is currently an issue of controversy. The smallest theoretically possible functional unit in the vascular system is a single capillary, and since precapillary sphincters anatomically do exist and since capillary walls contain some contractile elements (however no muscle cells) vasoregulation at the capillary level seems theoretically possible. As an extreme variant of vasoregulation at a capillary level, it has been claimed that complete opening and closing of capillaries and hence pronounced changes in capillary blood volume would represent a major mechanism of blood flow adjustment in the brain, the so-called capillary recruitment hypothesis (SHOCKLEY and LAMANNA 1988; WEISS 1988). However, a series of studies has now shown that already under resting conditions all cerebral capillaries are continuously perfused with plasma (GOBEL et al. 1989, 1990; VILLRINGER et al. 1994) and by far most of the capillaries also contain moving red blood cells (VILLRINGER et al. 1994; PAWLIK et al. 1981). It is concluded that capillary recruitment in the previously perceived yes or no sense is not a major mechanism for flow adjustment. Interestingly, capillaries, which were classically regarded as rigid tubes of fixed size, can change their diameter, e.g., during hypercapnia; thus, some minor change in capillary blood volume could be feasible during functional activation (DUELLI and KUSCHINSKY 1993; VILLRINGER et al. 1994).

Even if this classical concept of capillary recruitment has now been rejected, there may still be some regulation on the capillary level in a "more or less" fashion. Optical intrinsic signals, which are recorded by measuring the light reflected from exposed brain tissue, show functional maps at a precision of <100 µm, which is clearly below the vascular territory of one arteriole feeding capillaries. A detailed spectroscopic analysis of these optical signals has suggested that during the first seconds after stimulation onset beside a transient rise in [deoxy-Hb] there is also a rise in [oxy-Hb] which would mean an early change in capillary blood volume occuring before arteriorlar dilation (MALONEK and GRINVALD, 1996). This interesting finding, however, has been challenged recently (Mayhew et al., personal communication). Although this issue is by no means solved, presently there seems to be no convincing argument yet which seriously challenges the current textbook view, supported by a large body of previous work, that the smallest functional unit of vascular regulation in the brain is the feeding arteriole. Therefore the size of the vascular territory of one arteriole, which is on the order of >1 mm^3, is probably the smallest functional unit of the vascular response to brain activity.

1.2.3
Loss of Temporal Resolution

Whereas neuronal events occur on a time scale of milliseconds, metabolic and vascular events occur on a time scale of seconds. This sets limits to the possible temporal resolution of functional neuroimaging approaches based on metabolic/vascular imaging. The subsequent discussion refers to neurovascular coupling only, since there are no good data available on activity-metabolism coupling, due to the poor temporal resolution of the employed methods (e.g., autoradiography and PET). There are at least three types of temporal resolution to be considered:

1. The briefest possible neuronal event which induces a vascular response. It has been demonstrated that a visual stimulation as short as 30 ms still produced a vascular response. And although there is no systematic study on this issue, it seems quite likely, that even a very brief event on a millisecond time scale is associated with some metabolic/vascular response. The main limitation of whether this can be measured is probably the sig-

nal-to-noise ratio of the particular functional imaging method.
2. The second type of temporal resolution is the minimal separation in time of subsequent stimuli activating the same brain region. This temporal resolution is probably on the order of 1–2 s.
3. The third kind of temporal resolution refers to the temporal separation of events occurring in different brain regions. If the vascular response to neuronal activity has precisely the same temporal kinetics in every location in the brain, then this kind of temporal resolution could be much below 1 s. Recent data on hemifield visual stimulation seem to indicate that, for the temporal separation of activity in the left and right primary visual cortex, a temporal resolution on the order of 50–100 ms can be achieved (LUKNOWSKY et al. 1998).

The above mentioned shortcomings of metabolic/vascular imaging due to physiological events are further aggravated by limits in spatial and temporal resolution of the respective functional neuroimaging techniques, as outlined later in this chapter.

1.3
Changes in Cell Metabolism and Blood Flow During Functional Activation

Regarding the relationship between brain activity, metabolism and blood flow, based on studies in animals and human subjects, in the 1970s and 1980s a broad consensus was reached on a number of fundamental issues. These mainly related to a rest/baseline condition of the brain, and the answers which were given reflect the relationship between long-term (steady state) activity of a certain brain region and (long-term) adjustment of metabolism and blood flow. These long-term adjustments, however, may not necessarily reflect events occurring during short-term transient changes in brain activity, and in fact the confusion of these two situations has frequently confounded the discussion of these issues.

Concerning long-term adjustments of metabolism and blood flow, these are the generally accepted facts: Under normal conditions, the brain's almost exclusive source of energy is glucose (Clarke and Sokoloff 1994; Hasselbalch et al. 1994; Schwartz et al. 1979; Wree and Schleicher 1988). Therefore, local glucose uptake can be regarded as a very reliable

Table 1.2. Various physiological parameters are compared during different states of brain activity

	Long-term coupling[a]	Dynamic coupling[b]
Glucose consumption	↑	↑
Oxygen consumption	↑	→
Cerebral blood flow	↑	↑
Capillary density	↑	→
Blood velocity	→	↑
Cerebral oxygenation	→	↑
[Oxy-hemoglobin]	↑	↑
[Deoxy-hemoglobin]	↑	↓

[a] Two hypothetical brain regions of different long-term brain activity are compared. ↑, the respective parameter increases in the region with higher long-term activity.
[b] Two states of the same brain region are compared: transiently increased activation vs the resting state. ↑, during a transient increase in brain activity this physiological parameter increases.

marker of local metabolism and energy need, as measured by the deoxy-glucose method (Sokoloff 1981) used in autoradiography and PET (Phelps et al. 1979). Since by far most of the glucose is oxidatively metabolized (Hyder et al. 1997), local oxygen consumption is also proportional to local brain activity. The amount of local glucose consumption correlates highly with local CBF (Clarke and Sokoloff 1994; Iadecola et al. 1983; Kuschinsky et al. 1981, 1983; Mies et al. 1981, Sokoloff 1981). Beside these animal studies a high correlation between CBF and glucose consumption has also been shown in human subjects (Baron et al. 1982). The elevated level of cerebral blood flow is associated with an increase of local capillary density and blood volume (CBV) which both also correlate highly with local glucose metabolism (Gross et al. 1987; Klein et al. 1986). Hence, if one were to compare two brain regions with different long-term brain activity (see Table 1.2), the region with higher activity would have higher local glucose consumption (local cerebral metabolic rate of glucose, lCMRGlc), oxygen consumption (local cerebral metabolic rate of oxygen, lCMRO$_2$), capillary density, CBV and blood flow. Since local capillary density increases proportionally with local CBF, blood flow per capillary is not different between these two regions. (This statement is made by inference since the author is not aware of any systematic study on this issue.). Since lCMRGlc and lCMRO$_2$ are also proportionally increased, the oxygen extraction fraction would tend to be constant between different

brain regions (but see Weiss and Sinha 1993) as would be the local ratio of oxy-hemoglobin (oxy-Hb) and deoxy-hemoglobin (deoxy-Hb), i.e., local hemoglobin oxygenation.

Analogous to these findings for long-term adjustment, one has tried to model the dynamic changes which occur during a transient increase in brain activity, such as the one which is induced during a functional neuroimaging study. It has been shown that a transient increase in brain activity is associated with an increase in glucose consumption (Kennedy et al. 1976), and it was postulated that this goes along with a proportional increase in oxygen consumption. Regarding capillary density, it was clear that the density of capillaries could not change within seconds to minutes; however, a functional change of this density by opening and closing was suggested as a major mechanism of regulation of CBF (Weiss 1988), which, similar to the increase in local capillary density during long-term stimulation, would have allowed oxygen extraction fraction and hemoglobin oxygenation to remain constant (capillary recruitment hypothesis, see above for evidence against it). This picture was challenged by several studies (Fox and Raichle 1986; Fox et al. 1988; Madsen et al. 1995; Ueki et al. 1988) in which frequently the term "uncoupling" was used in order to emphasize the difference with the hitherto standard notion of "coupling."

In a series of PET studies, which essentially were confirmed by subsequent reports (except for Marrett and Gjedde 1997), Fox and Raichle (1986) and Fox et al. (1988) found: (1) a pronounced discrepancy between the large stimulus-induced increase in CBF and the relatively small (if any) increase in oxygen consumption, and (2) a pronounced discrepancy between the large stimulus-induced increase in glucose consumption and the much smaller (if any) increase in oxygen consumption. From these surprising and controversial findings, two testable hypotheses were derived: (1) If the increase in CBF much exceeds the increase in CMRO$_2$, then a local rise in blood oxygenation should occur. (2) If the increase in CMRGlc exceeds the increase in CMRO$_2$, then glucose metabolism should occur at least partially nonoxidatively. The evidence regarding these two hypotheses of Fox and Raichle (1986) is discussed below.

1.3.1.
The CBF/CMRO$_2$ Mismatch: ΔCBF>ΔCMRO$_2$

As mentioned above, the original finding of a mismatch between the increases in CBF and CMRO$_2$ has been confirmed by other studies (e.g., DAVIS et al. 1998, KUWABARA et al. 1992, SEITZ and ROLAND 1992). Furthermore, a number of studies have confirmed the expected consequence of this mismatch, namely the concomitant increase in cerebral blood oxygenation. In an early report (COOPER et al. 1966) oxygen availability was measured invasively in patients. During local brain activation a concomitant increase in oxygen availability was observed. Optical studies on the exposed brain surface of animals (MALONEK and GRINVALD 1996) have also indicated a rise in hemoglobin oxygenation occurring several seconds after activation onset. Using the noninvasive optical method of near-infrared spectroscopy (NIRS) the increase of hemoglobin oxygen-

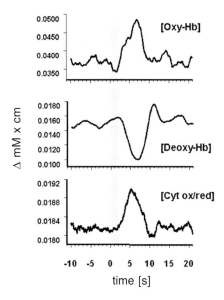

Fig. 1.2. Changes in the concentration of oxy-Hb, deoxy-Hb and cytochrome-oxidase redox state during functional activation. This study was performed with near-infrared spectroscopy (NIRS), an optical method (WENZEL et al. 1996). Light source and light receiver were connected to the subject's head via fiber optic bundles (optodes). The optodes were placed over the occipital cortex, and the subject looked at a computer monitor. Two-second periods (*shaded area*) of visual stimulation with an alternating checkerboard were alternated with 28 s of rest (*black screen*). Shortly after the activation, an increase in [oxy-Hb] and a decrease in [deoxy-Hb], and an increase in cytochrome-C-oxidase (Cyt-Ox) oxidation was seen. Note that the unit of concentration change is mM+cm, i.e., the concentration change times the (in this case unknown) optical path length

ation has also been confirmed during a variety of stimulation paradigms, such as visual activation (Fig. 1.2) (MEEK et al. 1995, VILLRINGER et al. 1993, WENZEL et al. 1996) (KATO et al. 1993) and the performance of motor (OBRIG et al. 1996) and cognitive tasks (VILLRINGER et al. 1993). While an increase in total hemoglobin concentration is usually observed during stimulation, the concentration of deoxy-Hb drops. The BOLD signal in fMRI, which depends on a drop in the concentration of paramagnetic deoxy-Hb during functional activation (BANDETTINI et al. 1992, FRAHM et al. 1992, KWONG et al. 1992, OGAWA et al. 1992), is another piece of evidence supporting these findings. Interestingly, using PET and BOLD fMRI, drops in signal intensity are frequently found during certain paradigms, which should reflect drops in CBF and increases in the concentration of deoxy-Hb ([deoxy-Hb]). Using a paradigm of acoustically cued saccades known to produce CBF drops in the occipital cortex (PAUS et al. 1995), we showed that BOLD-fMRI displays signal intensity decreases presumably suggesting increases in [deoxy-Hb]. This increase in [deoxy-Hb] was confirmed using NIRS, which showed a drop in [oxy-Hb] together with the [deoxy-Hb] increase.

During the first seconds of functional activation, the intrinsic signal study by MALONEK and GRINVALD (1996) reported a transient rise in [deoxy-Hb]; however, this finding is still discussed controversially (see above). Similarly, using fMRI, some reports have indicated an early drop in the BOLD signal during the first seconds of functional activation (MENON et al. 1995). However, this finding is also highly controversial, since a number of other groups have not been able to confirm it (FRANSSON et al. 1998).

Thus, there seems to be good evidence that, in many circumstances, as originally proposed by Fox and RAICHLE (1986), a pronounced mismatch between CBF and CMRO$_2$ leads to an increase in blood oxygenation. Controversies still exist whether: (1) during the early seconds of activation a transient deoxygenation does occur; (2) whether this mismatch occurs during all types of activation, since one study (MARRETT and GJEDDE 1997) has found a dependence on the type of stimulus; and (3) whether during prolonged stimulation this mismatch persists (HEEKEREN et al. 1997; HOWSEMAN et al. 1998; KRUGER et al. 1998).

It should be noted that a dissociation between blood flow and oxygen consumption does not necessarily imply that [deoxy-Hb] must drop. The behavior of [oxy-Hb] and [deoxy-Hb] depends on several

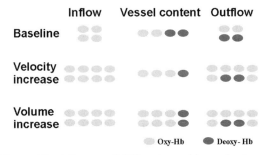

Fig. 1.3. The influence of different possible mechanisms of blood flow increase on hemoglobin oxygenation: increased blood volume vs blood flow velocity. The columns on the *left* (inflow) represent the number of oxygenated erythrocytes entering a capillary during a given time period. The column in the *middle* (vessel content) shows the number of oxygenated and deoxygenated erythrocytes in the capillary at a given time point, assuming a constant rate of oxygen consumption (two red cells change to a deoxygenated state in this time period). The rate of oxygen consumption is assumed to be constant. If blood flow doubles by increasing velocity (*second row*) the vessel content of deoxygenated hemoglobin decreases. If blood flow doubles by increasing blood volume (*third row*), the vessel content of deoxygenated hemoglobin stays constant

factors, including oxygen consumption, blood flow velocity and blood volume. In particular, it is frequently overlooked that it is important whether the blood flow change is mainly achieved by a blood volume change or by a change in blood velocity. This is illustrated in Fig. 1.3. If the blood flow increase is mainly achieved by an increase in blood volume, [deoxy-Hb] could remain constant despite a blood flow increase higher than the increase in oxygen consumption. If the main mechanism, however, is an increase in flow velocity, a drop in [deoxy-Hb] does occur. For many conditions it has now been shown that the main mechanism of blood flow increase at the capillary level is indeed a change in blood flow velocity rather than an increase in blood volume (ABOUNADER et al. 1995; BERECZKI et al. 1993; CHEN et al. 1995; VILLRINGER et al. 1994).

In conclusion, a disproportionate increase in CBF vs the increase in oxygen consumption leads to a rise in cerebral oxygenation, and since the rise in CBF is mainly achieved by changes in blood flow velocity (as opposed to blood volume), this is associated with a drop in [deoxy-Hb].

What could be the reason for this CBF/CMRO$_2$ mismatch (BUXTON and FRANK 1997, BUXTON et al. 1998)? Direct measurements of the kinetics of oxygen uptake in the brain (KASSISSIA et al. 1995) and the low concentration of oxygen which has been re-

ported for brain tissue (FENNEMA et al. 1989; LUBBERS et al. 1994, METZGER and HEUBER 1977) suggest that the rate of return of unmetabolized O$_2$ from the tissue to the intravascular space is small. Assuming that the capillary blood volume does not undergo major changes during functional activation, but rather that blood flow increases are mainly accomplished by a velocity increase, the gradient of intravascular/tissue oxygen tension is the driving force for oxygen transport into brain tissue. Due to the low tissue oxygen tension, the best way to make this concentration gradient steeper is to increase intravascular oxygenation. This can be achieved by a blood flow increase larger than the increase in oxygen consumption. A different way of describing the situation starts from the definition of the rate of delivery of oxygen to tissue as being proportional to the product of flow and oxygen extraction fraction. As mentioned above, during functional activation, CBF increases are mainly achieved by a velocity increase, therefore, capillary transit time decreases which, in turn, decreases oxygen extraction fraction. Therefore, oxygen delivery increases must be smaller than the flow increase.

This oxygen limitation model (BUXTON and FRANK 1997; BUXTON et al. 1998) provides a new interpretation of the mismatch between blood flow and oxygen metabolism changes during brain activation. In the light of this explanation, a larger increase of blood flow is needed to make increased oxygen uptake possible, i.e., the observed mismatch can be regarded as evidence for a tight coupling, rather than uncoupling, between metabolism and blood flow.

1.3.2.
The CMRGlc/CMRO$_2$ Mismatch: CMRGlc>ΔCMRO$_2$

This mismatch seems even more intriguing than the first part of the Fox and RAICHLE (1986) findings, since a logical conclusion seems to be that the additional energy requirements during increased brain activity are met by nonoxidative glucose metabolism. This would mean the generation of only 2 ATP per glucose molecule, as compared to 36 ATP in the case of oxidative glucose consumption.

Confirming the above mentioned PET studies, MADSEN et al. (1998) have shown a resetting of the global ratio of oxygen consumption/glucose consumption during functional activation in a study in awake rats as well as during performance of the Wisconsin Card Sorting test in human subjects (MADSEN et al. 1995). Whereas Fox and Raichle reported little, if any, increase in oxygen consumption, other studies have reported clear increases in oxidative glucose consumption (DAVIS et al. 1998, SEITZ and ROLAND 1992). Using localized NMR spectroscopy in the rat, HYDER et al. (1996, 1997) have shown that the tricarboxylic acid cycle flux increased approximately threefold during forepaw stimulation. By comparison with previous work for the same rat model, which measured total CMRGlc (UEKI et al. 1988), these authors concluded that oxidative CMRGlc supplies the majority of energy during sustained brain activation. Interestingly, the same group found the stoichiometry between oxidative glucose metabolism and glutamate-neurotransmitter cycling in the cortex to be close to 1:1. They concluded that the majority of cortical energy production supports functional (synaptic) glutamatergic neuronal activity and that brain activation studies, which map cortical oxidative glucose metabolism, provide a quantitative measure of synaptic glutamate release (SIBSON et al. 1998).

A number of studies have searched for lactate accumulation as a potential indicator of nonoxidative glycolysis occurring. Indeed, lactate accumulation has been observed in several studies (MADSEN et al. 1998; SHULMAN et al. 1993). However, the increase in lactate concentration is only transient (FRAHM et al. 1996; FRAY et al. 1996), and the amount of the lactate increase seems to be too small to account for all the additional glucose being metabolized (MADSEN et al. 1998). Furthermore, the lactate rise was not observed in anesthetized animals (KAUPPINEN et al. 1997).

It is not simple to draw a conclusion incorporating all these finding. On the one hand, a strong point can be made from several studies confirming the mismatch between the increase in glucose and oxygen consumption. On the other hand, a similarly strong point can be made against the most prominent interpretation of this finding, nonoxidative glucose consumption taking place. Therefore, we probably need a different explanation for the CMRGlc/CMRO$_2$ mismatch, which: (1) holds that for energy production glucose is metabolized oxidatively, and (2) explains the fate of the remaining glucose which is taken up by the cells. MADSEN et al. (1998) have suggested that a large share of the increase in glucose uptake serves an adjustment of intermediary substrate pools.

In conclusion, regarding both parts of the Fox and Raichle mismatch (uncoupling) suggestions, it seems that the basic findings of a mismatch between

CBF and CMRO$_2$ and between CMRGlc and CMRO$_2$ are confirmed; however, the most likely interpretations of these findings differ from the original ones:

1. It seems that a disproportionate increase in blood flow is needed in order to make an increase in oxygen consumption possible.
2. It seems that, despite a disproportionate increase in glucose vs oxygen consumption, oxidative glucose metabolism is the main mechanism of energy generation, leaving the fate of the remaining part of the increased glucose uptake unresolved.

1.3.3
The Current Picture

Brain activity, in particular presynaptic activity, is associated with increased energy requirements which are mostly met by oxidative glucose consumption. After onset of brain activity, a signal (see Chap. 3) is sent to the feeding arteriole which in turn dilates. The dilation of the feeding arteriole leads to an increase in CBF in downstream capillaries. All capillaries are already perfused during resting conditions, but the blood flow per capillary increases and heterogeneity of blood flow decreases. The increase in blood flow is larger than the increase in oxygen consumption, hence oxygenation increases especially at the venular side of the capillary and in the venous vessels. Furthermore, since the main mechanism of the blood flow increase is an increase in velocity, [deoxy-Hb] decreases. The latter is the basis of the BOLD contrast in fMRI.

It should be kept in mind that all considerations mentioned so far refer to healthy (in most studies young adult) human subjects. In all situations referring to other human subjects there may be considerable deviations. The vascular response to functional activation is known to be age-dependent. In neonates it was reported that [deoxy-Hb] does not decrease but rather increases with increased brain activity (MEEK et al. 1998). In adult subjects, the amount of blood flow increase during functional activation seems to attenuate with age (HOCK et al. 1995).

Furthermore, there is very little knowledge about alterations of metabolic and vascular responses in brain disease. After transient global ischemia, it is known that the vascular response is abolished for some time. In patients with carotid stenosis and decreased reserve capacity, the vascular response can be diminished. Furthermore, a number of drugs which are clinically used, such as theophylline and scopolamine, are know to inhibit the vascular response to functional activation (DIRNAGL et al. 1994; OGAWA et al. 1994). In all these (and probably many other) circumstances the integrity of the coupling between brain activity-metabolism and blood flow, which is the basis for the validity of metabolic/vascular functional neuroimaging methods, is not certain.

References

Abounader R, Vogel J, Kuschinsky W (1995) Patterns of capillary plasma perfusion in brains in conscious rats during normocapnia and hypercapnia. Circ Res 76:120–126

Bandettini PA, Wong EC, Hinks RS, Tikofsky RS, Hyde JS (1992) Time course EPI of human brain function during task activation. Magn Reson Med 25:390–397

Baron JC, Lebrun-Grandie P, Collard P, Crouzel C, Mestelan G, Bousser MG (1982) Noninvasive measurement of blood flow, oxygen consumption, and glucose utilization in the same brain regions in man by positron emission tomography: concise communication. J Nucl Med 23:391–399

Bereczki D, Wei L, Otsuka T, Acuff V, Pettigrew K, Patlak C, Fenstermacher J (1993) Hypoxia increases velocity of blood flow through parenchymal microvascular systems in rat brain. J Cereb Blood Flow Metab 13:475–486

Buxton RB and Frank LR (1997) A model for the coupling between cerebral blood flow and oxygen metabolism during neural stimulation. J Cereb Blood Flow Metab 17:64–72

Buxton RB, Wong EC, Frank LR (1998) Dynamics of blood flow and oxygenation changes during brain activation: the balloon model. Magn Reson Med 39:855–864

Chen JL, Wei L, Bereczki D, Hans FJ, Otsuka T, Acuff V, Ghersi-Egea JF, Patlak C, Fenstermacher JD (1995) Nicotine raises the influx of permeable solutes across the rat blood- brain barrier with little or no capillary recruitment. J Cereb Blood Flow Metab 15:687–698

Clarke DD, Sokoloff L (1994) Circulation and energy metabolism of the brain. In: Siegel GJ, Agranoff BW (eds) Basic neurochemistry. Raven, New York, pp 645–680

Cooper R, Crow HJ, Walter WG, Winter AL (1966) Regional control of cerebral vascular reactivity and oxygen supply in man. Brain Res 3:174–191

Davis TL, Kwong KK, Weisskoff RM, Rosen BR (1998) Calibrated functional MRI: mapping the dynamics of oxidative metabolism. Proc Natl Acad Sci USA 95:1834–1839

Dirnagl U, Niwa K, Lindauer U, Villringer A (1994) Coupling of cerebral blood flow to neuronal activation: role of adenosine and nitric oxide. Am J Physiol 267:H296-H301

Duelli R and Kuschinsky W (1993) Changes in brain capillary diameter during hypocapnia and hypercapnia. J Cereb Blood Flow Metab 13:1025–1028

Duffy FH and Burchfiel JL (1975) Eye movement-related inhibition of primate visual neurons. Brain Res 89:121–132

Duncan GE and Stumpf WE (1991) Brain activity patterns: assessment by high resolution autoradiographic imaging of radiolabeled 2-deoxyglucose and glucose uptake. Prog Neurobiol 37:365–382

Duncan GE, Stumpf WE, Pilgrim C (1987) Cerebral metabolic mapping at the cellular level with dry-mount autoradiography of [3H]2-deoxyglucose. Brain Res 401:43–49

Fennema M, Wessel JN, Faithful NS, Erdmann W (1989) Tissue oxygen tension in the cerebral cortex of the rabbit. Adv Exp Med Biol 248:451–60:451–460

Fox PT, Raichle ME (1986) Focal physiological uncoupling of cerebral blood flow and oxidative metabolism during somatosensory stimulation in human subjects. Proc Natl Acad Sci USA 83:1140–1144

Fox PT, Raichle ME, Mintun MA, Dence C (1988) Nonoxidative glucose consumption during focal physiologic neural activity. Science 241:462–464

Frahm J, Bruhn H, Merboldt KD, Hanicke W (1992) Dynamic MR imaging of human brain oxygenation during rest and photic stimulation. J Magn Reson Imaging 2:501–505

Frahm J, Kruger G, Merboldt KD, Kleinschmidt A (1996) Dynamic uncoupling and recoupling of perfusion and oxidative metabolism during focal brain activation in man. Magn Reson Med 35:143–148

Fransson P, Kruger G, Merboldt KD, Frahm J (1998) Temporal characteristics of oxygenation-sensitive MRI responses to visual activation in humans [In Process Citation]. Magn Reson Med 39:912–919

Fray AE, Forsyth RJ, Boutelle MG, Fillenz M (1996) The mechanisms controlling physiologically stimulated changes in rat brain glucose and lactate: a microdialysis study. J Physiol (Lond) 496:49–57

Gobel U, Klein B, Schrock H, Kuschinsky W (1989) Lack of capillary recruitment in the brains of awake rats during hypercapnia. J Cereb Blood Flow Metab 9:491–499

Gobel U, Theilen H, Kuschinsky W (1990) Congruence of total and perfused capillary network in rat brains. Circ Res 66:271–281

Gross PM, Sposito NM, Pettersen SE, Panton DG, Fenstermacher JD (1987) Topography of capillary density, glucose metabolism, and microvascular function within the rat inferior colliculus. J Cereb Blood Flow Metab 7:154–160

Hasselbalch SG, Knudsen GM, Jakobsen J, Hageman LP, Holm S, Paulson OB (1994) Brain metabolism during short-term starvation in humans. J Cereb Blood Flow Metab 14:125–131

Heekeren HR, Obrig H, Wenzel R, Eberle K, Ruben J, Villringer K, Kurth R, Villringer A (1997) Cerebral haemoglobin oxygenation during sustained visual stimulation–a near-infrared spectroscopy study. Philos Trans R Soc Lond B Biol Sci 352:743–750

Hock C, Muller-Spahn F, Schuh-Hofer S, Hofmann M, Dirnagl U, Villringer A (1995) Age dependency of changes in cerebral hemoglobin oxygenation during brain activation: a near-infrared spectroscopy study. J Cereb Blood Flow Metab 15:1103–1108

Howseman AM, Porter DA, Hutton C, Josephs O, Turner R (1998) Blood oxygenation level dependent signal time courses during prolonged visual stimulation. Magn Reson Imaging 16:1–11

Hyder F, Chase JR, Behar KL, Mason GF, Siddeek M, Rothman DL, Shulman RG (1996) Increased tricarboxylic acid cycle flux in rat brain during forepaw stimulation detected with 1H[13 C]NMR. Proc Natl Acad Sci USA 93:7612–7617

Hyder F, Rothman DL, Mason GF, Rangarajan A, Behar KL, Shulman RG (1997) Oxidative glucose metabolism in rat brain during single forepaw stimulation: a spatially localized 1H[13 C] nuclear magnetic resonance study. J Cereb Blood Flow Metab 17:1040–1047

Iadecola C, Nakai M, Mraovitch S, Ruggiero DA, Tucker LW, Reis DJ (1983) Global increase in cerebral metabolism and blood flow produced by focal electrical stimulation of dorsal medullary reticular formation in rat. Brain Res 272:101–114

Jueptner M, Weiller C (1995) Review: does measurement of regional cerebral blood flow reflect synaptic activity?-implications for PET and fMRI [In Process Citation]. Neuroimage 2:148–156

Kadekaro M, Crane AM, Sokoloff L (1985) Differential effects of electrical stimulation of sciatic nerve on metabolic activity in spinal cord and dorsal root ganglion in the rat. Proc Natl Acad Sci USA 82:6010–6013

Kassissia IG, Goresky CA, Rose CP, Schwab AJ, Simard A, Huet PM, Bach GG (1995) Tracer oxygen distribution is barrier-limited in the cerebral microcirculation. Circ Res 77:1201–1211

Kato T, Kamei A, Takashima S, Ozaki T (1993) Human visual cortical function during photic stimulation monitoring by means of near-infrared spectroscopy. J Cereb Blood Flow Metab 13:516–520

Kauppinen RA, Eleff SM, Ulatowski JA, Kraut M, Soher B, van ZP (1997) Visual activation in alpha-chloralose-anaesthetized cats does not cause lactate accumulation in the visual cortex as detected by [1H]NMR difference spectroscopy. Eur J Neurosci 9:654–661

Kennedy C, Des RM, Sakurada O, Shinohara M, Reivich M, Jehle JW, Sokoloff L (1976) Metabolic mapping of the primary visual system of the monkey by means of the autoradiographic [14C]deoxyglucose technique. Proc Natl Acad Sci USA 73:4230–4234

Klein B, Kuschinsky W, Schrock H, Vetterlein F (1986) Interdependency of local capillary density, blood flow, and metabolism in rat brains. Am J Physiol 251:H1333-H1340

Kruger G, Kleinschmidt A, Frahm J (1998) Stimulus dependence of oxygenation-sensitive MRI responses to sustained visual activation [In Process Citation]. NMR Biomed 11:75–79

Kuschinsky W, Suda S, Bunger R, Yaffe S, Sokoloff L (1983) The effects of intravenous norepinephrine on the local coupling between glucose utilization and blood flow in the rat brain. Pflugers Arch 398:134–138

Kuschinsky W, Suda S, Sokoloff L (1981) Local cerebral glucose utilization and blood flow during metabolic acidosis. Am J Physiol 241:H772-H777

Kuwabara H, Ohta S, Brust P, Meyer E, Gjedde A (1992) Density of perfused capillaries in living human brain during functional activation. Prog Brain Res 91:209–215

Kwong KK, Belliveau JW, Chesler DA, Goldberg IE, Weisskoff RM, Poncelet BP, Kennedy DN, Hoppel BE, Cohen MS, Turner R, et al (1992) Dynamic magnetic resonance imaging of human brain activity during primary sensory stimulation. Proc Natl Acad Sci USA 89:5675–5679

Lubbers DW, Baumgartl H, Zimelka W (1994) Heterogeneity and stability of local PO2 distribution within the brain tissue. Adv Exp Med Biol 345:567–74, 567–574

Luknowsky DC, Thomas CG, Gatley SJ, Menon RS (1998) Millisecond sequencing of neural activation in simple tasks determined by the BOLD fMRI neurovascular response. Neuroimage 7: S280–S280(Abstract)

Madsen PL, Hasselbalch SG, Hagemann LP, Olsen KS, Bulow J, Holm S, Wildschiodtz G, Paulson OB, Lassen NA (1995) Persistent resetting of the cerebral oxygen/glucose uptake ratio by brain activation: evidence obtained with the Kety-Schmidt technique. J Cereb Blood Flow Metab 15:485–491

Madsen PL, Linde R, Hasselbalch SG, Paulson OB, Lassen NA (1998) Activation-induced resetting of cerebral oxygen and glucose uptake in the rat. J Cereb Blood Flow Metab 18:742–748

Magistretti PJ, Pellerin L (1996) Cellular bases of brain energy metabolism and their relevance to functional brain imaging: evidence for a prominent role of astrocytes. Cereb Cortex 6:50–61

Malonek D, Grinvald A (1996) Interactions between electrical activity and cortical microcirculation revealed by imaging spectroscopy: implications for functional brain mapping. Science 272:551–554

Marrett S, Gjedde A (1997) Changes of blood flow and oxygen consumption in visual cortex of living humans. Adv Exp Med Biol 413:205–208

Mata M, Fink DJ, Gainer H, Smith CB, Davidsen L, Savaki H, Schwartz WJ, Sokoloff L (1980) Activity-dependent energy metabolism in rat posterior pituitary primarily reflects sodium pump activity. J Neurochem 34: 213–215

Meek JH, Elwell CE, Khan MJ, Romaya J, Wyatt JS, Delpy DT, Zeki S (1995) Regional changes in cerebral haemodynamics as a result of a visual stimulus measured by near infrared spectroscopy. Proc R Soc Lond B Biol Sci 261:351–356

Meek JH, Elwell CE, Firbank M, Noone MBO, Atkinson J, Wyatt JS (1998) Regional haemdoynamic changes in the occipital cortex of awake infants due to visual stimulation. Neuroimage 7: S311–S311(Abstract)

Menon RS, Ogawa S, Hu X, Strupp JP, Anderson P, Ugurbil K (1995) BOLD based functional MRI at 4 Tesla includes a capillary bed contribution: echo-planar imaging correlates with previous optical imaging using intrinsic signals. Magn Reson Med 33:453–459

Metzger H, Heuber S (1977) Local oxygen tension and spike activity of the cerebral grey matter of the rat and its response to short intervals of O2 deficiency or CO2 excess. Pflugers Arch 370:201–209

Mies G, Niebuhr I, Hossmann KA (1981) Simultaneous measurement of blood flow and glucose metabolism by autoradiographic techniques. Stroke 12:581–588

Nudo RJ, Masterton RB (1986) Stimulation-induced [14 C]2-deoxyglucose labeling of synaptic activity in the central auditory system. J Comp Neurol 245:553–565

Obrig H, Hirth C, Junge-Hulsing JG, Doge C, Wolf T, Dirnagl U, Villringer A (1996) Cerebral oxygenation changes in response to motor stimulation. J Appl Physiol 81:1174–1183

Ogawa M, Magata Y, Ouchi Y, Fukuyama H, Yamauchi H, Kimura J, Yonekura Y, Konishi J (1994) Scopolamine abolishes cerebral blood flow response to somatosensory stimulation in anesthetized cats: PET study. Brain Res 650:249–252

Ogawa S, Tank DW, Menon R, Ellermann JM, Kim SG, Merkle H, Ugurbil K (1992) Intrinsic signal changes accompanying sensory stimulation: functional brain mapping with magnetic resonance imaging. Proc Natl Acad Sci USA 89:5951–5955

Paus T, Marrett S, Worsley KJ, Evans AC (1995) Extraretinal modulation of cerebral blood flow in the human visual cortex: implications for saccadic suppression. J Neurophysiol 74:2179–2183

Pawlik G, Rackl A, Bing RJ (1981) Quantitative capillary topography and blood flow in the cerebral cortex of cats: an in vivo microscopic study. Brain Res 208:35–58

Phelps ME, Huang SC, Hoffman EJ, Selin C, Sokoloff L, Kuhl DE (1979) Tomographic measurement of local cerebral glucose metabolic rate in humans with (F-18)2-fluoro-2-deoxy-D-glucose: validation of method. Ann Neurol 6:371–388

Schwartz WJ, Smith CB, Davidsen L, Savaki H, Sokoloff L, Mata M, Fink DJ, Gainer H (1979) Metabolic mapping of functional activity in the hypothalamo- neurohypophysial system of the rat. Science 205:723–725

Seitz RJ, Roland PE (1992) Vibratory stimulation increases and decreases the regional cerebral blood flow and oxidative metabolism: a positron emission tomography (PET) study. Acta Neurol Scand 86:60–67

Shockley RP, LaManna JC (1988) Determination of rat cerebral cortical blood volume changes by capillary mean transit time analysis during hypoxia, hypercapnia and hyperventilation. Brain Res 454:170–178

Shulman RG, Blamire AM, Rothman DL, McCarthy G (1993) Nuclear magnetic resonance imaging and spectroscopy of human brain function. Proc Natl Acad Sci USA 90:3127–3133

Sibson NR, Dhankhar A, Mason GF, Rothman DL, Behar KL, Shulman RG (1998) Stoichiometric coupling of brain glucose metabolism and glutamatergic neuronal activity. Proc Natl Acad Sci USA 95:316–321

Sokoloff L (1981) Relationships among local functional activity, energy metabolism, and blood flow in the central nervous system. Fed Proc 40:2311–2316

Ueki M, Linn F, Hossmann KA (1988) Functional activation of cerebral blood flow and metabolism before and after global ischemia of rat brain. J Cereb Blood Flow Metab 8:486–494

Villringer A, Planck J, Hock C, Schleinkofer L, Dirnagl U (1993) Near infrared spectroscopy (NIRS): a new tool to study hemodynamic changes during activation of brain function in human adults. Neurosci Lett 154:101–104

Villringer A, Them A, Lindauer U, Einhaupl K, Dirnagl U (1994) Capillary perfusion of the rat brain cortex. An in vivo confocal microscopy study. Circ Res 75:55–62

Weiss HR (1988) Measurement of cerebral capillary perfusion with a fluorescent label. Microvasc Res 36:172–180

Weiss HR and Sinha AK (1993) Imbalance of regional cerebral blood flow and oxygen consumption: effect of vascular alpha adrenoceptor blockade. Neuropharmacology 32:297–302

Wenzel R, Brandt SA, Villringer A, Kwong KK (1997)Comparison of BOLD-contrast and blood flow during saccadic suppression. Neuroimage 5:S170–S170(Abstract)

Wenzel R, Obrig H, Ruben J, Villringer K, Thiel A, Bernarding J, Dirnagl U, Villringer A (1996) Cerebral blood oxygenation changes induced by visual stimulation in humans. J Biomed Opt 1:399–404

Wree A and Schleicher A (1988) The determination of the local cerebral glucose utilization with the 2- deoxyglucose method. Histochemistry 90:109–121

Yang TT, Gallen CC, Schwartz BJ, Bloom FE (1993) Noninvasive somatosensory homunculus mapping in humans by using a large- array biomagnetometer. Proc Natl Acad Sci USA 90:3098–3102

2 Regulation of Cerebral Blood Flow

W. KUSCHINSKY

CONTENTS

2.1 Introduction

Whereas the blood gases CO_2 and O_2 were once regarded as the – more or less – exclusive regulators of cerebral blood flow, the refinement of methods has now made it evident that a wide variety of factors is integrated into a highly differentiated system of local regulation of cerebral flood flow. These new findings clearly indicate that the principles of regulation of cerebral blood flow are comparable, at least qualitatively, to those which are active in other organs, allowing regulation of blood flow according to the functional and metabolic needs of the respective organ. However, when comparing the regulation of the vascular resistance of brain vessels with that of other organs, some features specific for brain vessels have to be considered: (1) In contrast to other blood vessels the brain vessels are equipped with a blood-brain barrier. This barrier is formed by the tight junctions of neighboring endothelial cells and it effectively prevents blood-borne polar substances of larger molecular weight from penetrating into the brain tissue (BRIGHTMAN and TAO-CHENG 1993) Therefore, vasoactive substances may be rather ineffective when offered from the blood side. (2) The interstitial fluid which surrounds the brain vessels is not just the result of filtration forces (hydrostatic and oncotic pressures) which act at the capillary membranes of other organs and result in an ultrafiltrate of the plasma. The interstitial fluid of the brain is formed by the cells of the choroid plexus and is therefore subject to a more differentiated fine regulation than the interstitial fluid of other organs. (3) Due to the localized activation and deactivation of neuronal circuits in the brain, the local demand for oxygen and nutrients varies parallel with the functional state; therefore, a highly localized regulation of blood flow is needed in the brain, including local actions of vasoactive substances. (4) Whereas the main effectors of blood flow regulation are the arterioles in all organs, the larger arterial vessels comprise a considerable part of the vascular resistance and its regulation in the brain.

The main factors which induce a regulatory adjustment of cerebral resistance vessels are shown in Fig. 2.1. Any activation or deactivation of neuronal circuits and neuronal connections induces changes in the ionic surroundings of the blood vessels. In addition, factors are released into the perivascular fluid depending on the metabolic activation of the surrounding cells. Whereas neuronal and metabolic factors are released and act from the perivascular side, other influences concern the blood side. Changes in intravascular pressure, flow and viscosity also induce regulatory adjustments of the vascular resistance.

More detailed descriptions of the factors which regulate cerebral blood flow and the mechanisms of action of these factors have been discussed in recent books and review articles (MRAOVITCH and SERCOMBE 1996; WELCH et al. 1997; FARACI and HEISTAD 1998).

W. KUSCHINSKY, MD, Professor, Department of Physiology, University of Heidelberg, Im Neuenheimer Feld 326, D-69120 Heidelberg, Germany

Supported by the Deutsche Forschungsgemeinschaft.

TRIGGERS OF REGULATION

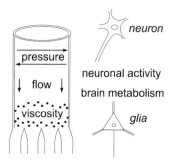

Fig. 2.1. Factors which induce regulatory adjustments of cerebral vessel. Adjustments can be triggered by intravascular and perivascular changes

2.2
Physical Factors: Autoregulation

2.2.1
Description

Autoregulation is a basic vascular phenomenon which exists in most organs, including the brain. (PAULSON et al. 1990). Autoregulation can be defined as the intrinsic ability of an organ to keep its blood flow relatively constant during changing perfusion pressures. The perfusion pressure is the difference between arterial pressure and either cerebrospinal fluid pressure or cerebrovenous pressure, whichever of these two is larger. Under physiological conditions, only arterial pressure is relevant. The brain, like other organs, maintains its blood flow largely, but not completely, constant by a vasodilatation, during decreases, and a vasoconstriction, during increases, in perfusion pressure. These vascular reactions have a time constant of many seconds, e.g., during an acute moderate hypertension blood flow increases first and then slowly comes returns to nearly its normotensive value (e.g., FLORENCE and SEYLAZ 1992). The resulting autoregulation curve, as depicted in Fig. 2.2, thus represents a steady state relationship. During the first few seconds after an acute change in perfusion pressure, the plateau part of the curve does not exist and a passive dependence of blood flow on perfusion pressure is found. This passive behavior of the vessels exists during pathophysiological conditions, such as ischemia, trauma or inflammation. Regarding ischemia, a gradual decline of autoregulatory reactions has been shown with increasing degrees of ischemia (DIRNAGL and PULSINELLI 1990). A more or less passive behavior of the cerebral resistance vessels is seen during very

high and very low perfusion pressures, as evident from the non-plateau part of the autoregulation curve. In these cases, the autoregulatory capacity is exhausted. At high perfusion pressures, vasoconstriction may alternate with passive distention of vessel segments, thus resulting in a "sausage string" appearance of the cerebral vessels, which does not represent vasospasm. It should be mentioned that the plateau part of the autoregulation curve is never complete, i.e., even here there is some degree of higher flow with higher perfusion pressure.

2.2.2
Sympathetic Influence

The inflection points where the autoregulation curve departs from its plateau part represent the upper and lower limit of the autoregulation curve. These limits have been determined as approximately 50 and 150 mm Hg. They can be shifted acutely and chronically. An acute shift to the right is found during an electrical stimulation of the cervical sympathetics. Conversely, sympathetic denervation induces a shift to the left. An acute increase in blood flow during the pressure rise is therefore blunted by sympathetic stimulation. From this, a protective effect of the sympathetic system has been deduced which, during acute increases in blood pressure, diminishes increases in cerebral blood flow. Severe hypertension also induces an increased permeability of the blood-brain barrier. This can be also attenuated by sympathetic stimulation, thus yielding an additional protective effect of the cervical

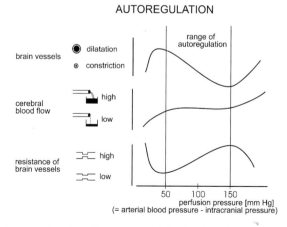

Fig. 2.2. Vascular adjustments which take place during autoregulation. Between the lower and the upper limit of autoregulation cerebral blood flow shows only minor long-term changes at different perfusion pressures

sympathetics. The protective effect at high perfusion pressures may change into a detrimental action at low perfusion pressures: a high sympathetic discharge during hypotension (e.g., during shock) may compromise the diminished blood flow by a constricting action of the sympathetics on the cerebral vessels. A chronic shift of the upper and lower limits of the autoregulation curve to the right is observed during chronic hypertension. Whereas the shift of the upper limit makes higher perfusion pressures tolerable and induces vascular hypertrophy, thus protecting cerebral vessels during hypertension (MAYHAN et al. 1987), the simultaneous shift of the lower limit can be detrimental during hypotensive periods, e.g., during a forced antihypertensive therapy. A moderate therapy is therefore necessary.

2.2.3
Renin-Angiotensin System

Besides the sympathetic nervous system, the renin-angiotensin system can also modulate autoregulatory reactions of cerebral vessels. This has been concluded from studies using the angiotensin converting enzyme inhibitor captopril, which shifts the limits of the autoregulation curve to lower blood pressure values in normotensive and spontaneously hypertensive rats (PAULSON et al. 1988). The effects appear to be less pronounced in humans (WALDEMAR et al. 1989) and cannot be abolished by acute sympathetic denervation. This points to the independence of mechanisms involving the sympathetic nervous system and the renin-angiotensin system in autoregulation (WALDEMAR 1990).

2.2.4
Possible Mechanisms

The basic mechanism which mediates autoregulatory adjustments of cerebral vessels has not yet been completely clarified. Metabolic, myogenic and endothelial mechanisms are under discussion; neurogenic mechanisms can probably be excluded since they only modulate, but do not cause, autoregulation.

2.2.4.1
Metabolic Mechanisms

The possibilities of directly verifying a metabolic mechanism of autoregulation are limited, because changes in metabolic factors at the resistance vessels are hard to detect during autoregulatory adjustments. Perivascular H^+ and K^+ activities have been measured close to pial arteries during their autoregulatory adjustments. The changes in these activities were small and can hardly explain the complete pial vascular reactions observed (WAHL and KUSCHINSKY 1979). Adenosine concentrations in brain tissue change inversely with blood pressure; however, a quantitative analysis of the interstitial concentrations of adenosine, using the brain dialysis technique, showed that adenosine could only be relevant at blood pressures of less than 50 mm Hg, thereby excluding all except an accessory role for adenosine in autoregulation (VAN WYLEN et al. 1988). Thus, although a metabolic component of the autoregulatory mechanism cannot be completely excluded, convincing evidence is lacking.

2.2.4.2
Myogenic Mechanisms

Myogenic mechanisms of autoregulation, i.e., stretch-dependent vasoconstriction and vasodilation with increasing stretch, have been demonstrated more convincingly, with the exception of one experimental model, the increase in cerebral venous pressure. If a myogenic component of autoregulation were effective, vasoconstriction should occur due to a raised intravascular pressure which could stimulate the myogenic response. The fact that an increased venous pressure does not change cerebral blood flow (e.g., McPHERSON et al. 1988) and induces dilation of pial arteries instead of constriction (e.g., WEI and KONTOS 1984) has been interpreted by some investigators to indicate the predominance of metabolic mechanisms in autoregulation. This indirect conclusion is opposed by the direct demonstration of myogenic mechanisms in autoregulatory cerebral vascular adjustment.

Myogenic mechanisms are reactions to changes in the transmural pressure of the vessel which oppose the passive behavior. In isolated middle cerebral arteries, autoregulatory reactions could be clearly demonstrated (KATUSIC et al. 1987; RUBANYI 1988; HARDER et al. 1989; McCARRON et al. 1989). Congruent with direct evidence for a myogenic mechanism of autoregulation in isolated cerebral vessels are in vivo experiments, in which the transmural pressure of pial arteries was altered at an unchanged perfusion pressure. This was achieved by putting the animal into a sealed box with the cranial cavity open to the atmosphere. With increased pressure in the box–

which means a vessel distention – pial arterioles constricted and with decreased pressure pial arteries dilated (BOHLEN and HARPER 1984). Altogether, most of the experimental evidence, with the exception of the experiments using increased venous pressure, argues for a myogenic component of autoregulation; indications exist for an additional metabolic component. The experiments employing increases in cerebrovenous pressure should not be taken as firm evidence against myogenic mechanisms; they may show that, under these special conditions, a metabolic component or the reaction to cerebral hypoxia overrides the myogenic mechanism. There are several mechanisms which mediate the reactions of blood vessels to physical distention or shear stress. They include: the extracellular matrix, integrins, ion channels, the sarcoplasmic reticulum, second messenger systems, length-dependent changes in contractile protein function and the cytoskeleton (MEININGER and DAVIS 1992; OSOL 1995).

2.2.4.3
Endothelial Mechanisms

Of the experiments which have been performed in isolated cerebral arteries, most have shown an endothelial component in the autoregulatory adjustment of cerebral blood flow (KATUSIC et al. 1987; RUBANYI 1988; HARDER et al. 1989) with one exception (MCCARRON et al. 1989). A calcium influx into endothelial cells during stretch appears to be the primary event (LANSMAN 1988). Nitric oxide (NO), whether released by endothelial cells or other sources in the brain, does not contribute to the autoregulatory adjustments (SAITO et al. 1994). These data support the hypothesis of a minor influence of the endothelium on autoregulatory reactions of cerebral vessels which appears to be confined to a modulation of basic reactions.

2.3
Brain Tissue Factors

In principle, cerebral blood flow can be adjusted to changing functional needs by factors which influence the smooth muscle cells of the resistance vessels from the perivascular or from the intravascular side. Of these factors those acting from the perivascular side and originating from the brain tissue appear to be of major importance. Tissue factors can be mainly divided into two groups: (1) local metabolic and ionic factors, (2) other perivascular factors.

2.3.1
Local Metabolic and Ionic Factors

In the brain, as in other organs, local blood flow is adjusted to the minute-by-minute functional activity and metabolic demands. This is achieved by the vasomotor action of the cerebral arteries and arterioles. The question arises which tissue factors could be regarded as coupling factors mediating an increase in cerebral blood flow with an increased neuronal activity. It appears to be justified to differentiate between neuronal activity and brain metabolism as they are two different entities either of which can trigger a regulatory change of vessel tone. As will be discussed in the context of Fig. 2.3, the vasoactive factors linked with neuronal activity and brain metabolism are not identical. The vasomotor response occurs within seconds and allows for rapid changes in regional blood flow. Its essentials are given in Fig. 2.3. Increased neuronal activity, as seen in a higher frequency of action potentials, leads to the

NEUROVASCULAR COUPLING

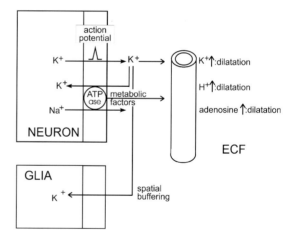

Fig. 2.3. Dynamic component of coupling between functional activity, metabolism and blood flow in the brain. Dynamic coupling consists of two elements: The function-dependent element is represented by K^+, the metabolic element by H^+ and adenosine. Increased concentrations of K^+, H^+, and adenosine dilate the cerebral resistance vessels. The release of K^+ depends on the frequency of action potentials (function-dependent element), whereas H^+ and adenosine concentrations increase if there is a mismatch between oxygen/glucose delivery and demand (metabolic element). The impact of both elements on the actual adjustment of vessel diameter may vary from situation to situation. *ECF*, extracellular fluid

release of cellular K^+ into the extracellular space. Since the extracellular space in the brain is small (about 15%) and the intra/extracellular K^+ concentration gradient high, the result is a considerable increase in the extracellular K^+ concentration, which in turn dilates the cerebral resistance vessels. This, together with the information forwarded by the action potential, results in the quick adjustment of blood flow to the increased functional activity.

The original extra/intracellular distribution of ions then has to be reestablished on a long-term basis. Pumps are activated to carry K^+ back into and Na^+ out of the cells. Increased pump activity is accompanied by increased metabolic activity. This is the basis for neuroimaging methods which make use of metabolic activity as an indicator of function. The signals for metabolically induced vasodilatation, of which H^+ and adenosine have been identified, continue to be released as long as a mismatch occurs between the oxygen/glucose demand and supply.

Vasodilation induced by these factors counteracts the mismatch and thus permits fine tuning of an adequate blood supply to the tissue. Hence, acute, dynamic coupling occurs by two mechanisms, the feedforward mechanism utilized by K^+, and the feedback mechanism used by H^+ and adenosine, which are key mechanisms in both circulatory and respiratory physiology.

For over a decade, controversies have persisted regarding the quantitative contributions of these regional factors to dynamic coupling. While K^+ is now accepted as an initial mediator of coupling, controversy persists regarding the quantitative contributions made by H^+ and adenosine to dynamic coupling. Some studies show that extracellular pH decreases immediately as neuronal activity increases, whereas others report a decrease in pH that lags behind the onset of neuronal activity by some seconds (for references see KUSCHINSKY 1982). However, increases in brain tissue lactate concentration have been measured using [^{1}H]NMR spectroscopic techniques during physiological activation states (PRICHARD et al. 1991) which have been taken as an indicator of anaerobic glycolysis under these conditions. With regard to adenosine, the situation is comparable to that of H^+ insofar as a number of negative data is more than balanced by a larger number of positive findings. Previous experiments have indicated an increase in brain tissue adenosine concentration during the starting phase of bicuculline-induced seizures (SCHRADER et al. 1980; WINN et al. 1980). As to the interstitial adenosine concentration, which is more relevant with regard to the effect on

vascular diameter (NGAI and WINN 1993), studies using the brain dialysis technique confirm an increase in adenosine release, although its extent is not overwhelming (PARK et al. 1987). The adenosine blocker theophylline has proven to be partly effective in reducing brain hyperemia during seizures (PINARD et al. 1990) and functional activation (Ko et al. 1990; DIRNAGL et al. 1994). However, the findings of Ko et al. (1990) could not be reproduced by NORTHINGTON et al. (1992).

The conditions under which K^+, H^+ and adenosine are active can be defined in the following way. While the release of K^+ is dependent on the neuronal firing rate, H^+ and adenosine accumulate in the tissue when a mismatch occurs between oxygen demand and delivery. Therefore, fine tuning by the H^+-adenosine metabolic mechanism is likely to become effective after a time lag and to have a greater effect in those cases in which the K^+ mechanism alone is not sufficient to yield an adequate O_2 supply. The effect of the H^+-adenosine mechanism, therefore, depends on the regional conditions. This impact is expected to be small where neural activation is accompanied by increased pO2. In contrast, it can be expected to play a major role in oxygen deficiency, e.g., during hypoxia and ischemia.

Local uncoupling has been postulated for somatosensory stimulation in humans (Fox and RAICHLE 1986). This postulate, derived from PET studies, appears to be a contradiction in terms, however. It is based on a greater percentage increase in local blood flow (+29%) than in local oxygen consumption (+5%) and on the maximal increase of these parameters measured in the contralateral brain hemisphere during cutaneous vibration of the finger pads of one hand. This notion of uncoupling, at first, seems plausible. However, the coupling sequence (i.e., neuronal activity-metabolism-blood flow) may not fully describe all aspects of the coupling procedure. The procedure may be cut short by the influence of neuronal activity on the cerebral vessels. The neuronal activity may be related directly to the interstitial K^+ concentration or to the cotransmission of vasoactive peptides, thereby modifying the metabolic link between neuronal activity and local hemodynamics. Dissociation, or partial dissociation, between regional oxygen consumption and blood flow would then be expected to result in a greater increase in blood flow than in metabolic rate. This, however, does not indicate uncoupling but rather a specific type of coupling. The greater increase in blood flow than in metabolism leads to regional hyperperfusion, the result being a smaller arteriovenous difference of substrates, e.g., glucose and oxygen. In conclusion, the coupling phenomenon is not fully described by relating blood flow rate to the metabolic rate only.

In a recent study the question of uncoupling was addressed by the Kety-Schmidt method (MADSEN et al. 1995). This approach has been verified by independent methodology and its basis is independent of the assumptions on which PET models for measurement of the cerebral metabolic rate for oxygen are based. The brains of healthy volunteers were activated by the Wisconsin Card Sorting Text. This study showed an unchanged global metabolic rate for oxygen during activation whereas global cerebral blood flow and global metabolic rate for glucose were increased by 12% each. Surprisingly, only a minor part of the increased glucose consumption could be ascribed to the production of lactate, which shows a smaller contribution of lactate production to metabolic changes than postulated from the [^{1}H]NMR studies by PRICHARD et al. (1991). Although this study confirms the dissociation of oxygen consumption and blood flow in the brain during functional activation, it remains open which pathway is taken by the additional glucose metabolized during activation. It appears tempting to ascribe a decisive role in this context to the astrocytes (see Chap. 3; PELLERIN and MAGISTRETTI 1994), which may be activated to redistribute the released K$^+$ to the resistance vessels (PAULSON and NEWMAN 1987).

2.3.2
Other Perivascular Factors

Whereas local metabolic and ionic factors appear to mediate the major part of the local coupling between function, metabolism and blood flow in the brain, several other factors can influence cerebral blood flow more globally by acting from the perivascular side. These factors are released by the vascular nerves and by perivascular mast cells. A recent review of this topic has been given by GOADSBY and SERCOMBE (1996). The main findings are summarized in Table 2.1.

Table 2.1. Morphology and major function of the brain vascular innervation

Innervation	Ganglia	Transmitters	Effect of activation on cerebral blood flow
Sympathetic	Superior cervical	Norepinephrine, neuropeptideY (NPY)	Decrease
Para-sympathetic	Sphenopalatine, otic, internal carotid	Acetylcholine, vasoactive intestinal poly-peptide (VIP), peptide histidine isoleucine (PHI)	Increase
Trigeminal	Trigeminal	Substance P, calcitonin gene-related peptide (CGRP), neuro-kinin A (NKA), cholecystokinin (CCK)	Increase

2.3.2.1
Perivascular Sympathetic Innervation

A rich sympathetic innervation has been demonstrated around the extraparenchymal cerebral vessels and the dura. The origin is located in the hypothalamus. After a synapse in the intermediolateral cell column of the spinal cord, the fibers pass to the superior cervical ganglion. Some innervation also comes from the stellate ganglion which reaches mainly the basilar and vertebral arteries and is less intense. The main transmitter of the sympathetic nerve fibers is norepinephrine which is stored in small vesicles. Neuropeptide Y (NPY) acts as a cotransmitter and is stored in large vesicles of the sympathetic nerve fibers. Activation of adrenergic α 1 and 2 receptors by either electrical stimulation of the sympathetic nerve fibers or by norepinephrine induces a moderate constriction of the extraparenchymal vessels (arteries and veins). The reduction of cerebral blood flow is moderate and heterogeneous (TUOR 1992). The constriction induced by stimulation of NPY receptors is stronger and longer lasting and has not yet been verified for veins. The tonic influence of the sympathetic nervous system on brain vessels appears to be rather small and insignificant during normal conditions. Its physiological and pathophysiological function is better defined as a protective action, e.g., during excessive increases in blood pressure. The shift of the upper limit of autoregulation to the left (lower blood pressures, see Sect. 2.2.3) prevents a detrimental increase in cerebral blood flow and simultaneously protects the blood-brain barrier from an extravasation of plasma fluid. Conversely, the same effect may be hazardous for the brain during hypotension, since it would tend to further decrease cerebral blood flow. Apart from the effects on brain vessels sympathetic stimulation has been shown to decrease the production of cerebrospinal fluid. Together with the vascular action, sympathetic stimulation therefore can decrease intracranial pressure. In addition to the acute effects of sympathetic transmitters on cerebrovascular resistance, chronic trophic actions have been ascribed to the sympathetic innervation which influence the composition and distensibility of cerebral arterioles (BAUMBACH et al. 1989).

2.3.2.2
Perivascular Parasympathetic Innervation

The parasympathetic innervation of the cerebral vessels originates from the superior salivary nucleus and takes the facial (VIIth cranial) nerve to distribute its fibers to the pterygopalatine (in humans) or sphenopalatine (in other species) and otic ganglia after passing through the greater superficial petrosal nerve. As in the sympathetic vascular system, at the brain vessels several transmitters are colocalized in the perivascular nerve fibers. The most significant transmitters appear to be acetylcholine, vasoactive intestinal polypeptide (VIP) and peptide histidine isoleucine (PHI). All these transmitters have dilating effects on cerebral vessels. Therefore, parasympathetic innervation represents an important system, as it has the ability to increase cerebral blood flow. This has also been shown by experiments in which different components of this system have been stimulated electrically, which is a rather complicated approach. The physiological significance of this dilator pathway is not evident. At least no modulating effect of stimulation is known in the standard tests of hypercapnia, hypoxia and autoregulation.

2.3.2.3
Perivascular Trigeminal Innervation

The trigeminovascular system represents the sensory afferent innervation of the cerebral vessels and dura mater. Its neuronal cell bodies are located in the trigeminal ganglion from where the information is passed to the medulla and high cervical cord until thalamic structures are reached. Therefore, there is no doubt concerning the important role of trigeminal innervation in the processing of pain information from the dura mater and brain vessels. However, such a purely afferent function may not describe totally the importance of the trigeminovascular system. Four neurotransmitter peptides have been found in the trigeminal neurons: Substance P, calcitonin gene-related peptide (CGRP), neurokinin A (NKA) and cholecystokinin (CCK). The major importance of these neuropeptides is ascribed to an action on brain vessels. This implies that these neuropeptides are released, during depolarization of the trigeminal neuron, to the outside of the brain vessels, although the normal direction of electrical excitation is from the vascular endings of the nerves to the neuronal cell bodies. Some indications exist that an excitation of some part of the perivascular nerve endings can be processed by an axon reflex-like mechanism to other parts of the perivascular nerve endings, which induces a release of neurotransmitter from these nerve endings to the vessel wall. All these neurotransmitters have a dilating action on cerebral vessels, although the extent of dilation varies with the different transmitters. Whereas the physiological role of the trigeminovascular system appears to be of minor importance, there are indications that excitation of this system induces inflammation of the blood vessels. Such a mechanism could be the basis of migraine and other headache-induced pain (GOADSBY and SILBERSTEIN 1997).

2.4
Factors of Mixed Origin

2.4.1
Serotonin, Histamine

For several vasoactive factors it is not possible to identify only one exclusive source in the brain. As an example, serotonin might be released by raphe-derived central serotonergic neurons, by perivascular mast cells or even by sympathetic perivascular nerve fibers after they have taken up serotonin. Another example is histamine, which has its sources in neurons, endothelial cells and mainly in perivascular mast cells.

Serotonin is a constrictor of major cerebral vessels and large pial arteries. In smaller arterioles it has either no vascular effect or even induces vasodilation. The receptors which mediate the effects of serotonin are of three main types: 5-HT$_1$, 5-HT$_2$ and 5-HT$_3$. Of these, the 5-HT$_1$ receptor has four subtypes: 5 HT$_{1A-D}$. Besides the variety of receptor types the release of norepinephrine and prostaglandins might contribute to the observed multiple actions of serotonin.

Similarly, histamine has, in principle, dilating and constricting actions on brain vessels. The constrictions appear to be mediated by H$_1$ receptors whereas dilations are mainly due to H$_2$ receptors although H$_1$ receptors sometimes are also involved. Although receptors and effects depend on the species investigated and the type of vessel, the dominating effect of histamine is a vasodilation. In addition to its vascular actions, histamine, like bradykinin, has been discussed as a mediator of an enhanced permeability of the blood-brain barrier which could result in the development of vasogenic brain edema.

2.4.2
Nitric Oxide, Eicosanoids

Nitric oxide is a powerful vascular dilator in many vascular beds. In the brain, there are at least three isoforms of the enzyme which catalyzes the synthesis of NO: constitutive neuronal (n-NOS, NOS-I) and endothelial (e-NOS, NOS-III) isoforms and an inducible isoform (i-NOS, NOS-II) originally isolated from macrophages. Therefore, NO in the brain is acting not only as an endothelium-derived relaxing factor (EDRF) but is also as a factor released by neurons. The most likely role of NO in the cerebral circulation is a facilitative effect supporting a general vasodilated state and the specific vasodilation which takes place during functional activation or hypercapnia. From knockout experiments it became apparent that the n-NOS isoform is more important than the other isoforms for these effects. From the residual activities of e-NOS and n-NOS in the different knockout mice it can be concluded that the total NOS activity in the brain is dominated by n-NOS. However, this does not exclude a local important role of e-NOS in the blood vessels.

Metabolites of arachidonic acid appear to be involved in a large number of vascular regulatory functions in the brain. In this respect they show similarities to the NO system. Of the prostaglandins, thromboxanes and leukotrienes formed by the cyclooxygenase pathway, prostacyclin (PGI$_2$) can be regarded as the most important vasodilator and

PGF$_{2\alpha}$ as its most important vasoconstrictor opponent. Two isoforms of cyclooxygenase have been described: cyclooxygenase-1 (COX-1) is the constitutive form and cyclooxygenase-2 (COX-2) the inducible form. As discussed for NO, a major role of prostaglandins appears to be a permissive action supporting the vasoactive effects of other substances. Prostacyclin also shares with NO the ability to reduce platelet aggregation of the blood passing by the vascular endothelial cells. An outline of the major features of NO and eicosanoids is given in Fig. 2.4.

NO AND PROSTACYCLIN : CEREBRAL VASODILATORS

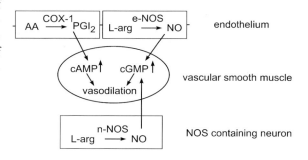

Fig. 2.4. Simplified outline of two major dilating systems in the brain. *AA*, arachidonic acid; *COX-1*, cyclooxygenase 1; *PGI$_2$*, prostacyclin; *L-arg*, l-arginine; *e-NOS*, endothelial nitric oxide synthase; *NO*, nitric oxide; *cAMP*, cyclic AMP; *cGMP*, cyclic GMP; *n-NOS*, neuronal nitric oxide synthase

2.5
Conclusion

Whereas regulation of cerebral blood flow could previously be explained as mainly the effect of the respiratory gases CO$_2$ and O$_2$ on brain vessels, the regulatory mechanisms have turned out to be much more complicated. It is often hard to separate a direct vascular action of a factor from a permissive and facilitative role. An interplay of all elements in the brain, i.e., endothelial cells, vascular smooth muscle cells, neurons and glial cells, makes it extremely difficult to find a simple causal relationship between an agent and its vascular action.

References

Baumbach GL, Heistad DD, Siems JE (1989) Effect of sympathetic nerves on composition and distensibility of cerebral arterioles in rats. J Physiol 416:123–140

Bohlen HG, Harper SL (1984) Evidence of myogenic vascular control in the rat cerebral cortex. Circ Res 55:554–559

Brightman MW, Tao-Cheng JH (1993) Tight junctions of brain endothelium and epithelium. In: Pardridge WM (ed) The blood-brain barrier. Raven, New York, pp 107–125

Dirnagl U, Pulsinelli W (1990) Autoregulation of cerebral blood flow in experimental focal brain ischemia. J Cereb Blood Flow Metab 10:327–336

Dirnagl U, Niwa K, Lindauer U, Villringer A (1994) Coupling of cerebral blood flow to neuronal activation: role of adenosine and nitric oxide. Am J Physiol 267:296–301

Faraci FM, Heistad DD (1998) Regulation of the cerebral circulation: Role of endothelium and potassium channels. Physiol Rev 78:54–97

Florence G, Seylaz J (1992) Rapid autoregulation of cerebral bood flow: A laser-Doppler flowmetry study. J Cereb Blood Flow Metab 12:674–680

Fox PT, Raichle ME (1986) Focal physiological uncoupling of cerebral blood flow and oxidative metabolism during somatosensory stimulation in human subjects. Proc Natl Acad Sci USA 83:1140–1144

Goadsby PJ, Sercombe R (1996) Neurogenic regulation of cerebral blood flow: extrinsic neural control. In: Sercombe R, Mraovitch S (eds) Neurophysiological basis of cerebral blood flow control: An introduction. John Libbey, London, pp 285–321

Goadsby PJ, Silberstein SD (1997) Headache. Butterworth-Heinemann, New York

Harder DR, Sanchez-Ferrer C, Kauser K, Stekiel WJ, Rubanyi GM (1989) Pressure releases a transferable endothelial contractile factor on cat cerebral arteries. Circ Res 65:193–198

Katusic ZS, Shepherd JT, Vanhoutte PM (1987) Endothelium-dependent contraction to stretch in canine basilar arteries. Am J Physiol 252:671–673

Ko KR, Ngai AC, Winn HR (1990) Role of adenosine in regulation of regional cerebral blood flow in sensory cortex. Am J Physiol 259:H1703–1708

Kuschinsky W (1982) Role of hydrogen ions in regulation of cerebral blood flow and other regional flows. In: Altura BM (ed) Ionic regulation of the microcirculation. Karger, Basel, pp 1–19

Lansman JB (1988) Going with the flow. Nature 331:481–482

Madsen PL, Hasselbalch SG, Hagemann LP, Olsen KS, Buelow J, Holm S, Wildschiodtz G, Paulson OB, Lassen NA (1995) Persistent resetting of the cerebral oxygen/glucose uptake ratio by brain activation: evidence obtained with the Kety-Schmidt technique. J Cereb Blood Flow Metab 15: 485–491

Mayhan WG, Werber AH, Heistad DD (1987) Protection of cerebral vessels by sympathetic nerves and vascular hypertrophy. Circulation 75:107–112

McCarron JG, Osol G, Halpern W (1989) Myogenic responses are independent of the endothelium in rat pressurized posterior cerebral arteries. Blood Vessels 26:315–319

McPherson RW, Koehler RC, Traystman RJ (1988) Effect of jugular venous pressure on cerebral autoregulation in dogs. Am J Physiol 255:H1516–1524

Meiniger GA, Davis MJ (1992) Cellular mechanisms involved in the vascular myogenic response. Am J Physiol 263:H647–659

Mraovitch S, Sercombe R (eds) (1996) Neurophysiological basis of cerebral blood flow control: An introduction. John Libbey, London, pp 1–408

Ngai AC, Winn HR (1993) Effects of adenosine and its analogues on isolated intracerebral arterioles. Extraluminal and intraluminal application. Circ Res 73:448–457

Northington FJ, Matherne GP, Coleman SD, Berne RM (1992) Sciatic nerve stimulation does not increase endogenous adenosine production in sensory-motor cortex. J Cereb Blood Flow Metab 12:835–843

Osol G (1995) Mechanotransduction by vascular smooth muscle. J Vasc Res 32:275–292

Park TS, van Wylen DGL, Rubio R, Berne RM (1987) Interstitial fluid adenosine and sagittal sinus blood flow during bicuculline-seizures in newborn piglets. J Cereb Blood Flow Metab 7:633–639

Paulson OB, Newman EA (1987) Does the release of potassium from astrocyte endfeet regulate cerebral blood flow? Science 237:896–898

Paulson OB, Waldemar G, Andersen AR, Barry DI, Pedersen EV, Schmidt JF, Vorstrup S (1988) Role of angiotensin in autoregulation of cerebral blood flow. Circulation 77:55–58

Paulson OB, Strandgaard S, Edvinsson L (1990) Cerebral autoregulation. Cerebrovasc Brain Metab Rev 2:161–192

PellerinL, Magistretti PJ (1994) Glutamate uptake into astrocytes stimulates aerobic glycolysis: A mechanism coupling neuronal activity to glucose utilization. Proc Natl Acad Sci USA 91: 10625–1062

Pinard E, Riche D, Puiroud S, Seylaz J (1990) Theophylline reduces cerebral hyperemia and enhances brain damage induced by seizures. Brain Res 511:303–309

Prichard J, Rothman D, Novotny E, Petroff O, Kuwabara T, Avison M, Howseman A, Hanstock C, Shulman R (1991) Lactate rise detected by [1H]NMR in human visual cortex during physiological stimulation. Proc Natl Acad Sci U S A 88:5829–5831

Rubanyi GM (1988) Endothelium-dependent pressure-induced contraction of isolated canine carotid arteries. Am J Physiol 255:H783–788

Saito S, Wilson DA, Hanley DF, Traystman RJ (1994) Nitric oxide synthase does not contribute to cerebral autoregulatory phenomenon in anesthetized dogs. J Auton Nerv Syst 49:S73–76

Schrader J, Wahl M, Kuschinsky W, Kreutzberg GW (1980) Increase of adenosine content in cerebral cortex of the cat during bicuculline-induced seizure. Pflugers Arch 387:245–251

Tuor U (1992) Acute hypertension and sympathetic stimulation: local heterogeneous changes in cerebral blood flow. Am J Physiol 263:H511–518

Wahl M, Kuschinsky W (1979) Unimportance of perivascular H^+ and K^+ activities for the adjustment of pial arterial diameter during changes of arterial blood pressure in cats. Pflugers Arch 382, 203–209

Waldemar G (1990) Acute sympathetic denervation does not eliminate the effect of angiotensin converting enzyme inhibition on CBF autoregulation in spontaneously hypertensive rats. J Cereb Blood Flow Metab 10:43–47

Waldemar G, Schmidt JF, Andersen AR, Vorstrup S, Ibsen H, Paulson OB (1989) Angiotensin converting enzyme inhibition and cerebral blood flow autoregulation in normotensive and hypertensive man. J Hypertens 7:229–235

Wei EP, Kontos HA (1984) Increased venous pressure causes myogenic constriction of cerebral arterioles during local hyperoxia. Circ Res 55:249–252

Welch KMA, Caplan LR, Reis DJ, Siesjö BK, Weir B (eds)(1997) Primer on cerebrovascular diseases. Academic, San Diego, pp 1–823

Winn HR, Welsh JE, Rubio R, Berne RM (1980) Changes in brain adenosine during bicuculline induced seizures in rats. Effects of hypoxia and altered systemic blood pressure. Circ Res 47:568–577

Wylen van DGL, Park TS, Rubio R, Berne RM (1988) Cerebral blood flow and interstitial fluid adenosine during hemorrhagic hypotension. Am J Physiol 255:H1211–1218

3 Regulation of Cerebral Energy Metabolism

P.J. MAGISTRETTI, L. PELLERIN

CONTENTS

3.1
Introduction

The techniques used for functional brain imaging are based on a simple physiological principle: neuronal activity requires energy. A corollary of this is that the increased energy demands, which are met by local increases in blood flow and metabolism, can be visualized. The first formulation of the principle delineating the coupling between neuronal activity and blood flow was provided by Charles Sherrington in a seminal article published about a century ago in *The Journal of Physiology* (ROY and SHERRINGTON 1890) . The cellular and molecular mechanisms that underlie activity-flow coupling have been reviewed

in the preceding chapter. The objective of the present chapter is to provide an overview of the current concepts on the mechanisms of the coupling between activity and metabolism, namely glucose utilization and oxygen consumption.

3.2
Glucose Metabolism in the Brain: An Overview

Except for a few particular conditions, glucose can be considered the major, if not exclusive, energy substrate for the brain (SOKOLOFF 1989). Overall, glucose metabolism in the brain is similar to other tissues, undergoing four principal metabolic pathways: glycolysis, the tricarboxylic acid cycle (TCA), the pentose phosphate pathway (PPP) and storage under the form of glycogen.

3.2.1
Glycolysis

Glycolysis (Embden-Meyerhof pathway) consists of the metabolism of glucose to pyruvate. It results in the net production of only two ATPs per glucose molecule . Under anaerobic conditions pyruvate is converted to lactate, allowing for the regeneration of nicotinamide adenine dinucleotide (NAD^+), which is essential to maintain a continued glycolytic flux. Another situation in which the end-product of glycolysis is lactate rather than pyruvate is when oxygen consumption does not match glucose utilization, implying that the rate of pyruvate production through glycolysis exceeds pyruvate oxidation by the TCA cycle. This metabolic pathway, known as aerobic glycolysis, is well described in muscle. As we will see below, the transient production of lactate under aerobic conditions may be consistent with observations made in the human cerebral cortex during activation using PET which suggest the exist-

P. J. MAGISTRETTI, MD, PhD; L. PELLERIN, PhD; Institut de Physiologie, 7 Rue du Bugnon, 1005 Lausanne, Switzerland

ence of an uncoupling between glucose utilization and oxygen consumption (Fox and Raichle 1986; Fox et al. 1988).

3.2.2
The Tricarboxylic Acid Cycle

Under aerobic conditions, pyruvate is oxidatively decarboxylated to yield acetyl coenzyme A, in a reaction catalyzed by the enzyme pyruvate dehydrogenase (PDH). Acetyl coenzyme A condenses with oxaloacetate to produce citrate. This is the first step of the TCA cycle, which through its coupling with the mitochondrial electron-transfer chain and the process of oxidative phosphorylation results in the production of 30 ATPs per glucose. Thus, under aerobic conditions, i.e.; when glucose is fully oxidized through the TCA cycle to CO_2 and H_2O, NAD^+ is regenerated, and glycolysis proceeds to pyruvate, not lactate. However, as soon as a mismatch, even transient, occurs between glucose utilization and oxygen consumption, lactate is produced. As will be discussed below, evidence has been provided through in vivo microdialysis and magnetic resonance spectroscopy studies that such a transient production of lactate is indeed occurring during activation (Schasfoort et al. 1988; Prichard et al. 1991; Sappey-Marinier et al. 1992; Fellows et al. 1993).

3.2.3
The Pentose Phosphate Pathway

Glycolysis, the TCA cycle and oxidative phosphorylation are coordinated pathways concerned with the production of ATP using glucose as a fuel. However, ATP is not the only form of metabolic energy. Indeed, for several biosynthetic reactions, in which the precursors are in a more oxidized state than the products, metabolic energy under the form of reducing power is needed in addition to ATP. This reducing power is provided by the reduced form of nicotinamide adenine dinucleotide phosphate (NADPH). The processing of glucose through the pentose phosphate pathway (PPP) produces NADPH. Particularly relevant to brain function is the necessity of NADPH reducing equivalents for the scavenging of reactive oxygen species (ROS). Among other processes, ROS are generated by the transfer of single electrons to molecular oxygen as by-products of certain physiological cellular processes, such as the electron-transfer chain associated with oxidative

phosphorylation (Boveris and Chance 1973; Chan and Fishman 1980; Cross and Jones 1991; Pou et al. 1992). ROS are highly damaging to cells since they can cause DNA disruptions and mutations as well as activation of enzymatic cascades involving proteases and lipases which can eventually lead to cell death (Coyle and Puttfarcken 1993; Greenlund et al. 1995).

3.2.4
Incorporation into Glycogen

Following phosphorylation to glucose-6-phosphate, glucose can be further metabolized and stored under the form of glycogen. Glycogen is the single largest energy reserve of the brain (Lajtha et al. 1981); it is mainly localized in astrocytes, although ependymal and choroid plexus cells as well as certain large neurons in the brain stem contain glycogen (Sotelo and Palay 1968; Vaughn and Grieshaber 1972). When compared to liver or muscle, the glycogen content of the brain is exceedingly small, about 100 and ten times inferior, respectively. However, glycogen turnover in the brain is extremely rapid (Watanabe and Passonneau 1973) and glycogen levels are finely coordinated with synaptic activity (Magistretti et al. 1993). For example, during general anesthesia, a condition in which synaptic activity is markedly attenuated, glycogen levels rise sharply (Phelps 1972); In addition, in vitro studies have demonstrated that glycogen levels are tightly regulated by various neurotransmitters such as the monoamines noradrenaline, serotonin and histamine, and the peptides vasoactive intestinal peptide (VIP) and pituitary adenylate cyclase activating peptide (PACAP) (Magistretti et al. 1993).

3.3
Brain Energy Metabolism: Regulation at the Global and Local Levels

While the brain represents only 2% of the body weight in humans, it accounts for approximately 25% of total body glucose utilization. Over four decades of in vivo studies at the organ level have unequivocally determined that – except under some particular ketogenic conditions such as fasting, lactation or diabetes – glucose is the obligatory energy substrate for the brain, where it is entirely oxidized to CO_2 and water (SOKOLOFF 1989; EDVINSSON et al. 1993).

The oxygen consumption of the brain, which accounts for almost 20% of the oxygen consumption of the whole organism, is 160 µmol/100 g brain weight per min and roughly corresponds to the value determined for CO_2 production. This O_2/CO_2 relation corresponds to what is known in metabolic physiology as a respiratory quotient of nearly 1 and provides the demonstration that carbohydrates, and glucose in particular, are the exclusive substrates for oxidative metabolism.

In normal adults, cerebral blood flow is approximately 57 ml/100 g of brain weight/min and the calculated glucose utilization by the brain is 31 µmol/100 g brain weight per min. Given a theoretical stoichiometry of 6 µmol of oxygen consumed for each µmol of glucose, glucose utilization by the brain should in theory be of 26.6 µmol/100 g per min. As indicated earlier, the measured glucose utilization is of 31 µmol/100 g per min, indicating that an excess of 4.4 µmol/100 g per min of glucose follows other metabolic fates. Glucose can be incorporated into lipids, proteins and glycogen and it is also the precursor of certain neurotransmitters such as γ-aminobutyric acid (GABA), glutamate and acetylcholine (SOKOLOFF 1989; EDVINSSON et al. 1993).

Studies carried out at the global, whole organ level, have allowed for the determination of the substrate requirements for the brain and its stoichiometry. However, such analyses failed to provide the appropriate level of resolution to appreciate two major features of brain energy metabolism, namely, its regional heterogeneity and its tight relationship with the functional activation of specific pathways. The autoradiographic 2-deoxyglucose (2-DG) method developed by Sokoloff and colleagues, and its subsequent extensions to humans with the advent of 2-(^{18}F)fluoro-2-deoxyglucose PET (FDG PET), have afforded a sensitive means to measure local rates of glucose utilization (SOKOLOFF et al. 1977; SOKOLOFF 1981). Basal glucose utilization of the gray matter, as determined by the 2-DG technique, varies depending on the brain structure, between 50 and 150 µmol/100 g wet weight per min (approximately 5–15 nmol/mg prot per min) in the rat (SOKOLOFF 1981) and approximately 50% lower in humans (HATAZAWA et al. 1988). Physiological activation by specific modalities (e.g., somatosensory, visual, cognitive) results in localized increases in glucose utilization of 10%–50% over basal levels (SHARP et al. 1975; KENNEDY et al. 1976; WOLF et al. 1983; MELZER et al. 1985; GINSBERG et al. 1987; SOKOLOFF et al. 1989).

3.4
Brain Energy Metabolism: Regulation at the Cellular Level

Brain energy metabolism is often considered to reflect predominantly, if not exclusively, neuronal energy metabolism. However other cell types, namely, glia and vascular endothelial cells, consume energy and play an active role in the flux of energy substrates from the circulation to neurons. Quantitatively, neurons contribute at most 50% of cerebral cortical volume (O'KUSKY and COLONNIER 1982; KIMELBERG and NOREMBERG 1989). The astrocyte:neuron ratio may be as high as 10:1, depending on the species, on brain areas and on developmental stages (O'KUSKY and COLONNIER 1982). This ratio increases with increasing brain size (TOWER and YOUNG 1973), an important consideration when approaching the study of the cellular bases of brain energy metabolism in humans.

3.4.1
The Central Role of Astrocytes in Coupling Activity to Metabolism

In addition to these quantitative considerations, the morphology and cytological relationship of astrocytes with the vasculature and the neuropil provide these cells with a strategic position between the "source and the sinks" of energy. Indeed, through specialized processes called end-feet, astrocytes surround virtually all intraparenchymal capillaries while other astrocytic processes ensheath synaptic contacts (PETERS et al. 1991). In addition to these cytological relationships which strongly suggest a possible role of astrocytes in coupling neuronal activity to energy metabolism, astrocytes possess receptors and reuptake sites for a variety of neurotransmitters, including the excitatory neurotransmitter glutamate (MURPHY 1993). In addition, astrocytic end-feet are enriched in the specific glucose transporter GLUT-1 (MORGELLO et al. 1995). Thus astrocytes possess the necessary functional armamentarium to sense synaptic activity, through receptors and reuptake sites for neurotransmitters, and to couple it with the entry of glucose into the brain parenchyma (TSACOPOULOS and MAGISTRETTI 1996).

This hypothesis has been tested and verified in purified cellular preparations of astrocytes, since the necessary cellular resolution cannot be achieved in vivo. These in vitro data have allowed for the elabo-

ration of a functional model for the coupling of neuronal activity to energy metabolism and, as will be
reviewed below, has found experimental verification
in in vivo paradigms.

3.4.2
Synaptically Released Glutamate Stimulates Glucose Uptake into Astrocytes

Glucose uptake can be monitored in primary astrocyte cultures using radiolabeled 2-DG as a tracer, in
analogy to what is monitored in vivo with PET
fluorodeoxyglucose (PHELPS et al. 1979). Neuronal
activity can in turn be mimicked by applying to astrocyte cultures glutamate, the predominant neurotransmitter released by excitatory pathways during activation of a given brain area. In the cerebral
cortex, activation of afferent pathways by specific
modalities (e.g., somatosensory, visual, auditory) or
of cortico-cortical association circuits results in a
spatially and temporally defined local release of
glutamate from the activated synaptic terminals
(FONNUM 1984). The released glutamate exerts profound effects on the excitability of target neurons,
which are mediated by specific subtypes of
glutamate receptors. The action of glutamate on
postsynaptic neurons is rapidly terminated by an
avid reuptake system present on astrocyte processes,
which ensheath synaptic contacts (ROTHSTEIN et al.
1994). This removal of glutamate from the synaptic
cleft is operated through specific glutamate transporters, two of which are predominantly, if not exclusively, glia-specific. These are GLT-1 and GLAST.
The third glutamate transporter subtype, EAAC-1, is
exclusively localized in neurons, but does not appear
to be involved in the clearance of synaptically released glutamate (ROTHSTEIN et al. 1994). Glutamate
uptake into astrocytes is driven by the electrochemical gradient of sodium, implying that it is a sodium-
dependent mechanism involving the co-transport of
glutamate with three sodium ions (Fig. 3.1). Once in
astrocytes glutamate is predominantly converted to
glutamine through an ATP-requiring reaction catalyzed by the astrocyte-specific enzyme glutamine
synthase (NOREMBERG and MARTINEZ-HERNANDEZ
1979). Glutamine is then released by astrocytes and
taken up by neurons to replenish the neurotransmitter pool of glutamate (NOREMBERG and MARTINEZ-
HERNANDEZ 1979).

The coupling between synaptic glutamate release
and its reuptake into astrocytes is so tight that determination of the Na^+ current generated in astrocytes

Stoichiometry of High Affinity Na^+-dependent Glutamate Transporters

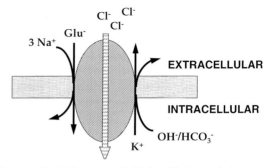

Fig. 3.1. Stoichiometry of high affinity Na^+-dependent
glutamate transporters. Five Na^+-dependent glutamate transporters have been identified so far with two (GLT1 and
GLAST) being exclusively expressed on glial cells. Glutamate
transport by these transporters is stoichiometrically coupled
with the transport of different ions. Thus, one glutamate
molecule is cotransported with three Na^+ while one K^+ and
one OH^- (or one HCO_3^-) are countertransported. Chloride is
also transported, as revealed by the chloride current recorded upon glutamate uptake

by the co-transport of glutamate and Na^+ through
the glutamate transporter provides an accurate reflection of glutamate release from the synapse
(BERGLES and JAHR 1997).

As shown in Fig. 3.2, glutamate stimulates 2-DG
uptake into astrocytes in a concentration-dependent
manner, with an EC_{50} of approximately 80 µM
(PELLERIN and MAGISTRETTI 1994). Interestingly,
this effect of glutamate is not mediated by specific
glutamate receptors, since agonists specific for each
glutamate receptor subtype do not mimic the effect
of glutamate, nor do antagonists inhibit it (PELLERIN
and MAGISTRETTI 1994). Rather, the effect of
glutamate on astrocytic glucose utilization is mediated by a glutamate transporter (PELLERIN and
MAGISTRETTI 1994). Similar conclusions have been
reached by Sokoloff and colleagues (TAKAHASHI et
al. 1995).

Thus, the glutamate-stimulated increase in glucose uptake and phosphorylation into astrocytes is
abolished in the absence of sodium in the extracellular medium (PELLERIN and MAGISTRETTI 1994;
TAKAHASHI et al. 1995), consistent with the necessity
of an electrochemical gradient for the ion to drive
glutamate uptake. In addition, L- and D-aspartate,
but not D-glutamate, mimic the effect of L-
glutamate, the physiological agonist. Such a specific
pharmacological profile provides the signature for a
phenomenon mediated by the glutamate transporter. Finally, the specific glutamate transporter in-

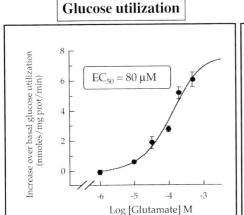

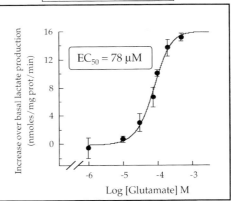

Fig. 3.2. Glutamate stimulates aerobic glycolysis in astrocytes. Both glucose utilization and lactate production are stimulated by glutamate with a similar EC_{50} of approximately 80 μM

hibitor THA inhibits also the glutamate-stimulated glucose utilization (PELLERIN and MAGISTRETTI 1994).

These data have been integrated in an operational model for the coupling between synaptic activity and glucose utilization (Fig. 3.3). Glutamate, released from excitatory synapses when neuronal pathways subserving specific modalities are activated, acts on postsynaptic neurons to modulate excitability, and through its reuptake into astrocytes causes glucose entry into these cells in register with neuronal activity.

Mechanism for Coupling Neuronal Activity to Glucose Utilization

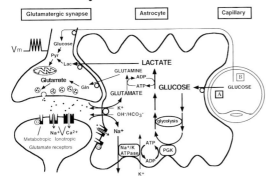

Fig. 3.3. Model for the coupling of synaptic activity to glucose utilization. At glutamatergic synapses, the action of glutamate is terminated by an efficient glutamate uptake system located in astrocytes. Glutamate is cotransported with Na^+, resulting in an increase in the intracellular concentration of Na^+, leading to the activation of the Na^+/K^+ ATPase. Lactate produced by the glutamate-stimulated glycolysis is released from astrocytes. Arrow labeled *A*, synaptic activation; direct glucose uptake into neurons under basal conditions is also shown. (Arrow labeled *B*, basal conditions). *Pyr*, pyruvate; *Lac*, lactate; *Gln*, glutamine; *G*, G-protein

3.4.3
Role of the Na^+/K^+-ATPase

The intracellular molecular mechanism(s) of this coupling involve the Na^+/K^+-ATPase since ouabain completely inhibits the glutamate-evoked 2-DG uptake by astrocytes (PELLERIN and MAGISTRETTI 1994, 1996). Indeed, the entry of Na^+ associated with glutamate uptake activates a subunit of the Na^+/K^+-ATPase, which is highly sensitive to ouabain, probably the α_2 subunit (PELLERIN and MAGISTRETTI 1997).

In a variety of cell types including smooth muscle cells and erythrocytes, increases in the activity of the Na^+/K^+-ATPase stimulate glucose uptake and glycolysis (PROVERBIO and HOFFMAN 1977; PAUL et al. 1979). Consistent with this view, glutamate stimulates the glycolytic processing of glucose in astrocytes, as indicated by the increase in lactate release (Fig. 3.2).

The overall stoichiometry of the molecular steps involved in the coupling between glutamate uptake and glucose utilization is the following: one glutamate is taken up with three sodium ions while one glucose consumed through glycolysis produces two ATPs. One ATP is used by the Na^+/K^+ ATPase for the extrusion of three sodium ions; the other ATP is used for the synthesis of glutamine from glutamate by the glutamine synthase. The glycolytic processing of glucose results in approximately two lactate molecules produced per one glucose molecule, i.e., a stoichiometrical relationship between glucose and lactate, as expected (Fig. 3.2).

To summarize, glutamate release from activated synaptic terminals is the key signal for coupling neuronal activity to glucose utilization. The cells that mediate this signaling are astrocytes, into which

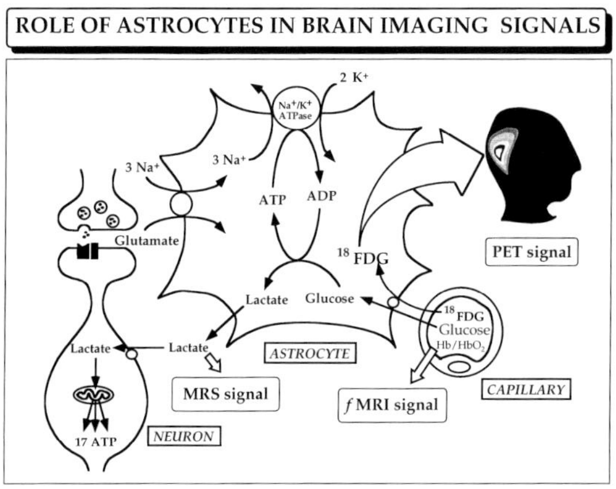

Fig. 3.5. Relevance of metabolic trafficking between astrocytes and neurons for brain imaging signals. The proposed model of glutamate-induced glycolysis in astrocytes implies that the activity-linked uptake of ^{18}FDG, monitored with PET, reflects primarily an astrocyte-based signal. Since neuronally released glutamate triggers the cascade of events that leads to glucose uptake, the ^{18}FDG-PET signal will faithfully reflect activation of neuronal circuits. In parallel to the glucose uptake and metabolism in astrocytes, an increase in blood flow occurs in the activated area. Such an increase in blood flow without an immediate increase in oxygen consumption will lead to a change in the ratio between oxy- and deoxy-hemoglobin, providing a signal detectable by fMRI. Finally, the formation and release of lactate by astrocytes, followed by its subsequent uptake and oxidation by neurons, give rise to a transient lactate peak in the activated area which is detected by MRS

References

Bergles DE, Jahr CE (1997) Synaptic activation of glutamate transporters in hippocampal astrocytes. Neuron 19:1297–308

Bignami A (1991) Glial cells in the central nervous system. In: Magistretti PJ (ed) Discussions in neuroscience, vol VIII/1. Elsevier, Amsterdam pp 1–45

Bittar PG, Charnay Y, Pellerin L, Bouras C, Magistretti PJ (1996) Selective distribution of lactate dehydrogenase isoenzymes in neurons and astrocytes of human brain. J Cereb Blood Flow Metab 16:1079–1089

Boveris A, Chance B (1973) The mitochondrial generation of hydrogen peroxide. Biochem J 134:707–716

Bröer S, Rahman B, Pellegri G, Pellerin L, Martin J-L, Verleysdonk S, Hamprecht B, Magistretti PJ (1997) Comparison of lactate transport in astroglial cells and monocarboxylate transporter 1 (MCT 1) expressing *Xenopus laevis* oocytes: expression of two different monocarboxylate transporters in astroglial cells and neurons. J Biol Chem 272:30096–30102

Chan PH, Fishman RA (1980) Transient formation of superoxide radicals in polyunsaturated fatty acid-induced brain swelling. J Neurochem 35:1004–1007

Coyle J, Puttfarcken P (1993) Oxidative stress, glutamate, and neurodegenerative disorders. Science 262:689–695

Cross AR, Jones OTS (1991) Enzymatic mechanisms of superoxide production. Biochim Biophys Acta 1057:281–298

Demestre M, Boutelle M, Fillenz M (1996) Stimulated release of lactate in freely moving rats is dependent on the uptake of glutamate. J. Physiol 499:825–832

Edvinsson L, MacKenzie ET, McCulloch J (1993) Cerebral blood flow and metabolism. Raven, New York, pp 161

Fellows LK, Boutelle MG, Fillenz M (1993) Physiological stimulation increases nonoxidative glucose metabolism in the brain of the freely moving rat. J Neurochem 60:1258–1263

Fonnum F (1984) Glutamate: a neurotransmitter in mammalian brain. J Neurochem 42:1–11

Fox PT, Raichle ME (1986) Focal physiological uncoupling of cerebral blood flow and oxidative metabolism during somatosensory stimulation in human subjects. Proc Natl Acad Sci USA 83:1140–1144

Fox PT, Raichle ME, Mintun MA, Dence C (1988) Nonoxidative glucose consumption during focal physiologic neural activity. Science 241:462–464

Fray AE, Forsyth RJ, Boutelle MG, Fillenz M (1996) The mechanisms controlling physiologically stimulated changes in rat brain glucose and lactate – a microdialysis study. J Physiol 496:49–57

Ginsberg MD, Dietrich WD, Busto R (1987) Coupled forebrain increases of local cerebral glucose utilization and blood flow during physiologic stimulation of a somatosensory pathway in the rat: demonstration by double-label autoradiography. Neurology 37:11–19

Greenlund LJS, Deckwreth TL, Johnson EM (1995) Superoxide dismutase delays neuronal apoptosis: a role for reactive oxygen species in programmed neuronal death. Neuron 14:303–315

Hatazawa J, Ito M, Matsuzawa T, Ido T, Watanuki S (1988) Measurement of the ratio of cerebral oxygen consumption to glucose utilization by positron emission tomography: its consistency with the values determined by the Kety-Schmidt method in normal volunteers. J Cereb Blood Flow Metab 8:426–432

Hu Y, Wilson GS (1997) Rapid changes in local extracellular rat brain glucose observed with an in vivo glucose sensor. J Neurochem 68:1745–1752

Hyder F, Chase JR, Behar KL, Mason GF, Siddeek M, Rothman DL, Shulman RG (1996) Increased tricarboxylic acid cycle flux in rat brain during forepaw stimulation detected with ^{1}H [^{13}C] NMR. Proc Natl Acad Sci USA 93:7612–7617

Izumi Y, Benz AM, Katsuki H, Zorumski CF (1997) Endogenous monocarboxylates sustain hippocampal synaptic function and morphological integrity during energy deprivation. J Neurosci 17:9448–9457

Kennedy C, Des Rosiers MH, Sakurada O, Shinohara M, Reivich M, Jehle JW, Sokoloff L (1976) Metabolic mapping of the primary visual system of the monkey by means of the autoradiographic [^{14}C]deoxyglucose technique. Proc Natl Acad Sci USA 73:4230–4234

Kimelberg HK, Norenberg MD (1989) Astrocytes. Sci Am 260:44–52

Lajtha AL, Maker H, Clarke DD (1981) Metabolism and transport of carbohydrates and amino acids In: Siegel GJ, Albers RW, Agranoff B, Katzman R (eds) Basic neurochemistry. Little Brown, Boston, pp 329–353

Larrabee MG (1995) Lactate metabolism and its effects on glucose metabolism in an excised neural tissue. J Neurochem 64:1734–1741

Magistretti PJ, Pellerin L (1996) Cellular bases of brain energy metabolism and their relevance to functional brain imaging: evidence for a prominent role of astrocytes. Cereb Cortex 6:50–61

Magistretti PJ, Sorg O, Martin J-L, (1993) Regulation of glycogen metabolism in astrocytes: physiological, pharmacological, and pathological aspects. In: Murphy S (ed) Astrocytes: pharmacology and function. Academic, San Diego, pp 243

Malonek D, Grinvald A (1996) Interactions between electrical activity and cortical microcirculation revealed by imaging spectroscopy: implications for functional brain mapping. Science 272:551–554

Marrett S, Meyer E, Kuwabara H, Evans A, Gjedde A (1995) Differential increases of oxygen metabolism in visual cortex. J Cereb Blood Flow Metab 15:S80

Mata M, Fink DJ, Gainer H, Smith CB, Davidsen L, Savaki H, Schwartz WJ, Sokoloff L (1980) Activity-dependent energy metabolism in rat posterior pituitary primarily reflects sodium pump activity. J Neurochem 34:213–215

McIlwain H, Bachelard HS (1985) Biochemistry and the central nervous system, vol. 5. Churchill Livingstone, New York, p. 54

Melzer P, Van der Loos H, Dörfl J, Welker E, Robert P, Emery D, Berrini JC (1985) A magnetic device to stimulate selected whiskers of freely moving or restrained small rodents: its application in a deoxyglucose study. Brain Res 348:229–240

Morgello S, Uson RR, Schwartz EJ, Haber RS (1995) The human blood-brain barrier glucose transporter (GLUT1) is a glucose transporter of gray matter astrocytes. Glia 14:43–54

Murphy S (1993) Astrocytes: Pharmacology and function. Academic Press, San Diego

Noremberg MD, Martinez-Hernandez A (1979) Fine structural localization of glutamine synthetase in astrocytes of rat brain. Brain Res 161:303–310

Ogawa S, Lee TM, Kay AR, Tank DW (1990) Brain magnetic resonance imaging with contrast dependent on blood oxygenation. Proc Natl Acad Sci USA 87:9868–9872

Ogawa S, Tank DW, Menon R, Ellermann JM, Kim SG, Merkle H, Ugurbil K (1992) Intrinsic signal changes accompanying sensory stimulation: Functional brain mapping with magnetic resonance imaging. Proc Natl Acad Sci

O'Kusky J, Colonnier M (1982) A laminar analysis of the number of neurons, glia and synapses in the visual cortex (area 17) of the adult macaque monkey. J Comp Neurol 210:278–290

Pardridge WM, Oldendorf WH (1977) Transport of metabolic substrates through the blood-brain barrier. J Neurochem 28:5–12

Paul RJ, Hardin DC, Raeymaekers L, Wuytack F, Casteels R (1979) Vascular smooth muscle: aerobic gycolysis linked to sodium and potassium transport processes. Science 206:1414–1416

Pellerin L, Magistretti PJ (1994) Glutamate uptake into astrocytes stimulates aerobic glycolysis: a mechanism coupling neuronal activity to glucose utilization. Proc Natl Acad Sci USA 91:10625–10629

Pellerin L, Magistretti PJ (1996) Excitatory amino acids stimulate aerobic glycolysis in astrocytes via an activation of the Na⁺/K⁺ ATPase. Dev Neurosci 18:336–342

Pellerin L, Magistretti PJ (1997) Glutamate uptake stimulates Na+,K+-ATPase activity in astrocytes via activation of a distinct subunit highly sensitive to ouabain. J Neurochem 69:2132–2137

Pellerin L, Pellegri G, Martin J-L, Magistretti PJ (1998) Expression of monocarboxylate transporter mRNAs in mouse brain: support for a distinct role of lactate as an energy substrate for the neonatal vs. adult brain. Proc Natl Acad Sci USA 95:3990–3995

Peters A, Palay SL, Webster H de F (1991) The fine structure of the nervous system: neurons and their supporting cells. WB Saunders, Philadelphia

Phelps CH (1972) Barbiturate-induced glycogen accumulation in brain. An electron microscopic study. Brain Res 39:225–234

Phelps ME, Huang SC, Hoffman EJ, Selin C, Sokoloff L, Kuhl DE (1979) Tomographic measurement of local cerebral glucose metabolic rate in humans with (F-18)2-fluoro-2-deoxy-d-glucose: validation of method. Ann Neurol 6:371–388

Poitry-Yamate CL, Poitry S, Tsacopoulos M (1995) Lactate released by Müller glial cells is metabolized by photoreceptors from mammalian retina. J Neurosci 15:5179–5191

Pou S, Pou WS, Bredt DS, Snyder SH, Rosen GM (1992) Generation of superoxide by purified brain nitric oxide synthase. J Biol Chem 267:24173–24176

Prichard J, Rothman D, Novotny E, Petroff O, Kuwabara T, Avison M, Howseman A, Hanstock C, Shulman R (1991) Lactate rise detected by ¹H NMR in human visual cortex during physiologic stimulation. Med Sci 88:5829–5831

Proverbio F, Hoffman JF (1977) Membrane compartmentalized ATP and its preferential use by the Na⁺-K⁺ ATPase of human red cell ghosts. J Gen Physiol 69:605–632

Rothstein JD, Martin L, Levey AI, Dykes-Hoberg M, Jin L, Wu D, Nash N, Kuncl RW (1994) Localization of neuronal and glial glutamate transporters. Neuron 13:713–725

Roy CS, Sherrington CS (1890) On the regulation of the blood supply of the brain. J Physiol 11:85–108

Sappey-Marinier D, Calabrese G, Fein G, Hugg JW, Biggins C, Weiner MW (1992) Effect of photic stimulation on human visual cortex lactate and phosphates using ¹H and ³¹P magnetic resonance spectroscopy. J Cereb Blood Flow Metab 12:584–592

Schasfoort EMC, DeBruin LA, Korf J (1988) Mild stress stimulates rat hippocampal glucose utilization transiently via NMDA receptors, as assessed by lactography. Brain Res 475:58–63

Schurr A, West CA, Rigor BM (1988) Lactate-supported synaptic function in the rat hippocampal slice preparation. Science 240:1326–1328

Sharp FR, Kauer JS, Shepherd GM (1975) Local sites of activity-related glucose metabolism in rat olfactory bulb during olfactory stimulation. Brain Res 98:596–600

Sibson NR, Dhankhar A, Mason GF, Rothman DL, Behar KL, Shulman RG (1998) Stoichiometric coupling of brain glucose metabolism and glutamatergic neuronal activity. Proc Natl Acad Sci USA 95:316–321

Sokoloff L (1981) Localization of functional activity in the central nervous system by measurement of glucose utilization with radioactive deoxyglucose. J Cereb Blood Flow Metab 1:7–36

Sokoloff L (1989) Circulation and energy metabolism of the brain. In: Siegel G, Agranoff B, Albers RW, Molinoff P (eds) Basic neurochemistry: Molecular, cellular, and medical aspects, 4th edn. Raven, New York, pp 565–590

Sokoloff L, Reivich M, Kennedy C, Des Rosiers MH, Patlak CS, Pettigrew KD, Sakurada O, Shinohara M (1977) The [^{14}C]deoxyglucose method for the measurement of local cerebral glucose utilization: theory, procedure, and normal values in the conscious and anesthetized albino rat. J Neurochem 28:897–916

Sokoloff L, Kennedy C, Smith CB (1989) The [^{14}C]deoxyglucose method for measurement of local cerebral glucose utilization. In: Boulton AA, Baker GB, Butterworth RF (eds) Neuromethods. Humana, Clifton, pp 155–193

Sotelo C, Palay SL (1968) The fine structure of the lateral vestibular nucleus in the rat. J Cell Biol 36:151–179

Takahashi S, Driscoll BF, Law MJ, Sokoloff L (1995) Role of sodium and potassium ions in regulation of glucose metabolism in cultured astroglia. Proc Natl Acad Sci USA 92:4616–4620

Tower DB, Young OM (1973) The activities of butyrylcholinesterase and carbonic anhydrase, the rate of anaerobic glycolysis, and the question of a constant density of glial cells in cerebral cortices of various mammalian species from mouse to whale. J Neurochem 20:269–278

Tsacopoulos M, Magistretti PJ (1996) Metabolic coupling between glia and neurons. J Neurosci 16:877–885

Vaughn JE, Grieshaber JA (1972) An electron microscopic investigation of glycogen and mitochondria in developing and adult rat spinal motor neuropil. J Neurocytol 1:397–412

Watanabe H, Passonneau JV (1973) Factors affecting the turnover of cerebral glycogen and limit dextrin in vivo. J Neurochem 20:1543–1554

Wolf NK, Sharp FR, Davidson TM, Ryan AF (1983) Cochlear and middle ear effects on metabolism in the central auditory pathway during silence: a 2-deoxyglucose study. Brain Res 274:119–127

Perfusion-Based Functional MRI

4 Use of Diffusible and Nondiffusible Tracers in Studies of Brain Perfusion

A.C. McLaughlin, F.Q. Ye, K.F. Berman, V.S. Mattay, J.A. Frank, D.R. Weinberger

CONTENTS

4.1 Introduction

Tracer kinetic theory is a powerful theoretical approach that allows the calculation of cerebral blood flow (CBF) from the time-course of an inert "tracer" in the brain (Lassen and Perl 1979). The theory deals with two kinds of tracers – diffusible tracers and nondiffusible tracers. Nondiffusible tracers (e.g., ^{131}I-labeled albumin) are assumed to remain within the vascular bed, while diffusible tracers (e.g., ^{133}Xe, $H_2^{15}O$) are assumed to equilibrate across the blood-brain barrier.

A.C. McLaughlin, PhD; F.Q. Ye, PhD; K.F. Berman, MD; V.S. Mattay, MD; D.R. Weinberger, MD, Clinical Brain Disorders Branch, National Institute of Mental Health, Building 10; Room B1D-125, National Institutes of Health, 9000 Rockville Pike, Bethesda, MD 20892, USA
J.A. Frank, MD, Laboratory of Diagnostic Radiology, Clinical Center, Building 10; Room B1N-256, National Institutes of Health, 9000 Rockville Pike, Bethesda, MD 20892, USA

Radioactive tracers have been extensively used for physiological or clinical measurements of CBF, but compounds that can be detected by MR imaging have recently been used as "MR tracers." Two MR tracers that have proved useful for human studies are magnetically "tagged" arterial water (a diffusible tracer) and paramagnetic MR "contrast agents" (nondiffusible tracers). This chapter briefly summarizes how tagged arterial water and paramagnetic contrast agents can be used to image CBF using classical tracer theory.

4.2 Perfusion Measurements with Steady State Arterial Spin Tagging

4.2.1 Theory

Steady state arterial spin tagging approaches (Detre et al. 1992; Williams et al. 1992) "tag" arterial blood as it moves up through the brain and follow the effect of tagged blood on the amplitude of the MRI signal from a given slice. The tag consists of a change in the longitudinal magnetic moment of arterial water protons. For example, using flow-induced adiabatic inversion approaches (Dixon et al. 1986; Williams et al. 1992), arterial water protons are inverted as they pass through a defined "tagging plane" (Fig. 4.1).

The effects of tagged arterial blood on the amplitude of MRI signals from brain tissue can be used to construct a quantitative image of cerebral blood flow, Q, using the following equation (Williams et al. 1992; McLaughlin et al. 1997):

$$\Delta M/M_{ss} = -\frac{2\alpha Q/\lambda}{1/T_1} \qquad (4.1)$$

where ΔM is the steady state change in the MRI signal from intracellular brain water when arterial spins are perturbed, M_{ss} is the steady state MRI sig-

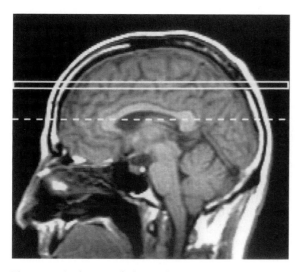

Fig. 4.1. Sagittal image of a human head, showing the approximate location of the imaging slice (*solid lines*) and the inversion plane (*dashed lines*) for a typical steady state arterial spin tagging experiment

nal from intracellular brain water, α is the degree of arterial spin inversion ($\alpha = 1$ for complete inversion), λ is the brain/blood partition coefficient for water, and $1/T_1$ is the observed longitudinal relaxation rate of brain water spins. Equation 4.1 should be applicable to most human studies, although it is strictly valid only if the off-resonance radio-frequency (RF) irradiation used to tag arterial water spins produces negligible saturation of macromolecular protons. More general expressions that are valid for arbitrary macromolecular saturation have been reported (McLaughlin et al. 1997).

The derivation of Eq. 4.1 assumes that water is a freely diffusible tracer, i.e., that water exchanges completely into brain tissue during transit through the capillary bed. However, both $H_2^{15}O$ PET (Eichling et al. 1974) and MR (Silva et al. 1997) studies have shown that water may not be freely diffusible at normal CBF rates found in humans. Under these conditions, CBF values estimated using Eq. 4.1 could be under-estimated by up to 10%.

One disadvantage of arterial spin tagging approaches is the presence of vascular artifacts (Ye et al. 1997a), which complicate the quantitation of CBF values calculated by Eq. 4.1. One vascular artifact arises from the fact that Eq. 4.1 pertains only to the effects of tagged water after it exchanges into brain tissue. A significant contribution to ΔM from tagged water in the arterial bed could cause an over-estimate of CBF. One approach for dealing with this artifact is to use "crusher" gradients, which reduce the amplitude of the MRI signal from moving arterial

water protons, but have little effect on the MRI signal from "static" brain water protons.

A second vascular artifact concerns longitudinal relaxation of tagged arterial blood during transit from the tagging plane to capillary exchange sites (Ye et al. 1997a). This relaxation reduces α by a factor $\exp(-\tau_a/T_{1a})$, where τ_a is the time required for tagged blood to move from the tagging plane to the capillary exchange sites in the imaging slice, and T_{1a} is the longitudinal relaxation time of arterial water spins. CBF values can be corrected for longitudinal relaxation during arterial transit if τ_a is known. One way to estimate τ_a is to measure the delay in the observed wash-in curve of tagged water into the brain. Figure 4.2 illustrates a delayed wash-in curve measured for a gray matter region of interest (ROI) (Ye et al. 1997a). The arterial transit time can be obtained from the fit of the delayed wash-in curve to a simple theoretical model. For the data shown in Fig. 4.2 the average arterial transit time for gray matter ($\tau_{a,gray}$) was ~1.0 s.

Figure 4.3 shows a ΔM image, and a CBF image calculated from the ΔM image using Eq. 4.1 and the calculated value of $\tau_{a,gray}$. Two problems with this approach are the extra time required (~30 min) to determine $\tau_{a,gray}$, and the fact that signal-to-noise limitations do not allow a calculation of τ_a for individual voxels. Both problems can be circumvented by using the mean value of $\tau_{a,gray}$ determined for a group of subjects as an estimate of τ_a for individual subjects in a similar group.

One difficulty with using a group mean value of

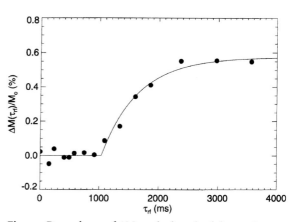

Fig. 4.2. Dependence of ΔM on the length of the tagging period. ΔM values were averaged for a large gray matter region of interest (ROI), and data were acquired in the presence of bipolar crusher gradients. The *solid curve* is the best fit of the data to a theoretical expression (Ye et al. 1997a): the arterial transit time estimated from the fit was 1.0 s. (Modified from Ye et al. 1997a)

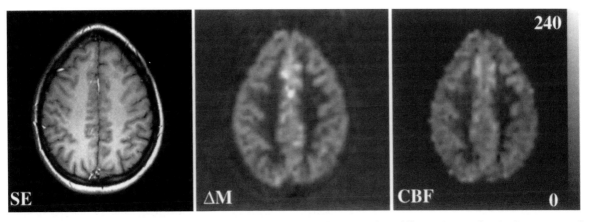

Fig. 4.3. Images of the slice shown in Fig. 4.1. *Left*, anatomical image (SE 500/20); *middle*, ΔM image taken in the presence of large bipolar crusher gradients with a tagging time of 3.6 s; *right*, cerebral blood flow (ml/100 g per min) image. (From Ye et al. 1997a)

$\tau_{a,gray}$ to calculate CBF is that deviations in τ_a from the group mean value could add significant error to the calculated CBF values. Alsop and Detre (1996) recently proposed that the sensitivity of calculated CBF values to variations in τ_a could be substantially reduced if acquisition of the MR images were delayed. Alsop and Detre (1996) used a two-compartment model (arterial bed and brain tissue) to interpret the delayed acquisition data. However, crusher gradients can be employed to reduce contributions from tagged water in the arterial bed, and a one-compartment model (brain tissue) can be used to interpret the data (Ye et al. 1997b). Both the one-compartment and the two-compartment delayed-acquisition approaches can be used to estimate CBF values using approximate estimates of the arterial transit time.

The single-compartment delayed-acquisition approach uses the following equation (Ye et al. 1997b):

$$\frac{\Delta M(\tau_{delay})}{M_o} = -\frac{2\alpha_o Q/\lambda}{R_{1o}} e^{-R_{1o}(\tau_{delay})} \{1 - \psi_1 - \psi_2\}\{\psi_3\}$$

$$(4.2)$$

where

$$\psi_1 = \left(1 - \frac{R_{1o}}{R_1(\omega_1,\Delta\omega)}\right) e^{-R_{1o}\tau_a} \qquad (4.3)$$

$$\psi_2 = \frac{R_{1o}}{R_1(\omega_1,\Delta\omega)} e^{-\left[R_{1o} - R_1(\omega_1,\Delta\omega)\right]\tau_a} e^{-R_1(\omega_1,\Delta\omega)\tau_{rf}}$$

$$(4.4)$$

$$\psi_3 = e^{\left[R_{1o} - R_{1a}\right]\tau_a} \qquad (4.5)$$

M_o is the equilibrium MRI signal from brain water, α_o is the value of α in the tagging plane, τ_{delay} is the delay between the end of the tagging period and the acquisition of data, R_{1o} and $R_1(\omega_1,\Delta\omega)$ are the relaxation rates of brain water protons in the absence and presence of the off-resonance RF irradiation used for tagging, and τ_{rf} is the length of the tagging period. Equation 4.2 assumes that $\tau_a < \tau_{delay}$.

4.2.2
Comparison with $H_2{}^{15}O$-PET

The accuracy of CBF values calculated using delayed-acquisition arterial spin tagging approaches can be tested by comparison with CBF values determined using $H_2{}^{15}O$-PET. Figure 4.4 shows two CBF images taken from the same slice in the same subject (but not at the same time). The middle image was determined using $H_2{}^{15}O$-PET, while the right-hand image was determined using a single-compartment delayed-acquisition arterial spin tagging approach (Ye et al. 1997c). Average CBF values determined by arterial spin tagging were ~10% higher than average CBF values determined by $H_2{}^{15}O$-PET for a group of control subjects (Ye et al. 1997c), which suggests that

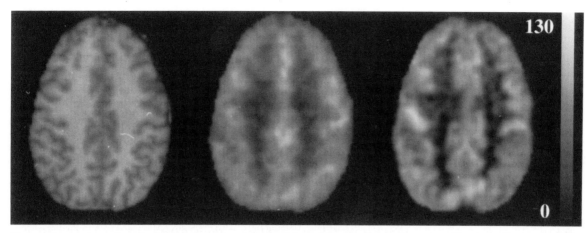

Fig. 4.4. Comparison of cerebral blood flow images obtained from the same slice in the same subject by $H_2^{15}O$ PET (*middle*) and steady state arterial spin tagging approaches (*right*). The scale is in ml/100 g per min. The image on the *left* is an anatomical image of the slice

the one-compartment delayed-acquisition arterial spin tagging approach provides accurate estimates of CBF.

4.2.3
Quantitative Regional Perfusion Changes During Motor Activation

Figure 4.5 shows quantitative CBF obtained from the same axial slice during rest (top, right) and during right-hand finger-tapping at approximately 2 Hz (top, left) (YE et al. 1997b). The difference image (bottom, left) shows the effect of finger tapping on CBF. The data in the difference image were processed using standard statistical methods to obtain the "activation" image shown in the bottom right of Fig. 4.5. Areas having a statistically significant increase in CBF during finger tapping are shown in red, superimposed on an anatomical image.

Finger-tapping paradigms would be expected to increase CBF in the contralateral primary sensorimotor cortex and the supplementary motor area (ROLAND et al. 1980). The data shown in Fig. 4.5 demonstrate activation in both areas. Similar results were observed for all subjects involved in the study. For example, activation was observed in the primary sensorimotor cortex for all subjects, while activation was observed in the supplementary motor area for five of seven subjects. The mean increase in CBF in activated primary sensorimotor region (averaged over all activated regions in all subjects) was 39 ± 6 ml/100 g per min ($63\%\pm22\%$).

CBF increases observed using steady state arterial spin tagging techniques can be compared with CBF increases observed using other approaches. If the difference in point-spread function are taken into account (YE et al. 1997b), the increases in CBF in the primary sensory motor cortex observed using arterial spin tagging approaches are consistent with increases in CBF observed using ^{133}Xe (ROLAND et al. 1980) and PET (COLEBATCH et al. 1991; SEITZ and ROLAND 1992; RAMSEY et al. 1996) approaches.

4.2.4
Quantitative Regional Perfusion Changes During Cognitive Tasks

Figure 4.6 shows a CBF activation map obtained for a simple "two-back" working memory task (YE et al. 1998a). Cognitive tasks that involve working memory components would be expected to produce focal increases in CBF in several cortical areas, especially prefrontal cortex (JONIDES et al. 1993; PAULESU et al. 1993; BERMAN et al. 1995). The data shown in Fig. 4.6 demonstrate activation in the prefrontal cortex region. Similar results were observed for all subjects involved in the study. For example, all subjects showed statistically significant increases in CBF in prefrontal cortex, although the pattern of activation varied widely among subjects. In addition, all subjects showed activation in the primary sensorimotor or premotor areas, presumably due to the finger motion involved in the responses. The mean increase in CBF in activated prefrontal cortex (averaged over all activated regions in all subjects) was 22 ± 5 ml/100 g per min ($23\%\pm7\%$).

Increases in prefrontal cortex blood flow observed during the working memory task ($\sim23\%$)

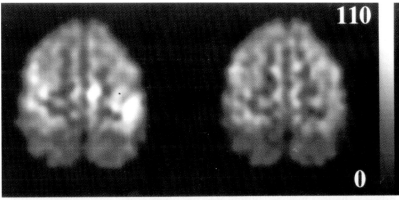

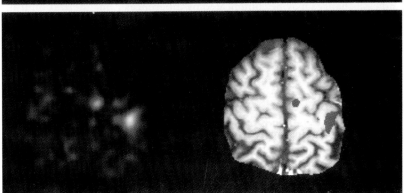

Fig. 4.5. Cerebral blood flow images of an axial slice through the primary sensorimotor cortex during rest (*top right*), and finger tapping conditions (*top left*). A difference image (*bottom left*) shows the effect of finger tapping on cerebral blood flow, and a cerebral blood flow activation image (*bottom right*) shows regions that had statistically significant differences in cerebral blood flow during finger tapping. The scale is in ml/100 g per min. (Modified from YE et al. 1998a)

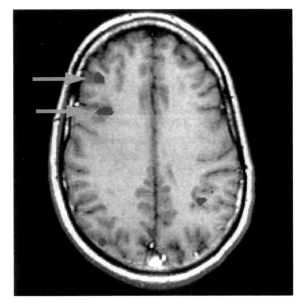

Fig. 4.6. A cerebral blood flow activation image for a two-back working memory task. Regions marked in *red* (superimposed on an anatomical image) had statistically significant differences in cerebral blood flow during the task. The *arrows* point to activated regions in the prefrontal cortex. (From YE et al. 1998a)

were substantially smaller than increases in primary sensorimotor cortex blood flow observed during motor tasks (~63%) using similar point-spread functions (5.6 mm). This observation is consistent with previous $H_2^{15}O$ PET results which suggest that focal CBF changes in prefrontal cortex during working memory tasks (PAULESU et al. 1993; DOLAN et al. 1995) are substantially smaller than focal CBF changes in primary sensorimotor cortex during motor tasks (COLEBATCH et al. 1991; RAMSEY et al. 1996). However, the reduced CBF increase in activated prefrontal cortex regions could be due to "partial volume" effects if the activated areas in the prefrontal cortex were substantially smaller than the voxel size.

4.2.5
Comparison with BOLD

Blood oxygen level-dependent (BOLD) changes are sensitive to CBF changes but are also sensitive to a number of other factors, e.g., cerebral oxygen consumption and cerebral blood volume (VAN ZIJL et al.

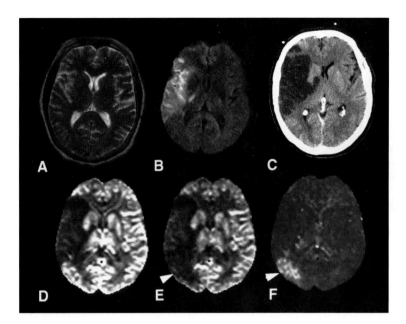

Fig. 4.8A–F. Images of a 53-year-old male, 3 h after onset of left hemiparesis. A T_2-weighted fast spin echo (**A**) showed minimal sulcal effacement in the right hemisphere. The isotropic diffusion-weighted image (**B**) correlated well with the size of the infarcted area at the follow-up CT scan 3 days later (**C**). The relative cerebral blood volume (**D**) and relative cerebral blood flow (**E**) maps showed a small region with low flow and high volume that survived the stroke (*arrow*). The region of flow-volume mismatch was clearly visible in the mean transit time map (*arrow*) (**F**). (From OSTERGAARD et al. 1996a, with permission)

arterial "curve", $\Delta R^*_{2art}(t)$, gives the deconvolved tissue "curve"

$$\frac{k^*_{tiss}}{k^*_{art}}\frac{Q}{V_{art}}\,\mathfrak{R}(t).$$

Since $\mathfrak{R}(0)=1$, the initial value of the deconvolved tissue curve is

$$\frac{k^*_{tiss}}{k^*_{art}}\frac{Q}{V_{art}}.$$

The initial value of the deconvolved tissue curve is thus proportional to the cerebral blood flow, Q (Ostergaard et al. 1996b).

4.3.2
Cerebral Blood Volume

Cerebral blood volume (V_b) is defined as the volume of blood in a brain voxel divided by the volume of the voxel. V_b for a specific brain voxel can be determined from a bolus tracking experiment using the equation (Larsen et al. 1994):

$$\frac{V_b}{V_{art}}=\frac{\int_0^\infty q_{tiss}(t)\,dt}{\int_0^\infty q_{art}(t)\,dt}\tag{4.8}$$

Using the definitions given above, Eq. 4.8 becomes:

$$\frac{V_b}{V_{art}}=\frac{k^*_{art}}{k^*_{tiss}}\frac{\int_0^\infty \Delta R^*_{2tiss}(t)\,dt}{\int_0^\infty \Delta R^*_{2art}(t)\,dt}\tag{4.9}$$

Equations 4.7 and 4.9 show that bolus tracking data, e.g., $\Delta R^*_{2tiss}(t)$ and $\Delta R^*_{2art}(t)$ can be used to calculate relative values of CBF and cerebral blood volume, but cannot be used to calculate absolute values of CBF and cerebral blood volume unless k^*_{tiss}/k^*_{art} and V_{art} are known. On the other hand, absolute values of the mean transit time, which is equal to V_b/Q, can be calculated without a knowledge of k^*_{tiss}/k^*_{art} or V_{art}.

4.3.3
Applications

Bolus tracking approaches have been used to follow regional cerebral activation during a number of different tasks, e.g., visual stimulation (BELLIVEAU et al. 1991), and can be used to study complex hemodynamic changes that take place in cerebral pathology. For example, Fig. 4.8 (taken from recent work by OSTERGAARD et al. 1996a) shows images of relative CBF, relative cerebral blood volume and mean transit time for an acute stroke patient. The cerebral blood volume and CBF maps both show reductions in the region that proceeds to infarction. In addition, CBF is also reduced in a region that has normal cerebral blood volume (see arrow in Fig. 4.8), and does not proceed to infarction. This region, which has a mismatch between CBF and cerebral blood volume, is shown as a bright area in the mean transit time map (see arrow in Fig. 4.8).

4.4 Summary

Arterial spin tagging approaches provide quantitative images of CBF and can be used to measure focal changes in CBF during motor and cognitive tasks. The disadvantage of arterial spin tagging techniques is the relative insensitivity of these approaches (compared, for example, to BOLD approaches), which necessitates relatively long exam times. Bolus tracking approaches provide images of relative CBF and relative cerebral blood volume, and are robust enough to be useful in the acute clinical environment. The disadvantage of bolus tracking techniques is the difficulty in providing absolute blood flow or blood volume measurements.

References

Alsop DC, Detre JA (1996) Reduced transit time sensitivity in noninvasive magnetic resonance imaging of human cerebral blood flow. J Cereb Blood Flow Metab 16:1236–1249

Alsop DC, Maccotta L, Detre JA (1997) Multislice perfusion imaging using adiabatic arterial spin labeling and an amplitude modulated control. Proc Int Soc Magn Reson Med 5:81

Belliveau JW, Kennedy DN, McKinstry RC, Buchbinder BR, Weisskoff RM, Cohen MS, Vevea JM, Brady TJ, Rosen BR (1991) Functional mapping of the human visual cortex by magnetic resonance imaging. Science 254:716–719

Berman KF, Ostrem J, Randolph C, Gold J, Goldberg TE, Coppola R, Carson RE, Herscovitch P, Weinberger DR (1995) Physiological activation of a cortical network during performance of the Wisconsin card sorting task: A positron emission tomography study. Neuropsychologia 33:1027–1046

Cohen JD, Forman SD, Braver TS, Casey BJ, Servan-Schreiber D, Noll DC (1994) Activation of prefrontal cortex in a nonspatial working memory task with functional MRI. Hum Brain Mapping 1:293–304

Colebatch JG, Deiber M-P, Passingham RE, Friston KJ, Frackowiak RSJ (1991) Regional cerebral blood flow during voluntary arm and hand movements in human subjects. J Neurophysiol 65:1392–1401

Detre JA, Leigh JS, Williams DS, Koretsky AP (1992) Perfusion imaging. Magn Reson Med 23:37–45

Dixon WT, Du LN, Faul DD, Gado M, Rossnick S (1986) Projection angiograms of blood labelled by adiabatic fast passage. Magn Reson Med 3:454–462

Dolan RJ, Fletcher P, Frith CD, Friston KJ, Frackowiak RKS, Grasby PM (1995) Dopaminergic modulation of impaired cognitive activation in the anterior cingulate cortex in schizophrenia. Nature 378:180–182

Edelman RR, Siewart B, Darby DG, Thangaraj V, Nobre AC, Mesulam MM, Warach S (1994) Qualitative mapping of cerebral blood flow and functional localization with echo-planar MR imaging and signal targeting with alternating radio frequency. Radiology 192:513–520

Eichling JO, Raichle ME, Grubb RL, Ter-Pogossian MM (1974) Evidence of the limitations of water as a freely diffusible tracer in brains of the rhesus monkey. Circ Res 35:358–364

Jonides J, Smith EE, Koeppe RA, Awh E, Minoshima S, Mintun MA (1993) Spatial working memory in humans as revealed by PET. Nature 363:623–625

Kim S-G (1995) Quantification of relative cerebral blood flow changes by flow-sensitive alternating inversion recovery (FAIR) technique: Application to functional mapping. Magn Reson Med 34:293–301

Kim SG, Tsekos NV (1997) Multislice perfusion-based functional MRI using the FAIR technique. Proc Int Soc Magn Reson Med 5:375

Kim S-G, Ugurbil K (1997) Comparison of blood oxygenation and cerebral blood flow effects in fMRI: Estimation of relative oxygen consumption change. Magn Reson Med 38:59–65

Kwong KK, Chesler DA, Weisskoff RM, Donahoue KM, Davis TL, Ostergaard L, Campbell TA, Rosen BR (1995) MR perfusion studies with T_1-weighted echo planar imaging. Magn Reson Med 34:878–887

Larson KB, Perman WH, Perlmutter JS, Gado MH, Ollinger JM, Zierler K (1994) Tracer kinetic analysis for measuring regional cerebral blood flow by dynamic nuclear magnetic resonance imaging. J Theor Biol 170:1–14

Lassen NA, Perl W (1979) Tracer kinetic methods in medical physiology, Raven, New York

McLaughlin AC, Ye FQ, Pekar JJ, Santha AKS, Frank JA (1997) Effect of magnetization transfer on the measurement of cerebral blood flow using steady state arterial spin tagging approaches: a theoretical investigation. Magn Reson Med 37:501–510

Ostergaard L, Sorenson AG, Kwong KK, Weisskoff RM, Glydensted C, Rosen BR (1996a) High-resolution measurement of cerebral blood flow using intravascular tracer bolus passage. Part II: Experimental comparison and preliminary results. Magn Reson Med 36:726–736

Ostergaard L, Weisskoff RM, Chesler DA, Gyldensted C, Rosen BR (1996b) High-resolution measurement of cerebral blood flow using intravascular tracer bolus passage. Part I: mathematical approach and statistical analysis. Magn Reson Med 36:715–725

Paulesu E, Frith CD, Frackowiak RSJ (1993) The neural correlates of the verbal component of working memory. Nature 362:343–345

Ramsey NF, Kirkby BS, van Gelderen P, Berman K, Duyn J, Frank JA, Mattay VS, van Horn JD, Esposito G, Moonen CTW, Weinberger DR (1996) Functional mapping of human sensorimotor cortex with 3D BOLD fMRI correlates highly with $H_2^{15}O$ PET rCBF. J Cereb Blood Flow Metab 16:755–764

Roland PE, Larsen B, Lassen NA, Skinhoj E (1980) Supplementary motor area and other cortical areas in organization of voluntary movements in man. J Neurophysiol 43:118–136

Rosen BR, Belliveau JW, Vevea JM, Brady TJ (1990) Perfusion imaging with NMR contrast agents. Magn Reson Med 14:249–265

Seitz RJ, Roland PE (1992) Learning of sequential finger movements in man: A combined kinematic and positron emission tomography (PET). Eur J Neurosci 4:154-165

Silva AC, Zhang W, Williams DS, Koretsky AP (1997) Estimation of water extraction fractions in rat brain using magnetic resonance measurement of perfusion with arterial spin labeling. Magn Reson Med 37:58–68

van Zijl PCM, Eleff SM, Ulatowski JA, Oja JME, Ulug AM, Traystman RJ, Kauppinen RA (1998) Quantitative assessment of blood flow, blood volume and blood oxygenation by functional magnetic resonance imaging. Nat Med 4:159–167

Wald LL, Carvajal L, Moyher SE, Nelson SJ, Grant PE, Barkovich AJ, Vigneron DB (1995) Phased array detectors and an automated intensity correction algorithm for high-resolution MR imaging of the human brain. Magn Reson Med 34:433-439

Weisskoff RM, Belliveau JW, Kwong KK, Rosen BR (1993) Functional imaging of capillary hemodynamics. In: Potchen EJ, Haake EM, Seibert JE, Gottschalk A (eds) Magnetic resonance angiography: concepts and applications. Mosby, St Louis, pp 473–484

Williams DS, Detre JA, Leigh JS, Koretsky AP (1992) Magnetic resonance imaging of perfusion using spin inversion of arterial water. Proc Natl Acad Sci U S A 89:212-216

Wong EC, Buxton RB, Frank LR (1998) Quantitative imaging of perfusion using a single substraction (QUIPSS and QUIPSS II). Magn Reson Med 39:702–708

Yang Y, Frank JA, Hou L, Ye FQ, McLaughlin AC, Duyn JH (1998) Multislice imaging of quantitative cerebral perfusion with pulsed arterial spin labelling. Magn Reson Med 39:825–832

Ye FQ, Pekar JJ, Jezzard P, Duyn J, Frank JA, McLaughlin AC (1996) Perfusion imaging of the human brain at 1.5 T using a single-shot EPI spin tagging approach. Magn Reson Med 36:219–224

Ye FQ, Mattay VS, Jezzard P, Frank JA, Weinberger DR, McLaughlin AC (1997a) Correction for vascular artifacts in cerebral blood flow values measured by using arterial spin tagging techniques. Magn Reson Med 37:226–235

Ye FQ, Smith AM, Yang Y, Duyn J, Mattay VS, Ruttimann UE, Frank JA, Weinberger DR, McLaughlin AC (1997b) Quantitation of regional cerebral blood flow increases during motor activation: A steady state arterial spin tagging study. NeuroImage 6:104–112

Ye FQ, Berman KF, Ellmore T, Esposito G, van Horn JD, Yang Y, Duyn J, Salustri C, Smith AM, Frank JA, Weinberger DR, McLaughlin AC (1997c) $H_2^{15}O$ PET validation of arterial spin tagging measurements of cerebral blood flow in humans. Proc Int Soc Magn Reson Med 5:87

Ye, FQ, Smith, AM, Mattay, VS, Ruttimann, UE, Frank, JA, Weinberger, DR, McLaughlin, AC (1998a) Quantitation of regional cerebral blood flow increases in the prefrontal cortex during a working memory task. NeuroImage 8:44-49

Ye FQ, Smith AM, Yang Y, Duyn J, Mattay VS, Frank JA, Weinberger DR, McLaughlin AC (1998b) 3-D imaging of cerebral blood flow changes during motor activation. Proc Int Soc Magn Reson Med 6:1467

Ye FQ, Frank JA, Weinberger DR, McLaughlin AC (1998c) Noise reduction in 3-D perfusion imaging using background suppression. Proc Int Soc Magn Reson Med 6:1210

Zhu X-H, Kim S-G, Anderson P, Ugurbil K, Chen W (1997) The correlation of BOLD and neuronal activity in primary visual cortex during photic stimulation at different frequencies. Proc Int Soc Magn Reson Med 5:742

Zierler KL (1965) Equations for measuring blood flow by external monitoring of radioisotopes. Circ Res 16:309–321

5 Perfusion fMRI with Arterial Spin Labeling

J.A. Detre, D.C. Alsop

CONTENTS

5.1 Introduction

The advent of 1H MRI has allowed unprecedented resolution to be obtained in a noninvasive imaging modality, without the use of ionizing radiation. Although proton MRI is generally considered to be a technique for anatomical imaging, it can be made sensitive to perfusion either by contrast agent administration (ROSEN et al. 1989; BELLIVEAU et al. 1991) or by electromagnetic labeling of the spins in the inflowing arterial water (DETRE et al. 1992).

J.A. DETRE, MD; D.C. ALSOP, MD, Departments of Neurology and Radiology, University of Pennsylvania, 3400 Spruce Street, Philadelphia, Pennsylvania 19104 USA

Studies in animal models and in human subjects have demonstrated that completely noninvasive, electromagnetic arterial spin labeling can be used as an endogenous tracer for quantitative perfusion imaging (DETRE et al. 1992, 1994; ROBERTS et al. 1994; SILVA et al. 1995; WILLIAMS et al. 1992; ZHANG et al. 1992, 1995). Such perfusion images were previously obtainable only with exogenous tracer methods and ionizing radiation using positron emission tomography (PET), single photon emission computed tomography (SPECT) or xenon enhanced X-ray computed tomography (XeCT). In the brain, perfusion images obtained with these methods are usually referred to as regional cerebral blood flow (CBF) images. MRI CBF images obtained with arterial spin labeling (ASL) are rapidly approaching the spatial resolution and image quality of these more established techniques. The short decay time of the ASL MRI label, approximately 1 s, permits far greater time resolution than with any other imaging technique. This property is particularly advantageous for brain activation studies, though it can be limiting in efforts to measure extremely low flow, particularly when associated with long arterial transit times.

ASL perfusion imaging is essentially a standard diffusible tracer method (KETY and SCHMIDT 1945). Water molecules in the tissue being imaged are constantly exchanging with those in the blood flowing through capillaries and venules. Electromagnetic labeling proximal to the tissue is used to modulate the magnetization of the protons in the arterial water. After the labeled protons reach the capillaries, they pass into the tissue and alter the total magnetization present. Since the MRI signal is proportional to the magnetization, images of the tissue are perturbed. An illustration of this concept is shown in Fig. 5.1. The behavior of the magnetization in the tissue is described by the modified Bloch equation (WILLIAMS et al. 1992):

$$\frac{dM_b}{dt} = \frac{M_b^0 - M_b}{T_{1b}} + \rho_b f (M_a - M_v)$$

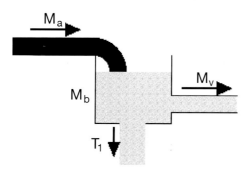

Fig. 5.1. The arterial spin labeling model. Spins, M_a, flow in from the arteries and move into the tissue. Nonequilibrium spins in the tissue, M_b, eventually disappear either by T_1 decay or by flowing out through the veins. Mb and perhaps some residual nonequilibrium spin in smaller arteries produce the signal used for perfusion imaging

where M_b, M_a and M_v are the magnetization of brain tissue, arterial blood and venous blood, M_b^0 is the equilibrium magnetization in the absence of radiofrequency (RF) excitation, T_{1b} is the T_1 of the brain and f is the flow or perfusion. T_1 is a magnetic resonance decay constant which is a function of tissue structure and magnetic field strength. ρ_b, the density of brain tissue, appears because flow is defined as the volume of blood flowing through a mass of tissue per unit time. Since the arterial magnetization can be altered with spatially selective RF irradiation, the impact of flow on the image intensity is under experimental control. ρ_b f is approximately 100 times smaller than the inverse of T_{1b}, so flow related effects usually cause image intensity changes on the order of 1%. Because T_{1b} cannot be known with this level of accuracy, it is virtually impossible to infer flow by observing just the time dependence of the signal. Instead, difference measurements are performed. For absolute flow measurement, two images with different M_a are subtracted. For activation studies (KWONG et al. 1992), subtraction of images in two different flow states can be used as long as M_a is made different from M_b. Because absolute quantification is often desirable and subtraction improves the temporal stability of the imaging (SIEWERT et al. 1996), we will focus primarily on the absolute flow measurement methods.

If we assume that the exchange of water molecules between the capillaries and the tissue is very fast, then the venous magnetization and the brain tissue magnetization are related by:

$$M_v = \frac{M_v^0}{M_b^0} M_b = \frac{1}{\lambda \rho_b} M_b$$

where λ is the brain-blood partition coefficient defined as the ml of water per mass of brain tissue divided by the ml of water per ml of blood. λ is a physiological quantity which is independent of MRI. The assumption of perfect capillary permeability to water is fairly accurate for normal flow rates but fails at higher flows (RAICHLE et al. 1976). We can rewrite the modified Bloch equation as:

$$\frac{dM_b}{dt} = \frac{M_b^0 - M_b}{T_{1app}} - \frac{f}{\lambda} 2\alpha(t) M_b^0$$

where we have defined:

$$\frac{1}{T_{1app}} = \frac{1}{T_1} + \frac{f}{\lambda}$$

$$\alpha((t)) = \frac{1}{2} \left(M_b^0 - \lambda \rho_b M_a(t) \right)$$

$\alpha(t)$ can range only between 0 and 1 and T_{1app} is constant for constant flow. All absolute perfusion imaging experiments involve the acquisition and subtraction of two or more images with different $\alpha(t)$. An example is the continuous arterial spin labeling (CASL) approach (DETRE et al. 1992; WILLIAMS et al. 1992) where α is a nonzero constant for one image and zero for the control image. If we wait for a long enough time, then a steady state is reached and the time derivative vanishes. The difference signal is then directly proportional to flow:

$$M_b^{control} - M_b^{label} = \frac{f}{\lambda} 2 T_{1app} \alpha_0 M_b^0$$

The CASL method is analogous to steady-state approaches used in PET and SPECT scanning in which a tracer with a relatively short half-life is administered continuously to the subject, and the regional accumulation, influenced by the regional blood flow and concomitant decay of the tracer, is measured (LAMMERTSMA et al. 1990; JONES et al. 1982). In CASL, continuous electromagnetic labeling of the proximal arterial supply to the brain using spatially selective excitation or inversion pulses provides a steady supply of tracer, while T_1 relaxation provides a measurable rate of decay. ASL techniques can also be used to image blood flow in organs other than brain (ROBERTS et al. 1995; WALSH et al. 1993; WILLIAMS et al. 1993a,b; TOUSSAINT et al. 1996).

5.2
Initial Validation of Arterial Spin Labeling

5.2.1
Rat Models

Experiments using alterations in arterial P_aCO_2 to alter CBF in rats, as well as a number of perturbations to produce focal changes in blood flow, have indicated that the technique does provide a quantitative measurement of CBF (DETRE et al. 1992; WILLIAMS et al. 1992), in excellent agreement with the literature (MORI et al. 1986). Independent validation of quantitative CBF values determined by the MR perfusion imaging technique against radioactive microspheres has also shown good agreement (WALSH et al. 1993). ASL MRI can be used to follow serial changes in CBF (WILLIAMS et al. 1993c).

5.2.2
Human Subjects

Initial studies of CASL perfusion MRI in humans were carried out at 1.5 Tesla using single slice technique employing a multishot, gradient echo pulse sequence (TR=100 ms, TE=5 ms, 64×256 matrix, 24 cm FOV) to acquire inversion and control images (ROBERTS et al. 1994). A single 5 mm axial slice through the centrum semiovale was imaged. ASL was accomplished using pseudocontinuous velocity-driven adiabatic inversion during the interscan interval with the duration of the labeling pulse corresponding to a 74% duty cycle. Signal averaging was performed to achieve a signal-to-noise ratio (SNR) greater than150:1, resulting in a typical acquisition time of 2–5 min per slice. For quantification, maps of T_1 were acquired using a two-point inversion recov-

ery measurement and required approximately 8 min of data acquisition.

The total imaging time to obtain inversion, control, and T1 images was12–18 min per slice. Average perfusion rates (mean±SD) in a set of nine volunteers determined by region of interest (ROI) analysis were 93±16 cc/100 g per min for gray matter, 38±10 cc/100 g per min for white matter and 52±8 cc/100 g per min for whole brain. Although these values were in reasonable agreement with literature values, the perfusion images were degraded by artifact due to inexact cancellation of scalp fat and the presence of bright spots representing intraluminal blood in which the spin label is highly concentrated ("transit artifact;" see below). Imaging was also highly sensitive to motion because arterial and control spin labeled images were obtained several minutes apart. This resulted in frequent motion degradation in perfusion images obtained from less cooperative patient populations. Further, acquisition was limited to a single slice at a time. Several recent improvements in ASL MRI have resulted in a dramatic improvement in image quality while reducing acquisition time and sensitivity to artifacts.

5.3
Strategies for Arterial Spin Labeling

As discussed above, any experiment which modifies the arterial input, $\alpha(t)$, can be used to obtain perfusion sensitive images. A number of different approaches to ASL have been developed in order to address hardware limitations or systematic errors. These approaches can be crudely divided into continuous or pulsed labeling experiments (Fig. 5.2).

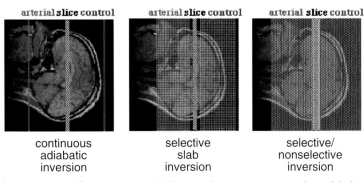

Fig. 5.2. Comparison of strategies used for arterial spin labeling. With continuous arterial spin labeling (CASL), *left*, inversion labeling is performed when blood flows past the labeling plane. With pulsed methods, all blood is labeled simultaneously with spatially selective pulsed inversion. In the original approach, *center*, pulsed inversion is applied inferior to the slice for labeling and superior to the slice for the control. Another approach, *right*, uses a nonselective inversion pulse to label all arterial spins and a selective inversion of the imaged slice as a control

5.3.1
Continuous Arterial Spin Labeling

Continuous arterial spin labeling (CASL) was the first method used for ASL imaging of perfusion. CASL can be implemented either with pseudo-continuous saturation or by flow-driven adiabatic inversion (DIXON et al. 1986; SARDASHTI et al. 1990). Since inversion produces twice the signal of saturation, it is generally preferred. Inversion is achieved by applying a constant magnetic field gradient and a constant RF irradiation at a frequency determined by the desired inversion plane. As spins flow across the inversion plane, they are very efficiently inverted (MACCOTTA et al. 1997). Adiabatic inversion is precise and simple to implement; however, it does have certain disadvantages. A practical limitation is that many MR scanners use pulsed RF amplifiers which cannot be operated continuously. Continuous irradiation with RF also deposits power in the subject. Although human perfusion scans can be performed within standard safety guidelines, RF deposition may be limiting as CASL is implemented at higher magnetic fields. Probably the greatest complication of adiabatic inversion labeling is the direct off-resonance saturation of the imaged tissue by labeling RF (Wolff and BALABAN 1989).

Application of off-resonance RF causes a decrease in signal and T_1 (YEUNG and SWANSON 1992) in tissues due to magnetization transfer. If the CASL imaging experiment is performed with adiabatic inversion for labeling and no RF for the control, a large systematic error will result because of the difference in off-resonance saturation. In the original implementation, the control image was acquired with labeling applied an equal distance distal to the slice by reversing the frequency offset of the RF (Fig. 5.3, left). Because off-resonance saturation is highly symmetric with frequency, this controls for differences in off-resonance saturation. More recently, cycling of the gradient amplitude has been proposed as a method to remove any residual errors due to small asymmetries in the off-resonance response (PEKAR et al. 1996). Unfortunately, the distal control method works for only one slice parallel to the labeling plane. An additional complication of off-resonance saturation is that the T_{1app} and M_b^0 of the brain tissue are reduced. A shorter T_{1app} decreases the observed signal, affecting quantification and reducing the SNR. For correct quantification, T_{1app} should be measured while the RF irradiation is on, but M_b^0 should be measured in its absence (ALSOP and DETRE 1996). Usually the reverse is done, but since the ratio of M^0 and T_1 in tissue is usually independent of off-resonance saturation (ALSOP and DETRE 1996; ZHANG et al. 1993), quantification is unaffected.

Because off-resonance saturation reduces signal and complicates multislice imaging, several modifications of the original CASL experiment have been proposed. A hardware approach to eliminating off-resonance saturation has been proposed by SILVA et al. (1995) and implemented for imaging of the rat. With this method a small coil placed proximal to the image slice is used to label the spins while a second volume coil is used for imaging. The labeling coil produces negligible RF power in the imaged tissue so off-resonance saturation is eliminated. This approach is attractive as long as the coil can be placed

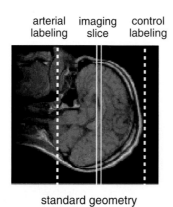

standard geometry

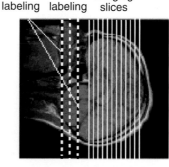

multislice geometry

Fig. 5.3. Comparison of single slice continuous arterial spin labeling (CASL) with multislice CASL using the amplitude modulated control. Both methods label spins identically. The control for the single slice method is placed an equal distance above the slice. With the amplitude modulated control, two effective inversion planes are created that doubly invert the inflowing spins while producing off-resonance saturation identical to the labeling radiofrequency (RF) across a large slab of tissue which can be imaged with multislice or 3D approaches

close enough to the tissue to minimize signal loss due to T_1 decay in transit. Off-resonance effects can also be reduced without hardware modifications if a delay is introduced between the labeling and control. Because this approach also affects the sensitivity to transit time, it will be discussed separately below.

5.3.2
Pulsed Arterial Spin Labeling

Arterial spin labeling using short RF pulses to invert or saturate the spins are attractive because they produce less off-resonance saturation and because some MRI scanners may be incapable of performing continuous labeling. A pulsed method for perfusion measurement was first introduced by EDELMAN et al. (1994). A slice selective RF pulse is used to invert the magnetization in a slab of tissue proximal to the imaged slice. Following the inversion, a period of time, TI, is allowed for the arterial blood that was originally in the inverted slab to flow into the tissue and then an image is acquired. The difference between an image without the inversion and one with the inversion reflects perfusion. A number of variations in this method have since been proposed (KWONG et al. 1995; WONG et al. 1997). One method (KWONG et al. 1995) employs the subtraction of two images obtained with slice selective or nonselective inversion recovery preparation. The signal difference in this experiment can be interpreted as a difference in the measured T_1 of the tissue as long as the T_1 of tissue and blood are equal and there is no delay between slice selective inversion and the arrival of uninverted blood from outside the inversion band in the imaged tissue.

A theoretical model for pulsed inversion ASL experiments was first reported by BUXTON et al. (1995). Assume that the labeled blood from outside the slice begins to arrive immediately after inversion and that labeled blood continues to arrive for a duration τ. As defined, this model neglects a dispersion in blood velocities and arrival times. This corresponds to:

$$\alpha(t) = \exp\left(\frac{-t}{T_{1a}}\right) \quad t < \tau$$

$$\alpha(t) = 0 \qquad\qquad t > \tau$$

where T_{1a} is the T_1 of arterial blood. The modified Bloch equation with this α inserted can be directly integrated (ALSOP and DETRE 1996). If T_{1app} and T_{1a} are comparable and the image is acquired before the

bolus has finished entering the slice (τ>TI), then the signal is given by:

$$M_b^{control} - M_b^{label} = \frac{f}{\lambda}\, 2M_b^0\, TI \exp\left(\frac{-TI}{T_{1app}}\right)$$

The maximum signal change, which occurs when TI equals T1app, is only 37% of the continuous labeling method, CASL. If the entire bolus enters the tissue, i.e. (τ<TI), and T_{1app} and T_{1a} are comparable then the signal is given by:

$$M_b^{control} - M_b^{label} = \frac{f}{\lambda}\, 2M_b^0\, \tau \exp\left(\frac{-TI}{T_{1app}}\right)$$

Since τ is not known, flow cannot be quantified without additional information.

5.4
Optimization of Arterial Spin Labeling Perfusion MRI

The ASL methods as outlined above can suffer from a number of errors in practical implementation. Most of these errors can be overcome but some issues remain outstanding. This topic is discussed in detail elsewhere in this volume.

5.4.1
Motion Artifact

Arterial spin labeling perfusion imaging involves the subtraction of two images almost 100 times larger than the difference between them. Small amounts of motion between scans can lead to large errors in the measured perfusion. The availability of single excitation imaging techniques such as echoplanar has helped to dramatically reduce motion related errors. Single excitation imaging reduces motion errors in two ways. First, the individual images are entirely free from the nonlocal phase artifacts that motion can produce in multi-excitation images. Second, the speed of the imaging permits interleaving of label and control images on the time scale of seconds. This rapid interleaving acts to attenuate the low frequency components of motion and other spurious signals which tend to be much larger than the higher frequencies (SIEWERT et al. 1996). Using echoplanar imaging, motion is rarely a problem except with the most uncooperative subjects. Echoplanar imaging itself does suffer from geometric distortion and chemical shift artifacts. Recently single shot RARE sequences have been evaluated for ASL perfusion imaging (CHEN et al. 1997).

5.4.2
Vascular Transit Time Errors

In the previous discussion, we have neglected the time delay between the application of labeling and the arrival of labeled blood at the image location. This arterial transit time, δ, can have important effects on the measured signal and consequently flow quantification. In addition, considerable evidence suggests that microvascular transit times are also highly variable . For the CASL experiment, δ enters because the labeled blood magnetization decays with T_{1a} in transit from the labeling plane to the tissue. The corrected equation is (WILLIAMS et al. 1992):

$$M_b^{control} - M_b^{label} = \exp\left(-\frac{\delta}{T_{1a}}\right)\frac{f}{\lambda} 2 T_{1app} \alpha_0 M_b^0$$

The signal decreases exponentially with the transit time. Likewise, for the pulsed experiment with (τ>TI), and T_{1app} comparable to T_{1a} the signal is given by (ALSOP and DETRE 1996):

$$M_b^{control} - M_b^{label} = \frac{f}{\lambda} 2 M_b^0 (TI-\delta) \exp\left(\frac{-TI}{T_{1app}}\right)$$

which depends linearly on δ. For humans, δ is approximately equal to T_{1a} so the effect on the signal can be quite large.

Transit time errors can be largely eliminated by slight modifications of the basic experiment. These modifications make use of the close similarity between the T_1s of blood and brain tissue, especially gray matter. If T_1 is similar in blood and tissue, then as long as the label ultimately ends up in the image the relative time the labeled spins spend in blood or tissue can be neglected. From this perspective, the transit time error can be viewed as an uncertainty in how much of the labeled blood remains in the feeding arteries outside of the tissue rather than in the tissue. This uncertainty can be eliminated if one

waits long enough after the labeling for all of the labeled blood to enter the tissue. With CASL, this involves introducing a delay, w, between labeling and image acquisition (ALSOP and DETRE 1996). In the absence of off-resonance saturation, the signal is then given by:

$$M_b^{control} - M_b^{label} =$$
$$\exp\left(\frac{-w}{T_{1app}} + \delta\left(\frac{1}{T_{1app}} - \frac{1}{T_{1a}}\right)\right)\frac{f}{\lambda} 2 T_{1app} \alpha_0 M_b^0$$

In the presence of off-resonance saturation, the expression becomes more complicated but retains the insensitivity to δ. An additional advantage of the delay is that T_{1app} is longer in the absence of the RF irradiation so the signal change is increased relative to the zero delay experiment.

For the pulsed experiment, we require $\tau+\delta$<TI in order for all of the blood to have entered the tissue. The signal is once again given by:

$$M_b^{control} - M_b^{label} = \frac{f}{\lambda} 2 M_b^0 \tau \exp\left(\frac{-TI}{T_{1app}}\right)$$

Unfortunately, τ is usually a function of the size of the inverted slab, the flow, and the geometry of the proximal vessels. WONG et al. (1997) proposed applying a saturation pulse at a time T_{sat} after the inversion to the same slab that was previously inverted. This saturation stops the inflow of any further labeled spins and externally defines a bolus duration $\tau = T_{sat}$.

With both of these techniques, the SNR need not be compromised as long as a fairly good estimate of the transit time is available. In order to insure transit time insensitivity over a wide range of transit delays, conservative values for w or T_{sat} must be selected which decrease SNR.

5.4.3
Vascular Volume Errors

Another source of error that is closely related to transit time errors is that induced by signal from labeled spins located within arterial vessels. Signal in larger vessels can degrade the spatial resolution and image quality by introducing bright linear or point-like artifacts in the perfusion images. Signal even in microscopically small vessels violates the assumptions of the above theory and the impact on the quantification must be considered.

The methods introduced above for eliminating transit time sensitivity also automatically eliminate vascular volume signal because they require that all of the labeled blood reach the tissue. It is difficult to verify that there is no label left in smaller vessels, however, since they are too small to produce artifacts or degrade resolution. It may also be too stringent a requirement that the all of the signal be in the tissue since this requires a longer post-labeling delay or a shorter T_{sat} that decreases the sensitivity of the measurement. Theoretical analyses using two transit times, one from the labeling plane to vessels within the image which are too small to degrade image resolution and a longer one to the tissue itself, suggest that labeled signal in small vessels need not degrade quantification (ALSOP and DETRE 1996). It is important to minimize any aspects of the imaging sequence which might differentially affect arterial blood and tissue spins. These aspects include T_2 weighting, since arterial blood T_2 is approximately twice that of brain, and flow attenuation as might be introduced by strong bipolar gradients. Strong bipolar gradients have in fact been used previously to eliminate the large vessel vascular volume artifacts in perfusion sensitive images without post-labeling delays (WILLIAMS et al. 1992; YE et al. 1997b). If bipolar gradients are necessary, it implies that the sequence is sensitive to transit time.

The methods outlined above have done much to improve the accuracy of perfusion quantification with ASL. Recently a quantitative validation of CASL perfusion MRI with ASL by comparison with ^{15}O-PET measurements of CBF was reported by YE et al. (1997a). This study was carried out in 12 volunteers and demonstrated an excellent correlation both in perfusion contrast and in quantitative CBF values across modalities.

5.5
Extension to Multislice Imaging

For clinical applications, a multislice technique is highly desirable both to increase coverage through the brain and because it is not always possible to know which slices are of interest prior to scanning. The extension of ASL MRI to a multislice modality has been a major technical advance which has greatly increased the feasibility of clinical use. The extension of the single slice methods to multiple slices faced two major obstacles. First, the acquisition of an image from one slice should not interfere with the flow of labeled blood into a more superior slice. This difficulty is conveniently addressed with

the approaches to transit time insensitivity. If the post-labeling delay or T_{sat} is chosen appropriately so that the first slice is insensitive to transit time, then there is no longer any labeled blood remaining in feeding vessels. Second, the off-resonance saturation and slice profile of the labeling RF has to be matched in the control image across a wide range of frequencies.

For CASL with adiabatic inversion, off-resonance saturation is the obstacle to multislice acquisition. The single slice approach of applying labeling an equal distance superior to the slice for the control image cannot be extended to multislice imaging. A second RF coil for labeling has been used successfully for multislice imaging in rat brain (SILVA et al. 1995). For human imaging, the second coil must be large enough to produce enough RF at the vessels for inversion while remaining small enough and distant enough to produce negligible RF in the imaged area. A two coil implementation for human perfusion imaging has been reported (ZAHARCHUK et al. 1997) but the labeling efficiency has not yet become competitive. We have reported a single coil approach using an alternative control irradiation which mimics the frequency dependent off-resonance effects of the labeling pulse. The control is an amplitude modulated version of the labeling (ALSOP and DETRE 1998). When a constant RF irradiation at a fixed frequency, f_0, is multiplied by a sine wave at frequency f_1, the signal produced is mathematically identical to continuous irradiation at two different frequencies, f_0+f_1 and f_0-f_1. The combined effect is that spins will be inverted twice resulting in no net effect. Because the average power and center frequency of the amplitude modulated control are identical to the labeling RF irradiation (Fig. 5.3, right), the off-resonance effects of the control are nearly identical to those of the labeling. This frequency independent matching of the off-resonance of labeling and control pulse make multislice CASL possible. Figure 5.4 shows an example of quantitative multislice perfusion imaging obtained using CASL with a post-labeling delay and amplitude modulated control labeling. Also shown are the T1 maps used for quantification.

For pulsed ASL, both the off-resonance saturation and the slice profile of the inversion can play a factor in systematic errors. FRANK et al. (1997) have evaluated the contribution of these two error sources to pulsed ASL imaging (WONG et al. 1997) and found that slice profile effects are the primary source of error. They also report pulse parameters capable of producing error free multislice images.

BOLD as well as perfusion sensitivity was present in the images; 45 labeled and 45 control images were obtained for each run. Four runs with post-labeling delays of 300, 600, 900, and1200 ms were obtained. Subjects were stimulated using flashing LED goggles at10 Hz. Subjects experienced 40 s of rest and 40 s of stimulation three times during each run. Some subjects also were asked to perform an additional finger opposition motor study with just the 300 ms post-labeling delay. All images were magnitude reconstructed and analyzed by linear fit to obtain an average ASL difference map, an ASL activation map and a BOLD activation map. The BOLD sensitivity was removed from the ASL images by subtraction of the control.

Activation was readily detectable in both the BOLD images and the ASL images. ASL activation intensity dropped rapidly with increasing post-labeling delay for all subjects. In all ASL images, including the short delay images, the activation regions were focal and did not display bright, long vascular features indicative of large vessel signal. The shape of the activation region did not change perceptibly with post-labeling delay. Despite the relatively short TE of the echoplanar images, BOLD intensity was greater than the ASL activation intensity. However, bright linear features were apparent in the BOLD activation images with especially prominent symmetric lines at the base of the occipital lobe suggestive of the transverse sinuses. The noise in the BOLD images was also higher presumably due to long term fluctuations in the background image intensity which we eliminated from the ASL images by subtracting the control.

Our results suggest that short post-labeling delays are optimal for detecting activation with continuous ASL imaging because signal intensity is higher while spatial distribution is unaffected. This observation is in sharp contrast to the situation for quantitative imaging of resting CBF. When the post-labeling delay is short or the transit time is very long, resting perfusion images demonstrate bright vascular features. Employing a short delay for activation imaging may not be possible if accurate quantification is desired. The spatial distribution of the multislice perfusion activation was more confined to visual cortex than the BOLD activation and did not display the prominent vascular features of the BOLD activation. If diffusion gradients or spin echoes must be used to attenuate these vascular signals in BOLD studies, the signal amplitude will be markedly lower and may be comparable to the ASL activation signal at 1.5 Tesla.

5.7.2
Global Activation

The cerebrovascular system can be modulated by alterations in blood oxygenation or carbon dioxide content. Such challenges may be used to validate flow measurements, or as a test of cerebrovascular reactivity (WIDDER et al. 1994; BAUMGARTNER and REGARD 1994). Figure 5.7 shows a map of percent change in CASL CBF obtained in a normal volunteer breathing 0% or 5% CO_2. Following hypercapnia, perfusion is globally increased consistent with the expected effects of hypercapnia on CBF.

5.8
Clinical Applications of Continuous Arterial Spin Labeling

5.8.1
Applications to Cerebrovascular Disease

Since hypoperfusion is the proximate cause of all stroke, it is an obvious application for a perfusion imaging methods. MRI methods for measuring perfusion offer the advantage of providing a direct comparison with high resolution structural imaging within the same modality. To assess the quality of CBF images obtained from patients with cerebrovascular disease using the multislice CASL method, and also to begin to evaluate the potential clinical role for this technique, we have studied patients who presented with stroke, transient ischemic attack (TIA), or severe carotid stenosis and were likely to have altered regional CBF, either focally or globally, based on clinical assessment (DETRE et al. 1998). Both the presence of arterial stenoses and the resulting prolonged transit times are potential sources of error or artifact in CASL perfusion MRI. We wished to determine whether perfusion could be reliably measured in patients with cerebrovascular disease using CASL, whether resting hemispheric perfusion asymmetries could be detected in such patients, and whether any such asymmetries correlated with the clinical presentation.

In our experience to date, abnormalities in cerebral perfusion are commonly observed in patients with high grade stenotic lesions of the cerebral vasculature both intracranially and extracranially. In regions of very low CBF with concomitant increased arterial transit times, bright intraluminal artifacts (transit artifacts) are sometimes observed. Transit artifacts are accentuated in CASL MRI as compared to PET CBF methods because the relatively short half-life of the electromagnetic tracer renders the technique particularly sensitive to transit time. At the same time, the increased spatial resolution of MRI allows the presence of transit artifacts to be readily identified, so that they can be considered in the interpretation of the results. Further, transit ab-

normalities detected by CASL MRI may have diagnostic significance in and of themselves.

In several patients with reduced blood flow and hemispheric asymmetries, T2-weighted structural imaging also revealed asymmetries in white matter signal intensities. An example of this is shown in Fig. 5.8. This patient had bilateral intracranial carotid stenosis and recurrent episodes of right hemiparesis, frequently associated with aphasia. Perfusion

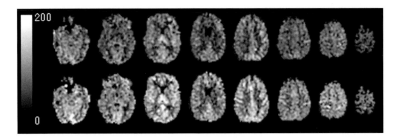

Fig. 5.7. Global activation using CO_2. Quantitative perfusion images acquired using continuous arterial spin labeling (CASL) in a normal volunteer breathing 0% (*top row*) or 5% CO_2 (*bottom row*). With CO_2 inhalation, perfusion was globally increased by 44%

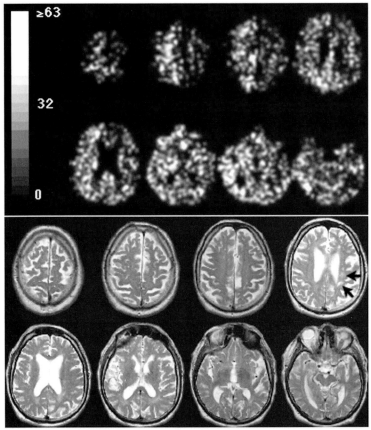

Fig. 5.8. Perfusion imaging and T2-weighted (fast spin-echo) imaging in a patient with bilateral significant carotid stenosis which was more severe on the left. *Top*, resting perfusion is globally low, but is visibly lower in the left hemisphere. *Bottom*, T2-weighted images of the same slices show patchy subcortical ischemic changes (*arrows*) likely representing internal border zone ischemia

imaging disclosed globally but also quite asymmetrically reduced flow (Fig. 5.8, top). T2-weighted images showed marked asymmetry in white matter lesions, which were much more evident in the left hemisphere (Fig. 5.8, bottom).

Under nonpathological conditions, CBF is maintained over a broad range of perfusion pressures (LASSEN 1974). This property of the cerebrovascular system is termed "autoregulation." Because autoregulatory mechanisms in the cerebral vasculature can maintain CBF through vasodilatation, it has been suggested that CBF alone is an inadequate measure of hemodynamic compromise (POWERS 1991). While resting reductions in perfusion are clearly abnormal, alterations in hemodynamic reserve are also significant because they suggest that the autoregulatory capacity of the cerebral vasculature may be exhausted. In the absence of intact autoregulation, cerebral perfusion becomes dependent on arterial blood pressure. Cerebrovascular reserve is tested by measuring the increase in CBF induced by carbon dioxide inhalation or acetazolamide administration (cerebrovascular reactivity). A number of studies have demonstrated that cerebrovascular reserve impairment is particularly significant in patients with border zone ischemia (BAUMGARTNER and REGARD 1994; RINGELSTEIN et al. 1994), and that abnormalities in augmentation are predictive of stroke (WIDDER et al. 1994; GUR et al. 1996; WEBSTER et al. 1995). CASL perfusion MRI provides a convenient method for quantitatively and noninvasively mea-

suring the effects of pharmacological augmentation throughout the brain. An example of an augmentation deficit in a patient with right middle cerebral artery stenosis is shown in Fig. 5.9. In this patient resting perfusion was normal in the right hemisphere and T2-weighted imaging was also normal. However, following administration of 1 g acetazolamide i.v., regional CBF failed to increase in the right middle cerebral artery distribution and actually decreased somewhat.

The measurement of cerebral perfusion and diffusion using MRI is becoming an important part of the evaluation of acute stroke (BAIRD et al. 1997; WARACH et al. 1992, 1995, 1996; SORENSEN et al. 1996). These data are used to confirm the diagnosis of stroke, to establish a baseline against which stroke therapies can be assessed, and to contribute to the prognosis in individual cases. Most cerebral perfusion studies in acute stroke have utilized a bolus-tracking approach in which the first-passage of an MRI contrast agent is imaged dynamically. Such data can be analyzed to yield maps of mean transit time and blood volume which are related to perfusion. Although the bolus-tracking methods provides a high SNR for perfusion abnormalities, its successful implementation requires administration of contrast through a relatively large bore i.v. catheter, often using a power injector. While ASL MRI requires a longer data acquisition, no contrast injection is required. This could result in a time savings for patients in whom i.v. access is difficult. The major chal-

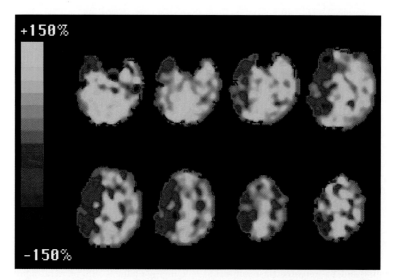

Fig. 5.9. Perfusion augmentation testing using intravenous acetazolamide in a patient with right middle cerebral artery stenosis. The regional percent change in perfusion between baseline and 10 min following 1 g i.v. acetazolamide is displayed. Following acetazolamide, a reduction in regional perfusion in the right middle cerebral artery is evident

lenge for ASL perfusion imaging in stroke relates to the short half-life of the spin label; if arterial transit times exceed 3 s, tracer delivery will be negligible. Although quantification is affected, a perfusion abnormality will still be identified. Initial studies suggest that ASL methods can faithfully identify focal perfusion deficits in acute stroke (SIEWERT et al. 1997).

5.8.2
Applications to Degenerative Disease

Functional imaging of Alzheimer's disease (AD) and frontotemporal dementia (FD) with PET and SPECT have demonstrated deficits in metabolism and flow in specific cortical association areas that are characteristic for the type of dementia. Structural MRI has also been used to quantify hippocampal and cortical atrophy. ASL perfusion imaging offers the possibility of obtaining both functional and structural information noninvasively during a single scanning session. SANDSON et al. (1996) have reported an initial evaluation of single-slice qualitative pulsed ASL imaging for functional studies of AD. They were able to detect temporoparietal flow deficits relative to controls. We have evaluated quantitative, multislice CASL in a cohort of patients with AD and FD. Brain registration between subjects was performed using features of the SPM96 software (FRISTON et al. 1995).

In severe AD subjects, pronounced temporoparietal and prefrontal deficits were observed, while in FD patients frontal deficits were dominant (Fig. 5.10). Very significant global flow deficits were also observed. Initial analysis of a very mildly demented cohort indicate a similar pattern of flow deficits but with reduced amplitude.

5.9
Conclusion

Over the past several years, the technical and theoretical foundations of ASL perfusion imaging techniques have evolved from feasibility studies into practical usage. Although ASL perfusion measures small changes in image signal intensity as compared to other functional imaging techniques, the ability to quantify results in well characterized physiological parameters along with the ability to sample these signal changes using a range of imaging techniques represent significant advantages. These techniques have a broad range of potential applications in clinical and basic research of brain physiology, as well as in other organs.

Acknowledgments. The authors acknowledge support from the National Institutes of Health, the American Heart Association, and the Whitaker Foundation.

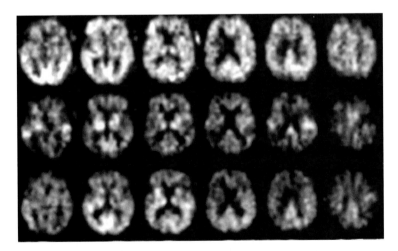

Fig. 5.10. Continuous arterial spin labeling (CASL) imaging of dementia. The average of images from three normal elderly subjects, *top row*, are compared to averages from three subjects with Alzheimer's disease, *second row*, and frontotemporal dementia, *bottom row*. AD patients demonstrate flow deficits in parietal and temporal areas as well as global flow deficits. FD patients have preserved posterior flow but decreased flow in frontal and anterior temporal areas

References

Alsop DC, Detre JA (1996) Reduced transit-time sensitivity in noninvasive magnetic resonance imaging of human cerebral blood flow. J Cereb Blood Flow Metab 16:1236–1249

Baird A, Lovblad K, Benfield A, Schlaug G, Siewert B, Edelman R, Warach S (1997) Correlation of diffusion/perfusion abnormalities and clinical outcome in acute stroke. Neurology 48 [Suppl 2]:A203

Baumgartner RW, Regard M (1994) Role of impaired CO2 reactivity in the diagnosis of cerebral low flow infarcts. J Neurol Neurosurg Psychiatry 57:814–817

Belliveau JW, Kennedy DW, McKinstry RC et al (1991) Functional mapping of the human visual cortex by magnetic resonance imaging. Science 254:716–718

Buxton RB, Frank LR, Siewert B et al (1995) A quantitative model for EPISTAR perfusion imaging. International Society for Magnetic Resonance in Medicine, 3rd Annual Meeting Book of Abstracts 132

Chen Q, Siewert B, Bly B, Warach S, Edelman R (1997) STAR-HASTE: Perfusion imaging without magnetic susceptibility artifact. Magn Reson Med 38:404–408

Detre JA, Alsop DC, Vives LR, Maccotta L, Teener JW, Raps EC (1998) Noninvasive MRI evaluation of cerebral blood flow in cerebrovascular disease. Neurology 50:633–641

Detre JA, Leigh JS, Williams DS, Koretsky AP (1992) Perfusion imaging. Magn Reson Med 23:37–45

Detre JA, Zhang W, Roberts DA et al (1994) Tissue specific perfusion imaging using arterial spin labeling. NMR Biomed 7:75–82

Dixon WT, Du LN, Faul DD, Gado M, Rossnick S (1986) Projection angiograms of blood labeled by adiabatic fast passage. Magn Reson Med 3:454–462

Edelman RR, Siewert B, Darby DG, Thangaraj V, Nobre AC, Mesulam MM, Warach S (1994) Qualitative mapping of cerebral blood flow and functional localization with echoplanar MR imaging and signal targeting with alternating radio frequency. Radiology 192:513–520

Frank LR, Wong EC, Buxton RB (1997) Slice profile effects in adiabatic inversion: application to multislice perfusion imaging. Magn Reson Med 38:558–564

Friston KJ, Ashburner J, Frith CD, Poline JB, Heather JD (1995) Spatial registration and normalization of images. Human Brain Mapping 3:165–189

Gur AY, Bova I, Bornstein NM (1996) Is impaired cerebral vasomotor reactivity a predictive factor of stroke in asymptomatic patients? Stroke 27:2188–2190

Jones SC, Greenberg JH, Reivich M (1982) Error analysis for the determination of cerebral blood flow with the continuous inhalation of 15O-labeled carbon dioxide and positron emission tomography. J Comput Assist Tomogr 6:116–124

Kety SS, Schmidt CF (1945) The determination of cerebral blood flow in man by the use of nitrous oxide in low concentrations. Am J Physiol 143:53–66

Kim SG (1995) Quantification of relative cerebral blood flow change by flow-sensitive alternating inversion recovery (FAIR) technique: application to functional mapping. Magn Reson Med 34:293–301

Kwong KK, Belliveau JW, Chesler DA et al (1992) Dynamic magnetic resonance imaging of human brain activity during primary sensory stimulation. Proc Natl Acad Sci USA 89:5675–5679

Kwong KK, Chesler DA, Weisskoff RM et al (1995) MR perfusion studies with T1-weighted echo planar imaging. Magn Reson Med 34:878–887

Lammertsma AA, Conningham VJ, Deiber MP, Heather JD, Bloomfield PM, Nutt J, Frackowiak RS, Jones T (1990) Combination of dynamic and integral methods for generating reproducible functional CBF images. J Cereb Blood Flow Metab 10:675–686

Lassen, NA (1974) Control of cerebral circulation in health and disease. Circ Res 34:749–760

Maccotta L, Detre JA, Alsop DC (1997) The efficiency of adiabatic inversion for perfusion imaging by arterial spin labeling. NMR Biomed 10:216–221

Mori, S, Ngai AC, Ko KR, Winn HR (1986) A venous outflow method for continuously monitoring cerebral blood flow in the rat. Am J Physiol 250:H304–H312

Pekar J, Jezzard P, Roberts DA, Leigh JS Jr, Frank JA, McLaughlin AC (1996) Perfusion imaging with compensation for asymmetric magnetization transfer effects. Magn Reson Med 35:70–79

Powers WJ (1991) Cerebral hemodynamics in ischemic cerebrovascular disease. Ann Neurol 29:231–240

Raichle ME, Eichling JO, Straatmann MG, Welch MJ, Larson KB, Ter-Pogossian MM (1976) Blood-brain barrier permeability of 11C-labeled alcohols and 15O-labeled water. Am J Physiol 230:543–552

Ringelstein EB, Weiller C, Weckesser M, Weckesser S (1994) Cerebral vasomotor reactivity is significantly reduced in low-flow as compared to thromboembolic infarctions: the key role of the circle of Willis. J Neurol Sci 121:103–109

Roberts D, Bolinger L, Detre JA, Insko E, Burgey P, Leigh JS (1992) Angiography by continuous inversion of arterial water. Magn Reson Med 29:631–636

Roberts DA, Detre JA, Bolinger L, Insko EK, Leigh JS Jr (1994) Quantitative magnetic resonance imaging of human brain perfusion at 1.5 T using steady-state inversion of arterial water. Proc Natl Acad Sci USA 91:33–37

Roberts DA, Detre JA, Bolinger L, Insko EK, Lenkinski RE, Pentecost MJ, Leigh JS (1995) Renal perfusion in humans: MR imaging with spin tagging of arterial water. Radiology 196:281–286

Rosen BR, Belliveau JW, Chien D (1989) Perfusion imaging by nuclear magnetic resonance. Magn Reson Q 5:263–281

Sandson, TA, O'Connor M, Sperling RA, Edelman RR, Warach S (1996) Noninvasive perfusion MRI in Alzheimer's disease: a preliminary report. Neurology 47:1339–1342

Sardashti M, Schwartzberg DG, Stomp GP, Dixon WT (1990) Spin labeling angiography of the carotids by presaturation and simplified adiabatic inversion. Magn Reson Med 15:192–200

Siewert B, Bly BM, Schlaug G, Darby DG, Thangaraj V, Warach S, Edelman RR (1996) Comparison of the BOLD- and EPISTAR-technique for functional brain imaging by using signal detection theory. Magn Reson Med 36:249–255

Siewert B, Schlaug G, Edelman RR, Warach S (1997) Comparison of EPISTAR and T2*-weighted gadolinium-enhanced perfusion imaging in patients with acute cerebral ischemia. Neurology 48:673–679

Silva AC, Zhang W, Williams DS, Koretsky AP (1995) Multislice MRI of rat brain perfusion during amphetamine stimulation using arterial spin labeling. Magn Reson Med 33:209–214

Sorensen AG, Buonanno FS, Gonzalez RG et al (1996) Hyperacute stroke: evaluation with combined multisection diffusion-weighted and hemodynamically weighted echo-planar MR imaging. Radiology 199:391–401

Talagala SL, Noll DC (1998) Functional MRI using strady state arterial water labeling. Magn Reson Med 39:179–183

Toussaint JF, Kwong KK, Mkparu FO, Weisskoff RM, LaRaia PJ, Kantor HL, M'Kparu F (1996) Perfusion changes in human skeletal muscle during reactive hyperemia measured by echo-planar imaging [published erratum appears in Magn Reson Med 37(1):152, 1997]. Magn Reson Med 35:62–69

Walsh EG, Minematsu K, Leppo J, Moore SC (1993) Radioactive microsphere validation of a volume localized continuous saturation perfusion measurement. Magn Reson Med 31:147–153

Walsh TR, Detre JA, Koretsky AP et al (1993) Response of normal and reperfused livers to glucagon stimulation: NMR detection of blood flow and high-energy phosphates. Biochem Biophys Acta 1181:7–14

Warach S, Chien D, Li W, Ronthal M, Edelman RR (1992) Fast magnetic resonance diffusion-weighted imaging of acute human stroke. Neurology 42:1717–1723

Warach S, Gaa J, Siewert B, Wielopolski P, Edelman RR (1995) Acute human stroke studied by whole brain echo planar diffusion-weighted magnetic resonance imaging. Ann Neurol 37:231–241

Warach S, Dashe JF, Edelman RR (1996) Clinical outcome in ischemic stroke predicted by early diffusion-weighted and perfusion magnetic resonance imaging; a preliminary analysis. J Cereb Blood Flow Metab 16:53–59

Webster MW, Makaroun MS, Steed DL, Smith HA, Johnson DW, Yonas H (1995) Compromised cerebral blood flow reactivity is a predictor of stroke in patients with symptomatic carotid artery occlusive disease. J Vasc Surg 21:338–344

Widder B, Kleiser B, Krapf H (1994) Course of cerebrovascular reactivity in patients with carotid artery occlusions. Stroke 25:1963–1967

Williams DS, Detre, JA Leigh JS, Koretsky AP (1992) Magnetic resonance imaging of perfusion using spin inversion of arterial water. Proc Natl Acad Sci USA 89:212–216

Williams DS, Zhang W, Koretsky AP, Adler S (1993a) MRI of perfusion in the kidney in vivo using spin inversion of arterial water. SMRM 12th Annual Meeting Book of Abstracts 641

Williams DS, Grandis DJ, Zhang W, Koretsky AP (1993b) Magnetic resonance imaging of perfusion in the isolated

rat heart using spin inversion of arterial water. Magn Reson Med 30:361–365

Williams DS, Detre JA, Zhang W, Koretsky AP (1993c) Fast serial MRI of perfusion in the rat brain using spin inversion of arterial water. Bull Magn Reson 15:60–63

Wolff SD, Balaban RS (1989) Magnetization transfer contrast (MTC) and tissue water proton relaxation in vivo. Magn Reson Med 10:135–144

Wong EC, Buxton RB, Frank LR (1997) Implementation of quantitative perfusion imaging techniques for functional brain mapping using pulsed arterial spin labeling. NMR Biomed 10:237–249

Ye FQ, Berman KF, Ellmore T et al (1997a) H215O PET validation of arterial spin tagging measurements of cerebral blood flow in humans. International Society for Magnetic Resonance in Medicine, 5th Scientific Meeting Book of Abstracts 1:87

Ye FQ, Mattay VS, Jezzard P, Frank JA, Weinberger DR, McLaughlin AC (1997b) Correction for vascular artifacts in cerebral blood flow values measured using arterial spin taggign techniques. Magn Reson Med 37:226–235

Ye F, Smith A, Yang Y et al (1997c) Quantitation of regional cerebral blood flow increases during motor activation: a steady-state arterial spin tagging study. Neuroimage 6:104–112

Yeung HN, Swanson SD (1992) Transient decay of longitudinal magnetization in heterogeneous spin systems under selective saturation. J Magn Reson 99:466–479

Zaharchuk G, Ledden PJ, Kwong KK, Rosen BR (1997) Multislice arterial spin labeling of perfusion territory and functional activation in humans using two coils. International Society for Magnetic Resonance in Medicine, 5th Annual Meeting Book of Abstracts 79

Zhang W, Williams DS, Detre JA, Koretsky AP (1992) Measurement of brain perfusion by volume-localized NMR spectroscopy using inversion of arterial water spins: accounting for transit time and cross relaxation. Magn Reson Med 25:362–371

Zhang W, Silva AC, Williams DS, Koretsky AP (1993) The effect of cross-relaxation on the measurement of perfusion by arterial spin labeling using two isolated RF coils. SMRM 12th Annual Meeting Book of Abstracts 617

Zhang W, Silva AC, Williams DS, Koretsky AP(1995) NMR measurement of perfusion using arterial spin labeling without saturation of macromolecular spins. Magn Reson Med 33:370–376

6 Potential and Pitfalls of Arterial Spin Labeling Based Perfusion Imaging Techniques for MRI

E.C. WONG

CONTENTS

6.1
The Potential of Arterial Spin Labeling in fMRI

As discussed in the previous chapters, imaging of cerebral blood flow (CBF) using arterial spin labeling (ASL) techniques provides a promising alternative to blood oxygen level-dependent (BOLD) contrast for fMRI. The primary benefits of ASL for fMRI are that it may provide more accurate localization of neuronal activity, allows for absolute measurement of CBF, and is less sensitive to subject motion than BOLD fMRI.

E.C. WONG, MD, PhD, Departments of Radiology and Psychiatry, University of California at San Diego Medical Center, 200 West Arbor Drive, San Diego, California 92103-8756 USA

6.1.1
Better Localization?

The BOLD fMRI signal arises from changes in blood oxygenation. Oxygen is extracted from blood in the capillaries, and the resulting deoxyhemoglobin travels into the venous circulation. While there is certainly a BOLD effect that arises from capillaries, the majority of the BOLD effect is venous in origin (see Sect. 6.3). Because of this, the BOLD signal may be localized to veins that may be removed by up to a few centimeters from the site of neuronal activity. Diffusion/flow weighting gradients that destroy intravascular signal cannot entirely alleviate this problem because the extravascular BOLD effect in tissues surrounding veins is not destroyed by such gradient pulses.

The ASL signal arises from the delivery of magnetically tagged arterial water into the imaging slice. The extraction of arterial water in the capillaries is nearly complete, allowing the tagged water to exchange into the tissue compartment. While the bi-directional exchange of water across the capillary is very rapid, the fact that the tissue compartment is much larger than the vascular compartment makes the time constant for clearance of tagged water by outflow into the venous system very slow. This time constant is essentially that of perfusion itself, and is on the order of 1 min. Thus, on the time scale of the ASL tagging and imaging process (<2 s), clearance of tag into the venous system is negligible, and the ASL tag behaves like a tracer that is delivered to brain tissue and stays there. The ASL signal is therefore localized to arteries, capillaries, and brain tissue. Brain tissue that receives increased perfusion is presumably the site of neuronal activity itself, and capillaries are embedded within those tissues, so the only component of the functional ASL signal that can be spatially removed from the site of brain activity is the intra-arterial component. However, the intra-arterial component of the ASL signal is simply proportional to the volume of tagged blood in the arteries at the time of image acquisition, as the concentration of the tag is not affected by the increases in flow that accompany activation. Arterial blood volume is small to begin with, and changes in arterial blood volume are likely to be undetectable through the ASL signal. It is possible that changes in transit times during activation (see Sect. 6.3.1) can affect the presence of tagged blood in arteries at the time of image acquisition, but this would be seen as a negative change in the ASL signal with activation. If the timing of the tag and imaging were such that in the rest condition the end of the tag was in an imaging voxel at the time of image acquisition, then with the higher flow rates that accompany activation, the end of the tag may clear that same voxel, resulting in a lower intra-arterial ASL signal with activation. While this is theoretically possible, it has not been reported experimentally. Even in the case that functional changes do occur in the intra-arterial ASL signal, it is relatively easy to destroy the intra-arterial ASL signal by simply introducing a delay between the application of the tag and image acquisition (ALSOP and DETRE 1996; WONG et al. 1998a) or applying diffusion/flow weighting gradients in the imaging process to destroy signal from flowing spins (YE et al. 1997).

Thus, on theoretical grounds it is reasonable to expect that the functional ASL signal maps closer in space to the true sites of neuronal activity than the BOLD signal. Unfortunately, there have not yet been studies that could provide direct evidence of this (such as BOLD and ASL fMRI combined with direct electrocorticography). However, there is fMRI evidence that the BOLD and ASL signals are only partially overlapping, and that the ASL signal is more

restricted to gray matter, while the BOLD signal clearly has a large intravenous component. In Fig. 6.1, functional correlation maps from a simultaneous ASL/BOLD finger tapping experiment show clearly different distributions of ASL and BOLD activations. On the left side, the ASL signal appears to lie within the gray matter on the anterior and posterior aspects of the central sulcus, while the BOLD signal lies primarily within the sulcus. On the right side the distinction is less clear, but demonstrates a typical finding from the motor area that the BOLD signal is more lateral than the ASL signal, again consistent with an ASL signal that is primarily parenchymal and a BOLD signal that is primarily intravenous.

6.1.2
Quantitation of Cerebral Blood Flow

The ASL signal is different from the BOLD signal in that it is quantitatively related to a well-defined physical parameter (CBF). Conversely, the BOLD signal reflects a complex combination of CBF, blood volume, and oxygen extraction.

It is generally assumed that CBF is directly (although probably not linearly) related to local neuronal activity. The details of this link have not been determined experimentally, but if and when this relationship is understood, ASL would then provide a quantitative measure of neuronal activity. Because the BOLD signal is critically dependent upon the local blood volume (which itself is dynamic), as well as the metabolic rate of oxygen, it will be much more difficult to quantify neuronal activity based on the BOLD signal.

6.1.3
Motion Insensitivity

In BOLD fMRI, the design of cognitive paradigms is significantly limited by the fact that the BOLD signal can only detect oxygenation changes related to the

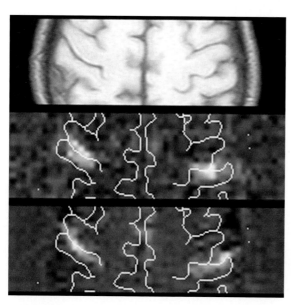

Fig. 6.1. Functional maps from a simultaneous arterial spin labeling (ASL)/blood oxygen level-dependent (BOLD) contrast finger tapping experiment. *Top,* anatomical reference; *middle,* ASL correlation map; *bottom,* BOLD correlation map. Note on the *left* that the ASL signal appears to map to the banks of the central sulcus while the BOLD signal lies within the sulcus. On the *right,* the ASL signal is more medial than the BOLD signal

difference between two states. The time scale of BOLD experiments is limited by the stability of the MRI signal relative to the amplitude of the BOLD related signal change. The stability of the MRI signal is usually limited primarily by subject motion and to a lesser degree by scanner stability. In all but the most highly motivated subjects, this places a practical upper limit on the time between task changes of a few minutes, beyond which signal drift due to motion is often difficult to distinguish from true functional activation. In ASL based fMRI, absolute values for CBF can be obtained from every pair of tag-control images. The effective decrease in long-term sensitivity to subject motion in ASL derives from the fact that the functional ASL signal is typically a 50%–100% increase in the ASL signal, while the BOLD signal is typically a 2%–4% change in the raw image intensity. Small subvoxel subject motion that changes the raw signal by a few percent can swamp the BOLD signal. However, because the ASL signal simply scales with the raw image intensity, such motion only changes the ASL signal by a few percent, and so does not swamp the large percentage changes in the ASL signal seen with activation.

In practice, even in combined ASL/BOLD experiments with interstimulus intervals in the common 40–60 s range, the ASL functional signal is typically much less contaminated by stimulus correlated motion than the BOLD functional signal. Figure 6.2 shows simultaneously acquired maps of BOLD signal change and ASL signal change for a simple finger tapping experiment. These correlation images demonstrate the typical findings of pronounced artifacts around the borders of the brain in the BOLD image, and a very clean subtraction with isolated regions of activation in the ASL correlation image.

This long-term insensitivity to subject motion makes ASL suitable for some types of studies that employ modulation of brain activity on a relatively long time scale and are therefore impractical with BOLD contrast. Examples include studies of sleep, vigilance, habituation, and the effects of drugs.

6.2
Limitations of Arterial Spin Labeling Relative to BOLD for fMRI

While ASL fMRI has many attractive properties, conventional BOLD contrast has several advantages that make it the appropriate choice for the majority of fMRI studies.

6.2.1
Smaller Functional Signal in Arterial Spin Labeling

The biggest advantage that BOLD has over ASL for fMRI is that the absolute BOLD signal change is usually two to four times as large as the change in the ASL signal with activation. While a typical BOLD signal is 2% of the raw image intensity, a typical baseline ASL signal (control–tag) is only 1% of the raw image intensity, and although the functional change in the ASL signal can be as high as 100%, this still represents only 1% of the raw image intensity. In fMRI, in which the signal to noise ratio critically af-

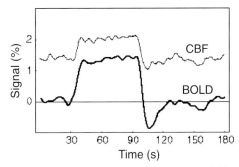

Fig. 6.3. Arterial spin labeling (ASL) (cerebral blood flow, *CBF*), and blood oxygen level-dependent (*BOLD*) time courses from a simultaneous ASL/BOLD finger tapping experiment. BOLD is shown as signal change relative to baseline, while CBF signal is absolute, but both are on the same scale. The amplitude of the BOLD signal change is approximately twice that of the ASL signal change. The BOLD signal also demonstrated a post-stimulus undershoot, while the ASL signal does not

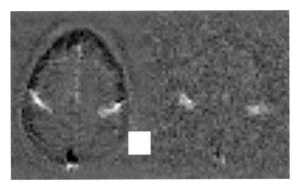

Fig. 6.2. Blood oxygen level-dependent (BOLD) (*left*) and arterial spin labeling (ASL) (*right*) correlation maps from a simultaneous ASL/BOLD finger tapping experiment, demonstrating relative motion insensitivity of ASL

fects the detectability of activated brain regions, a factor of two decrease in functional contrast makes functional ASL impractical in some cases. Signal averaging can make up the difference in functional contrast, but requires a factor of four increase in scan time, which is often prohibitively long. Figure 6.3 shows ASL and BOLD signal time courses for a region of interest from Fig. 6.1, selected for voxels demonstrating a functional ASL signal. In these voxels, the BOLD signal is approximately two times larger than the activation related change in the ASL signal. However, the region of the largest BOLD is spatially distinct from the region that has the largest ASL signal change (see Sects. 6.1.1), and the voxels with the largest BOLD signals have signal changes that are three to four times those of the ASL signal.

6.2.2
Temporal Resolution

Because of the time required to allow for tagged blood to flow into the imaging slices, even multislice ASL is limited in its maximum rate of image acquisition relative to BOLD imaging. In a typical ASL implementation, five to eight slices are acquired with a TR of 2–3 s. Both the minimum TR and the maximum number of slices is limited by the time required for a tagged bolus to be delivered to a slab of imaging slices. This represents a net image throughput of only two to three images per second, while in echo planar imaging (EPI) based BOLD imaging the throughput is typically limited by hardware to approximately ten images per second. For BOLD imaging, optimal sensitivity is achieved when the TR is no longer than about 1 s. At this TR, EPI based BOLD sequences can still cover about ten slices, each with two to three times as much signal averaging as in an ASL experiment.

6.2.3
Hardware Considerations

In BOLD imaging, the sensitivity of the imaging technique to functional changes is directly proportional to the B_1 sensitivity. In this case it is straightforward to optimize radiofrequency (RF) coils to cover only the areas of interest, and thus optimize the sensitivity to BOLD contrast. In ASL, RF is used both for image acquisition and for application of the inversion tag, and the dependence of sensitivity on the B_1 profile of the RF coil is somewhat more com-

plicated. If separate coils are used for transmit and receive, then it is straightforward to optimize each coil for its purpose: the receive coil to have high sensitivity over the region of interest, and the transmit coil to provide uniform B_1 in the tagging region. However, if a single coil is used for both transmit and receive, as is often the case, then the coil design will likely be larger than necessary for image acquisition in order to provide adequate coverage for tagging, and thus have a suboptimal signal-to-noise ratio (SNR) in the region of interest.

6.3
Issues in the Quantitation of Cerebral Blood Flow Using Arterial Spin Labeling

Absolute quantitation of CBF is a critical component in the development of ASL techniques for clinical applications such as acute stroke and can be important for fMRI if a quantitative link between CBF and neuronal activity can be established (see Sect. 6.1.2). ASL can potentially suffer from several sources of systematic errors, which have been the subject of intense study in the past few years. The most important of these are described below.

6.3.1
Transit Delay

After the application of the inversion tag in ASL, there is a transit delay before tagged blood begins to enter the imaging slices. This delay is typically between 500 ms and 1500 ms and can be highly variable even within a given imaging slice. In pathology, this delay can be significantly longer. Because the T_1 of blood is on the same order as this delay, it is necessary to acquire images as soon as possible after the arrival of tagged blood in the imaging slice in order not to lose too much of the ASL signal to T_1 decay. If the transit delay is not accounted for, then the ASL signal will be critically dependent upon the value of this delay. Recently, two modified ASL techniques have been introduced that greatly decrease sensitivity to the effects of the transit delay. In both techniques, a bolus of tagged blood of well defined time width is created and delivered to the imaging slices. If imaging is delayed until the entire bolus reaches the imaging slice, then the ASL is proportional to the width of the bolus+CBF, and CBF is thus easily calculated. One of the techniques is a pulsed ASL technique called QUIPSS II (WONG et al. 1997, 1998a). In this technique, a tag is produced using a slab selective inversion pulse, and at a time TI_1 later, a saturation pulse is applied in the tagging slab. In this manner, a known amount of tagged blood (TI_1+CBF) leaves the tagging region, and the remainder of the tag is destroyed by saturation. Imaging occurs after an additional delay to allow for the entire bolus to reach the imaging slice. An analogous technique uses continuous flow-dependent adiabatic inversion (ALSOP and DETRE 1996). In this technique the time width of the tag is simply equal to the duration of the inverting RF radiation, and a delay is inserted after the RF is turned off and before image acquisition.

If quantitation of CBF is required, these modified ASL techniques are particularly important for measuring activation induced changes in CBF, because the transit delay changes dynamically with activation. When brain activity increases, local CBF and flow velocities increase. Because of the increase in flow velocity, the transit delay decreases with activation. In Fig. 6.4, the ASL signal as a function of TI for an EPISTAR (EDELMAN et al. 1994) imaging sequence is shown for a motor cortex region of interest (ROI) in resting and active (finger tapping) states. The data clearly show a transition to shorter transit delays and increased ASL signal with activation. Also shown in the figure is the fit of the data to a kinetic model of the ASL inflow process (WONG et al. 1997; BUXTON et al. 1997, 1998). The transit delay as extracted from this fit decreases from 400 ms to 300 ms during activation. It should be noted that, if quantitative CBF information is not required, it is possible to use the decrease in transit delay to amplify the increase in the ASL signal with activation. If an ASL technique is employed with a short TI that is similar to or slightly longer than the resting transit delay, then with activation the ASL signal increases more than linearly with CBF. However, if too long a value for TI is used, there is the possibility that the ASL signal may not change, or may even decrease with activation. QUIPSS II (WONG et al. 1998a) and continuous ASL with an inserted delay (ALSOP and DETRE 1996) are not susceptible to this effect.

6.3.2
Intravascular Signal

Another source of systematic error is the inclusion of tagged intravascular signal in the perfusion measurement, some of which is in vessels that are passing through, but not perfusing, the imaging slice. Signal from these vessels are not properly interpreted as perfusion of the imaging slice because they will end in capillary beds in more distal slices. One approach that has been used for minimizing this source of artifact is the application of additional bipolar gradient pulses to dephase the magnetization of flowing spins in larger vessels. This has been shown to significantly increase the measured transit delay (YE et al. 1997), indicating that much of the tagged signal that appears at early TI is intravascular. However, it is difficult to determine what portion of this intravascular signal is destined for the imaging slice and what portion is flowing through to more distal slices. A second approach is to simply image at relatively long TI, so as to allow blood that is flowing through the imaging slice to do so before the image is acquired. With QUIPSS II or continuous ASL with an inserted delay, the tail of the tag is well defined, and it is possible to choose imaging parameters at which the tail of the tag has reliably flowed through the imaging slice before image acquisition.

6.3.3
BOLD Effects

A detailed discussion of the effects of BOLD contrast in ASL fMRI and inflow effects in BOLD imaging is in Chap. 17, Sect. 17.4.

6.3.4
Tagging Efficiency

Ideally, the tag pulses in ASL perfectly invert arterial blood in the tag condition and leave the arterial

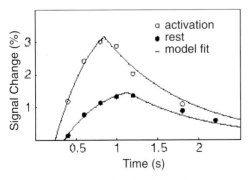

Fig. 6.4. Arterial spin labeling (ASL) signal vs TI for a region of interest in the motor cortex at rest and during finger tapping. The ASL signal amplitude increases and the transit delay decreases with activation

magnetization perfectly unperturbed in the control condition. Unfortunately, this is not the case, and the actual behavior of the tag and control RF radiation must be taken into account in the preparation of pulse sequences, and in the analysis of the results.

In pulsed ASL, the inversion efficiency is very high (>98%) even for very fast flowing blood (WONG et al. 1998b), but the slice profile at the edge of the tag is often significantly imperfect, and can contaminate the signal from static tissue in the imaging slices. Figure 6.5 shows the relationships between the tag and control pulses and the imaging slices for three pulsed ASL techniques: EPISTAR (EDELMAN et al. 1994), PICORE (WONG et al. 1997) and FAIR (KWONG et al. 1994, 1995; KIM et al. 1997). The inversion profile shown is the measured profile of a typical hyperbolic secant pulse used for ASL (SILVER et al. 1985). In these examples, the tag and control pulses modulate the magnetization in the imaging slices by up to a few percent, which can introduce significant artifacts in the ASL signal. This effect can be greatly alleviated by applying saturation pulses to the imaging planes immediately prior to the tag and control pulses. In this manner, magnetization in the imaging slices is destroyed before the tag and control pulses are applied and therefore cannot be modulated by imperfections in the tag and control pulses.

In continuous ASL techniques, the inversion efficiency is lower. For simple single slice applications, the inversion efficiency can be as high as 95%, but for multislice applications, generating an efficient control pulse that control for magnetization transfer (MT) effects and yet remains transparent is not straightforward. An effective technique for multislice control using an amplitude modulation scheme was recently introduced; it provides good control properties, but results in an inversion efficiency of only about 75% (WONG et al. 1998b; ALSOP et al. 1997).

6.4
Current Recommendations

Quantitative ASL techniques are an important adjunct to conventional BOLD fMRI for several reasons, as described above. However, primarily because of lower functional contrast and more limited slice coverage, BOLD contrast should remain the predominant technique for functional mapping. At the time of this writing, ASL based perfusion fMRI is a good choice for the following purposes:

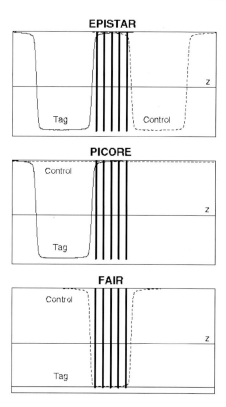

Fig. 6.5. Relationships between tag and control magnetization profiles and imaging slices for EPISTAR, PICORE, and FAIR. In all cases, imperfect slice profiles of the inversion pulses create imperfect subtraction of the static tissue signal between tag and control states

1. After coarse localization of regions of activation for a particular task, if precise localization is required, ASL can be used on a small set of slices to map the site of activation without contamination from downstream veins.
2. Simultaneous ASL and BOLD (see Chap. 17, Sect. 17.4) is a valuable tool for studying both the mechanism of BOLD contrast and the relative spatial distributions of the ASL and BOLD signals.
3. For functional studies in which the modulation of neuronal activity is naturally slow, such as those listed in Sect. 6.1.3, BOLD may not be a viable method, as the temporal stability of the BOLD signal over tens of minutes may not be sufficient for the reliable detection of functional signals.
4. For quantitative fMRI, it is almost certain that the ASL signal is more directly related to brain activity than the BOLD signal, as the latter is heavily influenced by cerebral blood volume (CBV) and the cerebral metabolic rate of oxygen ($CMRO_2$) in addition to CBF.

References

Alsop DC, Detre JA (1996) Reduced transit-time sensitivity in noninvasive magnetic resonance imaging of human cerebral blood flow. J Cereb Blood Flow Metab 16:1236–1249

Alsop DC, Maccotta L, Detre JA (1997) Multi-slice perfusion imaging using adiabatic arterial spin labeling and an amplitude modulated control. In: Fifth Meeting, International Society for Magnetic Resonance in Medicine, Vancouver, April 12-18, 1997, p. 81

Buxton RB, Frank LR (1997) A model for the coupling between cerebral blood flow and oxygen metabolism during neural stimulation. J Cereb Blood Flow Metab 17:64–72

Buxton RB, Frank LR, Wong EC, Siewert B, Warach S, Edelman RR (1998) A general kinetic model for quantitative perfusion imaging with arterial spin labeling. Magn Reson Med 40: 383–396

Edelman RR, Siewert B, Darby DG, Thangaraj V, Nobre AC, Mesulam MM, Warach S (1994) Qualitative mapping of cerebral blood flow and functional localization with echo-planar MR imaging and signal targeting with alternating radio frequency (STAR) sequences: applications to MR angiography. Radiology 192:513–520

Kim S-G, Tsekos NV (1997) Perfusion imaging by a flow-sensitive alternating inversion recovery (FAIR) technique: application to functional brain imaging. Magn Reson Med 37:425–435

Kwong KK, Chesler DA, Weisskoff RM, Rosen BR (1994) Perfusion MR imaging. In: Proceedings Society for Magnetic Resonance in Medicine, Second Meeting, San Francisco, August 6-12, 1994, p. 1005

Kwong KK, Chesler DA, Weisskoff RM, Donahue KM, Davis TL, Ostergaard L, Campbell TA, Rosen BR (1995) MR perfusion studies with T1-weighted echo planar imaging. Magn Reson Med 34:878–887

Silver MS, Joseph RI, Hoult DI (1985) Selective spin inversion in nuclear magnetic resonance and coherent optics through an exact solution of the Bloch-Riccati eqiation. Phys Rev A 31:2753–2755

Wong EC, Buxton RB, Frank LR (1997) Implementation of quantitative perfusion imaging techniques for functional brain mapping using pulsed arterial spin labeling. NMR Biomed 10:237–249

Wong EC, Buxton RB, Frank LR (1998a) Quantitative imaging of perfusion using a single subtraction (QUIPSS and QUIPSS II). Magn Reson Med 39:702–708

Wong EC, Buxton RB, Frank LR (1998b) A theoretical and experimental comparison of continuous and pulsed arterial spin labeling techniques for quantitative perfusion imaging. Magn Reson Med 40: 348–355

Ye FQ, Matay VS, Jezzard P, Frank JA, Weinberger DR, McLaughlin AC (1997) Correction for vascular artifacts in cerebral blood flow values measured by using arterial spin tagging techniques. Magn Reson Med 37:226–235

Flow-Based Functional MRI

7 Inflow-Based Functional MRI Using Time-of-Flight Angiographic Techniques

J.H. Duyn

CONTENTS

7.1
Introduction

In recent years, dedicated MRI techniques have been developed which allow the measurement of physiologic parameters in human brain in vivo. Examples of these techniques are spectroscopic imaging (BROWN et al. 1982; MAUDSLEY et al. 1983), diffusion MRI (TAYLOR and BUSHELL 1985; WESBEY et al. 1985; LeBIHAN ET AL.1986), angiography (MORAN 1982; SINGER and CROOKS 1983; WEHRLI et al. 1985; DIXON et al. 1986; DUMOULIN et al. 1989), perfusion MRI (ROSEN et al. 1989; DETRE et al. 1992; EDELMAN et al. 1994) and blood oxygen level-dependent contrast (BOLD) MRI (OGAWA et al. 1990, 1992; KWONG et al. 1992). The new information obtained with these techniques complements the structural information that is obtained with the conventional MRI

J.H. DUYN, PhD, Laboratory of Diagnostic Radiology Research, Clinical Center, Building 10, Room B1N256, National Institutes of Health, 9000 Rockville Pike, Bethesda, MD 20892, USA

examination, providing a window on the metabolic and functional state of the tissue.

A number of the new techniques, including perfusion and BOLD MRI, have demonstrated the ability to detect some of the physiologic changes which occur in human brain in response to task activation (BELLIVEAU et al. 1991; KWONG et al. 1992; OGAWA et al. 1992). Despite the fact that these functional MRI (fMRI) techniques do not measure synaptic activity directly, the measured perfusion and blood oxygenation increases with brain activation have provided valuable information in studies aimed at localizing functional neuronal clusters.

In current fMRI methodology, the functional contrast mechanism is not well defined. In fact, most methods are sensitive to a number of mechanisms, including BOLD and perfusion. Another, potentially important, fMRI contrast mechanism is the time-of-flight (TOF) effect (WEHRLI et al. 1985), which can occur during flow changes in the macrovasculature. TOF contrast often accompanies BOLD or perfusion contrast and can have confounding effects. Since TOF contrast enhances the functional effects in large vessels, it can compromise localization accuracy of neural activity. In the following we will take a closer look at the mechanisms behind TOF contrast in fMRI.

7.2
Time-of-Flight Contrast in MRI

7.2.1
Basis of Time-of-Flight Contrast

The TOF effect in MRI alludes to a signal enhancement which can be observed when magnetization is carried into the slice under study (observation slice) by flowing spins (SINGER 1959; SINGER and CROOKS 1983). A signal shift ΔS is generated when the magnetization level of stationary spins inside the obser-

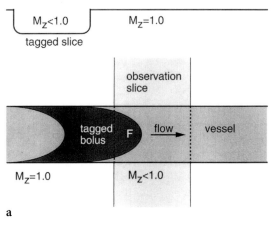

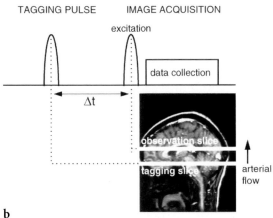

Fig. 7.1. a Example of time-of-flight (TOF) effect in a vessel traversing the image slice. A signal reduction is observed when a tagged intravascular bolus with a reduced magnetization level flows into the observation slice. **b** Example of a tagging pulse sequence. A slice selective pulse is used to magnetically label a region in the object. After a delay Dt, during which the intravascular spins move towards and into the observation slice, a second pulse excitation is used to acquire the image data

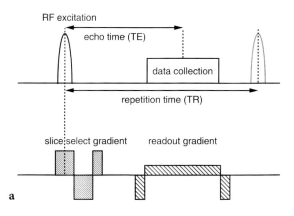

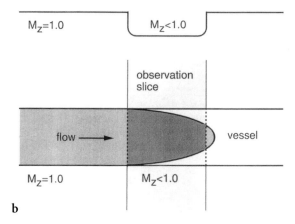

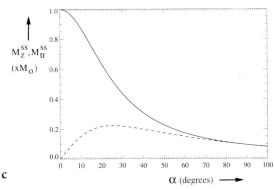

Fig. 7.2a–c. Fast gradient echo imaging time-of-flight (FLASH TOF) effect. **a** FLASH pulse sequence. The repetition time (TR) is generally well below the tissue relaxation time T_1. The particular gradient switching scheme of the slice select gradient (first order moment compensation) is designed to avoid flow-induced signal phase errors. **b** Generation of TOF effect. A signal increase is observed when intravascular blood with unsaturated magnetization flows into the observation slice. **c** Steady state magnetization level in RF-spoiled FLASH imaging (TR=0.1*TR). At RF flip angles well above the Ernst angle (α=25°), the longitudinal magnetization level (M_z *solid line*) is substantially reduced. The transverse magnetization (M_{tr}, *dashed line*) indicates the level of the measured signal originating from stationary tissue

vation slice (M_z^i) is different from outside areas (M_z^o) (Fig. 7.1a). This situation can be created by a simple "tagging" or "labeling" pulse sequence (Fig. 7.1b). The signal enhancement ΔS is proportional to the volume displacement F (see Fig. 7.1a) in the slice (WEHRLI et al. 1985):

$$\Delta S = F \cdot (M_z^o - M_z^i) \tag{7.1}$$

By performing a series of experiments with varying the labeling delay (Δt, Fig. 7.1b), information about the flow characteristics can be derived.

7.2.2
Time-of-Flight Contrast in Fast Gradient Echo Imaging

One of the simplest ways to generate TOF contrast in MRI is the use of a fast gradient echo imaging (FLASH) (HAASE et al. 1986) scan technique (Fig. 7.2a). The repetition time (TR) of the FLASH experiment is generally well below the tissue (and blood) relaxation time constant (T_1), leading to saturation (i.e., reduction) of the magnetization within the observation slice, while leaving the surrounding magnetization unperturbed (Fig. 7.2b). This saturation effect is particularly evident in radiofrequency (RF)-spoiled FLASH performed at high RF flip angle (a) and builds up over time after the start of the experiment. In case of perfect spoiling (ZUR et al. 1991; DUYN 1997) the steady state level of the longitudinal magnetization M^{SS} approaches (Fig. 7.2c):

$$M^{SS}_z = \frac{\cos\alpha \cdot (1 - e^{-\frac{TR}{T_1}})}{1 - e^{-\frac{TR}{T_1}} \cdot \cos\alpha} \qquad (7.2)$$

Spins flowing into the slice from its unsaturated surroundings have a higher magnetization level, resulting in an increase in signal. The size of this differential signal is dependent on the flow velocity v and can be calculated from computer simulations. An example of the calculated inflow enhancement as a function of v is given in Fig. 7.3 for three different settings of a. The signal enhancement increases with flow velocity, and can be substantial for flip angles above the Ernst angle:

$$\alpha = a\cos\left(e^{-\frac{TR}{T_1}}\right) \qquad (7.3)$$

which is the condition for optimum signal-to-noise ratio (SNR) of stationary tissue.

7.2.2.1
Maximization of Inflow Signal

By varying experimental parameters such as TR, α, and the slice thickness, one can control the inflow sensitivity of the FLASH experiment (Fig. 7.4). For faster flowing spins (v>10 cm/s), the inflow enhancement increases with α, until a maximum is reached around α=90° (Fig. 7.4a). The maximum enhancement is smaller for lower velocities and is reached at reduced values of α (Fig. 7.4b). Reduction of the slice thickness and increase of the TR both

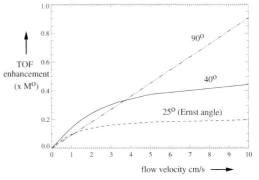

Fig. 7.3. Time-of-flight (TOF) enhancement in fast gradient echo imaging (FLASH) as a function of flow velocity. The differential signal change of flowing spins was calculated at flip angles at and above the Ernst angle (α=25°), with repetition time (TR)=0.1*T_1, and a slice thickness of 10 mm. The simulations assumed zero exchange of intravascular spins with the tissue magnetization. Note the strong TOF effects for fast flowing spins at α=90°

have the effect of shifting the curves (Figs. 7.3, 7.4a) to higher velocities. Note that in Figs. 7.3 and 7.4, the enhancement is given in units of M_0 and that, for a relative (percentage) enhancement, the stationary tissue signal needs to be taken into account.

7.2.2.2
Suppression of Stationary Spins

In order to selectively measure flowing spins, signal from spins stationary within the slice under study needs to be suppressed. For optimal suppression, phase spoiling of the RF excitation pulses needs to be performed (ZUR et al. 1991), combined with an appropriate choice of pulse sequence parameters. By using TR<<T_1 and choosing α well above the Ernst angle, a good amount of the stationary or "background" magnetization can be suppressed (see Fig. 7.2c) while maintaining high levels of inflow sensitivity.

7.2.3 Time-of-Flight Contrast in Angiography

The TOF effect has been extensively employed in angiographic studies, where it allows for a selective enhancement of arteries and veins. Original implementations used a spatially selective saturation or inversion preceding the image acquisition (SINGER and CROOKS 1983; WEHRLI et al. 1985; EDELMAN et al. 1994). An alternative method of "labeling" or "tagging" blood signal is the use of a flow-selective inversion, e.g., a flow-induced adiabatic inversion

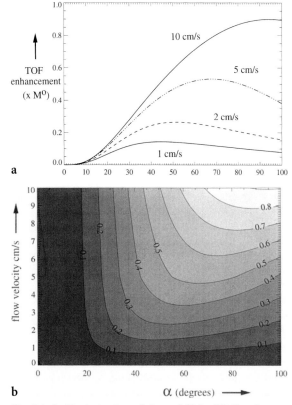

a

b   α (degrees) ⟶

Fig. 7.4a,b. Maximization of time-of-flight (TOF) enhancement. The differential signal enhancement of flowing spins was calculated as a function of α, with repetition time (TR)=0.1*TR, and a slice thickness of 10 mm. Both line plot (**a**) and contour plot (**b**) show that TOF effects increase with flow velocity and that the value of α at which TOF is maximized is different for different flow velocities

(Dixon et al. 1986). The TOF angiographic methods are a good alternative to phase contrast methods (Moran 1982; Dumoulin et al. 1989) for imaging of pulsatile or turbulent flow.

7.3
Time-of-Flight Contrast in fMRI

7.3.1
Time-of-Flight Contrast and Perfusion fMRI

A recent application of the TOF effect is the measurement of cerebral perfusion with continuous (Detre et al. 1992) or pulsed (Kim 1995; Kwong et al. 1995) spin labeling. These methods are known as ASL or AST, for "arterial spin labeling" or "arterial

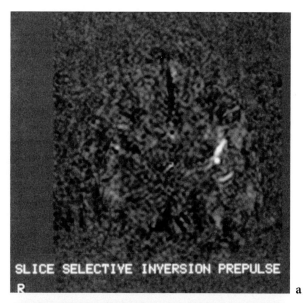

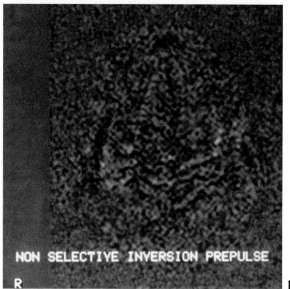

Fig. 7.5a,b. Time-of-flight (TOF) enhancement in motor cortex functional MRI (fMRI) experiment. The images were generated by subtracting rest stages from active stages, using a turbo spin echo scan technique. Labeling was performed by a slice selective inversion pre-pulse (**a**), while the nonlabeled control experiment used a nonselective inversion pre-pulse (**b**). The bright area in (**a**) represents a vessel in the motor cortex, demonstrating an increased TOF effect during activation. (Courtesy of Peter Luyten)

spin tagging." By following the fate of magnetically labeled intravascular water on its way to the observation slice and its exchange into the tissue, cerebral perfusion can be quantitatively estimated. Although the main objective of these techniques is not the measurement of the intravascular signal, the ASL perfusion pulse sequences are very similar to those used with the early angiographic techniques (SINGER and CROOKS 1983; DIXON et al. 1986). They use a separate labeling pulse, usually a spin inversion pulse, preceding the image acquisition. By adjusting experimental parameter settings, in particular the delay time between labeling and image acquisition, either the angiographic or the perfusion contrast can be selectively emphasized (KWONG et al. 1995; ALSOP and DETRE 1996; YE et al. 1997a; YANG et al. 1998). Additionally, for optimal suppression of the intra-arterial (angiographic) contribution, flow dephasing gradients can be used (YE et al. 1997a; YANG et al. 1998).

Both angiographic and perfusion experiments, based on ASL, have been used to measure the hemodynamic changes associated with neuronal activation (KWONG et al. 1992; KIM et al. 1995; YE et al. 1997b). By comparing a labeled activation experiment with a nonlabeled control activation experiment (Fig. 7.5), activation-related flow changes can be demonstrated (DUYN et al. 1994a). A potential problem in these studies is the inadequate suppression of the intravascular component, leading to enhancement of the larger arteries, which could be some distance away from the neuronal activation site (DUYN et al. 1994a). With appropriate arterial suppression techniques, a good spatial correspondence between perfusion-detected and BOLD-detected activation sites can be found (Fig. 7.6).

7.3.2
Time-of-Flight Contrast and BOLD fMRI

In a number of the early BOLD fMRI experiments, the blood oxygenation dependent contrast was often accidentally enhanced or overshadowed by TOF contrast. This was the result of the use of FLASH with short TR's (TR$<<$T$_1$), RF flip angles well above the Ernst angle, and a single-slice acquisition mode. Under these conditions, activation-related flow changes result in TOF-induced signal increases, particularly in the larger vessels (Fig. 7.7). Evidence for involvement of TOF contrast can be demonstrated by a reference experiment with suppression of the TOF effect either through explicit saturation of the areas outside the observation slice (DUYN et al. 1994a) or with true 3D acquisition (DUYN et al. 1994b) (Fig. 7.8). Alternatively, the relative contributions of BOLD and TOF effect can be studied by varying α (FRAHM et al. 1994) or echo time (TE) (GLOVER et al. 1996). The contribution of TOF contrast is generally much reduced in multi-slice experiments, because of the longer overall TR and the reduced spatial variation in saturation levels (DUYN et al. 1995).

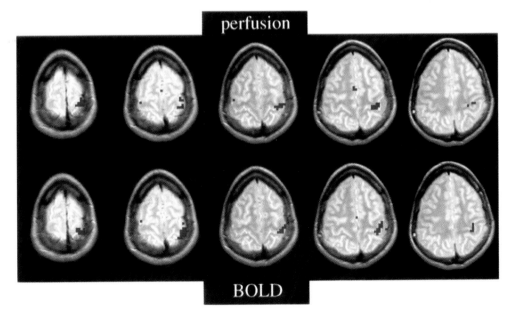

Fig. 7.6. Comparison of perfusion and blood oxygen level-dependent contrast (BOLD) effect in a motor cortex functional MRI (fMRI) (finger tapping with dominant hand). The perfusion data, obtained with a multislice pulsed labeling experiment, show locations of activation (indicated in *red*) that correspond closely to those obtained with the BOLD experiment

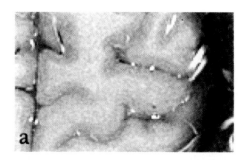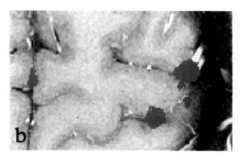

Fig. 7.7a, b. Time-of-flight (TOF) enhanced blood oxygen level-dependent contrast functional MRI (fMRI). This example of a motor cortex fMRI experiment, performed under saturating conditions (TR=80 ms, α=40°), is suspect for involvement of TOF contrast. The overlay of functional data on an angiographic MRI (**a**) with the result shown in (**b**) indicates that the activated areas corresponded closely to vessel locations

A potential problem with TOF contrast in BOLD fMRI is that it generally generates or enhances the activation-related signal changes in the larger supplying arteries or draining veins. An additional drawback, in, for example, FLASH experiments, is that the size of the TOF-related activation signal experiments is much dependent on the vascular geometry, its relation to the slice orientation, as well as the scan parameters. Therefore, in fMRI studies in which accurate localization or reproducible effects are required, large vessel enhancement through TOF contrast needs to be avoided.

7.3.3
Minimizing Time-of-Flight Contrast in fMRI

In order to avoid the TOF-related enhancement of the larger vessels in BOLD or perfusion fMRI studies, a number of techniques can be used. In single-slice FLASH studies, the use of low flip angles can reduce inflow enhancement (Gao et al. 1988; Frahm et al. 1994) (Figs. 7.3, 7.4). Another strategy is the use of a true 3D acquisition mode, in combination with thick slab-excitation (Duyn et al. 1994b), which reduces saturation differences between adjacent slices. This works well for the centrally located slices in the slab and generally eliminates TOF effects in all but the largest arteries. Furthermore, activation signal from intravascular spins can be suppressed by using flow sensitization gradients (Ye et al. 1997a; Yang et al. 1998), e.g., bipolar gradient pulses, which introduce a velocity-dependent phase shift to the NMR signal. The resulting phase dispersion over the vessel lumen, as well as the phase fluctuations over the course of the experiment, both result in a loss of intravascular signal. Finally, spin-echo acquisition

mode also can reduce signal from fast flowing spins; however, it is a less efficient way to obtain BOLD contrast as compared to gradient-echo techniques (Bandettini et al. 1994). Earlier suggested k-space phase encoded reordering techniques (Kim et al. 1994) do not guarantee significant reduction in TOF enhancement; this is because vessels that do not occupy much more than a single voxel have their signal intensity more or less equally distributed over k-space.

7.3.4
Maximizing Time-of-Flight Contrast in fMRI

The upper limit of the TOF effect in fMRI originating from the microvasculature is less than 1% of M_o for normal human brain, independent of MRI acquisition technique. This can be calculated from an estimated maximum activation-related perfusion change of 0.5 ml/g per min (Ye et al. 1997b), which is smaller than 1% fraction of the volume per second.

In the macrovasculature, by contrast, larger TOF effects can be expected, because of "pooling" effects. A larger artery or vein, supplying a sizable functional area, can give large effects in the voxel it traverses, the upper limit set by the volume fraction it occupies.

Nevertheless, the spatial accuracy and reliability of both BOLD and perfusion fMRI studies would benefit from a situation in which the TOF enhancement in the microvasculature is maximized, while at the same time TOF effects in the macrovasculature are suppressed. Unfortunately, simulations show (e.g. Fig. 7.4) that, for a FLASH experiment with $TR \ll T_1$, the signal increases to be expected from flow changes are relatively small for the low flow velocities typical for the microvasculature. For optimal effects in the microvasculature, TR values need to be increased to values close to the T_1 of blood (1.2 s at 1.5 T), a condition similar to that of ASL methods. However, at this long TR value, stationary tissue contributes significantly to the FLASH signal, which is undesirable since temporal fluctuations in the stationary tissue signal (whether they relate to the activation or not) can confound the perfusion-related signal. In this situation, ASL methods, which provide excellent suppression of stationary tissue signal, appear favorable over FLASH.

7.4
Future Directions

Most of the current fMRI methods are predominantly sensitized to BOLD contrast, with TOF effects playing only a secondary role. Unfortunately, BOLD measures of neuronal activation are only remotely related to synaptic activity. This is because the contrast is the result of a chain of physiologic events in response to neuronal activation, consisting of changes in metabolism, oxygen consumption, hemo-

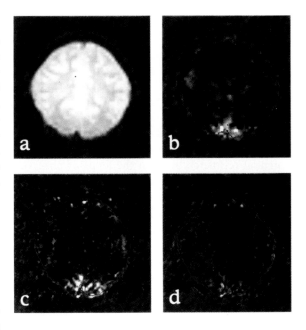

Fig. 7.8a–d. Suppression of time-of-flight (TOF) contrast in macrovasculature. This visual cortex experiment (alternating checkerboard), with baseline image shown in (**a**), was performed in 2D mode under saturating conditions (**b**), in 3D mode (**c**), and in 2D mode with inflow saturation (**d**). Note the reductions in area of activation in (**b**) and (**d**), suggesting an effective suppression of TOF effects

Fig. 7.9a–c. Motor cortex time-of-flight (TOF)-functional MRI (fMRI) with high temporal resolution. Shown is an example of a finger tapping fMRI experiment with alternating 10 s stages of rest and activity, performed with single shot spiral acquisition with a temporal resolution (TR) of 40 ms. The experiment was sensitized to TOF contrast (TE=8 ms, α=25°) to obtain adequate sensitivity to functional changes. The motor cortex area, encircled in the baseline image (**a**), as well as the difference image (activity-rest) (**b**), shows regions of activity-induced flow increase. The temporal characteristics of the signal within the primary sensory motor cortex is shown in (**c**)

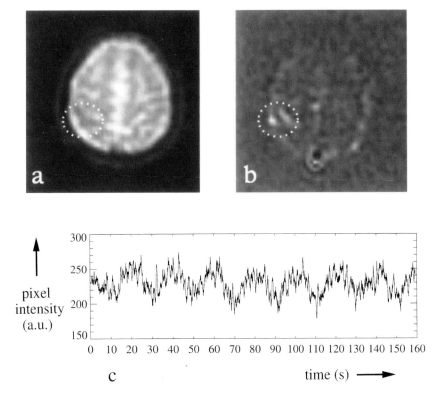

dynamics, and finally blood oxygenation. As of yet, the relationship between these changes has not been firmly established and is not necessarily uniform across individuals or even across functional brain regions. In this context, fMRI studies based on TOF contrast and specifically perfusion contrast can provide new information about the physiology of brain activation. TOF techniques that are sensitized to the larger arteries (or veins) have the disadvantage of a potential mismatch between the locus of observed signal change and the neuronal activation site. However, a potential advantage of these techniques is that they allow studies with high temporal resolution (Fig. 7.9), because of their high SNR (pooling effect). It remains to be seen how well the temporal characteristics of arterial flow changes correlate with the dynamics of changes in synaptic activity.

Acknowledgments. The author gratefully acknowledges Joe Frank, Yihong Yang, Chrit Moonen, Alan McLaughlin and Peter Luyten for their helpful suggestions and support.

References

Alsop DC, Detre JA 1996) Reduced transit-time sensitivity in noninvasive magnetic resonance imaging of human cerebral blood flow. J Cereb Blood Flow Metab 16:1236–1249

Bandettini PA, Wong EC, Jesmanowicsz A, Hinks RS, Hyde JS (1994) Spin-echo and gradient-echo EPI of human brain activation using BOLD contrast: A comparative study at 1.5 T. NMR Biomed 7:12–20

Belliveau JW, Kennedy DN, McKinstry RC, et al. (1991) Functional mapping of the human visual cortex by magnetic resonance imaging. Science 254:716–719

Brown TR, Kincaid B, Ugurbil K (1982) NMR chemical shift imaging in three dimensions. Proc Natl Acad Sci USA 79:3523–3526

Cohen MS, Vevea JM, Brady TJ, Rosen BR (1991) Functional mapping of the human visual cortex by magnetic resonance imaging. Science 254:716–719

Detre JA, Leigh JS, Williams DS, Koretsky AP (1992) Perfusion imaging. Magn Reson Med 23:37–45

Dixon WT, Du LN, Faul DD, Gado M, Rossnick S (1986) Projection angiograms of blood labeled by adiabatic fast passage. Magn Reson Med 3:454–462

Dumoulin CL, Souza SP, Walker MF, Wagle W (1989) Three-dimensional phase contrast angiography. Magn Reson Med 9:139–149

Duyn JH (1997) Steady state effects in fast gradient echo imaging. Magn Reson Med 37:559–568

Duyn JH, Moonen CTW, van Yperen GH, de Boer RW, Luyten PR (1994a) Inflow versus deoxyhemoglobin effects in 'BOLD' functional MRI using gradient echoes at 1.5 T. NMR Biomed 7:83–88

Duyn JH, Mattay VS, Sexton RH, et al. (1994b) 3-Dimensional functional imaging of human brain using echo-shifted FLASH MRI. Magn Reson Med 32:150–155

Duyn JH, Ramsey NR, Mattay VS, et al. (1995) Effect of large vessels in functional magnetic resonance imaging at 1.5 T. Int J Imag Syst Technol 6:245–252

Edelman RR, Siewert B, Darby DG, Thangaraj V, Nobre AC, Mesulam MM, Warach S (1994) Radiology 192:513–520

Frahm J, Merboldt KD, Hänicke W, Kleinschmidt A, Boecker H (1994) Brain or vein – oxygenation or flow? On signal physiology in functional MRI of human brain activation. NMR Biomed 7:45–53

Gao JH, Holland SK, Gore JC (1988) Nuclear magnetic resonance signal from nuclei in rapid imaging using gradient echoes. Med Phys 15:809–814

Glover GH, Lemieux SK, Drangova M, Pauly JM (1996) Decomposition of inflow and blood oxygen level dependent (BOLD) effects with dual-echo spiral gradient-recalled echo (GRE) fMRI. Magn Reson Med 35:299–308

Haase A, Frahm J, Matthaei D, Haenicke W, Merboldt KD (1986) Flash imaging. Rapid NMR imaging using low flip angle pulses. J Magn Reson 67:217–225

Kim S-G (1995) Quantification of relative cerebral blood flow change by flow-sensitive alternating inversion recovery (FAIR) technique: application to functional mapping. Magn Reson Med 34:293–301

Kim S-G, Hendrich K, Hu X, Merkle H, Ugurbil K (1994) Potential pitfalls of functional MRI using conventional gradient-recalled echo techniques. NMR Biomed 7:69–74

Kwong KK, Belliveau JW, Chesler DA et al. (1992) Dynamic magnetic resonance imaging of human brain activity during primary sensory stimulation. Proc Natl Acad Sci USA 89:5675–5679

Kwong KK, Chesler DA, Weisskoff RM et al. (1995) MR perfusion studies with T1-weighted echo planar imaging. Magn Reson Med 34:878–887

LeBihan D, Breton E, Lallemand D, Grenier P, Cabanis E, Laval-Jeantet M (1986) NMR imaging of intravoxel incoherent motions: Application to diffusion and perfusion in neurologic disorders. Radiology 161:401

Maudsley AA, Hilal SK, Perman WH, Simon HE (1983) Spatially resolved high-resolution spectroscopy by „four-dimensional" NMR. J Magn Reson 51:147–152

Moran PR (1982) A flow velocity zeugmatographic interlace for NMR imaging in humans. Magn Reson Imaging 1:197–203

Ogawa S, Lee TM, Ray AR, Tank DW (1990) Brain magnetic resonance imaging with contrast dependent on blood oxygenation. Proc Natl Acad Sci USA 87:9868

Ogawa S, Tank DW, Menon R, Ellerman JM, Kim S, Merkle H, Ugurbil K (1992) Intrinsic signal changes accompanying sensory stimulation: functional brain mapping using MRI. Proc Natl Acad Sci USA 89:5951–5955

Rosen BR, Belliveau JW, Chien D (1989) Perfusion imaging by nuclear magnetic resonance. Magn Reson Q 5:263–281

Singer JR (1959) Blood flow rates by nuclear magnetic resonance. Science 130:1652–1653

Singer JR, Crooks LE (1983) Nuclear magnetic resonance blood flow measurements in the human brain. Science 221:654–656

Taylor DG, Bushell MC (1985) Spatial mapping of translational diffusion coefficients by the NMR imaging technique. Phys Med Biol 30:345–349

Warrach S (1994) Qualitative mapping of cerebral blood flow and functional localization with echo-planar MR imaging and signal targeting with alternative radio frequency. Radiology 192:513–520

Wehrli FW, Shimakawa A, McFall JR, Axel L, Perman W (1985) MR imaging of venous and arterial flow by a selective saturation-recovery spin echo method. JCAT 9:537–545

Wesbey GE, Moseley ME, Ehman RL (1985) A new application of proton magnetic resonance imaging: Measurement of the translational diffusion coefficient. Invest Radiol 19:491–498

Yang Y, Frank JA, Hou L, Ye FQ, McLaughlin AC, Duyn JH (1998) Multislice imaging of quantitative cerebral perfusion with pulse arterial spin labeling. Magn Reson Med 39:825–832

Ye FQ, Mattay VS, Jezzard P, Frank JA, Weinberger DR, McLaughlin AC (1997a) Correction for vascular artifacts in cerebral blood flow values measured by using arterial spin labeling techniques. Magn Reson Med 37:226–235

Ye FQ, Smith AM, Yang Y, et al. (1997b) Quantitation of regional cerebral blood flow increases during motor activation: A steady-state arterial spin tagging study. NeuroImage 6:104–112

Zur Y, Wood ML, Neuringer LJ (1991) Spoiling of transverse magnetization in steady-state sequences. Magn Reson Med 21:251–263

8 Functional MR Angiography Using In-Flow and Phase-Contrast MR Acquisition Techniques

C. Segebarth, C. Delon-Martin, V. Belle, M. Roth, R. Massarelli, L. Lamalle, M. Décorps

CONTENTS

8.1
Introduction

Blood oxygen level-dependent (BOLD) contrasts (Ogawa et al. 1990a, b) in functional MRI (fMRI) reflect local mismatches between functional increases in blood flow and in oxygen consumption (Fox and Raichle 1986). The blood flow changes in the cortical areas involved with a particular task or stimulation induce concomitant downstream blood flow changes within the veins draining these areas. While MRI acquisition techniques may be more or less sensitive in detecting these flow changes, conventional gradient-recalled echo (GRE) techniques are extremely sensitive. This led to a debate, in the early days of fMRI, regarding the extent to which the signals observed in the experiments were due to BOLD phenomena in the cortex and to inflow phenomena in draining veins (Gomiscek et al. 1993; Lai et al. 1993; Belle et al. 1994, 1995; Duyn et al. 1994, Frahm et al. 1994; Haacke et al. 1994; Kim et al. 1994; Segebarth et al. 1994). It has turned out that, under certain experimental conditions, the fMRI signals from draining veins may largely predominate the functional responses. The goal of this chapter is to

review how these vascular contributions were identified by our group (Belle et al. 1994, 1995; Segebarth et al. 1994) and how they may be taken advantage of in order to obtain quantitative information about functional blood flow changes (Delon-Martin et al. 1999).

8.2
Venous Responses in Gradient-Recalled Echo fMRI

Figure 8.1 shows the functional responses obtained in an early single-slice fMRI experiment of motor activity, at 1.5 Tesla (Segebarth et al. 1994). The examination was performed on a right-handed, healthy volunteer. Sixty-four images were acquired sequentially. The paradigm alternated two task periods (6 images each) with three rest periods (respectively 8, 22 and 22 images). During the task periods, the subjects performed sequential opposition of the digits to the thumb, with the right hand during the first and with the left hand during the second task period. Functional responses are expressed relatively to the average signal intensity measured during the resting periods. A conventional GRE MR pulse sequence was applied. The major sequence parameters were the following: TR = 59 ms, TE = 40 ms, α = 30°, slice thickness=2 mm, field-of-view = 154×220 mm^3, scan matrix=90×128, acquisition time per slice 5.5 s. The imaging slice was oriented transversally and angled such that the intersection with the sagittal plane was parallel with the bicommissural axis. The slice was centered on the primary sensory and motor cortices, approximately at the level of the cortical representation of the hand. Functional areas were identified as those areas which exhibited signal increases in phase with any of the two task periods. These increases were conveniently detected on a series of "functional" images obtained by subtracting the first image acquired (during a resting period) from each of the images

C. Segebarth, PhD; C. Delon-Martin, PhD; V. Belle, PhD; M. Roth, PhD; R. Massarelli, PhD; L. Lamalle; M. Décorps PhD; INSERM U438 (RMN Bioclinique), Centre Hospitalier Universitaire, Pavillon B, BP 217, 38043 Grenoble Cedex 9, France

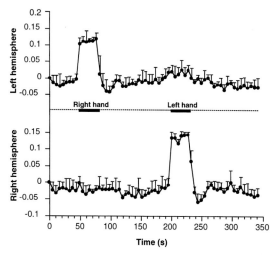

Fig. 8.1. Functional responses obtained from a right-handed healthy volunteer in a single-slice regular gradient-recalled echo (GRE) functional MRI (fMRI) experiment of motor activity (right hand followed by left hand finger tapping). Average values and standard deviations are shown of the relative signal increases obtained for five sequential, identical experiments performed. The responses shown are those from two areas located, respectively, in the left and right central sulci. Those areas correspond to the intersection of the imaging plane with superficial veins. (From Segebarth et al. 1994)

acquired subsequently. The responses shown in Fig. 8.1 are those from two such areas located, respectively, in the left and right central sulci. The graphs represent the average values and standard deviations of the relative signal increases obtained for five sequential, identical experiments performed on the subject. As anticipated, the right hand task induced a functional response in the left hemisphere, while the left hand task induced a functional response predominantly in the right hemisphere. The important observation here is the strength of the functional responses, ranging between 10% and 15% of the MR signal observed during resting conditions. These values are significantly higher than those anticipated from the cortex, on the basis of theoretical considerations (OGAWA et al. 1993; BOXERMAN et al. 1995). Furthermore, in our experience, minor modifications of the GRE MR pulse sequence could result in an increase of the functional responses, up to several tens of percent. Comparison with high resolution anatomical images has led us to suspect fMR responses from superficial veins rather than from the cortex.

8.3
Functional MR Angiography

In order to improve our insight into the origin of the functional responses detected in the previous experiment, we decided to explore the upper part of the brain in a slice per slice manner (Fig. 8.2A). The volume explored (26 adjacent slices of 2 mm thickness) was centered approximately at the same level as the single slice in the previous experiment. The paradigm consisted of a single resting period immediately followed by the task performance period (Fig. 8.2B). During task performance, finger tapping was performed either unilaterally or bilaterally. During each of the resting and task performance periods the volume was explored once, in a slice per slice manner. The GRE MR sequence described above was applied. Following a slice per slice subtraction of the images acquired during the resting period from the images acquired during the task period, a stack of 26 functional images was thus obtained for each finger tapping paradigm. As in the first experiment, those functional images exhibited small hyperintense areas suspected to correspond to vascular responses. Subsequent to the functional examination, a 3D, phase-contrast angiography, MR pulse sequence (DUMOULIN et al. 1989) was applied. The number of slices was set to 52 and the slice thickness to 1 mm. All other geometrical parameters matched those of the fMRI images acquired during the same session. Thus the volume of interest covered by this sequence was identical to the one explored in the fMRI experiment. Encoding velocity was set to 10 cm/s in the direction of the flow-sensitizing gradient. In three successively acquired flow-sensitive images, this

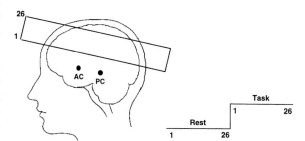

Fig. 8.2. A Scan planning in view of generating gradient-recalled echo (GRE) MR functional angiograms of the upper part of the brain. **B** Paradigm applied: a single resting period followed by a task performance period. During each of these periods the volume was explored once in a slice per slice manner (26 slices)

gradient was applied, respectively, in each of the two principal directions of the image planes and in the direction perpendicular to the latter. The flow sensitivity was nulled during acquisition of a fourth image and the phase-contrast MR angiography images derived from the set of four images.

Maximum intensity projections were then obtained from each of the sets of 26 fMRI images derived from the functional MR experiments and from the set of 52 phase-contrast angiography MR images. The maximum intensity projections derived from the functional MR experiments were eventually superimposed on the conventional MR angiograms.

Figure 8.3 shows a typical result obtained for bilateral finger tapping during the task period of the functional examination. The maximum intensity projections in the transverse plane were obtained by projecting perpendicularly to the image planes. The regular MR angiogram is shown in black and white. The maximum intensity projection derived from the set of functional images is superimposed in color. This figure demonstrates that the hyperintensities detected in the functional MR images correspond to a number of tributary veins of the sagittal sinus which may be identified in the regular MR angiogram. Similar results were obtained for unilateral finger tapping, with vascular responses predominantly located in the hemisphere contralateral to the hand involved in the motor task (BELLE et al. 1994, 1995; SEGEBARTH et al. 1994). Thus the maximum intensity projections derived from the sets of functional MR images represent those vessels which exhibit a functional response. The maximum intensity projections are therefore referred to as "functional angiograms."

Similar functional MR angiograms were generated when exploring the volume slice per slice by means of short echo-time SE rather than by means of GRE MR sequences (BELLE et al. 1995). The functional responses obtained with SE MR sequences are equally due mainly to task-induced increases in venous flow velocities. For both the GRE and SE MR sequences, the inflow sensitivity to the functional blood flow velocity increases depends on the relationships between slice thickness Δz, repetition time T_R and blood flow velocity v_{Rest} under rest conditions.

Consider, for the sake of simplicity, that the excitation pulse angle is 90°, that the velocity profile is constant over the vessel section ("plug flow") and that the vessel is oriented perpendicularly to the imaging plane (Fig. 8.4A). Two regimes may then be distinguished. In the first (regime A, Fig. 8.4B), the

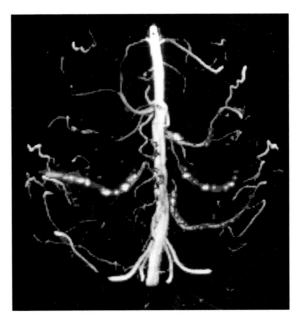

Fig. 8.3. Gradient-recalled echo (GRE) functional MR angiogram. Transverse view. A bilateral hand motor task was performed. The functional MR angiogram (*in color*) is superimposed onto a regular MR angiogram (*in white*)

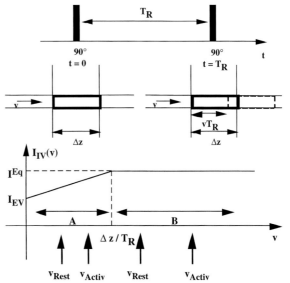

Fig. 8.4. Principles of inflow-sensitivity of the functional MRI (fMRI) experiment. **A** For the sake of simplicity, one assumes the repeated application of 90° radiofrequency (RF) pulses, which are slice-selective (slice thickness Δz). One also assumes "plug flow," i.e., constant blood velocity (*v*) throughout the vessel lumen. During the time lapse T_R between successive pulses, "refreshment" of the spins flowing into the slice occurs. **B** Intravascular signal intensity (I_{IV}) as a function of the blood velocity. If refreshment of the blood within the slice is partial in resting conditions (regime A: $v_{Rest} < \Delta z / T_R$), the functional experiment exhibits inflow sensitivity. If refreshment is total in resting conditions (regime B: $v_{Rest} + \Delta \psi << z / T_R$), the functional experiment exhibits no inflow sensitivity

velocity v_{Rest} is smaller than a critical velocity $v_c = \Delta z / T_R$. The functional increase in blood flow velocity will then result in an increase of the intravascular signal intensity I_{IV}. In the second (regime B, Fig. 8.4B), the velocity v_{Rest} is equal or greater than the critical velocity v_c. The functional increase in blood flow velocity will then result in no intravascular signal increase. Signal intensity will then remain constant between conditions, and equal to the thermal equilibrium intensity I_{Eq}. In the experimental conditions applied in the fMRI measurements described earlier ($\Delta z = 2$ mm, $T_R = 77$ ms), the critical velocity is 2.6 cm/s. This value lies within the range of mean blood velocities typically encountered in superficial veins draining the cortex. Thus, the inflow sensitivity of the fMRI measurement may depend upon details of the MR acquisition sequence as well as on the particular veins considered. Thus, when generating SE or GRE fMR angiograms on different subjects, we sometimes had to enlarge slice thickness in order to increase the value of the critical flow velocity in those cases in which the mean resting flow velocities were above 2.6 mm/s. In addition, because of the lower pulse angles applied in the GRE MR pulse sequences, the variations in flow velocity contribute less to fMR signal intensity in GRE than in SE fMR imaging. However, in SE fMR angiography, outflow phenomena should, in principle, be taken into account. But they play a minor role in practice (BELLE et al. 1995).

The possibility to generate functional MR angiograms by maximum intensity projecting of the functional images derived from two sets of GRE MR images (one measured during resting conditions and the other during performance of a motor task) illustrates that the responses from superficial veins predominate with the GRE MR sequences applied under certain experimental conditions (corresponding to inflow sensitivity). The possibility to derive functional MR angiograms from SE MR images acquired under experimental conditions similar to the GRE MR images (in terms of repetition times and slice thicknesses) further illustrates the inflow-sensitivity of both techniques.

The responses from the superficial veins are due to functional increase of the blood flow velocity in these vessels. This velocity increase may also be detected by means of phase-contrast MR techniques. We have applied these techniques, as a first step, as an alternative approach for generating functional MR angiograms. The volume described in Fig. 8.2A was then explored by means of 3D phase-contrast MRI, first during resting conditions and then during performance of the hand motor task discussed earlier. The major sequence parameters of the 3D phase-contrast MR scans were the following: TR=67 ms, TE=30 ms, $\alpha = 30°$, field-of-view=132×220 mm^2, number of slices=35 (reconstruction onto 70 slices by means of Fourier interpolation), slice thickness at acquisition=2 mm, in-plane scan matrix=38×128, in-plane reconstruction matrix=154×256, total acquisition time=7.5 min. A stack of functional MR angiography images was subsequently obtained by subtracting the phase-contrast MR images measured during rest from those measured during task performance. The functional angiograms were eventually generated by maximum intensity projecting of these difference images. A regular MR angiogram from the volume functionally examined was obtained by calculating maximum intensity projections from the phase-contrast MR images acquired during the rest period.

Figure 8.5 shows a functional and a regular MR angiogram thus obtained in the sagittal orientation from the right hemisphere of the subject who was also depicted in Fig. 8.3. A left hand motor task was performed. As in the functional MR angiogram obtained from the single slice GRE MR images in the

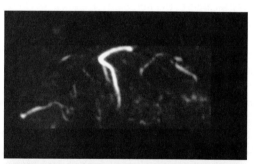

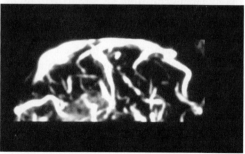

Fig. 8.5. Phase-contrast functional MR angiogram. Sagittal view of the right hemisphere. Same subject as in Fig. 8.3. A left hand motor task was performed. *Right,* phase-contrast regular MR angiogram obtained during resting conditions. *Left,* phase-contrast functional MR angiogram. (From BELLE et al. 1994)

previous experiments, one vein centered on the central sulcus is singled out in the right hemisphere. The position of this vein with respect to the central sulcus may be appreciated on the MR image shown in Fig. 8.6.

8.4
Quantification of the Venous Blood Flow Changes

In a second step, the phase-contrast MR techniques were applied in order to measure the blood flow changes induced by a motor task in the superficial veins draining the motor cortex (DELON-MARTIN et al. 1999). Measurements were performed by means of a small circular surface coil (8 cm diameter) centered on the vein of interest. The imaging plane was oriented perpendicularly to the vein, so that flow encoding could be set in the slice selection direction only. The major parameters of the high resolution, 2D phase-contrast MR acquisition technique were the following: TR=46 ms, TE=22 ms, α=20°, slice thickness=3 mm, field-of-view=50×50 mm^2, scan matrix=154×256 (nominal in-plane resolution of 325×200 μm^2), reconstruction matrix 512×512, number of averages=12, total acquisition time about 3 min. Velocity profiles were fitted by means of a paraboloid, permitting us to obtain estimates of blood flow and vessel section. Ten healthy volunteers who presented a superficial vein centered on the central sulcus in at least one hemisphere were included in the study. Measurements were performed in resting conditions and during mental imagery and actual execution of a motor task with the hand contralateral to the vein considered. Excellent intra-subject reproducibility was obtained for the estimates of blood flow as well as of vessel section. While no differences in vessel section were detected, blood flow increases between resting conditions and actual execution of the hand motor task were found that ranged between 1.7 and 14.0 ml/min, corresponding respectively to 32% and 72% of the values measured in resting conditions. Relative blood flow changes ranged between 26% and 72% (44%±18%). The large inter-subject variability of the task-induced blood flow changes measured in a single vein centered on the Rolandic sulcus reflects both the variability of the cerebral blood flow changes in response to a particular task and the variability of individual vascular architecture. It should be pointed out that, with this approach, the functional blood

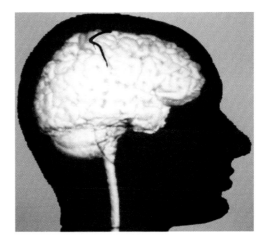

Fig. 8.6. Lateral view of right hemisphere. Same subject as in Figs. 8.3 and 8.5

flow changes in a single vein are quantified, but not the overall task-related blood flow changes.

The venous flow changes reflect the regional cerebral blood flow (rCBF) changes upstream in the cortex drained. Functional changes in rCBF may be determined by MRI by means of arterial spin labeling techniques (KIM 1995; KIM and TSEKOS 1997; YE et al. 1997) or by PET (ORRISON et al. 1995). For motor tasks, these changes range typically between 20% and 38%, as estimated with the latter technique (ROLAND 1993). Arterial spin labeling MRI techniques have led to relative rCBF changes of 53%±17% (KIM and TSEKOS 1997) and of 42%±15% if spatial filtering was matched with that typically encountered in PET studies (YE et al. 1997).

The brain volume drained upstream of the site where blood flow measurements are performed with the 2D phase-contrast method is significantly larger than the voxel sizes encountered in PET or in MRI perfusion studies. One would thus expect that the partial volume effects between tissues involved and tissues uninvolved in the task would be more important with the former than with the latter two methods. The comparable values of the relative rCBF changes in the cortex, as determined with the latter two methods, and the relative blood flow changes in the draining veins, as determined by means of the phase-contrast MR methods, is therefore surprising. It would suggest that the veins centered on the central sulcus and on which the flow measurements have been carried out drain mainly cortical territories involved in the performance of the motor task (or, conversely, that the contribution of blood flow from noninvolved territories is low). Alternatively, it

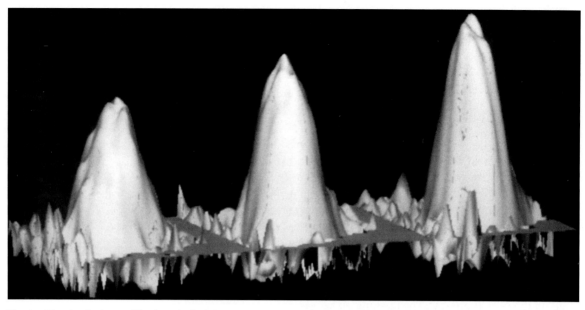

Fig. 8.7. Blood velocity profiles in vein draining motor cortex. Velocity profiles were measured in resting conditions (*left*), during mental imagery (*center*) and actual execution (*right*) of finger tapping task. Mean blood velocity is 3.14 cm/s, 3.94 cm/s, and 4.69 cm/s, respectively. Vein section is 6.5 mm^2

would suggest that the perfusion imaging methods provide underestimated functional flow changes.

8.5
Conclusions

It has been illustrated in this chapter that, in the presence of inflow sensitivity, the signals from draining veins may predominate the functional responses to motor activity detected with regular 2D GRE MR techniques. The signals from draining veins have been used to generate functional MR angiograms. The possibility to generate such angiograms provides further demonstration of the predominance of the venous signals, when 2D GRE MR acquisition is performed under (in)appropriate conditions of inflow sensitivity. It has further been shown that functional angiograms may be derived from 2D SE as well as from 3D phase-contrast MR acquisition. The application of 2D phase-contrast MRI furthermore provides the possibility to measure the functional blood flow changes occurring within the veins detected in the functional angiograms. Those blood flow changes reflect the rCBF changes occurring upstream within the cortical areas drained by the vein considered.

References

Belle V, Delon-Martin C, Massarelli R, Decety R, Le Bas JF, Benabid AL, Segebarth C (1994) Intracranial functional MR angiography in humans. MAGMA 2:343–345

Belle V, Delon-Martin C, Massarelli R, Decety J, Le Bas JF, Benabid AL, Segebarth C (1995) Intracranial gradient-echo and spin-echo functional MR angiography (fMRA) in humans. Radiology 195:739–746

Boxerman JL, Bandettini PA, Kwong KK, Baker JR, Davis TL, Rosen BR, Weiskoff RM (1995) The intravascular contribution to fMRI signal change: Monte Carlo modeling an diffusion-weighted studies in vivo. Magn Reson Med 34:4–10

Delon-Martin C, Roth M, Morand S, Massarelli R, Belle V, Decety J, Felblinger J, Décorps M, Segebarth C (1999) MRI measurement of the functional blood flow changes in large superficial vein draining the motor cortex. NMR Biomed, in press

Dumoulin CL, Souza SP, Walker MF, Wagle W (1989) Three dimensional phase-contrast angiography. Magn Reson Med 9:139–149

Duyn JH, Moonen CTW, van Yperen GH, de Boer RW, Luyten PR (1994) Inflow versus deoxyhemoglobin effects in BOLD functional MRI using gradient echoes at 1.5 T. NMR Biomed 7:83–88

Fox PT, Raichle ME (1986) Focal physiological uncoupling of cerebral blood flow and oxidative metabolism during somatosensory stimulation in human subjects. Proc Natl Acad Sci USA 83:1140–1144

Frahm J, Merboldt KD, Hänicke W, Kleinschmidt A, Boecker H (1994) Brain or vein – Oxygenation or flow? On signal physiology in functional MRI of human brain activation. NMR Biomed 7:45–53

Gomiscek G, Beisteiner R, Hittmair K, Mueller E, Moser E (1993) A possible role of in-flow effects in functional MR imaging. MAGMA 1:109–113

Haacke EM, Hopkins A, Lai S, Buckley P, Friedman L, Meltzer H, Hedera P, Friedland R, Klein S, Thompson L, Detterman D, Tkach J, Lewin JS (1994) 2D and 3D high resolution gradient echo functional imaging of the brain: Venous contributions to signal in motor cortex studies. NMR Biomed 7:54–62

Kim SG (1995) Quantification of relative cerebral blood flow change by flow-sensitive alternating inversion recovery (FAIR) technique: Application to functional mapping. Magn Reson Med 34:293–301

Kim SG, Tsekos NV (1997) Perfusion imaging by a flow-sensitive alternating inversion recovery (FAIR) technique: Application to functional brain imaging. Magn Reson Med 37:425–435

Kim SG, Hendrich K, Hu X, Merkle H and Ugurbil K (1994) Potential pitfalls of functional MRI using conventional gradient-recalled echo techniques. NMR Biomed 7:69–74

Lai S, Hopkins AL, Haacke EM, Li D, Wasserman BA, Buckley P, Friedman L, Meltzer H, Hedera P, Friedland R (1993) Identification of vascular structures as a major source of signal contrast in high resolution 2D and 3D functional activation imaging of the motor cortex at 1.5 T: Preliminary results. Magn Reson Med 30:387–392

Ogawa S, Lee TM, Kay AR, Tank DW (1990a) Brain magnetic resonance imaging with contrast dependent on blood oxygenation. Proc Natl Acad Sci USA 87:9867–9872

Ogawa S, Lee TM, Nayak AS, Glynn P (1990b) Oxygenation-sensitive contrast in magnetic resonance imaging of rodent brain at high fields. Magn Reson Med 14:68–78

Ogawa S, Menon RS, Tank DW, Kim SG, Merkle H, Ellermann JM, Ugurbil K (1993) Functional brain mapping by blood oxygenation level-dependent contrast magnetic resonance imaging. A comparison of signal characteristics with a biophysical model. Biophys J 64:803–812

Orrison WW, Lewine JD, Sanders JA, Hartshorne MF (1995) Functional brain imaging. Mosby, St Louis

Roland PE (1993) Brain activation. Wiley-Liss, New York

Segebarth C, Belle V, Delon C, Massarelli R, Decety J, Le Bas JF, Décorps M, Benabid AL (1994) Functional MRI of the human brain. Predominance of signals from extracerebral veins. Neuroreport 5(7):813–816

Ye FQ, Smith AM, Yang Y, Duyn J, Mattay VS, Ruttimann UE, Frank JA, Weinberger DR, McLaughlin AC (1997) Quantitation of regional cerebral blood flow increases during motor activation: A steady-state arterial spin tagging study. Neuroimage 6:104–112

9 Principles of Susceptibility Contrast-Based Functional MRI: The Sign of the Functional MRI Response

C.S. Springer, Jr., C.S. Patlak, I. Pályka, W. Huang

CONTENTS

9.1 Introduction

Changes in the magnetic susceptibility parameter of the bulk blood phase, bulk magnetic susceptibility (BMS), inside vessels during neuronal activation lie at the heart of most modern MRI studies of brain function, colloquially referred to, inaptly (Springer 1995), as functional MRI (fMRI). However, the path from the BMS change to the measured fMRI response is not a simple one. A consideration of the determinants of the *sign* of the response is particularly instructive with regard to an understanding of the BMS principles involved.

The initial 1992 papers on the contrast agent-free detection of brain function by MRI (Bandettini et al. 1992; Frahm et al. 1992; Kwong et al. 1992; Ogawa et al. 1992) each reported positive changes (i.e., signal *increases*). Almost all of the subsequent reports, now surely exceeding 100, have shown the same thing. On careful examination of the time dependence of the response, one does often see a negative-going signal at its end (an "undershoot") – clearly after the stimulus has ceased. There have

been only very sporadic reports of completely negative changes. We have listed some of these (Huang et al. 1996). It will be shown below that these cannot be necessarily attributed simply to neuronal deactivation. As one example, we have observed some negative fMRI changes in the brains of anesthetized mice in response to a flashed, point light source provided inside the bore of a 9.4 T magnet (Huang et al. 1996). Intriguingly, they seem to arise from the region of the pineal gland, which, in the mouse, is much too tiny to be directly resolved.

There is, however, another rarely observed negative change that has engendered much more excitement (Barinaga 1997a, b). In work completed in 1994, the Minneapolis group reported a very small negative-going spike in the first few seconds of the response from some regions of the visual cortex of the awake human subject (Menon et al. 1995) – the so-called early, or (more poorly) fast, response. Even at the highest value of magnetic field strength (reported as flux density, B_0) then used for humans, 4 T, the early response is so small (–1.2% at approx. 2 s) that in the initial study the responses from several stimulations and several subjects had to be averaged in order to demonstrate it clearly (Menon et al. 1995). The strength of the fMRI response generally varies supralinearly with B_0 (Turner et al. 1993) – a signature of its BMS origin (vide infra). The observed early response goes back through zero at approx. 4 s, and then appears normal (approx. 2% positive) for the remainder of its duration, including a small undershoot at the end. More extensive regions of the visual cortex showed the more normal initial response, i.e., an only positive change (Menon et al. 1995). This early response was likely also detected in a non-mapping ^1H_2O time-domain MR signal experiment at B_0=2 T (Ernst and Hennig 1994). Though these results generated considerable controversy, the Minneapolis group has now considerably refined its fMRI techniques to the point where the early response is unambiguously and reproducibly evident for individual subjects (Hu et al. 1997). Moreover, its essential features (time dependence

C.S. Springer, Jr., PhD; I. Pályka, PhD; Chemistry Department, Brookhaven National Laboratory, Building 555, Upton, New York 11973, USA; Department of Chemistry, State University of New York, Stony Brook, New York 11794, USA
C.S. Patlak, PhD, Department of Surgery, State University of New York, Stony Brook, New York 11794, USA
W. Huang, PhD, Department of Radiology, State University of New York, Stony Brook, New York 11794, USA

and spatial extent) have been reproduced in another 4 T laboratory (McIntosh et al. 1996; Moore et al. 1997; Tweig et al. 1997), and now at a 3 T laboratory (Vasquez et al 1997). This response scales with B_0 just as the positive fMRI change, and is, at best, – 0.6% at 3 T (Vasquez et al. 1997). Thus, it is unlikely to be detectable in conventional fMRI experiments at clinical field strengths of 2 T or less.

9.2
A Functional MRI Network

What is the significance of the sign of the fMRI response? To get at this question, we must first remember the nature of the signal measured in fMRI studies. The quantity that is mapped is the intensity of the water ^1H magnetic resonance. In the fMRI case, changes in this quantity are surely due only to changes in one and/or the other of the two ^1H NMR relaxation rate constants (not rates); $(T_1{}^*)^{-1}$, for the longitudinal magnetization recovery, and $(T_2{}^*)^{-1}$, for the transverse magnetization decay. (The quantities $T_1{}^*$ and $T_2{}^*$ are the respective apparent relaxation times. The symbols T_1 and T_2 are reserved for the "intrinsic" relaxation times.) In almost all of the fMRI (radiofrequency and field gradient) pulse sequence protocols employed, a *positive* response signifies an *increase* in the $(T_1{}^*)^{-1}$ value, and/or a *decrease* in the $(T_2{}^*)^{-1}$ value, or one of these dominating the opposite of the other: for a *negative* response, the opposite changes in the relaxation rate constants obtain. This is shown at the top of the network seen in Fig. 9.1 (relationships b and a). In this network, a plus sign on an arrow indicates that the quantities connected are proportional to each other; a minus sign means that they bear a reciprocal relationship. The degree of the weighting of an fMRI response toward the $T_1{}^*$ or $T_2{}^*$ effect can be adjusted over almost the entire range by the choice of pulse sequence.

9.3
Physicochemical Effects

The second step is to recognize the physicochemical changes that can give rise to such (fMRI) changes in the water ^1H $(T_1{}^*)^{-1}$ and $(T_2{}^*)^{-1}$ values. There are two major effects. There is general consensus that, in fMRI studies, an increase in the $(T_1{}^*)^{-1}$ value of the

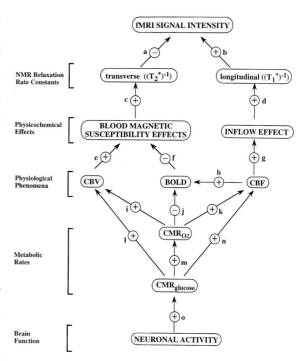

Fig. 9.1. An fMRI network is shown. This scheme attempts to distinguish the various mechanisms that influence the sign of the fMRI response. Here, a *plus sign* on an *arrow* signifies that the quantities linked have a proportional relationship. A *negative sign* represents an inverse proportionality. If one quantity increases, the other decreases, and vice versa

water ^1H signal from a voxel is caused by an increase in the flow rate of blood entering (perfusing) the tissue region represented by that voxel (the inflow effect, Fig. 9.1d) (Kwong et al. 1992; Lee et al., 1999). Similarly, an *increase* in the $(T_2{}^*)^{-1}$ value of this signal is thought to be due to an *increase* in the BMS effect caused (in an agent-free study) by an increase in the small fraction of paramagnetic deoxygenated hemoglobin iron atoms (bearing four unpaired electrons) in the blood present in the voxel (Fig. 9.1c). How is this so?

9.4
Bulk Magnetic Susceptibility Effects

From almost the very beginning of NMR, it was recognized that the BMS value of the sample could have an effect on the resonant frequency of an observed nuclear spin it contained (Dickinson 1951). The volume magnetic susceptibility (χ) of a substance is the (dimensionless) measure of the extent to which the substance modifies the strength of the magnetic field passing through it (Springer 1994a; Schenck

1996).[1] For many years, however, such effects were never formally developed or organized, probably for the reasons suggested below. Eventually, experimenters began to notice seemingly adverse results that could be attributed only to BMS effects. These include: image artifacts (LÜDEKE et al. 1985; SCHENCK 1996) caused because a BMS-induced frequency shift was encoded as a spatial shift by the MRI-processing, line-broadening of spectral peaks arising from lung tissue (CHRISTMAN et al. 1996) and from solid powder samples (BARBARA 1994), and even dynamic BMS effects that necessarily occur during the recovery of nuclear magnetization after an RF pulse (LEVITT 1996).

In our efforts to organize and systematize the phenomena of BMS effects in NMR (CHU et al. 1990; XU et al. 1990; XU 1990; SPRINGER and XU 1991; ALBERT et al. 1993a,b; SPRINGER 1994a,b; PALYKA et al. 1995; WAGSHUL et al. 1996), we have emphasized a first principle that we find to be extremely useful. This is a separation (originally made without comment by ZIMMERMAN and FOSTER 1957) of effects into what we refer to as homogeneous and inhomogeneous contributions (CHU et al. 1990; SPRINGER 1994a). The homogeneous term (we call it D, for Dickinson) includes effects due to the size, shape, and orientation (in $\mathbf{B}_0$) of the macroscopic compartment containing the nuclear spin. The inhomogeneous term (I) includes, in addition, effects due to the position of the spin within the compartment, and especially its proximity to an adjacent compartment with a different χ value. XU (1990) analytically solved for each of these terms in the general case of spins both inside and outside an ellipsoid of revolution suspended in a medium. He included the compartmental demagnetization effect as well as, extremely importantly, the cavity demagnetization effect modeled by the imaginary, microscopic Sphere of Lorentz.

Why did BMS theory remain disorganized for so long? Our separation into D and I terms offers an answer. Much of the first 50 year period of NMR was given over to chemical and biochemical applications.

These are characterized mostly by homogeneous samples (solutions) in single compartments (NMR tubes). The early introduction of the use of an internal reference solute eliminated the D term. The use of an RF transceiver coil smaller than the appropriately positioned cylindrically shaped sample eliminated the I term. It was essentially only when researchers started studying samples that were necessarily multi-compartmented (with different χ values) and/or smaller than the transceiver coil – tissues, solid powders, etc. – that these early methods failed, and systemization became necessary. Of course, MR researchers are very adept at turning adversity into advantage by learning to exploit what was initially considered an artifact. The most spectacular example of this for BMS is the fMRI story, which began with the recognition by the Massachusetts General Hospital (MGH) group that certain vascular MRI effects had a BMS origin (VILLRINGER et al. 1988; BELLIVEAU et al. 1991).

For fMRI (as well as for many other situations), the special case when Xu's ellipsoid is a cylinder is the most useful because this is the appropriate model for a blood vessel (XU 1990; SPRINGER and XU 1991; SPRINGER 1994a). Thus, we have shown that the inhomogeneous (I_e) and homogeneous (D_v) contributions to the resonance frequencies, $\nu(=\partial\phi/\partial t; \phi$ is the spin precession phase angle), of spins located outside and inside of a cylindrical vessel, respectively, are given by Eqs. (9.1) and (9.2) where: χ_v is the BMS value of the medium in the vessel lumen,

$$I_e = \mathbf{B}_0 \cdot \{(\chi_v - \chi_e)/2\} + \{\sin^2\Phi \cdot R^2\} + \{\cos2\theta \cdot (r'')^{-2}\} \quad (9.1)$$

$$D_v = \{(\chi_v - \chi_e)/6\} + \{(3\cos^2\Phi) - 1\} + (\chi_e/3) \quad (9.2)$$

χ_e is the BMS value of the extravascular medium, Φ is the angle between the vessel axis and the direction of $\mathbf{B}_0$, R is the radius of the vessel, r'' is the perpendicular distance of the (external) spin from the vessel axis, and θ is the angle between r'' and the plane defined by $\mathbf{B}_0$ and the vessel axis. Thus, θ and r'' are properties of the position of an outside spin with reference to the vessel, whereas Φ and R are parameters that characterize the cylinder orientation and size. It is therefore obvious that the BMS effects depend on the orientation of the vessel relative to the direction of the magnetic field. Note that the factor $\sin^2\Phi$ in Eq. 9.1 is zero when Φ is zero. They also depend on the proximity of other vessels (Springer 1994b).

---

[1] The dimensions and units of bulk magnetism can be extremely confusing. We employ the rationalized SI (MKSA) system of units (Chu et al. 1990; Albert et al. 1993a, b; Springer 1994a), because it considerably simplifies the equations for BMS effects in NMR. In the CGS system, the rationalization factor of 4π (=12.57) is usually not made implicit in the susceptibility value. Thus, for example, the value of χ for pure water at 37°C, though dimensionless (and thus unitless) in both, is −9.05 ppm in the SI system and −0.72 ppm in the CGS system. Beware the 4π factor! For an excellent discussion of these issues, see (Schenck 1996).

A pictorial representation of aspects of the I_e term is presented in Fig. 9.2, which combines modifications of parts of Figs. 7, 13, and 16 of SPRINGER (1994a). Figure 9.2a is a cartoon version of the mechanism underlying the famous acronym coined by OGAWA et al. (1990), BOLD, for blood oxygenation level-dependent (HUANG et al. 1996). It shows a transverse cross-section of a cylindrical vessel oriented perpendicular to B_0 (i.e., $\Phi = 90°$), which is represented by the horizontal flux lines. "Before" the increase in activity of neurons near this vessel, the value of χ inside the vessel is slightly greater than that of χ outside the vessel. This is because of the small fraction of paramagnetic hemoglobin iron atoms present in resting state blood. Actually, χ_{in} is slightly "less negative" than χ_{out}, which is ~-9.10 ppm (SPRINGER 1994a). The distortion of the flux lines outside the vessel is due to the I_e term of Eq. 9.1 because $\Delta\chi[=(\chi_v-\chi_e)]$ is nonzero, positive here. An inhomogeneous magnetic field is characterized by flux lines that are not parallel, and it increases the precessional dephasing of the spin moments in this region (shown with dots in Fig. 9.2). If the fraction of hemoglobin iron atoms that are paramagnetic de-

creases "during" the increased neuronal activity, the value of $\Delta\chi$ will decrease (shown going to zero in Fig. 9.2a), and the flux lines will become more parallel. (Physiological and metabolic reasons why such an increase in the blood oxygenation level could occur will be discussed below.) This means a transient decrease in $(T_2^*)^{-1}$ for the signal from the spins outside the vessel and a positive fMRI response (Fig. 9.1a). This is the so-called extravascular (EV) BOLD mechanism. For an isolated vessel, the value of I_v is zero (SPRINGER 1994a). Side views (longitudinal cross-sections) of the vessel, projecting past parenchymal cells, lined with endothelial cells, and containing erythrocyte cells, are also suggested in Fig. 9.2a for the "before," "during," and "after" conditions.

The physical source of χ is the sum of interactions of the nuclear spin magnetic dipole with all other magnetic dipoles in the sample (SPRINGER 1994a; LEVITT 1996). The cartoon in Fig. 9.2b attempts to suggest these latter. It represents the same transverse vessel cross-section as in Fig. 9.2a. For solutions, the major effect is due to the magnetic moments in the paired electron distributions of the solvent and diamagnetic solute molecules that are induced by B_0.

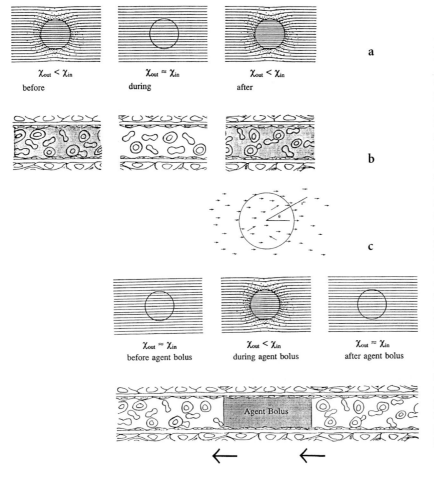

Fig. 9.2a–c. Inhomogeneous BMS aspects are depicted. In the *top* parts of **a** and **c**, and in **b**, a transverse cross-section of a cylindrical vessel oriented perpendicular to the magnetic field is shown. In the *bottom* parts of **a** and **c** a longitudinal cross-section of the same vessel is shown. **a** The BOLD (blood oxygenation level-dependent), or Ogawa, mechanism. The magnetic susceptibility of blood is transiently decreased by a small amount during neuronal activation. **c** The BALD (blood agent level-dependent), or Rosen, mechanism. Here, the magnetic susceptibility of the blood is transiently elevated by a large amount during the passage of a bolus of a paramagnetic agent. **b** The magnetic dipolar origin of susceptibility. Induced (diamagnetic) magnetic moments are shown, and unpaired electron magnetic moments are present only inside the vessel. For further details, see text. (Modified from Figs. 7, 13, 16 of SPRINGER 1994a)

These are represented in Fig. 9.2b by the small arrows oriented parallel to B_0. The small nuclear magnetization itself is ignored in Fig. 9.2b. The much larger magnetic moments of the few unpaired electrons present have quantized orientations in $\mathbf{B}_0$, and a tiny population mismatch at Boltzmann equilibrium. (They are symbolized by the larger arrows inside the vessel.) The resulting higher value for χ inside the vessel than outside is what causes the relative concentration of flux lines inside the vessel seen in Fig. 9.2a. The compartmental demagnetization aspect can be imagined from Fig. 9.2b. The outside vessel wall on the right has a preponderance of arrow tails. If these are considered as monopolar magnetic charges (say, souths, for example), then the outside vessel wall on the right has an excess south charge. Conversely, the outside vessel wall on the left has an excess north charge. The vessel walls on the top and bottom are relatively magnetically neutral. These compartmental space (magnetic) charges affect the magnetic field that is actually sensed by a resonant nuclear magnetic moment. The coordinates of such a moment (r'' and θ) are also indicated in Fig. 9.2b. From this picture, it is easy to appreciate why the compartmental demagnetization effect should be dependent on the size and orientation (Φ value) of the vessel.

A pictorial representation of aspects of the D_v and D_e terms is presented in Fig. 9.3. The situation in two limiting cases is depicted in the cartoon tissue ^1H_2O spectra sketched there. The stick spectra on the right represent a hypothetical case in which the region of interest (ROI) contains only two vessels, one oriented parallel to $\mathbf{B}_0$ ($\Phi=0°$), and one oriented perpendicular to B_0 ($\Phi=90°$). The spectrum in the center is drawn for a situation in which χ_e is –9.10 ppm, χ_v is –8.70 ppm, and the volume fraction due to the vessel lumens is approx. 0.4. The BMS values represent a case of noticeably deoxygenated (~30%) blood (ALBERT et al. 1993b; SPRINGER 1994a) and the intravascular volume fraction – proportional to the cerebral blood volume (CBV) – is also exaggerated for the purposes of clarity. Equation 9.2 tells us that D_v is –2.90 ppm for the parallel vessel and –3.10 ppm for the perpendicular vessel. There are lines drawn at the positions of these frequencies (given in dimensionless units). The D_e value ($=\chi_e/3$) for the parenchymal (extravascular) spins is –3.03 ppm (SPRINGER 1994a), and a line at that frequency is indicated with an "e". It is very important to note that the fact that the two D_v values are dispersed to either side of D_e is due to the cavity demagnetization effect modeled by the Sphere of Lorenz (SPRINGER 1994a). If one ignores cavity demagnetization (as in

SCHENCK 1996), this crucial feature of BMS effects is missed (SPRINGER 1994a). With our formalism, the Sphere of Lorentz contribution is contained within the D term. That is why we could ignore it in Fig. 9.2, which is concerned with the I terms.

The earliest type of fMRI experiment actually involved a bolus injection of a paramagnetic contrast reagent (CR) (BELLIVEAU et al. 1991) – an approach that we have labeled the BALD (blood agent level-dependent) technique (ALBERT et al. 1993a; SPRINGER 1994a). The bottom spectrum on the right of Fig. 9.3 represents a situation at the peak of the

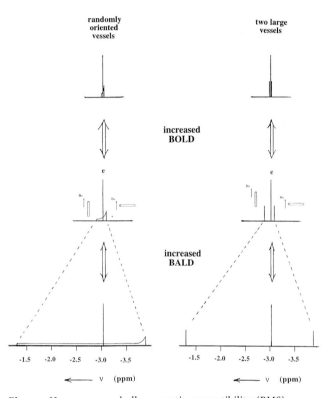

Fig. 9.3. Homogeneous bulk magnetic susceptibility (BMS) aspects of tissue ^1H_2O MR spectra. These represent the changes in a spectrum from a region of interest (ROI) containing vascular and extravascular (*e*) water that are expected when the BMS of the medium in the vessels changes. For clarity, the spectral lines are presented as if they have infinitely narrow intrinsic line widths (δ-functions). The spectra on the *right* represent a hypothetical case in which only two vessels are present: one parallel to $\mathbf{B}_0$ and one perpendicular. On the *left* is a more realistic situation in which there is a very large number of vessels, with random orientations relative to the magnetic field direction. The lower changes to the intravascular lines are those that would obtain if the BMS of the vessel media were to increase – by the passage of a bolus of a paramagnetic contrast reagent, for example. The upper changes are those occurring if the vessel media BMS decreases – by increasing the level of oxygenation of blood, for example. These are calculated from Eq. 9.2. Quantitative details are given in the text

first pass of the CR through the vessels in the ROI. In this case, the value of χ_v has transiently increased to -4.00 ppm. According to Eq. 9.2, the two D_v values disperse dramatically, to -1.30 ppm and -3.88 ppm as shown. A cartoon depiction of the passage of an idealized BALD bolus is also shown in Fig. 9.2c. We have also referred to this as the Rosen mechanism (SPRINGER 1994a). In Fig. 9.2c, the small value of $\Delta\chi$ present during the pre- and post-bolus states is ignored. This is the same as the resting state $\Delta\chi$ value in Fig. 9.2a. However, we can ignore it in Fig. 9.2c because the $\Delta\chi$ value reached at the peak of the bolus passage is much larger (ALBERT et al. 1993a; SPRINGER 1994a). Thus, for a BALD experiment, the EV increase in $(T_2^*)^{-1}$ caused by the large $\Delta\chi$ value is much greater than the decrease in $(T_2^*)^{-1}$ normally seen in a BOLD study. Thus, the *negative* fMRI response expected in a BALD protocol is much greater than the *positive* fMRI response for the equivalent BOLD experiment. Unfortunately, the BALD protocol requires a separate bolus CR injection for each brain activation state of interest (ALBERT et al. 1993a; SPRINGER 1994a).

The more practical agent-free fMRI experiment, however, depends on much smaller intrinsic changes in the blood BMS value caused by brain activation. As we will see below, the blood oxygenation level is often found to increase, and thus the value of χ_v to decrease. Thus, the top spectrum on the right of Fig. 9.3 depicts the case when the value of χ_v has transiently decreased to -9.00 ppm (from -8.70 ppm). Equation 9.2 tells us that the D_v values move much closer to D_e. With a sufficiently large vessel, one can study an ROI contained completely within the vessel lumen. Then, there is only one D_v line in the spectrum. Recently this was accomplished with pial veins (HOOGENRAAD et al. 1998), and Eq. 9.2 was used to convert the accumulated phase (ϕ) – the precession time integral of ν [D_v] – into the decreased value of χ_v exhibited during motor activation. This was used in turn to calculate the level of blood oxygenation during the activated state (HOOGENRAAD et al. 1998).

Of course, in most fMRI studies, the ROI contains a large ensemble of vessels with distributions of orientations in $\mathbf{B}_0$ and sizes. Thus, there will be distributions of D_v and I_e values for the spins within the ROI – even if the ROI is a single voxel (LABADIE et al. 1994). The spectra on the left of Fig. 9.3 depict the same increased BALD and increased BOLD changes, except that the ROI more realistically contains an ensemble of vessels of random orientations, with a fractional CBV value more like

0.2. Thus, the vessel D_v values are rendered into the classic axial powder pattern-like dispersion (SPRINGER 1994a,b) by the second-rank spherical harmonic factor in Eq. 9.2. The edge at low frequency is more intense because the perpendicular orientation is more probable.

An increase in the width of a frequency distribution in Fig. 9.3 means an increase in the rate of loss of precessional phase coherence of intravascular spins experiencing the different frequencies, and therefore an increase in the $(T_2^*)^{-1}$ value of the resulting signal. Changes in the D_v distributions in Fig. 9.3 are thus the sources of the so-called intravascular (IV) BMS contribution to an fMRI change (BOXERMAN et al. 1995a; VAN ZIJL et al. 1998). Of course, the intravascular ^1H_2O spectral lines are not really δ-functions, as depicted on the right in Fig. 9.3 for clarity, but have finite intrinsic linewidths.[2]

The much more intense extravascular ^1H_2O spectral lines in Fig. 9.3 are also not really δ-functions, though their line widths are narrowed to some extent by the diffusional motion of water molecules

---

[2] Sometimes, the blood ^1H_2O spectrum, arising from within the vessel, has been modeled as resulting from a two-site equilibrium exchange of ^1H_2O between the plasma and erythrocyte cytoplasmic spaces (Gasparovic and Matwiyoff 1992; van Zijl et al. 1998). However, we have shown that this is incorrect (Springer 1994b). In important aspects, the exchange-less blood ^1H_2O spectrum is very much like that in the center on the left in Fig. 9.3, with the intracellular signal replacing the intravascular signal. The important point is that the intracellular signal is a powder pattern dispersed about the extracellular signal (though reversed from Fig. 9.3), with its average frequency at exactly the same value as that of the extracellular signal (Springer 1994a, b). Equilibrium exchange between a single line and a powder pattern is most definitely not a two-site process. (Even if it were, in this particular case the two sites would have identical frequencies.) Intermediate exchange situations here would result in very complicated inhomogeneous line shapes. In general, our theory informs us that, for ensembles of spherical cells, or nonspherical cells with random orientations, BMS effects do not allow the quantitative discrimination of the intra- and extracellular resonance frequencies of spins on molecules present in both spaces (Albert et al. 1993b; Springer 1994a). Though nonspherical erythrocytes can be aligned by a magnetic field (Kuchel et al. 1997), this is unlikely to happen in the rough and tumble of passage through vessels that, at the smallest sizes, are randomly oriented within even the smallest voxels employed for fMRI. There are certainly situations in biology in which there is a significant net orientation of nonspherical cells. In regions of human skeletal muscle tissue in vivo (Boesch et al. 1997), and sections of plant tissue in vitro (Shachar-Hill et al. 1997), our equations for D_V (Eq. 9.2) and D_e have been found to accurately account for baseline spectral splittings of resonances that can be observed or induced for spins in oriented intra- and extracellular compartments having different χ values. This is very gratifying.

about the vessel. Furthermore, Eq. 9.1 indicates that the width of the I_e distribution will change as well during brain activation, if any of the variables on the right hand side change. The trigonometric factors of the I_e expression always give rise to symmetrical spectral dispersions (CHU et al. 1990; SPRINGER 1994b), but the central one will still lead to ensemble bias by the probability distribution of Φ values. Changes in the width of such a dispersion are the sources of the extravascular (EV) BMS contribution (Fig. 9.2) to an fMRI change.

Now, we can complete our considerations of Fig. 9.1. Equations 9.1 and 9.2 are the bases of the most realistic Monte Carlo modeling of fMRI responses due to the EV and IV BMS effects of vessel ensembles (OGAWA et al. 1993; BOXERMAN et al. 1995a, b). Since an increase in the width of the distribution of either D_v or I_e leads to an increase in $(T_2{}^*)^{-1}$, relationship c in Fig. 9.1 has a plus sign. Since the contributions expressed in Eqs. 9.1 and 9.2 are constant in the dimensionless ppm unit, their importance increases with field strength (measured as flux density, $\mathbf{B}_0$). This is why fMRI studies come into greater advantage with increasing field (HUANG et al. 1996).

9.5
Physiological Phenomena

The third step in Fig. 9.1 is to identify the relevant physiological phenomena. There are three of these. Changes in the blood magnetic susceptibility itself are caused by changes in the concentration of deoxygenated hemoglobin iron (HUANG et al. 1996). Since the oxygenated hemoglobin iron atom is diamagnetic, the blood BMS value, χ_v, is reciprocally related to the blood oxygenation level. If we recall that the quantity $(\chi_v - \chi_e)$ in Eqs. 9.1 and 9.2 is $\Delta\chi$, we can state that $\Delta\chi$ is never negative; because χ_v is never more negative than χ_e. If blood is fully oxygenated, $\Delta\chi$ is essentially zero. If there is any degree of deoxygenation, $\Delta\chi$ is positive (ALBERT et al. 1993b; SPRINGER 1994a). Thus, the relationship between blood BMS and BOLD must have a negative sign, as shown in Fig. 9.1f. The relationships of the other two physiological parameters – the CBV, and the cerebral blood flow (CBF) – are also depicted in Fig. 9.1. The proportional relationship of CBF to the inflow effect (Fig. 9.1g) is obvious. However, the other two relationships (e and h) require some elaboration.

Let us consider the CBV influence on the blood BMS effect (relationship 1e). The CBV is increased by dilation of resistance arterioles and/or venules (probably not capillary recruitment; HUANG et al. 1996). It is quite clear that the number of spins experiencing D_v increases with vessel size, because there will be more intravascular spins. Thus, the area under the D_v distribution (Fig. 9.3) increases. It is also clear that I_e increases with R^2 (Eq. 9.1). Thus, relationship 1e has a plus sign.

It may be useful to recap the last two paragraphs. There are two ways that physiological changes can change the blood BMS effects described by Eqs. 9.1 and 9.2, and of relevance here. An increase in CBV increases the BMS effect (relationship 1e), whereas an increase in the blood oxygenation level decreases the blood BMS (χ_v) itself (relationship 1f). These are important distinctions. Of course, both phenomena can occur simultaneously.

9.6
Metabolism

How can the CBF influence the concentration of oxygenated hemoglobin iron atoms in the blood (BOLD, relationship 1h)? To understand this, we must recall that this concentration is a steady state quantity, depending on the balance of two opposing kinetic processes. A cartoon depiction of this is shown in Fig. 9.4. Panel a represents a single brain capillary (vessel with diameter ≤ 10 μm) with erythrocytes (ovals) flowing from left to right. The state of oxygenation of the hemoglobin iron atoms is indicated inside the ovals: apFeO$_2$ signifies an oxygenated atom (ap stands for the apoprotein), while apFe signifies a deoxygenated atom. We refrain from using HgbO$_2$ and Hgb because it is the concentration of iron atoms in a given state of oxygenation that matters (HUANG et al. 1996). The concentration of totally deoxygenated hemoglobin (Hgb) is almost never significant in vivo. Erythrocytes bearing some deoxygenated iron are represented as stippled ovals. The endothelial cells are suggested in the capillary walls. Below the capillary are suggested some brain parenchymal cells; neurons (star-shaped), and glia (square-shaped). Besides erythrocytes, the blood also delivers glucose ($C_6H_{12}O_6$). Its metabolic processes are indicated by arrows. It is the aerobic metabolism of glucose (CMR$_{O2}$) that ultimately produces the paramagnetic apFe as a product. As we have seen, this can affect the value of the blood BMS (χ_v). No other paramagnetic species in the blood (O_2, NO) has a concentration high enough to have any significant effect. The value of χ_v increases with [apFe], i.e., it becomes less negative (SPRINGER

1994a). Thus, the value of [apFe], and therefore χ_v, increases as one progresses down the capillary (panel b) because the capillary has passed an increasing number of cells with some baseline amount of CMR_{O2} activity. However, apFe is removed from the capillary by the blood flow (CBF), and replaced with diamagnetic $apFeO_2$. Thus, the value of [apFe] at any point in the capillary is a steady state balance caused by the competing CMR_{O2} and CBF processes. With constant CBF, the value of $[apFeO_2]$ must concomitantly fall, down the capillary (panel b), but since it is diamagnetic this has no influence on χ_v (ALBERT ET AL 1993b).

If CBF were to rise with no accompanying increase in CMR_{O2}, the $[apFeO_2]$ line in Fig. 9.4b would have a less negative slope while that for [apFe] would have a less positive slope. Thus, the value of χ_v at any point would decrease. In hypercapnia, the value of CBF increases due to dilation of the larger vessels supplying and draining the capillaries (CHEN et al. 1994). When transient hypercapnia causes a positive fMRI response (JEZZARD et al. 1994), it must be that pathway h→f→c→a (and/or pathway g→d→b) in Fig. 9.1 dominates pathway e→c→a. Each of the former has a net positive sign while the latter has a net negative sign. In such an event, the effect of the dilation of the diamagnetic arterioles dominates that of the dilation of the less diamagnetic venules in the same ROI. Another way of saying this is that the reduction of χ_v in the venule caused by the increase in CBF is more important than the effect due to increasing its size (pathway e→c→a).

Now, we must move to the level of the metabolic rates (CMR_{O2} and $CMR_{glucose}$) themselves. There are many relationships in Fig. 9.1 stemming from these (i, j, k, l, m, n). Let us consider the aerobic metabolism, first as if it occurs alone. Here, we are talking about the pathway that includes relationship m. If the value of CMR_{O2} increases without (or before) a concomitant increase in CBF (n; possibly inextricably due to an increase in CBV, l) – say, in response to increased neuronal activity (o), the consequences are very interesting. The pathway o→m→j→f→c→a has a net negative sign. Thus, it would cause a negative fMRI change. The key is relationship j, which has a negative sign. If CMR_{O2} increases with no increase in CBF, it is clear from Fig. 9.4 that the [apFe] line will have a more positive slope and the $[apFeO_2]$ line will have a more negative slope (the blood oxygenation level will decrease). Imagine a decreased BOLD, a small extent in the direction of the increased BALD in Fig. 9.3. Thus, χ_v at any point will increase (become less negative). It seems mechanically sensible that in-

creases in CBV and thus CBF (relationships i, k, l, n) would be somewhat slower to respond to neuronal activity than the enzyme catalyzed chemical reactions of aerobic metabolism (o, m). The great excitement about the initial negative fMRI dip is that it may very well reflect this situation. It does appear to correspond to an early increase in the steady state value of [apFe] that is detected by light microscopy experiments (MALONEK and GRINVALD 1996). If this holds true, it promises a route to avoid the delay imposed on the fMRI response by the lag time required to increase blood flow, and also to avoid the inflow effect contribution (d) (HU et al. 1997).

When the CBF has finally increased sufficiently, the positive 1h relationship then overwhelms the negative 1j relationship to obliterate the negative dip and produce a large positive fMRI response. The ultimate decrease in apFe is possibly three times the initial increase in apFe (HU et al. 1997). Why is this? It has often been characterized as an "overcompensation" of flow for CMR_{O2}, an "imbalance" or, worse, a "decoupling" of CBF and CMR_{O2}. However, BUXTON and FRANK (1997) have shown that this can be considered a necessary consequence simply of decreased *efficiency* of the extraction of O_2 from the blood into the tissue (Fig. 9.4) with increasing capil-

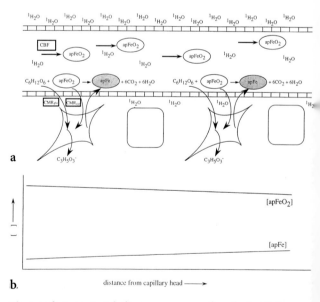

Fig. 9.4a, b. Some metabolic consequences of cerebral activity are suggested. **a** A single capillary blood vessel. Blood is flowing from left to right. Oxygenated hemoglobin iron atoms ($apFeO_2$) and deoxygenated hemoglobin iron atoms (apFe) are shown within *ovals* representing erythrocytes. Glycolytic metabolic processes in neurons (*star-shaped*) and glia (*square-shaped*) are suggested. **b** The spatial dependence of the concentrations of $apFeO_2$ and apFe as one moves downstream in the capillary lumen. More details are given in the text

lary blood velocity, a sensible likelihood. Restated, this means that a disproportionately larger increase in CBF is required just to compensate a smaller increase in CMR_{O2}.

In their paper, BUXTON and FRANK (1997) do not attempt to model the early response. They seem to make the perhaps troubling assumption that the increase in CBF has causal influence on CMR_{O2}. Employing familiar pharmacokinetic modeling concepts for blood-brain barrier transport (SAWADA et al. 1989; KNUDSEN et al. 1990), the early response (initial negative dip) has been mathematically simulated by the MGH group (DAVIS et al. 1994), and by BUXTON et al. (1997)in other work. Using many of the MGH parameters, we have begun to survey the behavior of such models ourselves. Figure 9.5 shows curves that can be produced. In this particular case, the ordinate measures relative values of averaged amounts of apFe (<apFe>) in the venule and capillary (includes arteriole) compartments of an ROI that does not contain any large vessels. The venules occupy 1%, and the capillaries and arterioles 1.5% of the ROI volume, respectively. At time zero, there is slightly more (13%) apFe in venule compartments than in capillary compartments because its concentration in the arterioles and at the capillary heads is zero. The 10 s increase of 20% (DAVIS et al. 1994) in CMR_{O2} is made to begin instantly at time zero (step function at the bottom of the Fig. 9.5). Just as in DAVIS et al. (1994), the flow is also caused to increase, but only after a delay time of 1 s, and a time to ramp to maximum (70%) of 2 s. In the essentials of most of the other parameters as well, our values were the same as those of DAVIS et al. (1994). It is obvious that there are initial increases in the amounts of apFe in both the capillary and venule compartments very soon after the onset of increased aerobic metabolism, peaking slightly later for the venule (2.3 s) than for the capillary (1.0 s) compartment. These are due to the o→m→j pathway of Fig. 9.1. Later, the amounts decrease below their resting values because of the increase of pathway h. After the CMR_{O2} returns to its resting level at 10 s, the apFe amounts begin to return slowly to their resting levels. Other simulations show that this happens by ~35 s. In the case of Fig. 9.5, the maximum increase in total apFe is approx. 3% (at 1.6 s) and the maximum decrease is approx. 21% (at 11.6 s). However, the increase is dominated by the venule compartment and the decrease is dominated by the capillary compartment.

The anaerobic glycolysis metabolism can also effect an fMRI response. Consider pathways o→l→e→c→a and those that begin o→n→h→ or

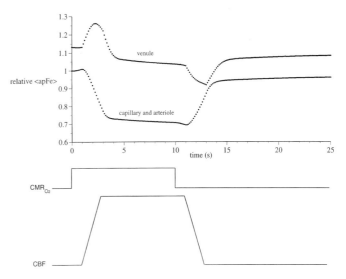

Fig. 9.5. The results of a simulation of the time course of apFe levels during a burst of increased aerobic glycolytic activity. The *vertical axis* measures the relative amounts of the average levels of apFe in venule compartments, and in capillary and arteriole compartments, of a region of interest (ROI) that does not contain any large vessels. The 10 s period of increased metabolic activity is shown as a step function below. As is also shown, the larger, concomitant increase in cerebral blood flow (CBF) is made to lag behind the increase in aerobic metabolism of glucose (CMR_{O2}). Details are given in the text

o→n→g→ in Fig. 9.1, which admit the possibility that anaerobic glycolysis can cause vessel dilation and increased flow. While the first has a net negative sign, the latter two have net positive signs. The increased production of lactate within a few seconds of photic stimulus onset has now been confirmed in an MR spectroscopic experiment (MENON and GATI 1997). Though the lactate ($C_3H_5O_3^-$) shown produced in Fig. 9.4 appears as though by neuronal metabolism, the cartoon is not meant to be that literal. Certainly cerebral metabolism occurs in both neurons and glia, and various metabolic pathways may very well be partitioned between them (BARINAGA 1997a, b). Certainly also, aerobic and anaerobic glycolysis metabolic processes can be increased simultaneously.

As discussed above, each of the many pathways in Fig. 9.1 can, and likely do, have different time courses. It is also true that they can, and likely do, have different spatial loci. Figure 9.6 is a modification of a cartoon that we have published elsewhere (PALYKA et al. 1995). It depicts an extremely idealized pair of capillary beds supplied by the same arteriole and drained by the same venule. This is meant to represent the essence of the necessarily fractal nature of vasculature in tissue – there are more small

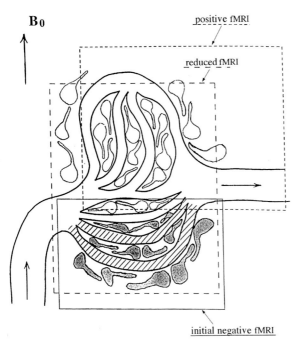

Fig. 9.6. A pair of capillary beds fed by one arteriole and drained by one venule is suggested. The bottom capillary bed supplies cerebral cells that are active (*stippled*). The time course of the fMRI response can depend on the particular region of interest (ROI) measured. Three cases are considered. (Modified from PALYKA et al. 1995)

because it focuses the spatial resolution more directly on the region of brain tissue experiencing the increased activity (HU et al. 1997).

It is hoped that the network presented in Fig. 9.1 will provide a general framework for analyzing fMRI results. Let us conclude with an example from one of the mouse findings with which we began. What could be a mechanism for a negative only response such as that we have also reported elsewhere (HUANG et al. 1996)? Suppose there was a tissue that was stimulated (directly or indirectly) to aerobic metabolic activity by photic stimulation, but which was serviced by arterioles that could not dilate. Then pathway o→m→j→f→c→a in Fig. 9.1 would be the only one available. One would see an only negative response. Perhaps the pineal gland is just such a tissue.

Acknowledgments. We thank Professors Paul Adams, Joseph Fenstermacher, and Xiaoping Hu, Drs. Lawrence Latour, Jing-Huei Lee and Nora Volkow, and Mr. Charles Landis for many stimulating discussions, and a reviewer for very insightful comments. Professor Hu generously supplied us with a video tape showing the early response. We also thank the Department of Energy, contract DE-AC02-98CH10884 with the Office of Biological and Environmental Research to BNL, and the National Institutes of Health, grant RO1-GM32125, for supporting this work.

vessels than there are large vessels. In this cartoon, the neurons supplied by one of the capillary beds exhibit increased activity, and they are shown as stippled. Thus, an ROI that contains essentially only that capillary bed could show an fMRI response with an initial negative dip, followed by a positive image intensity increase – pathway o→m→j→f→c→a in Fig. 9.1 followed, for example, by pathway o→m→k→h→f→c→a. On the other hand, an ROI containing a group of neurons that are not activated but that are supported by a capillary bed supplied by the same arteriole would also exhibit an fMRI response. Since the former pathway is not possible, a response with no initial negative dip could be produced by pathway h→f→c→a. Our model simulations for such a capillary bed indeed show no initial increase in <apFe> such as that seen in Fig. 9.5. A larger ROI that contains both capillary beds might show a reduced early fMRI response, due to a partial volume effect. The general finding, reported above, that the image areas exhibiting the early negative dip are not as diffuse as those that do not, is probably reflective of aspects like these. Thus, the early response is important not only because it avoids the time lag caused by the hemodynamic effect but also

References

Albert MS, Huang W, Lee J-H, Patlak CS, Springer CS (1993a) Susceptibility changes following bolus injections. Magn Reson Med 29:700–708

Albert MS, Huang W, Lee J-H, Balschi JA, Springer CS (1993b) Aqueous shift reagents for high-resolution cation NMR. VI: Titration curves for *in vivo* ^{23}Na and ^{1}H$_2$O MRS obtained from rat blood. NMR Biomed 6:7–20

Bandettini PA, Wong EC, Hinks RS, Tikofsky RS, Hyde JS (1992) Time course EPI of human brain function during task activation. Magn Reson Med 25:390–397

Barbara TM (1994) Cylindrical demagnetization fields and microprobe design in high-resolution NMR. J Magn Reson A 109:265–269

Barinaga M (1997a) What makes brain neurons run? Science 276:196–198 (and references therein)

Barinaga M (1997b) New imaging methods provide a better view into the brain. Science 276:1974–1976 (and references therein)

Belliveau JW, Kennedy DN, McKinstry RC, Buchbinder BR, Weisskoff RM, Cohen MS, Vevea JM, Brady TJ, Rosen BR (1991) Functional mapping of the human visual cortex by magnetic resonance imaging. Science 254:716–719

Boesch C, Slotboom J, Hoppeler H, Kreis R (1997) In vivo determination of intra-myocellular lipids in human muscle by means of localized ^{1}H-MR-spectroscopy. Magn Reson Med 37:484–493

Boxerman JL, Bandettini PA, Kwong KK, Baker JR, Davis TL, Rosen BR, Weisskoff RM (1995a) The intravascular contribution to fMRI signal change: Monte Carlo modeling and diffusion-weighted studies *in vivo*. Magn Reson Med 34:4–10

Boxerman JL, Hamberg LM, Rosen BR, Weisskoff RM (1995b) MR contrast due to intravascular magnetic susceptibility perturbations. Magn Reson Med 34:555–566

Buxton RB, Frank LR (1997) A model for the coupling between cerebral blood flow and oxygen metabolism during neural stimulation. J Cerebr Blood Flow Metab 17:64–72

Buxton RB, Wong EC, Frank LR (1997) A biomechanical interpretation of the BOLD signal time course: the balloon model. Proc Int Soc Magn Reson Med 5:743

Chen J-L, Wei L, Acuff V, Bereczki D, Hans F-J, Otsuka T, Finnegan W, Patlak C, Fenstermacher J (1994) Slightly altered permeability-surface area products imply some cerebral capillary recruitment during hypercapnia. Microvasc Res 48:190–211

Christman RA, Ailion DC, Case TA, Durney CH, Cutillo AG, Shioya S, Goodrich KC, Morris AH (1996) Comparison of calculated and experimental NMR spectral broadening for lung tissue. Magn Reson Med 35:6–13

Chu SC-K, Xu Y, Balschi JA, Springer CS (1990) Bulk magnetic susceptibility shifts in NMR studies of compartmentalized samples: Use of paramagnetic reagents. Magn Reson Med 13:239–262

Davis TL, Weisskoff RM, Kwong KK, Boxerman JL, Rosen BR (1994) Temporal aspects of fMRI task activation: Dynamic modeling of oxygen delivery. Proc Soc Magn Reson Med 2:69

Dickinson WC (1951) The time average magnetic field at the nucleus in nuclear magnetic resonance experiments. Phys Rev 81:717–731

Ernst T, Hennig J (1994) Observation of a fast response in functional MR. Magn Reson Med 32:146–149

Frahm J, Bruhn H, Merboldt KD, Hänicke W (1992) Dynamic MRI of human brain oxygenation during rest and photic stimulation. J Magn Reson Imaging 2:501–505

Gasparovic C, Matwiyoff NA (1992) The magnetic properties and water dynamics of the red blood cell: A study by proton-NMR lineshape analysis. Magn Reson Med 26:274–299

Hoogenraad FGC, Reichenbach JR, Haacke EM, Lai S, Kuppusamy K, Sprenger M (1998) In vivo measurement of changes in venous blood-oxygenation with high resolution functional MRI at 0.95 tesla by measuring changes in susceptibility and velocity. Magn Reson Med 39:97–107

Hu X, Le T-H, Ugurbil K (1997) Evaluation of the early response in fMRI in individual subjects using short stimulus duration. Magn Reson Med 37:877–884

Huang W, Palyka I, Li H-F, Eisenstein EM, Volkow ND, Springer CS. (1996) Magnetic resonance imaging (MRI) detection of the murine brain response to light: Temporal differentiation and negative functional MRI changes. Proc Natl Acad Sci USA 93:6037–6042

Jezzard P, Heineman F, Taylor J, DesPres D, Wen H, Balaban RS, Turner R (1994) Comparison of EPI gradient-echo contrast changes in cat brain caused by respiratory challenges with direct simultaneous evaluation of cerebral oxygenation via a cranial window. NMR Biomed 7:35–44

Knudsen GM, Pettigrew KD, Paulson OB, Hertz MM, Patlak CS (1990) Kinetic analysis of blood-brain barrier transport of D-glucose in man: Quantitative evaluation in the presence of tracer backflux and capillary heterogeneity. Microvasc Res 39:28–49

Kuchel PW, Coy A, Stilbs P (1997) NMR "diffusion-diffraction" of water revealing alignment of erythrocytes in a magnetic field and their dimensions and membrane transport characteristics. Magn Reson Med 37:637–643

Kwong KK, Belliveau JW, Chesler DA, Goldberg IE, Weisskoff RM, Poncelet BP, Kennedy DN, Hoppel BE, Cohen MS, Turner R, Cheng H-M, Brady TJ, Rosen BR (1992) Dynamic magnetic resonance imaging of human brain activity during primary sensory stimulation. Proc Natl Acad Sci USA 89:5675–5679

Labadie C, Lee J-H, Vetek G, Springer CS (1994) Relaxographic imaging. J Magn Reson B 105:99–112

Lee J-H, Li X, Sammi MK, Springer CS. (1999) Using flow relaxography to elucidate flow relaxivity J Magn Reson 136:

Levitt MH (1996) Demagnetization field effects in two-dimensional solution NMR. Concepts Magn Reson 8:77–103

Lüdeke KM, Röschmann P, Tischler R (1985) Susceptibility artefacts in NMR imaging. Magn Reson Imaging 3:329–343

Malonek D, Grinvald A (1996) Interactions between electrical activity and cortical microcirculation revealed by imaging spectroscopy: Implications for functional brain mapping. Science 272:551–554

McIntosh J, Zhang Y, Kidambi S, Harshbarger T, Mason G, Pohost GM, Tweig D (1996) Echo-time dependence of the functional MRI "fast response." Proc Int Soc Magn Reson Med 4:284

Menon RS, Gati JS (1997) Two second temporal resolution measurements of lactate correlate with EPI BOLD fMRI timecourses during photic stimulation. Proc Int Soc Magn Reson Med 5:152

Menon RS, Ogawa S, Hu X, Strupp JP, Anderson P, Ugurbil K (1995) BOLD based functional MRI at 4 tesla includes a capillary bed contribution: Echo-planar imaging correlates with previous optical imaging using intrinsic signals. Magn Reson Med 33:453–459

Moore GG, Zhang YT, Tweig DB (1997) Assessment of the fast response spatial distribution. Proc Int Soc Magn Reson Med 5:377

Ogawa S, Lee TM, Kay AR, Tank DW (1990) Brain magnetic resonance imaging with contrast dependent on blood oxygenation. Proc Natl Acad Sci USA 87:9868–9872

Ogawa S, Tank DW, Menon R, Ellermann JM, Kim S-G, Merkle H, Ugurbil K (1992) Intrinsic signal changes accompanying sensory stimulation: Functional brain mapping with magnetic resonance imaging. Proc Natl Acad Sci USA 89:5951–5955

Ogawa S, Menon RS, Tank DW, Kim S-G, Merkle H, Ellermann JM, Ugurbil K (1993) Functional brain mapping by blood oxygenation level-dependent contrast magnetic resonance imaging: Comparison of signal characteristics with a biophysical model. Biophys J 64:803–812

Palyka I, Huang W, Springer CS (1995) The effects of bulk magnetic susceptibility in NMR. Bull Magn Reson 17:46–53

Sawada Y, Patlak CS, Blasberg RG (1989) Kinetic analysis of cerebrovascular transport based on indicator diffusion technique. Am J Physiol 256:H794-H812

Schenck JF (1996) The role of magnetic susceptibility in magnetic resonance imaging: MRI magnetic compatibility of the first and second kinds. Med Phys 23:815–850

Shachar-Hill Y, Befroy DE, Pfeffer PE, Ratcliffe RG (1997) Using bulk magnetic susceptibility to resolve internal and external signals in the NMR spectra of plant tissues. J Magn Reson 127:17–25

Springer CS (1994a) Physicochemical principles influencing magnetopharmaceuticals. In: Gillies RJ (ed) NMR in physiology and biomedicine. Academic, New York, pp. 75–99

Springer CS (1994b) Bulk magnetic susceptibility frequency shifts in cell suspensions. NMR Biomed 7:198–202

Springer CS (1995) What's in a name? NMR Biomed 8:233–234

Springer CS, Xu Y (1991) Aspects of bulk magnetic susceptibility in in vivo MRI and MRS. In: Rinck PA, Muller RN (eds) New developments in contrast agent research. European Magnetic Resonance Forum, Blonay, Switzerland, pp. 13–25

Turner R, Jezzard P, Wen H, Kwong KK, Le Bihan D, Zeffiro T, Balaban RS (1993) Functional mapping of the human visual cortex at 4 and 1.5 Tesla using deoxygenation contrast EPI. Magn Reson Med 29:277–279

Tweig DB, Moore GG, Zhang YT (1997) Estimating fast response onset time. Proc Int Soc Magn Reson Med 5:1645

van Zijl PCM, Eleff SM, Ulatowski JA, Oja JME, Ulug AM, Traystman RJ, Kauppinen RA (1998) Quantitative assessment of blood flow, blood volume and blood oxygenation effects in functional magnetic resonance imaging. Nat Med 4:159–167

Vazquez A, Peltier S, Davis D, Noll D (1997) Evidence of the fast response at 3.0 T. Proc Int Soc Magn Reson Med 5:726

Villringer A, Rosen BR, Belliveau JW, Ackerman JL, Lauffer RB, Buxton RB, Chao Y-S, Wedeen VJ, Brady TJ (1988) Dynamic imaging with lanthanide chelates in normal brain: Contrast due to magnetic susceptibility effects. Magn Reson Med 6:164–174

Wagshul ME, Button TM, Li H-F, Liang Z, Springer CS, Zhong K, Wishnia A (1996) In vivo MR imaging and spectroscopy using hyperpolarized ^{129}Xe. Magn Reson Med 36:183–191

Xu Y (1990) Implications of multiple quantum coherences and bulk magnetic susceptibility effects for NMR studies of biological systems. PhD Dissertation. State University of New York, Stony Brook, New York

Xu Y, Balschi JA, Springer CS (1990) Magnetic susceptibility shift selected imaging: MESSI. Magn Reson Med 16:80–90

Zimmerman JR, Foster MR (1957) Standardization of N.M.R. high resolution spectra. J Phys Chem 61:282–289

10 Principles of BOLD Functional MRI

W. Chen, S. Ogawa

CONTENTS

10.1
Introduction

Like other functional neuroimaging methods such as positron emission tomography (Raichle 1987) and optical imaging (Malonek and Grinvald 1996), BOLD (blood oxygenation level-dependent) fMRI is based on physiological responses related to brain activation. To start with, there is the fact that brain function is spatially segmented and compartmentalized. Such functional specialization can be mapped via measuring secondary hemodynamic and metabolic changes in response to alterations in neuronal activity. The spatial resolution of fMRI, although limited, can provide significant and useful information on functional compartmentalization. The coupling between the physiological response and neuronal activation is tight and well localized, but the response time is relatively slow, in seconds, rather than the time constant of neuronal activity which is in tens or hundreds of milliseconds.

W. Chen, PhD, Center for Magnetic Resonance Research, Radiology Department, University of Minnesota, School of Medicine, 3021 6th Street SE, Minneapolis, MN 55455, USA
S. Ogawa, PhD, Biological Computation Research, Bell Laboratories, Lucent Technologies, Murray Hill, NJ 07974, USA

BOLD imaging uses the endogenous MRI contrast agent deoxyhemoglobin as the source of the contrast. The ferrous iron on the heme of deoxyhemoglobin is paramagnetic, but diamagnetic in oxyhemoglobin (i.e., heme with a bound oxygen molecule). Although unbounded oxygen molecule in water is paramagnetic, its effect on the MRI water signal in tissue is very small. In the presence of one atmospheric pressure of oxygen, the dissolved oxygen induced change in water proton relaxation times becomes barely detectable. When the red cells containing deoxyhemoglobin are placed in the magnetic field used for MRI, there is some field distortion induced by the difference in the magnetic susceptibility relative to the surrounding. This susceptibility induced field shift or field distortion related to deoxyhemoglobin is the source of BOLD contrast, and the change in the deoxyhemoglobin content associated with the functional activation can be detected in the MRI signal.

The T_2 relaxation time of blood water has been known to be dependent on the degree of deoxygenation of the blood (Thulborn et al. 1982) due to the above described field shift. In the MR images of the rat brain at 7 Tesla, the susceptibility effect is visible even in the extravascular spaces (Ogawa et al. 1990b; Ogawa and Lee 1990). BOLD contrast varies with the physiological state, especially with hemodynamic changes, and was postulated to be useful for functional study (Ogawa et al. 1990a). The effect of a lack of oxygen in the blood in an ischemic episode can be observed as a decrease in the MRI signal due to the tissue T_2^* shortening (Turner et al. 1991). The feasibility of using the MRI technique based on BOLD contrast for mapping neuronal activation was first demonstrated in the human brain during simple visual perception task (Kwong et al. 1992; Ogawa et al. 1992) and motor task (Bandettini et al. 1992) performances in 1992. These studies opened a totally new dimension regarding visualizing functional activation in the human brain using BOLD based fMRI (Ugurbil et al. 1994). Furthermore, recent efforts in fMRI have shown the way to measuring and mapping cerebral blood flow (CBF) itself and has been further extended to image cerebral perfusion – one of the most important aspects of cerebral physiology.

Various aspects of BOLD fMRI are discussed in many chapters in this book. In this chapter, we present only a general description of BOLD fMRI.

10.2
Functional MRI Signal

10.2.1
Activation Induced MRI Signal

The MRI signal commonly acquired with a single pulse sequence can be expressed in a simple way such as:

$$S = M(T_1{}^*) \cdot A(T_2{}^*) \qquad (10.1)$$

where M is the sampled magnetization which is the signal intensity at echo time zero. The magnitude of M is determined by $T_1{}^*$ (T_1 with inflow) and is also dependent on the method of NMR signal acquisition in terms related to T_1. The term A, the signal attenuation, is the $T_2{}^*$ decay of the in-plane magnetization. BOLD contrast contributes to the $T_2{}^*$ decay process and the echo time is the parameter one can vary to examine the transverse relaxation process. The compartments in an image voxel, such as tissue, blood and bulk cerebrospinal fluid (CSF), have signals that are added together vectorially. As discussed in the chapters on perfusion, in capillary beds the water exchange across the capillary wall is relatively fast compared with T_1 and the blood transit time through the capillary bed. Therefore the longitudinal magnetization for blood water and tissue water in capillary beds can be summed together as a single entity. The venous blood from the capillaries and beyond has a magnetization quite similar to the tissue water. $T_2{}^*$ decay, on the other hand, occurs at a much faster rate than water exchange, and thus blood and tissue have different contributions to the attenuation, A.

When there is an activation induced MRI signal in a capillary bed, the signal change is the sum of the changes in M due to $T_1{}^*$ and in A due to the $T_2{}^*$ attenuation, as described by:

$$\Delta S/S = \Delta M/M + \Delta A/A \qquad (10.2)$$

The first term is the inflow effect and is zero if the magnetization at the sampling time is maintained at a fully relaxed condition. At a steady state of continuous imaging sampling with single pulse MRI acquisition, a repetition time of $\sim T_1$ or shorter and the sampling pulse at Ernst's angle:

$$\Delta M/M = \sim 0.4\Delta(1/T_1{}^*)/(1/T_1{}^*) \qquad (10.3)$$

where $1/T_1{}^* = 1/T_1 + CBF/\alpha$ and $\Delta(1/T_1{}^*) = \Delta CBF/\alpha$. With water partition α of 0.92 and when ΔCBF is as high as 50 ml blood/100 g tissue per min, the inflow contribution $\Delta M/M$ is ~ 0.0035. Therefore, in capillary beds, the inflow effect due to the CBF increase is small relative to a BOLD signal change, $\Delta A/A$, of a few percent or larger. Actually, when the activation signal detected by fMRI is measured with varying echo times (te), extrapolation to echo time zero shows a very small remaining activation signal (Menon et al. 1993). In contrast, with the inversion recovery type of signal acquisition used for perfusion measurements, the coefficient in Eq. 10.3 is ~ 3, in stead of 0.4, at TI (flow-in time after inversion) $=\sim T_1$ with a sufficiently long recovery time.

If A is described by a simple $T_2{}^*$ decay (or T_2 decay for spin echo sampling), $A = \exp(-te/T_2{}^*)$ and $\Delta A/A = -te\Delta(1/T_2{}^*)$. Estimated values of $\Delta(1/T_2{}^*)$ decreases from fMRI experiments are $\sim 1\ s^{-1}$ depending on B_0 field strength (Menon et al. 1993; Bandettini et al. 1994). With a typical echo time of 20–40 ms, $\Delta A/A$ is a few percent at the tissue.

One of the major features of the fMRI method is its capability to follow dynamic physiological changes in real time. The limiting temporal resolution is the echo time, ten to several tens of milliseconds, although the actual physical limit may be the scanning time needed to cover the image k-space. In perfusion measurements, the inflow signal response to the change in CBF may lag slightly behind the actual CBF change because of the water exchange process, which is only slightly shorter than 1 s and which takes some time to reach steady state. With these time resolutions of BOLD fMRI, one can follow the changes in the physiology induced by neuronal activation. Recently, significant progress has been made in mapping temporal BOLD changes in response to a single task trial or averaging single task trials (Buckner et al. 1996; Richter et al. 1997). These studies will provide more information about dynamic BOLD changes that may reflect neuronal events. The success of these experiments is a result of the high sensitivity of BOLD measurement. Figure 10.1 demonstrates the BOLD time course (at 4 T) of a

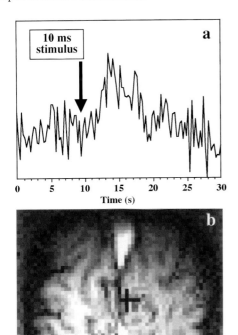

Fig. 10.1. a Time course of blood oxygen level-dependent (BOLD) signal from a single pixel in the activated V1 areas induced by a single trial of 10 ms photic stimulation. b The *cross marker* depicts the pixel position on the coronal image. The temporal resolution of BOLD time course is 0.25 s

single pixel ($3.1 \times 3.1 \times 5.0$ mm^3) in the primary visual cortex (V1) of the human brain in response to an extremely short burst of red light of 10 ms duration. The time course is from a single trial without any averaging. The task-induced BOLD change can be easily identified from the baseline level of the time course. The high sensitivity of BOLD contrast provides a general neuroimaging tool for mapping brain activation, from large cortical areas near the brain surface to the small nuclei located in deepest brain.

10.2.2
Red Cell Induced Susceptibility Effect

BOLD contrast is solely due to the susceptibility difference of red cells with paramagnetic deoxyhemoglobin relative to their surrounding. Interaction of water molecules with deoxyhemoglobin itself does not cause any significant field shift in the bulk of water to be imaged. This has been clearly shown in blood water NMR signals that lose the deoxyhemoglobin induced shift or in a shortened T_2^* condition generated by lysing red cells without oxygenating hemoglobin.

As described in the chapter on susceptibility contrast (see Chap. 9, this volume), the bulk susceptibility variation of red cells, which is due to the hemoglobin deoxygenation level, changes the field shift inside and outside these red cells. In the blood, water molecules diffuse through the plasma and exchange across the red cell membrane between intra- and extracellular spaces at relatively fast rates compared with the imaging echo time. The water exchange across the blood vessel wall is slow in this time scale and the extravascular tissue water senses the spatially dependent field shift which is smaller than the intravascular shift.

For magnetic resonance, the z component of this field shift or the local field distortion along the static B_0 field is the relevant physical quantity. The observed MR signal is the sum of the resonance signal with phase factor $\exp(i\phi)$, $\phi = \omega t$ and ω is the field shift in angular frequency and t is the observation time or the echo time. The value of ω is proportional to the deoxygenation level and B_0 field strength. The MRI signal of a voxel is a spatial and temporal average of the phase factor, $<\exp(i\phi)>$, within the voxel. The temporal average means averaging due to the movement of water molecules during the observation period by diffusion through space or exchange between red cell and plasma. Averaging with the range of ϕ values present in the voxel leads to signal attenuation in addition to other T_2^* decay processes and it also leaves some residual phase shift in the averaged signal. The residual phase shift is expected for the blood water signal but not for extravascular tissue water. The quantity of this attenuation is the subject of the following chapter in this book. In general, the T_2^* attenuation or $(1/T_2^*)$ rate is larger at higher B_0 field and deoxygenation level (proportional or more than proportional) and increases with more red cells in a voxel (blood volume fraction).

The quantitative description of the activation signal, $\Delta S/S$ or $\Delta A/A$ in Eq. 10.2, in terms of the measurable physiological parameters (blood oxygenation level Y, ΔCBF or the changes of cerebral blood volume, ΔCBV) and the MRI parameters (B_0, te, etc.) is of great interest because of the involvement of the oxygen consumption rate in determining the blood oxygenation level. A model used some time ago to fit the Y dependence of the MRI signal of rat brain at high magnetic field strength, as shown below, may be too simple to cover such multiple parameter-dependent phenomena:

$$\Delta A/A = a.te.\Delta(1/T_2^*) = a.te\Delta(v.B_0.(1-Y)) \qquad (10.4)$$

where a, v and Y are a constant, blood volume fraction and venous blood oxygenation level, respectively. Efforts are being made to calibrate BOLD signal as a function of CBF change in the same brain using hypercapnia conditions, in which the oxygen consumption rate does not change much from the basal state (Rostrup et al. 1994; Bandettini et al. 1997; Davis et al. 1998). Measurements of CBF and BOLD signal under hypercapnia may allow more reliable spatial correlation of the BOLD signal to Y.

10.2.3
Extra- and Intravascular BOLD Contribution

Since the T_2^* decay rates of intra- and extravascular water are fairly different, the T_2^* attenuation A in Eq. 10.2 has to be separated into two terms.

$$A = \{f A(T_2^*)\}_{blood} + \{f A(T_2^*)\}_{tissue} \qquad (10.5)$$

where f is the volume fraction of the compartment. In general, the susceptibility-dependent part of the T_2^* decay rate is larger for the blood water than the tissue water, which senses the red cell susceptibility effect at more distant sites than the blood water in the red cell and the blood plasma. However, the blood volume fraction f_{blood} is much smaller than the tissue water f_{tissue}.

It has been shown that most BOLD signals in the motor cortex during a finger tapping task disappeared at 1.5 Tesla when a relatively small dipolar diffusion gradient (b-factor of 42 s/mm^2) was applied during the signal acquisition (Song et al. 1996). With this diffusion gradient, intravascular signals from noncapillary vessels with blood flow velocities of above several millimeters per second would be dispersed out. This indicated that these fMRI signals were intravascular and mostly contributed by noncapillary vessels. The extravascular signal by the susceptibility change at this B_0 field is small, especially around capillaries. At higher magnetic fields of 3 Tesla (Song et al. 1995) and 4 Tesla, however, substantial fMRI BOLD signals in gradient echo acquisition persisted even with dipolar diffusion gradient of b=400 s/mm^2, showing that the extravascular BOLD contribution becomes more dominant at higher magnetic field strength. The relative importance of the intravascular component at very high magnetic field strength likely depends on the echo time, because the attenuation A_{blood} itself at resting and activated conditions is fairly smaller than A_{tissue}. Therefore with a long echo time the high sensitivity to susceptibility changes does not contribute so much to the overall BOLD signal.

10.3
Uncoupling between Changes of CMR_{O2} and Cerebral Blood Flow

The major determinant of the deoxyhemoglobin content in the blood is the supply and demand of oxygen at the tissue. The oxygenation level of the venous blood is related to the oxygen extraction (or cerebral metabolic rate of oxygen consumption, CMR_{O2}) and CBF by Fick's principle of oxygen balance between arterial and venous blood. Changes in CBF and/or CMR_{O2} cause a change in Y (oxygenation of venous blood) as related by:

$$oxygen\ extraction\ factor=$$
$$CMRO_2/(CBF \cdot Ch)=(1-Y) \qquad (10.6)$$

and

$$\{(\Delta CMR_{O2}/CMR_{O2})+1\}/\{(\Delta CBF/CBF)+1\}=$$
$$-\Delta Y/(1-Y)+1 \qquad (10.7)$$

where Ch is heme concentration and the oxygenation level in arterial blood is taken as 1. Once the Y dependence of the BOLD signal is known, $\Delta CMR_{O2}/CMR_{O2}$ can be calculated using Eq. 10.7. BOLD and $\Delta CBF/CBF$ data can be accurately determined from NMR measurements, and one can use the known relationship between $\Delta CBF/CBF$ and $\Delta CBV/CBV$ to estimate ΔY (Grubb et al. 1974; Kim and Ugurbil 1997b; Davis et al. 1998; Ogawa et al. 1998). Since the *in vivo* spatial mapping of $\Delta CMR_{O2}/CMR_{O2}$ is very difficult and laborious, the BOLD and CBF MRI measurements will be very valuable to characterize the metabolic response of a particular brain area to particular functional activation.

In the case of complete coupling between CMR_{O2} and CBF, as occurs in the resting state of brain (Siesjo 1978) ($\Delta CMR_{O2}/CMR_{O2}=\Delta CBF/CBF$), ΔY in the above equation is zero and the susceptibility change does not accompany the CBF increase. In order for the BOLD signal change generated by functional activation to be as positive as the CBF change (ΔY is positive in Eq. 10.7), the fractional CMR_{O2} change should be sufficiently smaller than the CBF fractional change. This forms the basis of BOLD-based fMRI, thought to result from the uncoupling between CBF and CMR_{O2} changes during elevated neuronal activity. This argument is consistent with the findings by Fox and Raichle and other groups, that the increases of CMR_{O2} (0%–5%) were much less than those of CBF and cerebral metabolic rate of glucose (CMR_{glc}) (40%–51%) in the human brain during functional activation elevated by visual and somatosensory stimuli (Fox et al. 1988; Fox and RAICHLE 1986; RIBEIRO et al. 1993). The findings suggested involvement of nonoxidative pathway of glucose utilization and were supported by: (1) the observation of increased lactate in the primary visual cortex (V1) in the human brain during visual stimulation (PRICHARD et al. 1992; SAPPEY-MARINIER et al. 1992; FRAHM et al. 1996), and (2) an animal autoradiographic study using dual-radiolabeled flurodeoxyglucose and glucose traces (ACKERMANN and LEAR 1989). How this inefficient utilization of energy through nonoxidative glucose metabolism can be the mode of the metabolic response to functional activation is discussed elsewhere in this volume.

10.4
BOLD Response to Neuronal Activation

One important question for functional brain mapping using fMRI is how well the BOLD response is correlated with neuronal activation. Since the BOLD signal is closely related to the change in CBF, which is known to be closely coupled to functional activation, the BOLD response in space is expected to represent the site of activation. However, the BOLD change is complicated by the multiple contributions from both the metabolic change in CMR_{O2} and hemodynamic changes in CBF and CBV (OGAWA et al. 1990a). Whether the magnitude of the BOLD change is quantitatively correlated with alterations in CBF and/or neuronal activity needs to be examined. Since neuronal and vascular responses to activation are expected to vary among subjects as well as across different regions in a given brain, a close examination of CBF and BOLD changes in the same activation region with stimuli in different modes and without inter-subject averaging is warranted. This can be accomplished in studies of the visual cortex by varying the degree of neuronal activity with graded visual stimulation.

Previous neuroimaging studies have demonstrated that neuronal activity in V1 is sensitive to the temporal frequency of photic stimulation, showing a maximal response at approximately 8 Hz in the human brain (Fox and RAICHLE 1985a, b; KWONG et al.

1992). Similar observations have also been demonstrated in the visual pathway by evoked potential (REGAN 1977) and neuronal recording with electrodes (MOVSHON et al. 1978) studies. We have applied the multislice flow-sensitive alternating inversion recovery (FAIR) technique (KWONG et al. 1995; KIM et al. 1997) to measure BOLD and CBF changes simultaneously at 4 T during checkerboard visual stimulations flashing at 2, 4, 6, and 8 Hz frequencies in single subjects (ZHU et al. 1998). In the FAIR technique, multislice coronal images with echo-planar imaging (EPI) acquisition preceded by slice-selective inversion recovery (ssIR) and nonslice-selective IR (nsIR) are obtained in an interleaved way. The BOLD-based fMRI maps were generated by nsIR images alone, which are dominated by the BOLD changes; the FAIR images were generated by paired subtraction between the nsIR and ssIR images on a pixel-by-pixel basis and they were further used to generate the CBF-based fMRI maps (KIM and UGURBIL 1997). This technique has been used to examine the dynamic correlation between BOLD and CBF changes in V1 as a function of visual stimulation frequency (ZHU et al. 1998). In this study, only the common activation pixels in V1 which passed a statistically significant threshold for both the BOLD and CBF maps across all visual stimulation tasks were utilized for calculating and comparing the average BOLD and CBF changes. The FAIR sequence parameters were chosen for optimizing perfusion component in the microvascular areas and suppressing the macrovascular contributions (KIM 1995). Therefore, the pixels common to images based on both BOLD and CBF changes will not suffer from the macrovascular component that can be present in the BOLD map alone. The common BOLD/CBF activation pixels were located mainly in the gray matter areas of the primary visual cortex areas in the absence of obvious large vessels, as demonstrated from a single subject in Fig. 10.2. Figure 10.3 shows the plots of BOLD and CBF changes as a function of visual stimulation frequency from an individual subject (Fig. 10.3a) and the average results of six subjects (Fig. 10.3c). Both BOLD and CBF changes behave similarly as a function of stimulus frequency, reach a peak at 8 Hz visual stimulation frequency and decline at high frequency (>8 Hz), as demonstrated in Fig. 10.3a. These results are consistent with previous reports (Fox and RAICHLE 1985a, b; KWONG et al. 1992). Figures 10.3b and 10.3d are the plots of BOLD change vs CBF change at different visual stimulation frequencies from an individual subject and inter-subject averaged results, respectively.

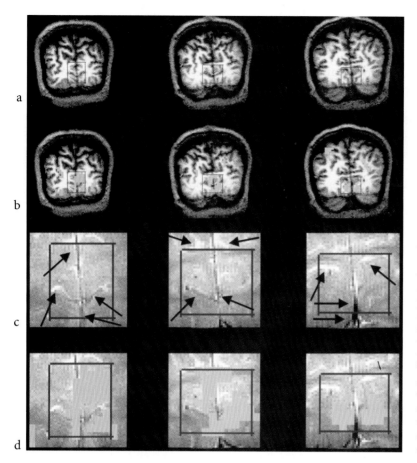

Fig. 10.2a–d. Functional maps created from common activation pixels which are statistically significant for both blood oxygen level-dependent (BOLD) and cerebral blood flow (CBF) maps and all visual tasks at 2, 4, 6 and 8 Hz visual stimulation frequency. Three coronal slice images are illustrated from a representative subject. The regions of interest (ROI), highlighted by *red line boxes*, mainly cover the primary visual cortex around the calcarine fissure and only the common activation pixels within the ROIs were used for quantitative comparisons. **a,b** T_1-weighted anatomic images and the common activation maps superimposed on the T_1 weighted anatomic images. **c,d** T_2^*-weighted high resolution fast gradient echo (FLASH) images and the common activation maps superimposed onto the T_2^*-weighted image. The *arrows* in **c** depict the relatively dark and bright areas in the T_2^*-weighted image which mainly reflect obvious large vessels and CSF areas that are spatially dissociated from the common activation pixels. (From Zhu et al. 1998)

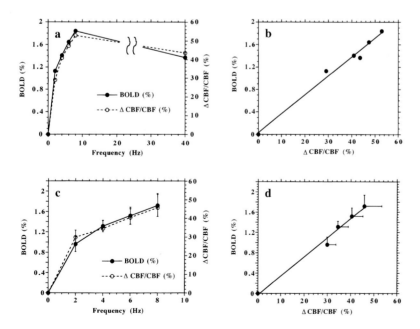

Fig. 10.3a–d. Blood oxygen level-dependent (BOLD) and cerebral blood flow (CBF) changes in the primary visual cortex as a function of visual stimulation frequency from **a** one representative subject and **c** average results of six inter-subjects. Both BOLD and CBF change as a unimodal function of stimulus frequency and reach a maximal value at 8 Hz. **b,d** The relationship between BOLD and CBF changes with varying stimulus frequency from **b** a representative subject and **d** average results of six inter-subjects. Linear correlation fitting between the BOLD and CBF changes is demonstrated for both individual and average data. *Error bars* indicate standard error of inter-subject measurements. (From Zhu et al. 1998)

A significant linear correlation between BOLD and CBF changes was obtained for both cases. This supports the hypothesis that task-induced BOLD changes associated with the microvasculature are well correlated with the CBF changes which presumably reflect metabolic alterations corresponding to variations in neuronal activity itself (YAROWSKY and INGVAR 1981; RAICHLE 1987). Therefore, the magnitude of BOLD change can be used to evaluate variations in neuronal activity within the same activation areas. However, such a relationship may be not valid for comparing different activation areas during the same task performance because of the complex characteristics of the vasculature and hemodynamics in different cortical areas. In this study, it was also found that the linear correlation for intra-subject comparisons was more significant than those for inter-subject comparisons (ZHU et al. 1998). This suggests that using intra-subject comparisons for quantitative studies of neuronal activity related to different task stimuli and task performances should be more reliable than using inter-subject comparisons.

Animal studies also demonstrated a consistency of the activation locations between microflow and BOLD functional maps in the somatomotor cortex during somatosensory stimulation (KERSKENS et al. 1996) and a close relationship among CBF, BOLD and evoked potentials in response to the stimulus frequency (LENIGER-FOLLERT and HOSSMANN 1979; GYNGELL et al. 1996). This suggests that the BOLD signal may quantitatively reflect neuronal events.

10.5
Spatial Specificity of BOLD fMRI

Generally, the activation locations detected by BOLD-fMRI in cortical areas were found to be consistent with CBF-based functional maps generated by PET (CONNELLY et al. 1995; RAMSEY et al. 1995) or perfusion MRI techniques (EDELMAN et al. 1994; KIM 1995; KIM et al. 1996). However, the spatial specificity that can be achieved with fMRI and how well the activation location detected by fMRI correlated to the actual sites of neuronal activity remain debatable. This question is particularly salient for methods such as PET and fMRI, in which functional maps are not based on monitoring neuronal activity directly but rather indirectly through the secondary metabolic and hemodynamic changes in response to neuronal activity. With respect to fMRI, this indirect detection raises questions about the contributions

of macrovascular inflow effects, macrovascular BOLD effects, and the spatial correspondence between the actual site of neuronal activity and the extent of the metabolic and hemodynamic response. These points will be discussed in other chapters. One efficient way to address this issue is to map functionally distinct structures with a much finer spatial scale (e.g., millimeter) and well defined organization and topography in the human brain.

The lateral geniculate nucleus (LGN), located posteriorly and ventrally within the thalamus, provides an excellent case for evaluating the question whether structures which are only a few millimeter in size can be accurately mapped by fMRI methodology. The relay function of the LGN in the visual pathway is well known. The LGN is a primary target of retinal afferents connected by optic tracts and, in turn, it projects to the primary visual cortex V1. Therefore, LGN activation must be present during visual stimulation because of the retinal input. Whether LGN activation in the human brain can be robustly detected during photic stimulation and resolved from activation that may be expected in adjacent structures within the thalamus, such as the pulvinar nucleus, was recently examined at high (4 Tesla) magnetic field (CHEN et al. 1998a). In this effort, the multislice capability of fMRI to generate a three-dimensional functional map of the entire brain was utilized so as to resolve the LGN from adjacent relevant structures based on the anatomical information in three orientations. Figure 10.4 illustrates fMRI maps showing V1 and bilateral LGN activation in three different orientations. These maps were generated from one participant in a single experiment. In the axial image illustrated in Fig. 10.4, the optic tract is seen clearly in both hemispheres near the optic chiasm, anterior to the mid-brain; proceeding posteriorly from the optic chiasm, it appears to merge with the mid-brain and is no longer visualized with clarity as it runs along the cerebral peduncle. Following this curved tract should directly lead to the LGN which is where the activated loci identified as the LGN are located. In the coronal and parasagittal views, this activated area appears superior to the hippocampal formation as expected for the LGN. Figure 10.5 demonstrates the comparison between the LGN locations assigned from a brain atlas and those mapped from fMRI in three identical planes with different orientations. They are virtually identical. The LGN activation is well defined in space without surrounding large vessel contribution and the activation sizes are in agreement with the size of the LGN body. In addition, activation in the pulvinar nucleus in the thalamus was

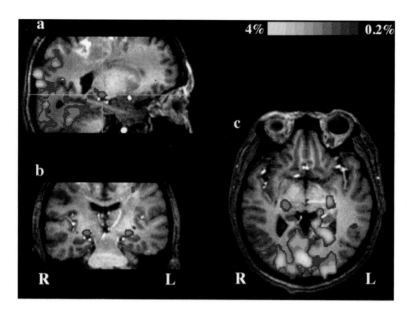

Fig. 10.4a–c. Functional MRI maps of the lateral geniculate nucleus (LGN) activation (*color*) superimposed on anatomical images (*gray scale*) in three orientations from a single subject during a 8 Hz visual stimulation task. The fMRI map with a sagittal orientation located in the right hemisphere is illustrated in (**a**). The intersection point of the two lines identifies the positions of the coronal and axial fMRI maps presented in (**b**) and (**c**). Bilateral LNG activation superior to the hippocampal formation in the coronal view in (**b**) and lateral to the midbrain in the axial view in (**c**) was clearly shown. Extensive visual cortex activation is also shown in these fMRI maps. *L,R*, left and right hemispheres. (From CHEN et al. 1998a)

also observed during visual stimulation and was well resolved from the adjacent LGN based on the three-dimensional reconstructed maps (CHEN et al. 1998a). These results indicate that BOLD-fMRI has the sensitivity to detect small neuronal organizations in a few millimeter spatial domain, such as thalamic nuclei (KLEINSCHMIDT et al. 1994; GUIMARAES et al. 1996; BUCHEL et al. 1997; CHEN et al. 1998a). Recently, progress has been made in studying the visual field topography and sub-organizations of the LGN in the human brain using high resolution fMRI at high magnetic field strength (CHEN et al. 1998b). This may lead to a better understanding of neuronal circuitry involving both thalamic nuclei and cortical activation.

In high resolution functional MRI of the rat brain, the activation in somotosensory cortex induced by a single whisker stimulation has been demonstrated. The spatial distribution of the BOLD signal coincided well with electrical activity in the rat whisker barrels (YANG et al. 1996, 1997). Recently, high spatial resolution fMRI has been applied to visualize the activation in the human ocular dominance columns (~ 0.5–1 mm cross-section) during interleaved visual tasks between left eye and right eye photic stimulation (MENON et al. 1997). Although the spatial resolution of fMRI is dictated by the vasculature of the activated site, these results provide evidence that the main activation detected by fMRI (excluding apparent artifacts) represents brain activation sites of interest. It is unlikely that the spatial extent of the BOLD response is much farther beyond the sites of neuronal activity.

10.6 Summary

The original type of BOLD contrast, based on the field distortion of deoxyhemoglobin in blood, is well known. Functional MRI-based on BOLD contrast is a promising method for mapping brain activation in terms of sensitivity, spatial specificity and correlation of BOLD change related to neuronal events. In addition, compared with other neuroimaging techniques, such as magneto-electroencephalography (MEG) and optical imaging, BOLD-fMRI provides a more isotropic technique for mapping brain activation from the cortical surface to the deepest brain structures. It is becoming one of the most powerful and popular neuroimaging techniques, allowing mapping of neuronal pathways including large cortical and small nucleus activation in the entire human brain. Recently, there has been much progress in clarifying the quantitative aspect of the BOLD signal related to hemodynamic and metabolic changes in response to elevated neuronal activity (e.g., BUXTON et al. 1997; KIM and UGURBIL 1997; DAVIS et al. 1998; VAN ZIJL et al. 1998). This will lead to a better understanding of BOLD-fMRI and provide a tool for mapping $CMRO_2$ associated with functional activation.

Acknowledgements. We thank Drs. Kamil Ugurbil, Xiao-Hong Zhu, Seong-Gi Kim, Toshinori Kato and other colleagues and collaborators for their support, Peter Andersen, John Strupp, and Gregor Adriany for technical assistance. This work was supported in part by NIH grants P41 RR08079 (National Research Resource grant) and NS38071.

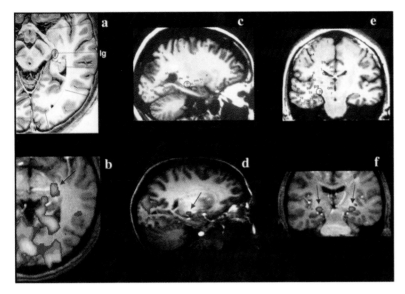

Fig. 10.5a–f. Comparison of anatomical identification of lateral geniculate nucleus (LGN) and the functional activity detected by fMRI in three orthogonal planes. *Top row*, three anatomical images taken from human brain anatomy references (DUVERNOY 1991; NOLTE 1993). *lg*, lateral geniculate nucleus (*circled in red*). *Lower row*, three fMRI images in three different planes from two different subjects (**b** and **f** are from one). The *arrows* depict the sites of LGN activation. Bilateral LGN activation during visual stimulation is clearly demonstrated. (From CHEN et al. 1998a)

References

Ackermann RF, Lear J (1989) Glycolysis-induced discordance between glucose metabolic rates measured with radiolabeled fluorodeoxyglucose and glucose. J Cereb Blood Flow Metab 9:774–785

Bandettini PA, Wong EC, Hinks RS, Tikofsky RS, Hyde JS (1992) Time course EPI of human brain function during task activation. Magn Reson Med 25:390

Bandettini PA, Wong EC, Jesmanowicz A, Hinks RS, Hyde JS (1994) Spin-echo gradient-echo EPI of human brain activation using BOLD contrast: a comparative study at 1.5 T. NMR Biomed 7:12–20

Bandettini PA, Luh W, Davis TL, van Kylen J, Forster H et al (1997) Simultaneous measurement of cerebral perfusion and oxygenation changes during neuronal activation and hypercapnia. 5th annual meeting of the International Society for Magnetic Resonance in Medicine, Vancouver, Canada, p 740

Buchel C, Turner R, Friston K (1997) Lateral geniculate activations can be detected using intersubject averaging and fMRI. Magn Reson Med 38:691–694

Buckner RL, Bandettini PA, O'Craven KM, Savoy RL, Petersen SE, Raichle ME et al (1996) Detection of cortical activation during averaged single trials of a cognitive task using functional magnetic resonance imaging. Proc Natl Acad Sci USA 93:14878–14883

Buxton RB, Wong EC, Frank LR (1997) Dynamics of blood flow and oxygenation changes during brain activation: the balloon model. Magn Reson Med 39:855–864

Chen W, Kato T, Zhu XH, Strupp J, Ogawa S, Ugurbil K (1998a) Mapping of lateral geniculate nucleus activation during visual stimulation in human brain using fMRI. Magn Reson Med 39:89–96

Chen W, Voyvodic JT, Martin C, Davis D, Ugurbil K, Thulborn KR (1998b) Functional organization of lateral geniculate nucleus in human brain: a fMRI study at 3.0 T. 6th annual meeting of the International Society for Magnetic Resonance in Medicine, Sydney, Australia, p 511

Connelly A, Dettmers C, Stephan KM, Turner R, Friston KJ, Frackowiak RSJ et al (1995) Quantitative comparison of functional magnetic resonance imaging and positron emission tomography using a controlled-force motor paradigm. 3rd annual meeting of the Society for Magnetic Resonance, Nice, p 786

Davis TL, Kwong KK, Weisskoff RM, Rosen BR (1998) Calibrated functional MRI: mapping the dynamic of oxidative metabolism. Proc Natl Acad Sci USA 95:1834–1839

Duvernoy HM (1991) The human brain: surface, three-dimensional sectional anatomy and MRI. Springer, Vienna New York

Edelman RR, Siewet B, Darby DG, Thangaraj V, Nobre AC, Mesulam MM et al (1994) Qualitative mapping of cerebral blood flow and functional localization with echo-planar MR imaging and signal targeting with alternating radio frequency. Radiology 192:513–520

Fox PT, Raichle ME (1985a) Stimulus rate dependence of regional cerebral blood flow in human striate cortex, demonstrated by positron emission tomography. J Neurophysiol 51:1109–1120

Fox PT, Raichle ME (1985b) Stimulus rate determines regional brain blood flow in striate cortex. Ann Neurol 17:303–305

Fox PT, Raichle ME (1986) Focal physiological uncoupling of cerebral blood flow and oxidative metabolism during somatosensory stimulation in human subjects. Proc Natl Acad Sci USA 83:1140–1144

Fox PT, Raichle ME, Mintun MA, Dence C (1988) Nonoxidative glucose consumption during focal physiologic neural activity. Science 241:462–464

Frahm J, Kruger G, Merboldt KD, Kleinschmidt A (1996) Dynamic uncoupling and recoupling of perfusion and oxidative metabolism during focal brain activation in man. Magn Reson Med 35:143–148

Grubb RL, Raichle ME, Eichling JO, Ter-Pogossian MM (1974) The effects of changes in Paco2 on cerebral blood volume, blood flow, and vascular mean transit time. Stroke 5:630–639

Guimaraes AR, Melcher JR, Talavage TM, Baker JR, Rosen BR, Weisskoff RM (1996) Detection of inferior colliculus activity during auditory stimulation using cardiac gated functional MRI with T_1 correction. Neuroimage 3:S9

Gyngell ML, Bock C, Schmitz B, Hoehn-Berlage M, Hossmann KA (1996) Variation of functional MRI signal in response to frequency of somatosensory stimulation in a-chloralose anesthetized rats. Magn Reson Med 36:13–15

Kerskens CM, Hoehn-Berlage M, Schmitz B, Busch E, Bock C, Gyngell ML et al (1996) Ultrafast perfusion-weighted MRI of functional brain activation in rats during forepaw stimulation: comparison with T2*-weighted MRI. NMR Biomed 8:20–23

Kim S-G (1995) Quantification of relative cerebral blood flow change by flow-sensitive alternating inversion recovery (FAIR) technique: application to functional mapping. Magn Reson Med 34:293–301

Kim SG, Ugurbil K (1997) Comparison of blood oxygenation and cerebral blood flow effects in fMRI: estimation of relative oxygen consumption change. Magn Reson Med 38:59–65

Kim SG, Sidtis JJ, Strother SC, Anderson JR, Rehm K, Ugurbil K et al (1996) Comparison of functional activation studied by whole-brain BOLD- and CBF-based fMRI and [^{15}O] water PET during sequential finger opposition. 26th annual meeting of the Society for Neuroscience, Washington DC, p 569

Kim S-G, Tsekos NV, Ashe J (1997) Multi-slice perfusion-based functional MRI using the FAIR technique: comparison of CBF and BOLD effects. NMR Biomed 10:191–196

Kleinschmidt A, Merboldt KD, Anicke W, Steinmetz H, Frahm J (1994) Correlational imaging of thalamocotical coupling in the primary visual pathway of the human brain. J Cereb Blood Flow Metab 14:952–957

Kwong KK, Belliveau JW, Chesler DA, Goldberg IE, Weisskoff RM, Poncelet BP et al (1992) Dynamic magnetic resonance imaging of human brain activity during primary sensory stimulation. Proc Natl Acad Sci USA 89:5675–5679

Kwong KK, Chesler DA, Weisskoff RM, Donahue KM, Davis TL, Stergaard L et al (1995) MR perfusion studies with T_1-weighted echo planar imaging. Magn Reson Med 34:878–887

Leniger-Follert E, Hossmann KA (1979) Simultaneous measurements of microflow and evoked potentials in the somatomotor cortex of the cat brain during specific sensory activation. Pflugers Arch 380:85–89

Malonek D, Grinvald A (1996) Interactions between electrical activity and cortical microcirculation revealed by imaging spectroscopy-implications for functional brain mapping. Science 272:551–554

Menon RS, Ogawa S, Tank DW, Ugurbil K (1993) 4 tesla gradient recalled echo characteristics of photic stimulation-induced signal changes in the human primary visual cortex. Magn Reson Med 30:380–386

Menon RS, Ogawa S, Strupp JP, Ugurbil K (1997) Ocular dominance in human V1 demonstrated by functional magnetic resonance imaging. J Neurophysiol 77:2780–2787

Movshon JA, Thompson ID, Tolhurst DJ (1978) Spatial and temporal contrast sensitivity of neurons in areas 17 and 18 of the cat's visual cortex. J Physiol (Lond) 283:101–120

Nolte J (1993) The human brain. An introduction to its functional anatomy. St Louis, Mosby Year Book

Ogawa S, Lee TM (1990) Magnetic resonance imaging of blood vessels at high fields: in vivo and in vitro measurements and image simulation. Magn Reson Med 16:9–18

Ogawa S, Lee T-M, Kay AR, Tank DW (1990a) Brain magnetic resonance imaging with contrast dependent on blood oxygenation. Proc Natl Acad Sci USA 87:9868–9872

Ogawa S, Lee T-M, Nayak AS, Glynn P (1990b) Oxygenation-sensitive contrast in magnetic resonance image of rodent brain at high magnetic fields. Magn Reson Med 14:68–78

Ogawa S, Tank DW, Menon R, Ellermann JM, Kim S-G, Merkle H et al (1992) Intrinsic signal changes accompanying sensory stimulation: functional brain mapping with magnetic resonance imaging. Proc Natl Acad Sci USA 89:5951–5955

Ogawa S, Menon RS, Kim S-G, Ugurbil K (1998) On the characteristics of functional magnetic resonance imaging of the brain. Annu Rev Biophys Biomol Struct 27:447–474

Prichard J, Rothman D, Novotny E, Petroff O, Kuwabara T, Avison M et al (1992) Lactate rise detected by ^{1}H NMR in human visual cortex during physiologic stimulation. Proc Natl Acad Sci USA 88:5829–5831

Raichle ME (1987) Circulatory and metabolic correlates of brain function in normal humans. In: Mountcastle VB, Plum F, Geiger SR (eds) Handbook of physiology – the nervous system. American Physiological Society, Bethesda, pp 643–674

Ramsey NF, Kirby B, Van Gelderen P, Berman K, Monen CTW, Mattay VS et al (1995) A direct comparison of 3D BOLD fMRI and H$_2^{15}$O PET imaging of primary sensory motor cortex in humans. 3rd annual meeting of the Society for Magnetic Resonance, Nice, p 1324

Regan D (1977) Steady-state evoked potentials. J Opt Soc Am 67:1475–1489

Ribeiro L, Kuwabara H, Meyer E, Fujita H, Marrett S, Evans A et al (1993) Cerebral blood flow and metabolism during nonspecific bilateral visual stimulation in normal subjects. In: Uemura K (ed) Quantification of brain function in tracer kinetics and image analysis in brain PET. Elsevier Science, New York, pp 229–236

Richter W, Georgopoulos AP, Ugurbil K, Kim SG (1997) Time-resolved fMRI of mental rotation. Neuroreport 8:3697–3702

Rostrup E, Larsson HBW, Toft PB, Garde K, Thomsen C, Ring P et al (1994) Functional MRI of CO_2 induced increase in cerebral perfusion. NMR Biomed 7:29–34

Sappey-Marinier D, Calabrese G, Fein G, Hugg JW, Biggins C, Weiner MW (1992) Effect of photic stimulation on human visual cortex lactate and phosphates using ^{1}H and ^{31}P magnetic resonance spectroscopy. J Cereb Blood Flow Metab 12:584–592

Siesjo BK (1978) Brain energy metabolism. Wiley, New York

Song AW, Wong EC, Jesmanowicz A, Tan S, Hyde JS (1995) Diffusion weighted fMRI at 1.5 T and 3 T. 3rd annual meeting of the Society for Magnetic Resonance, Nice, France, p 457

Song AW, Wong EC, Tan S, Hyde JS (1996) Diffusion weighted fMRI at 1.5 T. Magn Reson Med 35:155–158

Thulborn KR, Waterton JC, Mattews PM, Radda GK (1982) Oxygenation dependence of the transverse relaxation time of water protons in whole blood at high field. Biochem Biophys Acta 714:265–270

Turner R, Le Bihan D, Moonen CT, Despres D, Frank J (1991) Echo-planar time course MRI of cat brain oxygenation changes. Magn Reson Med 22:159–166

Ugurbil K, Ogawa S, Menon R, Kim S-G, Hu X, Hinke R et al (eds) (1994) Mapping brain function non-invasively by nuclear magnetic resonance. New Horizons in Neuropsychology. Elsevier Science, Amsterdam

van Zijl PC, Eleff SM, Ulatowski JA, Oja JM, Ulug AM, Traystman RJ et al (1998) Quantitative assessment of blood flow, blood volume and blood oxygenation effects in functional magnetic resonance imaging. Nature Med 4:159–167

Yang X, Hyder F, Shulman RG (1996) Activation of single whisker barreal in rat brain localized by functinal magnetic resonance imaging. Proc Natl Acad Sci USA 93:475–478

Yang X, Hyder F, Shulman RG (1997) Functional MRI BOLD signal coincides with electrical activity in the rat whisker barrels. Magn Reson Med 38:874–877

Yarowsky P, Ingvar DH (1981) Neuronal activity and energy metabolism. Fed Proc 40:2353–2363

Zhu XH, Kim SG, Andersen P, Ogawa S, Ugurbil K, Chen W (1998) Simultaneous oxygenation and perfusion imaging study of functional activity in primary visual cortex at different visual stimulus frequency: quantitative correlation between dynamic BOLD and CBF changes. Magn Reson Med 40:703–711

11 Basic Theoretical Models of BOLD Signal Change

R.M. WEISSKOFF

CONTENTS

11.1
Introduction

Blood oxygenation level-dependent (BOLD) contrast relies on macroscopic detection of changes in the microscopic magnetic fields surrounding red blood cells. When the hemoglobin in the red cell changes from the oxygenated to the deoxygenated state, there is a profound change in its magnetic properties (PAULING and CORYELL 1936) as the red cell transforms from being isomagnetic to paramagnetic with respect to the surrounding tissue. While this physical change is relatively simple to describe, its impact on MRI contrast can be quite complicated. In any small piece of cortex, blood will exist at a variety of oxygenations, and, more importantly, the water, which is the primary probe of these magnetic field distortions for fMRI, dances randomly among the different magnetic environments both inside and outside of the blood vessels, and inside and outside the red cells. The resulting changes in contrast depend on this intricate dance, and thus the quantitative interpretation of these changes depends on an understanding of the formation of these signal changes.

In this chapter, we describe a physical model and results from a variety of simulation and analytic techniques that attempt to model these BOLD changes due to neuronal activation. Developing these models is still an active area of research in a number of laboratories, and there is some controversy underlying the specifics of the models. However, the goal of this chapter is not to provide a comprehensive review of these models, but rather to present a specific biophysical picture of the underlying contrast mechanism. This picture, we believe, demonstrates how the simple magnetic field shifts can produce signal changes in a variety of ways, and how understanding these different mechanisms may help understand aspects of experimental design and interpretation in fMRI.

In addition, no model of the signal changes can be complete without an understanding of the other physiological changes that occur during activation, including the nonlinear coupling between flow and oxygen consumption, flow and volume changes, and the dynamics of this coupling. These subjects, which are also controversial, form complete topics within this book. Thus this chapter has a much more limited focus: describing the relationship between oxygenation changes in the blood and macroscopic image contrast in fMRI.

This chapter has two main parts. In the first, we review the physical hierarchy of the vascular bed in the cortex. In the second, we break down the BOLD effect into three sub-effects, each of which contributes to the BOLD mechanism. These effects, roughly, are: (1) direct signal loss in a single blood vessel, (2) signal loss due to incoherent combinations of the signals from different blood vessels, and (3) signal loss due to extravascular protons diffusing around these blood vessels. Finally, we conclude with a discussion of the (relatively limited) experimental evidence supporting this model and point to a number of unresolved questions in this contrast.

R. M. WEISSKOFF, PhD, Massachusetts General Hospital NMR Center, Department of Radiology, CNY 2301, Massachusetts General Hospital, 149 13th Street, Charlestown, MA 02129, USA

11.2
The Big Picture

In order to generate a biophysical model of the BOLD-related signal changes, we first need a model of the tissue and the magnetic field changes that occur when one compartment of a heterogeneous system changes its magnetic properties. This model has two fundamental components: the red cells, which affect the magnetic field, and the tissue water, which senses this field. The MR signal changes comes from the interaction of these two parts.

11.2.1
The Red Cell, Vessels and Paramagnetism

"Magnetic susceptibility" refers to the general magnetic response of a material when it is placed in an external magnetic field. This response occurs when some of the many infinitesimal magnetic constituents of the material (called dipoles), which are usually randomly oriented, line up with or against the magnetic field. Nearly all materials have some interaction with a magnetic field. The nuclear interaction, though critical for MRI, is one of the weakest. In general, the electrons are responsible for the more important interactions.

All materials have a slight tendency to counteract the presence of an applied magnetic field, and thus slightly decrease the magnetic field's effect inside them. This effect, which usually distorts the applied field by less than ten parts per million, is called "diamagnetism." Most proteins, tissue water, and other biological constituents, per gram of tissue, are similarly diamagnetic. In some materials, however, the dipoles tend to line up with the magnetic field, producing an additive internal field. These materials are called "paramagnetic." If this effect sounds suspiciously like the phenomena underlying MRI, it is: sometimes NMR is referred to as nuclear paramagnetism. Hemoglobin, when it is saturated with oxygen, acts like a typically diamagnetic protein and has roughly the same magnetic characteristics of the tissue surrounding the blood. However, because of the difference in iron chemistry, when the heme releases its oxygen, the hemoglobin becomes much more paramagnetic. Since hemoglobin makes up nearly 15 gm/100 cm^3 of normal blood (BERNE and LEVY 1988), the deoxygenated red cells and blood vessels themselves thus become little magnets in the body, distorting the magnetic field around them.

As described in Chap. 8, the field shifts caused by these bulk magnetic susceptibility (BMS) effects depend very strongly on shape and orientation (CHU et al. 1990; SPRINGER and XU 1991). That is, the same degree of deoxygenation will produce a different magnetic field outside an isolated red cell, inside a vein packed with red cells aligned with the main magnetic field of the imager, or inside a vein perpendicular to the field.

The red blood cell (RBC) is one of the smaller cells in the body, and in its healthy form is a flattened disk, approximately 6 μm wide and 1–2 μm thick, making up about 40% by volume of the blood. If we consider in particular human cortex, these red cells are delivered almost completely oxygenated (typically 97%) at the arteriolar end of the cortex microvascular bed. These arterioles are approximately 25 μm in diameter and make up less than 15% of the blood volume in the cortex. They feed the primary exchange vessels: the capillaries. The capillaries, although they make up only 5%–7% of the blood volume of the body (GUYTON 1991), make up closer to 40% of the blood volume of an MRI cortical voxel (PAWLIK et al. 1981), or roughly 2% of the net volume of the voxel. These capillaries are typically 8 μm in diameter (i.e., about the size of the RBC), and in brain cortex form a randomly oriented network of paths (BAR 1980). Oxygen diffuses out of the capillaries along their length. Because of the much greater effective solubility of oxygen in the blood due to hemoglobin binding (BUXTON and FRANK 1997; BUXTON et al. 1998), oxygen transport behaves as if it were diffusion limited, and thus the relative oxygenation of the blood decreases linearly down the length of the capillaries. In human cortex, the typical blood oxygenation is about 60% at the end of the capillary bed (GUYTON 1991).

When we model the BOLD signal changes, we care more about the average oxygenation in the capillary bed. While somewhat model-dependent, this average oxygenation can be estimated by integrating the oxygen extraction along a normalized capillary segment (e.g., BOXERMAN et al. 1995a; LARSSON et al. 1990). The average capillary oxygenation, $\bar{Q}_c$, can be estimated as:

$$\bar{Q}_c = Q_a - (Q_a - Q_v) \left[\frac{1}{E} + \frac{1}{\ln(1-E)} \right] \qquad (11.1)$$

where Q_a is the oxygenation at the arteriolar end, Q_v is the end capillary oxygenation, and E is the oxygen extraction fraction, which is roughly 0.5 (ALPERT et al. 1988). In fact, this expression is very close to

$(Q_a+Q_v)/2$ – i.e., the average of the venous and arterial oxygenation – for any extraction less than about 0.8. Thus the average oxygenation in the cortical capillary bed is about 80% saturated.

These capillaries drain into venules, which are somewhat larger at 25–50 μm and which also form about 40% of the blood volume in a cortical voxel. As described above, the venules are about twice as deoxygenated as the capillary average, and thus twice as magnetic. While discussed in greater detail below, one immediate implication of this algebra is that, under normal circumstances, the venules have a greater opportunity to contribute to the BOLD effect: they have approximately the same blood volume as the capillary, but are twice as magnetic.

Finally, these venules flow into collecting veins. To give some sense of the numbers of these microvessels in a typical gray matter MRI cortical voxel, the net total blood volume is about 4% (LEENDERS et al. 1990). Considering a 3×3×3 mm voxel, there are about 10 meters of capillary length and about 50 mm of venular length. This translates into around 20,000–50,000 capillary segments, and 50–150 venular segments in the voxel. In cortex, these segments are roughly randomly oriented.

As described in previous chapters, local neuronal activation causes blood flow increases that, after the first second or two, are proportionally larger than the average oxygen consumption change of the tissue. Since the increased vascular delivery of oxygen at the arteriolar end of the tissue bed is greater than the increased consumption of oxygen within the tissue, and since no oxygen is stored in the tissue, the blood leaving the tissue bed at the venous end has a greater concentration of oxygen during the activation.

We can express algebraically this increase in the venous oxygenation, and thus by Eq. 11.1, the average capillary oxygenation. Using conservation of oxygen (Fick's principle) and assuming the arterial end is 100% oxygenated and the hematocrit remains unchanged during activation, the end capillary oxygen content will be:

$$1 - fO_2^{post} = (1 - fO_2^{pre}) \frac{CMRO_2^{post}}{CMRO_2^{pre}} \frac{F_{pre}}{F_{post}} \qquad (11.2)$$

where fO_2 is the fraction of saturation of the venous blood, $CMRO_2$ is the metabolic oxygen consumption rate, F is the blood flow, and the sub- and superscripts "pre" and "post" refer to pre- and post-stimulation. (This expression also ignores dissolved oxygen, which under normal physiological conditions is

an excellent approximation.) Since $1-fO_2$ is also the fraction of reduced (deoxygenated) hemoglobin, Eq. 11.2 directly relates the change in the magnetism of the blood. For particularly vigorous activation, the flow changes can be as large as 70%, the $CMRO_2$ changes roughly 20% and thus end-capillary (venular) oxygen saturation can change from its resting level of 60% to 72% oxygenated; the average capillary oxygen saturation would change from 80% to 86%.

11.2.2
Tissue Water

In the preceding section, we described the vascular network, which in fMRI creates changes in the magnetic field distortion. However, we detect these change indirectly, through water protons diffusing through these field nonuniformities. Water is always in motion in the body, whether through diffusive processes, like Brownian motion, or convective processes in the cells. While this motion can be very complicated, we will simplify its description in order to get some theoretical handle on the BOLD signal changes.

First, we consider water when it is in the vessels. Even though blood has many constituent components, for the purposes of fMRI modeling we focus on just the RBCs and the general plasma. Free water, at body temperature, diffuses randomly with a diffusion coefficient of about $D=3$ μm^2/ms. That is, two water molecules that originally start next to one another move in a random walk away from each other so that they separated at a time T later by about $\sqrt{6DT}$. In the whole blood, $D\sim1$ μm^2/ms, so that in 50 ms (roughly the time MRI samples this movement), the "average" water molecule travels about 25 μm. Thus water in a capillary will encounter both many red cells as well as the boundary of the capillary (i.e., the endothelium) in this time.

From a number of experiments, including MRI which offers some of the most biologically accessible measurement, it appears that the cell membrane of the RBC offers little resistance to the flow of water. The residence time for a water molecule in an RBC is about 5 ms (KONISHI et al. 1996; WRIGHT et al. 1992), which is fairly close to the time that it takes water to diffuse across the diameter of cell. Thus water diffuses readily in and out of the these red cells.

However, the capillary endothelium appears to offer much more resistance to water transport across it. This may seem surprising, especially given the assumptions of most of the water labeling MR methods for measuring perfusion. However, the much shorter relevant evolution time (50 ms for BOLD vs 1000 ms for water labeling) explains this difference. The permeability-surface area (PS) product for water in the capillary bed is in the range of 100–300 ml/ 100 g per min (Berne and Levy 1988). While this PS product allows for 90%–95% extraction under normal conditions, it does require the 1–3 s it takes water to move from the arteriolar to venular side of the capillary bed. In the mere 50 ms of evolution time allowed in the BOLD experiment, however, less than 5% of the water that starts in the capillary bed can diffuse out of the bed into the tissue. For the purposes of the rest of this chapter, then, we will consider water that starts in the vascular bed to remain in the vascular bed and, conversely, water that starts in the tissue to remain in the tissue.

Summarizing: water moves freely between the RBCs and the plasma, but remains within the vascular space for the BOLD experiment.

The extravascular space in the brain is much more complicated, but for the purposes of the BOLD experiment, on time scales of 50 ms, water diffuses fairly uniformly in the gray matter with $D \sim 1\ \mu m^2/ms$ (e.g., LeBihan et al. 1990; McKinstry et al. 1992) apparently moving with relative ease between the various intracellular and extracellular spaces.

11.3
Multiple Sites of the BOLD Effect

Thus for the purposes of the BOLD experiment, we have two completely separated pools of water that can sense the magnetic changes in the blood. One homogenous pool is outside the vessels, which senses the inhomogeneous field changes of these vessels, and a second much smaller pool is inside the vessels themselves. We now link the magnetic changes, the water pools, and the resulting MRI detectable changes together. In this section, we follow the treatment in Boxerman et al. (1995a).

Since the intravascular and extravascular pools are separate, we can consider their effects separately; that is, the MRI signal comes from the sum of the two compartments: $S = |S_t + S_b|$, where S refers to the total normalized MRI signal, the "t" subscripts refer to tissue, and the "b" refers to blood. As we will describe below, there are three main effects that modulate these signals when the blood oxygenation changes. First, in the blood compartment, the water rapidly moving in and around the red cells loses coherence because the deoxyhemoglobin creates field inhomogeneities in the blood. Second, the *average* frequency sensed by all protons in any given vessel segment depends on that vessel's orientation to the imager's magnetic field. Thus, the random orientation of the thousands of capillaries or hundred of venules causes destructive interference between the signals coming from different vessels. Finally, for the vast majority of protons outside of the vessels, the field nonuniformity caused by the randomly oriented vessels creates signal loss in the extravascular space. We can summarize these effects:

$$S \sim \left| e^{-TE/T2_t^*} S_t + e^{-TE/T2_b^*} S_t \left(f_c S_c + f_v S_v \right) \right|, \qquad (11.3)$$

where the "c" refers to the capillary, "v" to the venules, "f" refers to the volume fraction, TE to the echo time, and T2 to the intrinsic (i.e., non-BOLD-related) transverse relaxation times of the tissue components. The capillary and venules have separate signal attenuations, S, both because they have different oxygenations (Eq. 11.1) and because their different sizes will cause the combination of the first and second effects described above to be different. S_t, which describes the extravascular attenuation, multiplies both the extravascular and intravascular term. (The addition of this term is not particularly significant, but is there to account for the fact that each vessel individually is in a magnetic environment that includes both its own intravascular fields as well as the combined extravascular fields of all the other vessels.) We now discuss these terms separately.

11.3.1
T2 Changes in Blood Itself

Blood T2 is directly affected by its oxygenation (Thulborn et al. 1982). This has been measured extensively, and has been proposed as a method for measuring blood oxygenation quantitatively in vivo (Wright et al. 1992).

In the most general case, the observed blood attenuation is a complicated function of pulse sequence, echo time and field strength. However, in the limiting case of relatively long (>20 ms) echo time gradient echo, or spin echo sequences with long times between the refocusing pulse(s) (>20 ms), blood behaves very much like a material with a simple T2 that depends on the oxygenation of the blood:

$$1/T2 \approx 1/T2_o + K \cdot (1-Y)^2 \qquad (11.4)$$

where $T2_o$ is the intrinsic T2 of the blood (about 240 ms at 1.5 T), Y is the oxygen saturation of the hemoglobin, and K is a constant that depends on the hematocrit and field strength, but at 1.5 T with normal blood is about 40/s. This equation comes from fitting empirical data (Wright et al. 1992) to a simple Luz-Meiboom model (Luz and Meiboom 1963) of the water exchange in and out of the RBCs, but is also found from simple Monte Carlo estimates of signal change around perfectly diffusible spheres (Boxerman et al. 1995a) with magnetization given by deoxygenated blood's susceptibility (Weisskoff and Kiihne 1992). K depends roughly on the field strength squared and linearly with hematocrit.

Thus, in a draining venule from an activated vessel, where Y shifts from 60% to 72%, we could expect a direct T2 change of 95 ms to 135 ms at 1.5 T. The average effect in the capillary would be more subtle, shifting from about 175 ms to about 200 ms.

At very high field (>4 T) strength, this relationship would be expected to break down, since the T2s begin to become short compared to the 5 ms water residence time in the RBC.

11.3.2
T2' Effect Due to Vessel Orientations

In addition to the net dephasing that shortens T2, the deoxygenated RBCs also, on average, change the magnetic fields that the protons sense. While the heterogeneity of the field within an individual vessel caused the T2 effect described in Sect. 11.3.1, there is also an average frequency shift for all the protons in a given vessel segment. For a large vessel, this frequency shift is given by:

$$\Delta f = K'(3\cos^2 \theta - 1)(1-Y) \qquad (11.5)$$

where K'=10 Hz at 1.5 T, and scales linearly with field strength. Since all the protons see the same frequency shift, it does not affect the T2 of the protons within the vessel. However, when the signal from different vessels are combined, either from the multiple microvessels in a given voxel or when a single, larger vessel is partial volumed with tissue outside the vessel (Yablonskiy and Haacke 1994), signal loss will

occur for a gradient echo scan. In the case of a spin-echo scan, assuming that the water does not move into a vessel with a different orientation in 50 ms, this effect is completely refocused. (The assumption that water does not shift between vessel segments in this time seems fairly conservative. Blood has a velocity of about 0.1–0.5 µm/ms in the capillary bed, and thus in 50 ms moves 5–25 µm; much less than the length of a typical capillary segment.)

However, Eq. 11.5 is actually an oversimplification for the microvessels in the brain. This is because the red cells are large enough – or the vessels are small enough – that the water in the vessels does not see the full dipole field of the deoxygenated RBCs. That is, some of the field distortion caused by the RBC is outside the blood vessel where the vascular protons cannot sense it. In addition, in the capillaries, where the RBCs line up one after the other to get through, the average distance between RBCs is actually larger than it is in venules and larger veins, where the RBCs can pack more tightly together. This distance can become significant compared to the water diffusion distance, so the simplified form in Eq. 11.5 is not necessarily relevant.

To deal with these subtleties and account for the "direct" T2 effects described in Sect. 11.3.1, Boxerman et al. (1995a) used Monte Carlo techniques to simulate the water diffusion inside the vascular tree. By using simplified RBC shapes and randomized vessel orientations this calculation produced attenuation estimates as a function of vessel size for different levels of RBC oxygenation. Figure 11.1 shows the results of these calculations. In this figure, we show the log of the signal attenuation divided by the echo time (equivalent to 1/T2 for monoexponential decay) for normal blood in a randomly oriented (Fig. 11.1A) capillary bed, and (Fig. 11.1B) venular bed, both ignoring diffusion (to show the effect of intravascular phase shift) and including diffusion. (Obviously, imaging in the absence of diffusion is not physical: the data are just included to demonstrate the effect.) While not shown in this figure, the simulated attenuations are complex numbers; that is, they could contain a net overall phase shift as well as a magnitude reduction. In practice, ensembles of vessels from random orientations do not show significant average frequency shifts at the blood oxygenation-based magnetization shifts relevant for BOLD fMRI (Boxerman et al. 1995a). Figure 11.1 thus shows the relevant S_v and S_c for Eq. 11.3.

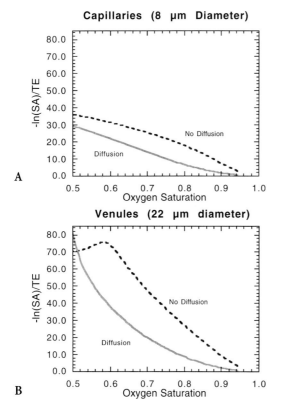

Fig. 11.1A, B. The intravascular BOLD effects. Comparison of signal loss in **A** capillaries and **B** venules as a function of oxygen saturation at 1.5 T. The *dotted lines* shows the effect in the absence of diffusion, the *solid lines* shows the effect in the presence of physiological diffusion

11.3.3
Extravascular Effects

In addition to these two intravascular effects, the extravascular protons also lose coherence in BOLD experiments. This effect, which has also been exploited for blood volume and blood flow mapping with exogenous contrast agents (e.g., ROSEN 1992), has been explored extensively (e.g., BOXERMAN et al. 1995a; FISEL et al. 1991; HARDY and HENKELMAN 1989; WEISSKOFF et al. 1994; YABLONSKIY and HAACKE 1994) using Monte Carlo and analytic methods.

While the estimation of these signal changes in the absence of diffusion is tractable analytically, a complete analytic expression in the presence of water motion has not been derived for the extravascular attenuation. As a result, Monte Carlo simulations, or equivalent numerical integration of the Bloch-Torrey equation (WONG and BANDETTINI 1993), currently seem the best way to estimate these signal changes.

The results of such simulations, as an example for spin and gradient echo sequences at 1.5 T at different oxygenations, are shown in Fig. 11.2. Gradient echo sequences tend to favor signal changes outside the larger microvessels (venules and beyond), while the spin echo sequences favor the microvessels over the macrovessel. Unlike contrast agent-based studies, which typically work in a regime in which capillary contribution in maximum (WEISSKOFF et al. 1994), BOLD at clinical field strength appears to weigh smaller venules and capillaries approximately equally. At higher fields (>4.0 T), there should be a shift towards weighting the smaller vessels.

By considering a weighting of different sized vessels (BOXERMAN et al. 1995b), a composite extravascular signal attenuation, S_t, can be constructed for use in Eq. 11.3.

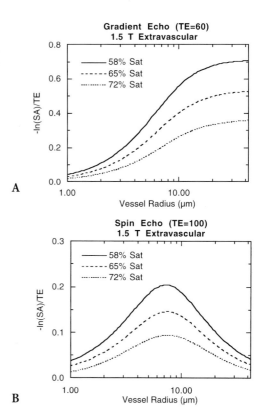

Fig. 11.2A, B. The extravascular BOLD effect. Comparison of signal attenuation at different oxygenation for 2% by volume randomly oriented vessels for **A** gradient echo and **B** spin echo pulse sequences. The simulations are via random walk Monte Carlo estimates at 1.5 T. (After BOXERMAN 1994)

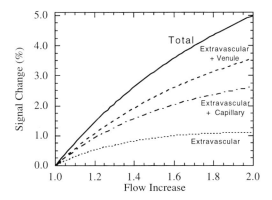

Fig. 11.3. Estimated BOLD related signal changes at 1.5 T from different signal mechanisms. (Adapted from BOXERMAN et al. 1995a)

11.3.4
Putting It All Together

By separately considering the intravascular and extravascular effects, the appropriate signal attenuation as a function of blood oxygenation can be computed. Using the Fick relationship, Eqs. 11.1 and 11.2, the relationship between blood flow, oxygen consumption, and resulting venular and capillary oxygenations can be computed. Finally, by assuming a relationship between blood volume and blood flow (e.g., GRUBB et al. 1974), the volume fraction changes needed for Eq. 11.3 can be estimated as well. Thus for a given field strength and assumed resting blood oxygenation, the blood volume and oxygenation changes can be computed as a function of blood flow change, and thus the change in BOLD-based MRI signal can be estimated.

In BOXERMAN et al. (1995a), for example, the blood volume was assumed to vary as the 0.4 power with blood flow, and changes in $CMRO_2$ were ignored. The resulting 1.5 T BOLD predictions, separated into the intravascular and extravascular parts, are shown in Fig. 11.3. This figure shows a relatively linear response at first, though it tends to show signs of saturation at higher flows. This non-linearity is due a combination of two effects: (1) the nonlinearity of deoxygenation with flow in Eq. 11.2, and (2) the nonlinearity of signal change with blood oxygenation, as seen in Figs. 11.1 and 11.2. However, the predicted response is monotonic, and, at least in parenchymal voxels, shows significant change over the whole range of physiologically important flow changes for the brain. This relative linearity, though, is much less preserved in voxels with significant large vessel contamination. Because of the dramatic

changes in venous blood T2 with activation, and the blood's long T2 compared to brain, it is possible with sequences using TE~T2$_{\text{brain}}$ to lose their sensitivity exponentially to changes in oxygenation.

11.4
Selected Experimental Evidence and Questions

The direct experimental evidence that supports the model presented in Sect. 11.3 is fairly sparse. The extravascular Monte Carlo simulations have been validated against nuclear methods in small animal models (e.g., BOXERMAN et al. 1995b), and the direct blood T2 changes have been measured against models numerous times (e.g., WRIGHT et al. 1992). However, the exact distribution of blood sizes, orientations, resting oxygenation level, $CMRO_2$ changes, blood volume changes, etc. are very difficult to measure in vivo in normal subjects.

The best evidence that at least the model hierarchy is correct is that: (a) the signal changes are approximately correct at 1.5 T, and (b) experiments that attempt to distinguish the intra- and extravascular have shown approximately the right ratio and generally correct field dependence.

As an example of the latter, BOXERMAN et al. (1995a) presented results from visual stimulation experiments in which an additional bipolar gradient was added to dephase the flowing spins in the microcirculation (LEBIHAN et al. 1988). Those data are adapted into Fig. 11.4, taken from experiments at 1.5 T. By increasing the duration of the bipolar gradient, spins with smaller and smaller velocity ranges are dephased. The x-axis in this figure shows the inverse velocity spread required to dephase the signal. Thus, adding minimal velocity spoiling eliminates about one third of the signal at velocity spreads greater than about 10 mm/s (venular flows), and increasing this dephasing so that velocity spreads of greater than 0.5 mm/s (capillary flows) eliminates another one third of the signal, in relatively good agreement with Fig. 11.3.

At increasing field strength, less of the signal should come from the intravascular water both because the extravascular mechanisms becomes more potent and because the blood T2s become short enough that even in the activated state the blood is dark. Data from activation at 3 T (R. Buxton, personal communication) show that velocity spoiling

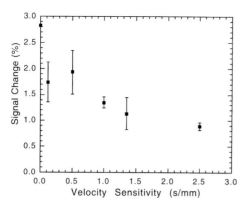

Fig. 11.4. Visual stimulation results from *n*=5 subjects, demonstrating signal attenuation due to velocity spoiling gradients. The velocity sensitivity is in inverse units corresponding to roughly 1/velocity dispersion required to attenuate most of the MR signal from flowing spins. (Adapted from BOXERMAN et al. 1995a)

only eliminates about one half of the signal. Animal data at 9.4 T (K. Ugurbil, personal communication) show that velocity spoiling has no effect on the BOLD signal.

The line broadening mechanism (Sect. 11.3.2) helps explain one peculiar finding from early fMRI research. HOPPEL et al. (1993) measured the changes in both spin echo and gradient echo experiments due to hypercapnia and a large bolus of an exogenous contrast agent that magnetized the blood vessel by another factor of 10–20 beyond the BOLD effects. In comparing these measurements to those performed on oxygenated and deoxygenated blood samples, they found the ratio between gradient echo and spin echo contrast for hypercapnia was more like the contrast agent study (i.e., a factor of 3) than the blood (i.e., a factor of 1.2). It would appear from these finding that the BOLD effect was thus primarily extravascular at 1.5 T, i.e., more like the contrast agent susceptibility contrast effect than like the intravascular effect. However, this conclusion ignored the heterogeneity of vessel orientation, which, as described above, produces line broadening that is only detectable on gradient echo scans. Thus nearly all experimental evidence points to an intravascular source for the BOLD effect at clinical field strengths, but an increasing extravascular contribution at increasing field strength.

While this model seems to explain a number of experimental observations, there are still several open questions for quantitatively understanding the BOLD signal changes. It is not clear what happens locally when the blood volume increases. The model presented above assumes that the proton density increases, rather than displacing other material. While a subtle effect (perhaps 1%), this change could be a significant contributor to apparent BOLD changes. The susceptibility contrast models, in addition, are not completely clear about whether RBC motion in the capillary bed has some impact on BOLD contrast. That is, while the model above assumes no direct modulation of BOLD by flow increases, the theoretical data are a bit ambiguous. BOXERMAN et al. (1995b) showed that RBCs in the contrast agent experiments (with larger magnetic perturbations) have negligible effect, but the results were less clear at BOLD levels of magnetic perturbation. Finally, there could be other sources of susceptibility contrast that are not included in this model formulation, for example, due to the average magnetic differences between two adjoining regions of the brain, or within macroscopic, but still subvoxel, regions within a given brain area. Molecular oxygen itself is paramagnetic, though most estimates show that its concentrations seem too low to cause significant perturbations.

11.5 Conclusions

In conclusion, we have presented a relatively brief model of the BOLD effect in the brain. This model assumes that the signal from the extravascular and intravascular water pools are separate and that we can consider the effects in the different pools independently, combining them together to estimate BOLD signal changes. There are three primary mechanisms of contrast: signal loss within a single vessel, signal loss due to interference between the signals of different orientations of different vessel (or with the tissue), and loss of coherence of the extravascular water due to the magnetic changes in the vessels.

References

Alpert N, Buxton R, Correia J, Katz P, Ackerman R (1988) Measurement of end-capillary pO2 with positron emission tomography. J Cereb Blood Flow Metab 8:403–410

Bar T (1980) The vascular system of the cerebral cortex. Advances in anatomy, embryology and cell biology. Springer, Berlin Heidelberg New York

Berne R, Levy M (1988) Physiology. Mosby, Washington DC

Boxerman J (1994) Non-invasive measurement of physiology using dynamic susceptibility contrast NMR imaging, PhD thesis, MIT

Boxerman, J, Bandettini P, Kwong K, Baker J, Davis T, Rosen B, Weisskoff R (1995a) The intravascular contribution to fMRI signal change: Monte Carlo modeling and diffusion-weighted studies in vivo. Magn Reson Med 34:4–10

Boxerman J, Hamberg L, Rosen B, Weisskoff R (1995b) MR contrast due to intravascular magnetic susceptibility perturbers. Magn Reson Med 34:555–566

Buxton R, Frank L (1997) A model for the coupling between cerebral blood flow and oxygen metabolism during neural stimulation. J Cereb Blood Flow Metab 14:365–372

Buxton R, Wong E, Frank L (1998) Dynamics of blood flow and oxygenation changes during brain activation: the balloon model. Magn Reson Med 39:855–864

Chu SCK, Xu Y, Balschi JA, Springer CS (1990) Bulk magnetic susceptibility shifts in NMR studies of compartmentalized samples: use of paramagnetic reagents. Magn Reson Med 13:239–262

Fisel CR, Ackerman JL, Buxton RB, Garrido L, Belliveau JW, Rosen BR, Brady TJ (1991) MR contrast due to microscopically heterogeneous magnetic susceptibility: numerical simulations and applications to cerebral physiology. Magn Reson Med 17:336--347

Grubb RL, Raichle ME, Eichling JO, Ter-Pogossian MM (1974) The effects of changes in PaCO2 on cerebral blood volume, blood flow, and vascular mean transit time. Stroke 5:630–639

Guyton A (1991) Textbook of medical physiology. Saunders, Philadelphia

Hardy PA, Henkelman RM (1989) Transverse relaxation rate enhancement caused by magnetic particulates. Magn Reson Imag 7:265–275

Hoppel B, Weisskoff R, Thulborn K, Moore J, Kwong K, Rosen B (1993) Measurement of regional blood oxygenation and cerebral hemodynamics. Magn Reson Med 30:715–723

Konishi S, Yoneyama R, Itagaki H et al (1996) Transient brain activity used in magnetic resonance imaging to detect functional areas. Neuroreport 8:19–23

Larsson HBW, Stubgaard M, Frederiksen JL, Jensen M, Henriksen O, Paulson OB (1990) Quantitation of blood-brain barrier defect by magnetic resonance imaging and gadolinium-DTPA in patients with multiple sclerosis and brain tumors. Magn Reson Med 16:117–131

LeBihan D, Breton E, Lallemand D, Aubin ML, Vignaud J, Laval JM (1988) Separation of diffusion and perfusion in intravoxel incoherent motion MR imaging. Radiology 168(2):497–505

LeBihan D, Turner R, Douek P (1990) Is water diffusion restricted in human brain? Society of Magnetic Resonance in Medicine, 9th annual scientific meeting and exhibition 1:377

Leenders K, Perani D, Lammertsma A et al (1990) Cerebral blood flow, blood volume and oxygen utilization: normal values and effect of age. Brain 113:27–47

Luz Z, Meiboom S (1963) NMR study of the protolysis of trimethylammonium ion in aqueous solution: order of the reaction with respect to the solvent. J Chem Phys 39:366–370

McKinstry R, Weisskoff R, Belliveau J (1992) Ultrafast MR imaging of water mobility: animals of altered cerebral perfusion. J Magn Reson Imag 2:337–384

Pauling L, Coryell C (1936) The magnetic properties and structure of hemoglobin, oxyhemoglobin and carbon monooxyhemoglobin. Proc Natl Acad Sci USA 22:210–216

Pawlik G, Rackl A, Bing RJ (1981) Quantitative capillary topography and blood flow in the cerebral cortex of cats: an in vivo microscopic study. Brain Res 208:35–58

Rosen B (1992) MR studies of perfusion in the brain. Current practice in radiology. Mosby Yearbook, Philadelphia

Springer CS, Xu Y (1991) Aspects of bulk magnetic susceptibility in In Vivo MRI and MRS. New developments in contrast agent research. Eur Workshop Magn Res Med, Blonay, Switzerland

Thulborn KR, Waterton JC, Matthews PM, Radda GK (1982) Oxygenation dependence of the transverse relaxation time of water protons in whole blood at high field. Biochim Biophys Acta 714:265–270

Weisskoff RM, Kiihne S (1992) MRI susceptometry: image-based measurement of absolute susceptibility of MR contrast agents and human blood. Magn Reson Med 24:375–383

Weisskoff RM, Zuo C, Boxerman J, Rosen B (1994) Microscopic susceptibility variation and transverse relaxation: theory and experiment. Magn Reson Med 31:601–610

Wong E, Bandettini P (1993) A deterministic method for computer modeling of diffusion effects in MRI with application to BOLD contrast imaging. 12th Annu Sci Meeting SMRM 10

Wright G, Hu B, Macovski A (1992) Estimating oxygen saturation of blood in vivo with MR imaging at 1.5 T. J Magn Reson Imag 1:275–283

Yablonskiy D, Haacke E (1994) Theory of NMR signal behavior in magnetically inhomogeneous tissues: the static dephasing regime. Magn Reson Med 32:749–763

Scanning Techniques for BOLD Functional MRI

12 Gradient Echo and Spin Echo Methods for Functional MRI

R.P. Kennan

CONTENTS

12.1 Introduction

Blood oxygen level-dependent (BOLD) contrast has been a subject of great interest since it was first demonstrated by Ogawa et al. (1990) that varying levels of oxygen saturation can change contrast in T_2^* weighted images. Though these effects have been successfully exploited in the development of functional MRI (fMRI) techniques there are still many questions concerning the relationship between cerebral hemodynamics and signal changes induced in MR images. In functional imaging a complex array of mechanisms may affect image contrast including alterations of blood flow, blood volume and intravascular magnetic susceptibility. Among the factors influencing the effectiveness of susceptibility based contrast are the strength of the field perturbations and the size and relative spacing of the field perturbers (Kennan et al. 1994; Yablonskiy et al. 1994; Boxerman et al. 1995) Equally important factors are the type of sequence and sequence parameters used to obtain an image. Mechanisms which affect transverse relaxation can be probed by both spin echo and gradient echo imaging sequences. While the image contrast in these sequences have been documented for a large variety of anatomical studies (Glover 1993; Plewes et al. 1993), it is not clear how these sequences are sensitive to the physiologic alterations associated with neuronal activation. It is known that the generation of microscopic field gradients can have different effects on both gradient echo and spin echo based sequences (Kennan et al. 1994; Boxerman et al. 1995). Spin echo sequences are sensitive to BOLD effects through time irreversible diffusion in inhomogeneous magnetic field distributions whereas gradient echo based sequences are also sensitive to time reversible dephasing that is caused by the spatial distribution of magnetic field within a voxel. Spin echo and gradient echo sequences may also have different sensitivity to inflow effects which could change the resultant activation patterns observed in fMRI. It has been shown that in many cases pure inflow based activation maps can differ significantly from BOLD based activation maps (Kim et al. 1994).

12.2 Contrast in Gradient Echo Imaging

For single slice gradient echo images the signal for stationary spins within the imaging slice is given by (Glover 1993):

R.P. Kennan, PhD, Departments of Diagnostic Radiology and Biomedical Engineering, Yale University School of Medicine, 333 Cedar Street, Fitkin B, New Haven, CT 06510, USA

$$S_{GE}(TE,TR) \cong \rho_H \exp\left(-\frac{TE}{T_2^*}\right)\sin(\alpha)\frac{1-2\exp\left(-\frac{TR-TE/2}{T_1}\right)}{1+\cos(\alpha)\exp\left(-\frac{TR}{T_1}\right)}$$

(12.1)

where ρ_H denotes the proton density, and T_2^* is the gradient echo relaxation time which includes both inhomogeneous (time reversible) and homogeneous (time irreversible) broadening contributions. This signal is optimized when the flip angle is adjusted to the Ernst angle [$\cos(\alpha)=\exp(-TR/T_1)$]. When the repetition time is chosen to be shorter than T_1 the Ernst angle will be less than 90° and the stationary spins in the imaging plane will be driven to a steady state that is reduced from the equilibrium state.

12.3 Contrast in Spin Echo Imaging

The signal from a voxel for a spin echo sequence can be written in terms of the echo time (TE), repetition time (TR), longitudinal relaxation time (T_1), transverse relaxation time (T_2), and proton density (ρ_H) as (PLEWES et al. 1993):

$$S_{SE}(TE,TR) = \rho_H\left[1-2\exp\left(-\frac{TR-TE/2}{T_1}\right)+\exp\left(-\frac{TR}{T_1}\right)\right]\exp\left(-\frac{TE}{T_2}\right)$$

(12.2)

For most imaging applications TR>>TE so Eq. 12.2 reduces to:

$$S_{SE}(TE,TR) \cong \rho_H\left[1-\exp\left(-\frac{TR}{T_1}\right)\right]\exp\left(-\frac{TE}{T_2}\right)$$

(12.3)

As before, T_1 weighting is controlled through the repetition time whereas T_2 weighting is controlled by the echo time. Throughout the rest of this chapter we shall use the transverse relaxation rates ($R_2^*=1/T_2^*$, $R_2=1/T_2$) to describe the effects of blood oxygenation changes on the MR image. While relaxation times may be more familiar to many readers it is the relaxation rate which is more directly calculated and provides more insight into the relaxation process.

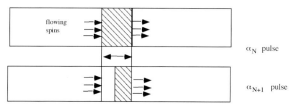

A   Inflow Effects in Gradient Echo Sequence

Fresh spins enter during repetition time between partial flip angle α pulses replacing spins that have been partially saturated. Fresh spins *increase* NMR signal.

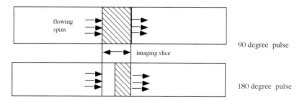

B   Inflow Effects in Spin Echo Sequence

Fresh spins enter during time between 90 and 180 degree pulses (TE/2). Only spins that were originally within the slice are refocused by the 180 pulse. Fresh spins *decrease* NMR signal.

Fig. 12.1. Effects of inflow on gradient echo and spin echo sequences. The figures above represent a region of tissue in which fresh spins can flow into the imaging slice (*shaded area*)

12.4 Gradient Echo/Spin Echo Sensitivity to Inflow

Gradient echo sequences generally depict moving spins with greater intensity than spin echo sequences (AXEL 1984). In particular, short TR gradient echo sequences show contrast between partially saturated tissues in the imaging plane and unsaturated blood flowing into the imaging plane. This will lead to a disproportionately intense blood signal. This should only occur for spins with a sufficient velocity such that a significant number can enter the imaging plane over several TR intervals, as illustrated in Fig. 12.1a. If the repetition time becomes longer these partial saturation effects are reduced since spins can return to equilibrium and flowing spins will not be relatively enhanced. Conversely, the refocusing pulse in spin echo sequences provides time-of-flight selection for moving spins. Flowing spins which enter the slice between the slice selection and refocusing pulses will be suppressed since they will only be exposed to the 180° pulse leaving no transverse component, as illustrated in Fig. 12.1b. In addition the 180° pulses from adjacent slices in multiple slice techniques can serve as presaturation filters for the blood signal (GLOVER 1993; PLEWES et al. 1993). As a consequence spin echo sequences may suffer less from pulsatility artifacts since the flow signal is suppressed. It is important to note that the time scale for inflow is different for the gradient echo and spin echo sequences. For the gradient echo the important time interval is the repetition time between image acquisitions (TR) while for the spin echo it is the time between the selection and refocusing pulses (TE/2). Usually the echo time is much shorter than the repetition time so inflow suppression in a spin echo sequence would occur for spins with a relatively high flow velocity.

12.5
Susceptibility Contrast in Gradient Echo and Spin Echo Sequences

The loss of transverse magnetization in the presence of magnetic inhomogeneities can be separated into three regimes which are determined by the magnetic, geometric and dynamic properties of the system. These regimes (which we shall term motionally averaged, intermediate, and static) are most easily defined in terms of the diffusive correlation time of the water molecules in the presence of the magnetic inhomogeneity τ_D and the characteristic variation in Larmor frequency due to the field perturbation, $\delta\omega$ (GILLIS and KOENIG 1987). For magnetic impurities that are localized τ_D is the time required for diffusion past the field perturber (a magnetic particle or a capillary), and $\delta\omega$ is the change in frequency on the surface of the magnetic region. For a spherical magnetic particle these quantities can be written as (GILLIS and KOENIG 1987; CALLAGHAN 1991; KENNAN ET AL 1994):

$$\tau_D = k_D R^2 / D \tag{12.4a}$$

$$\delta\omega = \gamma B_{eq}(R) \tag{12.4b}$$

where R is the radius of the sphere, and $B_{eq}(R)$ is the equatorial magnetic field evaluated on the surface of the particle, and the factor k_D represents a proportionality constant which is related to the volume fraction and spacing of the perturbers.

When the diffusion rate $1/\tau_D$ is much greater than $\delta\omega$ (i.e., $\delta\omega\tau_D <<1$) then diffusion is fast with respect to the spatial variations of the field perturbations and the system is said to be in a motionally narrowed regime. In this case standard "outer sphere" relaxation theory may be applied. GILLIS et al. (1987) have shown that under these conditions the relaxation rate due to a spherical magnetic impurity may be written as:

$$R_{2^{sus}} = 16\tau_D(\delta\omega)^2 / 135, \qquad \delta\omega\tau_D << 1 \tag{12.5}$$

which varies quadratically with magnetization (i.e., quadratically with magnetic field and susceptibility) and inversely with D. When diffusion is slow, such that $\delta\omega\tau_D >>1$ the relaxation can be described in terms of an ensemble of spins moving through a static distribution of linear gradients. Majumdar and Gore (1988) have shown that under these conditions the transverse relaxation in a spin echo experiment is well described by:

$$R_{2^{sus}} = (\gamma\sigma_G TE)^2 D / 12, \qquad \delta\omega\tau_D >> 1 \tag{12.6}$$

where σ_G^2 denotes the variance of the internal gradient distribution induced by the perturbation. Under these circumstances the relaxation rate increases linearly with diffusion and quadratically with the magnetization. When the diffusion is slow enough, such that the spin echo effectively refocuses the magnetization (also $\delta\omega\tau_D >>1$), there still is dephasing seen in a gradient echo due to the field inhomogeneities introduced by the perturber. Recent work has also shown that the signal decay in a gradient echo sequence in the absence of diffusion can be calculated in terms of the field distribution. Under these conditions the NMR signal does not demonstrate monoexponential decay but rather undergoes a transition from Gaussian to Lorentzian decay (YABLONSKIY et al. 1994).

A general treatment of both spin echo and gradient echo attenuation in the presence of spatially varying local fields can be accomplished using the mean field treatment developed by ANDERSON and WEISS (1953). The application of the model assumes that there is a static spatially dependent field distribution which induces a spatially varying Larmor frequency distribution. Random motion of water molecules through these fields leads to modulations in the local field experienced by the water molecules. These fluctuations are described by the field correlation function (ANDERSON and WEISS 1953; HAZELWOOD et al. 1974; KENNAN et al. 1994).

$$g_\omega(\tau) = \frac{<\Delta\omega(t)\Delta\omega(t+\tau)>}{<\Delta\omega_0^2>} = e^{-|\tau|/\tau_c} \tag{12.7}$$

where $<\Delta\omega_0^2>$ is the mean square frequency fluctuation, τ_c is the corresponding correlation time for these fluctuations, and $\Delta\omega(t)$ is the instantaneous frequency deviation at time t. Assuming the distribution of frequencies is Gaussian, the signal amplitudes in a spin echo, E(TE), and a gradient echo, G(TE), are given by (ANDERSON et al. 1953; HAZELWOOD et al. 1974):

$$E(TE) = \exp\left(-<\Delta\omega_0^2>\tau_c^2\left\{4\exp\left(\frac{-TE}{2\tau_c}\right) - \exp\left(\frac{-TE}{\tau_c}\right) + \frac{TE}{\tau_c} - 3\right\}\right)$$
(12.8a)

$$G(TE) = \exp\left(-<\Delta\omega_0^2>\tau_c^2\left\{\exp\left(\frac{-TE}{\tau_c}\right) - 1 + \frac{TE}{\tau_c}\right\}\right)$$ (12.8b)

If we assume that $\Delta\omega$ has a Gaussian distribution, then the resulting signal decay is also Gaussian for long correlation times. Identifying the correlation time as that due to diffusion past the field perturbation, i.e., $\tau_c = \tau_D$, the relaxation rate can be computed for different frequency fluctuations. Figure 12.2 shows the effective relaxation rate as a function of correlation time for a system with a mean square frequency of $400(rad/s)^2$ (corresponding to field variations of 0.75 mGauss). When the correlation time is short compared to the echo time there is little difference between the gradient echo and spin echo rates. However as the correlation time is increased, the spin echo relaxation rate reaches a peak and then begins to decrease as refocusing becomes more effective, while the gradient echo relaxation rate approaches the static limit, R_2^*. These results have be

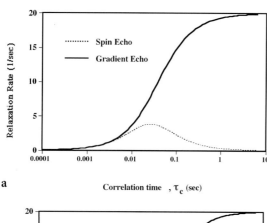

a

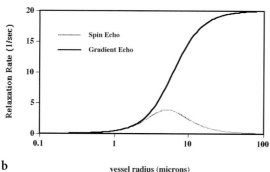

b

Fig. 12.2. a Anderson Weiss mean field theory prediction for transverse relaxation rate as a function of correlation for gradient echo (*solid*) and spin echo (*dotted*) sequences. b Anderson Weiss mean field theory prediction for transverse relaxation rate as a function of vessel size ($D = 1e^{-5} cm^2/s$, $k_D = 1$) for gradient echo (*solid*) and spin echo (*dotted*) sequences

validated by a wide range of computer simulation and experimental data (KENNAN et al. 1994; (BOXERMAN et al. 1995).

12.5.1
T_2 Sensitivity

It is immediately apparent that spin echo based sequences produce the largest degree of susceptibility based contrast for objects with a size scale on the order of 5–10 µm. For BOLD imaging this length scale is on the order of capillary and red blood cell sizes.

12.5.2
T_2^* Sensitivity

Gradient echo based sequences will show maximal contrast for structures which are larger than 20 µm such as venules and veins. A further result is that gradient echo sequences will of course be most sensitive to large scale inhomogeneities such as cavities and sinuses within the brain whereas a spin echo sequence can effectively refocus these effects.

12.6
Optimal Pulse Sequence Parameters for Gradient Echo and Spin Echo BOLD Imaging

In general it has been shown that imaging methods which are more sensitive to inhomogeneous broadening, such as gradient echo or asymmetric spin echo techniques, will be more sensitive to susceptibility changes than spin echo methods. However, some other considerations should be accounted for in the choice of imaging strategies. As illustrated previously T_2^* sensitive methods are preferentially sensitive to large field perturbations such as larger vessels or venules which may not always be associated with localized neuronal activation while a spin echo sequence in preferentially weighted in favor of true capillary type effects. A second consideration comes when determining which technique will provide the maximal signal change in an activation measurement. In a typical activation experiment one forms parametric maps based on the difference between a series of images with and without stimulus. This signal difference, ΔS, can be described as:

$$\Delta S = S_0 \exp(-R_0 TE) - S_{act} \exp(-R_{act} TE) \qquad (12.9)$$

To determine the maximal absolute signal change as a function of echo time one can differentiate Eq. 12.9 with respect to TE. For a gradient echo measurement it can be shown that the optimal echo time to produce the maximal signal change is given by $TE=T_2^*$ (the static relaxation rate) (Menon et al. 1993), whereas for a spin echo the maximal signal change is produced when the echo time equals the true T_2 of the tissue, $TE=T_2$ (Bandettini et al. 1994). This provides the following criteria to determine which imaging method will be more useful.

$$\frac{\Delta R_2^{GE}}{R_2^{GE}} > \frac{\Delta R_2^{SE}}{R_2^{SE}}$$ Gradient echo is more sensitive (12.10a)

$$\frac{\Delta R_2^{GE}}{R_2^{GE}} < \frac{\Delta R_2^{SE}}{R_2^{SE}}$$ Spin echo is more sensitive (12.10b)

where ΔR_2^{GE} and ΔR_2^{SE} are the relaxation rate changes in a spin echo a gradient echo sequence caused by activation. Generally speaking it is known that gradient echo sensitivity to blood oxygenation changes will always be greater than spin echo response. We must also note that for regions near cavities where the field is significantly more inhomogeneous the intrinsic T_2^* may be sufficiently short that a spin echo technique is preferable. An extreme example is the recent use of BOLD imaging techniques to monitor blood oxygenation response in the kidney (Fabry et al. 1996). In this abdominal region long TE gradient echo methods were not applicable since the intrinsic T_2^* of the region was much shorter than the true T_2. Further examples would be the recent use of fMRI techniques to monitor activation in the spinal cord (Collins et al. 1994, 1995; Rudin et al. 1995; Poraszasz et al. 1997). In these cases spin echo methods were chosen in preference to gradient echo methods because of the increased signal to noise obtained through the elimination of static dephasing effects of from nearby bone tissue interfaces.

12.7
Intravascular BOLD Contrast Mechanisms

The susceptibility contrast mechanisms discussed throughout this chapter can be broadly termed as a combination of an extravascular susceptibility contrast mechanism in which effects are generated by blood vessels in the surrounding parenchyma, and intravascular contrast caused by blood cell effects on the blood plasma within vessels. Recent experiments have supported this hypothesis by showing that by suppressing intravascular contributions to signal the degree of functional activation is decreased (Boxerman et al. 1995; Song et al. 1996; Zhong et al. 1997). In this case blood oxygenation changes can influence the relaxation by changing both the field gradients in which the plasma water traverses and the true T_2 of the blood pool through direct paramagnetic effects with hemoglobin mediated by exchange of water in and out of erythrocytes. High resolution activation studies at 1.5 T have shown a strong correlation between activated pixels and draining veins in the motor cortex (Lai et al. 1993; Belle et al. 1995). A second possible dephasing mechanism is intravoxel dephasing of water confined in vessels with different orientations. As described earlier, the field within a uniform vessel is constant and depends on the orientation of the vessel axis with the applied magnetic field. If the voxel of interest contains many of these types of vessels they will all precess with slightly different Larmor frequencies and therefore will cause dephasing in gradient echo measurements. For isolated vessels these dephasing effects can be exploited to measure the venous blood susceptibility changes caused by neuronal activation (Lai et al. 1996). These static effects will be completely refocused in the spin echo measurement.

12.8 Imaging Sequences (Pros and Cons)

1. Spin echo: Easy to implement but imaging time is too slow (several minutes) for most fMRI studies.
2. Gradient echo (GRASS/FLASH): Faster imaging time (several seconds to a minute). Multi-slice is difficult to implement without significant increase in imaging time. These sequences will usually have heightened inflow sensitivity due to the short repetition time (which leads to in slice saturation) required for rapid imaging. Flow sensitivity can be decreased using magnetization prepared turbo flash sequences (Kim et al. 1994).
3. Fast spin echo/RARE: Multi-shot spin echo sequences decrease imaging time for spin echo to tens of seconds, but will have large power deposition for multi-slice complex activation paradigms that require many images.
4. Echo planar: Requires gradient hardware but allows easy implementation of both spin echo and gradient echo multi-slice imaging.

12.9
Experimental Comparisons
of Gradient Echo and Spin Echo
Techniques with BOLD Models

In order to compare the relative efficacy of spin echo and gradient echo methods researchers have used respiratory challenges such as anoxia and hypercapnia to modulate blood flow and general global BOLD responses through the brain (HOPPEL et al. 1993; PRIELMEIR et al. 1994; KENNAN et al. 1997; PRINSTER et al. 1997; Table 12.1). An important study in this regard used an asymmetric spin echo based echo planar imaging (EPI) sequence (HOPPEL et al. 1993) to measure changes in both time reversible and time irreversible relaxation rates in response to hypercapnia and anoxia. The asymmetric spin echo (ASE) sequence is a hybrid of the spin echo sequence in which the gradient echo at the center of the readout is shifted in time relative to the center of the spin echo. This shift introduces time reversible dephasing such as would occur in a gradient echo sequence. It is interesting to note that this essentially the same pulse sequence as the Dixon method for performing chemical shift based fat/water imaging (DIXON 1984). Previous work has suggested that since the (ASE) sequence is selectively sensitive to a range of both time reversible and time irreversible effects, it could be used to characterize the source of the vascular response (capillary or vein) in an fMRI experiment. Table 12.2 summarizes results for regions of cortical gray matter in both rabbits and dogs in response to anoxia, hypercapnia, and bolus injection

Table 12.1. 1.5 Tesla BOLD results

	$\Delta R_2/\Delta R_2'$
Anoxia (dog)	0.34±0.21
Anoxia (rabbit)	0.33±0.11
Hypercapnia (dog)	0.36±0.18
Hypercapnia (rabbit)	0.33±0.04
Intravascular contrast agent (dog)	0.39±0.13
Intravascular contrast agent (rabbit)	0.35±0.07

Table 12.2. Comparison of tissue and vessel in a cat model (hypercapnia/hypoxia): 2.0 T results

	$\Delta R_2/\Delta R_2'$
Hypercapnia gray matter	0.44±0.04
Hypercapnia vessel	0.158±0.014

of superparamagnetic contrast agent (HOPPEL et al. 1993). ΔR_2 denotes the change in spin echo relaxation rate, while $\Delta R_2'$ denotes the change in the inhomogeneous component of the relaxation rate (which is analogous to the gradient echo relaxation rate).

It is interesting to note that in both animals for a wide range of stimuli the inhomogeneous (refocusable) contribution to the relaxation rate is about three times greater than the homogeneous (nonrefocusable) contribution. According to mean field theory and computer simulations this ratio of relaxation rates is consistent with the dominant source of relaxation occurring at the capillary and venule level (see Fig. 12.2b). In order to examine the effects of vessel size more closely another study has employed a cat model of hypercapnia and hypoxia in order to compare gradient echo and spin echo relaxation rate changes in a variety of tissue and vasculature throughout the brain (PRINSTER et al. 1997). The authors correlated the response of respiratory challenges to flow weighted angiograms. Pure gray matter regions, which were devoid of vessels and CSF, were taken in the basal ganglia, whereas vessel related regions of interest (ROIs) were chosen from the angiograms. Table 12.2 shows results obtained at 2.0 T.

This result is consistent with the mean field theory predictions presented earlier, that the ratio spin echo to gradient echo relaxation rates should decrease in the presence of larger structures. However the authors note that the absolute magnitude of the relaxation rate changes were actually larger for both spin echo and gradient echo near the large vessels (by almost a factor of 2). Some possible explanations for this effects are: The higher diffusion coefficient of the CSF that is often proximal to large vessels can reduce the effective correlation time of water molecules near the vessel and thus increase spin echo relaxation. Intravascular effects may be heightened in the presence of large vessels. This points out that the acquisition of T2 weighted EPI data using a spin echo sequence does not differentiate signal changes from parenchyma from those occurring near large vessels but the ratio of spin echo and gradient echo relaxation does. As mentioned previously short repetition time gradient echo based methods can also be sensitive to inflow of blood into the partially saturated imaging plane. Hypercapnia models have shown that for TR<1 s significant signal changes due to inflow can be detected (RIGHINI et al. 1995).

12.10
Experimental Comparisons of Gradient Echo and Spin Echo Techniques in fMRI

12.10.1
Comparison of FSE and GRE Sequences for Visual Activation

As an example of the different contrasts obtainable in gradient echo and spin echo sequences we demonstrate brain activation studies using both a T_2^* weighted gradient echo sequence and the same activation paradigm using a heavily T_2 weighted fast spin echo sequence (CONSTABLE et al. 1994). Activation maps were obtained at 1.5 T using a hemi-field visual stimulation task (a flashing 16 Hz checkerboard). The gradient echo sequence used an optimal echo time of 45 ms while the fast spin echo images used an effective echo time of 210 ms (the time at which the zero order phase encoded gradients are placed) with an interecho spacing of 14 ms. In each case 20 pairs of left right stimulation were acquired sequentially. The image pairs were processed using a split t test method which essentially determines the level of significance of signal changes with respect to noise fluctuations in each data set. The activation maps were thresholded with a t value of 2 (corresponding to $\simeq$ 0.0025 level of significance).

Figures 12.3a and 12.3b demonstrate activation of the visual cortex upon hemi-field stimulation. Two adjacent axial-oblique slices running next to the calcerine fissure are shown. It is apparent from these images that the gradient echo activation maps show greater activation than the corresponding spin echo maps. For the gradient echo dataset shown we found the average percent change of signal $\Delta S/S$ is 4.3%, while for the fast spin echo sequence the change $\Delta S/S$ is only 2.32%. The corresponding relaxation rate changes associated with the stimulus are given in Table 12.3. We note that the spin echo images show a more localized activation within the visual cortex, while the gradient echo data sets show more widespread activation, which may be attributable to the presence of large vessels, from which extravascular effects are effectively refocused and intravascular effects are suppressed in the spin echo measurement.

Another study was reported using fast spin echo methods to monitor visual stimulation at 1.9 T (GAO et al. 1995) in which the authors found somewhat larger spin echo relaxation rate changes than those reported at 1.5 T ($\Delta R_2^{FSE} = 0.26 \pm 0.09/s$). This could be attributable to the higher field strength used or the longer interecho spacing ($\tau = 20$ms) used in the fast spin echo (FSE) sequence.

12.10.2
Echo Planar Imaging: Gradient Echo vs Spin Echo Contrast

A recent study used gradient echo and spin echo based echo planar imaging (EPI) to characterize the changes in relaxation rates due to motor activation at 1.5 T (BANDETTINI et al. 1994). Separate image data

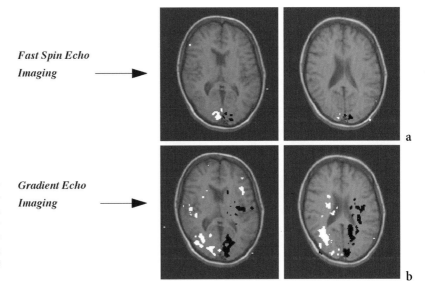

Fast Spin Echo Imaging

Gradient Echo Imaging

Fig. 12.3. a *Upper* images show anatomic images with overlaid activation maps derived from fast spin echo (FSE) images for visual stimulation. **b** *Lower* images show the corresponding gradient echo activation maps at the same level of significance ($p<0.0025$)

Table 12.3. Selected fMRI studies using gradient echo and spin echo methods

Field strength (T)	Paradigm	Imaging sequence	$\Delta R_2/\Delta R_2^*$
1.5 T	Visual stimulation	GE: spoiled GRASS SE: fast spin echo (τ=14 ms)	0.16±0.05
1.5 T	Motor stimulation	GE: EPI SE: EPI	0.28 ± 0.04
2.0 T	Motor stimulation (rat)	GE: EPI SE: EPI	0.42 ± 0.08
3.0 T	Motor stimulation	GEEPI SE EPI	0.28 ±0.042

sets of 100 images were recorded at different echo times. For each spin echo time course series TE was varied from 40 ms to 200 ms whereas for each gradient echo series TE ranged from 20 ms to 120 ms. By varying echo time one can easily separate transverse relaxation effects from inflow. For regions which showed significant activation the resting and active transverse relaxation rates could be evaluated (BANDETTINI et al. 1994) The resulting changes are shown in Table 12.3. In general it was found that the gradient echo relaxation rate change was approximately 3.5±0.6 times larger than that for the spin echo. The authors also derived the optimal signal changes for the gradient echo and spin echo sequences by using the baseline values of the regional relaxation times as the optimal echo time (TE=T_2^*, TE=T_2, as discussed earlier). Under optimal conditions they found that the gradient echo signal difference was 1.9±0.4 times greater than the optimal spin echo difference. Asymmetric spin echo sequences have also been used to compare the dynamic response of ΔR_2 and $\Delta R_2'$ during visual stimulation. At 1.5 T it was found that the ratio of $\Delta R_2/\Delta R_2'$ was 0.12±0.02 (HOPPEL et al. 1993b). A possible reason that the asymmetric spin echo sequence shows less response than gradient echo sequences is that the intravascular signal from blood will be diminished relative to the gradient echo sequence as discussed previously. Similar experiments on a rat model for somatosensory activation of the motor cortex (SCANLEY et al. 1997) at 2.0 T have shown somewhat higher spin echo to gradient echo relaxation rate ratios.

Studies utilizing crusher gradients to null vascular signal have also indicated that the efficacy of gradient echo sequences is enhanced relative to spin echo sequences in regions of large scale vasculature. This effect was demonstrated at 4.0 T using photic stimulation (MENON et al. 1994). When crusher gradients were applied in the imaging sequence a large portion of the activation signal was suppressed which was attributed to large vessels. The authors assessed that the ratio of the fractional signal change for spin echo and gradient echo sequences with optimal echo times $(\Delta S/S)_{SE}/(\Delta S/S)_{GE}$ were 0.13±0.05 in regions with strong diffusive attenuation (denoted as vasculature) and was 0.38±0.10 in regions of weak diffusive attenuation (denoted as tissue). This result is consistent with those reported earlier for the animal model of hypercarbia in which vascular regions were explicitly mapped through angiographic techniques (PRINSTER et al. 1997).

12.10.3
Field Dependence for Spin Echo and Gradient Echo Relaxivities

There is not a great deal of experimental results for evaluating the field dependence of gradient echo and spin echo relaxivities. Theoretical models have indicated that one may expect the spin echo relaxation rate to have a somewhat stronger dependence on field strength than the corresponding gradient echo, though this depends on the precise source of BOLD contrast (KENNAN et al. 1994; BOXERMAN et al. 1995). Studies of motor response at 1.5 T (BANDETTINI et al. 1994) and 3.0 T (JESMANOWICZ et al. 1993) have shown a similar field dependence for both spin echo and gradient echo response, as illustrated in Table 12.3. To date the exact field dependence of the BOLD signal remains unknown for both gradient echo and spin echo methods A more important consideration is the contrast to noise at different field strengths since both T_2^* and T_2 will be shortened to different degrees as field strength is increased. Unfortunately there are no comparative studies to date for spin echo and gradient echo methods. It is also noteworthy that one can expect different field dependencies from different vascular sources. Gradient echo based field dependence studies have shown that contrast to noise increases greater than linearly in tissue regions while it increases sublinearly in identifiable vessel regions (GATI et al. 1997).

12.11
Summary

For most cases studied to date the ratio of spin echo to gradient echo relaxivity for fields at or below 2.0 T has ranged from approximately 0.2 to 0.4. This indicates that at these field strengths gradient echo based sequences will generally be more sensitive to BOLD based signal changes. At 1.5 T it has been determined that the optimal signal change for motor stimulation will be greater in a gradient echo experiment by almost a factor of 2. The most likely utility of spin echo methods at lower field would be in regions of poor shim such as those near sinuses or in the lower brain. At higher field strength it is known that the intrinsic T_2 will decrease somewhat. For example the transverse relaxation time for gray matter in the rat brain varies from 80–100 ms at 1.5 T to approximately 50 ms at 4.7 T (LING and BENDEL 1992). The corresponding field dependence of T_2^* will be more dependent on the specifics of the magnet system and cannot be generalized easily. Studies have furthermore suggested that the ratio of gradient echo to spin echo relaxivities may be useful as a means for interpreting the vascular origin of the fMRI signal. This is because the ratio of spin echo to gradient echo relaxation rate changes are dependent on the exact nature of the vascular source. Spin echo sequences will be more sensitive to changes in smaller vessels which may be more closely associated with regions of neuronal activation whereas gradient echo sequences should be most sensitive to larger vessels which include draining veins (LAI et al. 1993). Due to the increased sensitivity of gradient echo methods to inflow effects of blood the gradient echo methods also have shown increased sensitivity to intravascular effects which are reduced in both spin echo and asymmetric spin echo methods. Further studies need to be performed at higher field strength, where the intrinsic gradient echo and spin echo relaxation times will be shortened and the corresponding BOLD effects should be increased.

References

Anderson PW, Weiss PR (1953) Exchange narrowing in paramagnetic resonance. Rev Mod Phys 25:269

Axel L (1984) Blood flow effects in magnetic resonance (MR) imaging. AJR 143:1157–1166

Bandettini PA, Wong EC, Jesmanowicz A, Hinks RS, Hyde JS (1994) Spin-echo and gradient echo EPI of human brain activation using BOLD contrast. A comparative study at 1.5 T. NMR Biomed 7:12–20

Belle V, Delon-Martin C, Massarelli R, Decety J, Le Bas JF, Benaibid AL, Segabarth C (1995) Intracranial gradient echo and spin echo functional MR angiography in humans. Radiology 195:739–746

Boxerman JL, Bandettini PA, Kwong KK, Baker JR, Davis TL, Rosen BR, Weisskoff RM (1995a)The intravascular contribution to fMRI signal change: Monte Carlo modeling and diffusion-weighted studies in vivo. Magn Reson Med 34:4

Boxerman JL, Hamberg LM, Rosen BR, Weisskoff RM (1995b)MR contrast due to intravascular susceptibility perturbations. Magn Reson Med 34:555–566

Callaghan PT (1991) Principles of nuclear magnetic resonance microscopy. Oxford University, New York

Collins JG, Kennan RP (1995) Functional magnetic resonance imaging of human spinal cord activation by noxious stimuli. Society for Neuroscience Annual Meeting, San Diego CA, abstract 155.1, pp 377

Collins JG, Kennan R, Kaneko M, Tsukamoto T (1994) Functional magnetic resonance imaging of rat spinal cord following hindpaw formalin injection. Society for Neuroscience Annual Meeting, Miami FLA, abstract 134.9, pp 306

Constable RT, Kennan RP, Puce A, McCarthy G, Gore JC (1994) Functional NMR imaging using fast spin echo at 1.5T. Magn Reson Med 31:686–690

Dixon WT (1984) Simple proton spectroscopic imaging. Radiology 153:189–194

Fabry ME, Kennan RP, Paszty C. Constantini F, Rudin EM, Gore JC, Nagel RL (1996) Magnetic resonance evidence of hypoxia in a homozygous alpha knockout model of a transgenic mouse model for sickle cell disease. J Clin Invest 98:11, 2450–2455

Gao JH, Xiong J, Li J, Schiff J, Roby J, Lancaster JL, Fox PT (1995) Fast spin echo characteristics of visual stimulation induced signal changes in the human brain. J Magn Reson Imaging 5:709–714

Gati JS, Menon RS, Ugurbil K, Rutt BK (1997) Experimental determination of the BOLD field strength dependence in vessels and tissue. Magn Reson Med 38:296–302

Gillis P, Koenig SH (1987) Transverse relaxation of solvent protons induced by magnetized spheres: application to ferretin, erythrocytes, and magnetite. Magn Reson Med 5:323–345

Glover GH (1993) Gradient echo imaging. In: Bronskil MJ, Sprawls P (eds) The physics of MRI: 1992 AAPM summer school proceedings, medical monograph 21. American Institute of Physics, New York, pp 125–140

Hazelwood CF, Chang DC, Nichols BL, Woessner DE (1974) Nuclear magnetic resonance transverse relaxation time of water protons in skeletal muscle. Biophys J 14:584

Hoppel BE, Baker JR, Weisskoff RM, Rosen BR (1993a)Dynamic response of DR_2 and DR_2' during photic activation.12th Annual Meeting of the Society for Magnetic Resonance in Medicine, pp 1384

Hoppel BE, Weisskoff RM, Thulborn KR, Moore JB, Kwong KK Rosen BR (1993b)Measurement of regional blood oxygenation and cerebral hemodynamics. Magn Reson Med 30:715–723

Jesmanowicz A, Bandettini PA, Wong EC, Tan G, Hyde JS, (1993) Spin echo and gradient echo EPI of human brain function at 3.0 T. 12th Annual Meeting of the Society for Magnetic Resonance in Medicine, pp 1390

Kennan RP, Zhong J, Gore JC (1994) Intravascular susceptibility contrast mechanisms in tissue. Magn Reson Med 31:9–31

Kennan RP, Scanley BE, Gore JC, (1997) Physiologic basis for BOLD MR signal changes due to hypoxia/hyperoxia: separation of blood volume and magnetic susceptibility effects. Magn Reson Med 37:953–956

Kim SG, Hendrich K, Hu X, Merkle H, Ugurbil K (1994) Potential pitfalls of functional MRI using conventional gradient recalled echo techniques. NMR Biomed 7:69–74

Lai S, Hopkins AL, Haacke EM, Li D, Wasserman BA, Buckley P, Friedman L, Meltzer H, Hedera P, Friedland R (1993) Identification of vascular structures as a major source of signal contrast in high resolution 2D and 3D functional activation imaging of the motor cortex. Magn Reson Med 30:387–392

Lai S, Haacke M, Reichenbach JR (1996) In vivo quantification of brain activation-induced change in cerebral blood oxygen saturation using MRI. Proc ISMRM 4th Annual Meeting, New York, April 29–May3, 1996, p. 1756

Ling YL, Bendel P (1992) Thin section MR imaging of rat brain at 4.7 T. J Magn Reson Imaging 2:393–399

Majumdar S, Gore JC (1988) Studies of diffusion in random fields produced by variations in susceptibility. J Magn Reson 78:41–55

Menon RS, Ogawa S, Tank DW, Ugurbil K (1993) 4 Tesla gradient recalled echo characteristics of photic stimulation-induced signal changes in the human primary visual cortex. Magn Reson Med 30:380–386

Menon RS, Hu X, Adriany G, Andersen P, Ogawa S, Ugurbil K (1994) Comparison of spin echo EPI and conventional EPI applied to functional neuroimaging: The effect of flow crushing gradients on the BOLD signal. Proceedings of the 2nd Annual Meeting of the Society for Magnetic Resonance San Francisco, August 6–12, 1994, p. 622

Ogawa S, Lee TM, Nayak AS, Glynn P (1990) Oxygenation sensitive contrast in magnetic resonance imaging of rodent brain at high magnetic fields. Magn Reson Med 14:68–78

Plewes DB, Bishop J (1993) Spin echo imaging. In: Bronskil M.J, Sprawls P (eds) The physics of MRI: 1992 AAPM summer school proceedings, medical physics monograph 21. American Institute of Physics, New York

Porszasz R, Rudin M, Beckman N, Bruttel K, Urban L (1997) Functional magnetic resonance imaging of spinal cord activation induced by subcutaneously administered formalin: sensitivity to lidocaine. Proceedings ISMRM 5th Annual Meeting, Vancouver British Columbia, April 12–18, 1997, p. 237

Prielmeir F, Nagatomo Y, Frahm J (1994) Cerebral blood oxygenation in rat brain during hypoxic hypoxia: quantitative MRI of effective relaxation rates. Magn Reson Med 31:678–681

Prinster A, Pierpaoli C, Turner R, Jezzard P (1997) Simultaneous measurement of DR_2 and DR_2^* in cat brain during hypoxia and hypercapnia. Neuroimage 6:191–200

Righini A, Pierpaoli C, Barnett AS, Waks E, Alger JR, (1995) Blue blood or black blood: R1 effects in graded echo planar functional neuroimaging. Magn Res Imaging 13:369–378

Rudin M, Beckman N, Urban L, Dray A (1995) Visualization of spinal cord activation in rats after injections of formalin into the hindpaw using functional magnetic resonance imaging. Proceedings ISMRM 3rd Annual Meeting, Nice France, August 19–25, 1997, p. 780

Scanley B E, Kennan RP, Cannan S, Skudlarski P, Innis RB, Gore JC (1997) Functional magnetic resonance imaging of median nerve stimulation in rats at 2.0 T. Magn Reson Med 37:969–972

Song AW, Wong EC, Tan SG, Hyde JS (1996) Diffusion weighted fMRI at 1.5 T. Magn Reson Med 35:155–158

Yablonskiy DA, Haacke EM (1994) Theory of NMR signal behavior in magnetically inhomogeneous tissues: the static dephasing regime. Magn Reson Med 32:749–763

Zhong J, Kennan RP, Fullbright RK, Anderson AW, Gore JC (1997) Intra and extra- vascular contributions to signal changes induced by inspired oxygen or intravascular contrast agents. Proc ISMRM 5th Annual Meeting, Vancouver, British Columbia, April 12–18, 1997, p. 159

13 Echo-Planar Imaging and Functional MRI

M.S. Cohen

CONTENTS

13.1 Introduction

Since the first days of human NMR imaging, reaching back to the late 1970s (e.g., MANSFIELD et al. 1978; DAMADIAN et al. 1977; PYKETT and MANSFIELD 1978), imaging time has presented a serious practical limitation. The practical reality of ordinary structural imaging is that normal subjects are willing to tolerate perhaps an hour of lying inside of the imaging magnet, and are able to stay still for little more than 15 min. Both NMR contrast and signal to noise ratio, however, are time-dependent phenomena. As a result, imaging time and image quality have traditionally been at odds for all manner of magnetic resonance imaging. Figure 13.1 shows the relationship between imaging time and a variety of interesting biological phenomena. Figure 13.1B, conceived by Van J. Wedeen at Harvard University, shows the steady decrease in practical MR imaging times that took place over the first decade of human imaging and demonstrates the remarkably steady logarithmic improvements in imaging speed that have characterized the field. It is perhaps even more remarkable, therefore, that today's fastest practical imaging method, echo-planar imaging (EPI) was conceived in 1977 (MANSFIELD 1977), before the veritable explosion in clinical use of MRI. EPI achieved largely novelty status, however, until it found a driving application – namely functional MRI and especially functional neuroimaging. A major factor in the relatively slow acceptance of EPI is that it is just plain hard to implement, as we will see below.

13.2 What is Echo Planar Imaging?

While MRI, as practiced conventionally, builds up the data for an image from a series of discrete signal samples, EPI is a method to form a complete image from a single data sample, or a single "shot." The speed advantages can be astonishing. For example, a typical T2-weighted imaging series (to form an image whose contrast depends predominantly on the intrinsic tissue magnetization parameter, T2) requires that the time between excitation pulses, known as TR, be two to three times longer than the intrinsic tissue magnetization parameter, T1. The T1 of biological samples is typically on the order of a second or so (cerebrospinal fluid can have much longer T1s of several seconds); TR must therefore be 3 s or more. A more or less typical MR image is formed from 128 repeated samples, so that the imaging time for our canonical T2-weighted scan is about 384 s, or more than 6.5 min. By comparison, the EPI approach collects all of the image data, for an image of the same resolution, in 40–150 ms (depending on hardware and contrast considerations). This reflects a nearly 10,000-fold speed gain.

M.S. COHEN, PhD, UCLA School of Medicine, Ahmanson-Lovelake Brain Mapping Center, Room 215A, 604 Charles E Young Drive South, Los Angeles, CA 90095-7085, USA

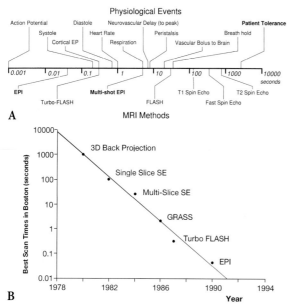

Fig. 13.1. A Comparison of physiological processes and imaging speeds of common magnetic resonance imaging methods. To avoid image artifacts, scan times must not be longer than the duration of motion. To study the dynamics of these processes, the imaging times must be substantially shorter. Echo-planar imaging (EPI) and multi-shot EPI, the methods discussed in this chapter, are indicated in *bold type*. **B** Fastest MRI scan times in Boston (as conceived by Van Wedeen) as a function of year and technology

Although, as we will discuss below, there are myriad variations, EPI is fundamentally just a trick of spatial encoding. To understand the difference between EPI and conventional imaging, it is necessary therefore, to have some understanding of spatial encoding in MRI.

13.2.1
MRI Spatial Encoding

Tomographic image formation requires spatial encoding in three dimensions. In most cases, one dimension is determined by slice selective excitation (MANSFIELD and MAUDSLEY 1977; see Fig. 13.2 for axis labels). Briefly, a radiofrequency (RF) excitation pulse with a narrow frequency range is transmitted to the subject in the presence of a spatial magnetic field gradient. Because the magnetic resonance phenomenon depends on an exact match between the RF excitation pulse frequency and the proton spin frequency, which depends, in turn, on the local magnetic field, this pulse will excite the MR signal over a correspondingly narrow range of locations: an imaging *slice*. The differences between EPI and conventional imaging occur in the remaining "in-plane" spatial encoding.

When a magnetic field gradient is applied across this excited slice, it will cause the spin frequency to be a function of position. The pixel size, or spatial resolution, of an MR image depends on the product (actually the integral) of the imaging gradient amplitudes and their "on" duration. Specifically, the pixel size is equal to $1/\gamma Gt$, where γ is the Larmor constant (4258 Hz/gauss), G is the gradient amplitude, usually expressed in Gauss/cm, and t is the gradient "on" time. A gradient of 0.5 Gauss/cm, left on for 10 ms, for example, yields a spatial resolution of 0.47 mm. This, however, reflects spatial encoding along one in-plane dimension only – the "readout" direction. In ordinary two-dimensional Fourier transform imaging, the encoding for the second in-plane dimension is created by applying a brief gradient pulse (along a second gradient axis) before each readout line. For 128 lines of resolution in this axis, 128 separate lines must be acquired, each for 10 ms. The total readout duration is therefore 128×10 ms, or 1.28 s. Unfortunately, the MR signal lasts for only about 100 ms (limited by T2) and over the course of a 1.28 s readout duration (spatial encoding period) the signal will have decayed to nothing.

In EPI, much larger gradient amplitudes are used. A gradient of about 2.5 Gauss/cm is typical, but human imagers with gradient amplitudes in excess of 5 Gauss/cm are achievable. With five times the gradient amplitude, the encoding duration can be reduced by fivefold, to 2 ms/line, so that the total spatial encoding time for our reference image is reduced from 1.28 s to 256 ms. The human brain has a T2 of about 100 ms at typical imaging field strengths. Thus, a 256 ms readout might be marginally realistic. In

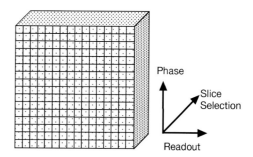

Fig. 13.2. The three axes used for spatial encoding of MR images. One dimension of spatial encoding is achieved by slice selective excitation (the slice selection axis). The other two are encoded by phase and frequency. Some texts will refer to the slice selection axis as the "z" axis. The Readout axis is variously labeled the "frequency" or "x" axis; the phase encoding axis is sometimes labeled the "y" axis

Fig. 13.3 A, B. K-space traversal patterns (heavy lines) used in conventional imaging (**A**, *left*) and echo-planar imaging (**B**, *right*). *Small circles* represent the required data samples. In conventional imaging, each raw data line is separately acquired after a radiofrequency (RF) excitation. As a result, TR elapses between the collection of each data line. In echo-planar imaging (EPI), the lines are acquired continuously, in a raster-like pattern, with as little as 300 μs elapsing from line to line

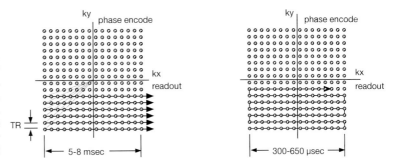

Fig. 13.3 A, B. K-space traversal patterns (heavy lines) used in conventional imaging (**A**, *left*) and echo-planar imaging (**B**, *right*). *Small circles* represent the required data samples. In conventional imaging, each raw data line is separately acquired after a radiofrequency (RF) excitation. As a result, TR elapses between the collection of each data line. In echo-planar imaging (EPI), the lines are acquired continuously, in a raster-like pattern, with as little as 300 μs elapsing from line to line

practice, however, for reasons discussed below, this is not a practical configuration. Most significantly, the gradients cannot instantly reach such large magnitudes, and the rise time therefore becomes a significant fraction of the readout duration. Secondly, the decay of the MR signal during readout introduces blurring into the images (FARZANEH et al. 1990) Because of these tradeoffs, most EPI studies are performed at somewhat lower resolution. In-plane voxel sizes between 1.5 and 3 mm are typical.

In many cases all of this is somewhat easier to understand in terms of k-space, which is a representation of the MRI raw data before it has been Fourier-transformed in order to make an image (TWIEG 1983, 1985; LJUNGGREN 1983; BROWN et al. 1982). The signal location in k-space is the integral of the gradient amplitude and "on" time:

$$k_i(t) = \gamma \int G_i(t)dt, \qquad (13.1)$$

where k_i is the location in k-space along the i axis, $G_i(t)$ is the gradient amplitude along the i axis as a function of time, γ is the Larmor constant, and t is the gradient "on" time. As the gradient time product increases, that is, as the signal is encoded to higher k values, the image resolution increases. Thus, in order to make an MR image of any desired final resolution, we must collect MR data over a corresponding area of k-space.

In conventional MRI, k-space is covered line by line, as suggested in Fig. 13.3A. Following each RF excitation, a single line of raw data is collected along k_x (the readout axis), with sequential lines acquired at different displacements along the k_y axis. Because a separate excitation step is required prior to the collection of each data line, the total imaging time depends on the time between excitations (TR) as well as on the total number of data lines collected. The latter depends on the desired resolution and field of view in the final images.

Figure 13.3B shows the k-space trajectory used in EPI. Here, the sequential raw data lines are acquired immediately after one another. In modern imagers,

the collection of each data line can be as rapid as 300 μs. Figure 13.4 shows the gradient encoding scheme needed for the EPI k-space trajectory. The rapid back and forth traversal of the readout axis is preformed by using an oscillating readout gradient. Following each readout excursion, a brief pulse of the phase encoding gradient is used to move to the next line in the phase encode direction.

Figure 13.4 suggests also that the echo-planar encoding portion of the sequence can be encapsulated as a module that is somewhat independent of the RF pulse sequence. As we will see below, this is important, as the image contrast is determined largely by the RF sequence, rather than the gradient spatial encoding.

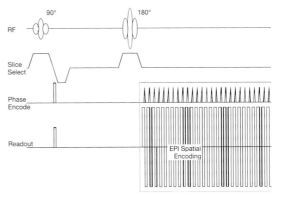

Fig. 13.4. Echo-planar pulse sequence corresponding to the k-space trajectory shown in Fig. 13.3B

13.3
Signal-to-Noise Ratio

Signal-to-noise ratio (SNR) in MRI is a function of:
1. Available transverse magnetization (pulse sequence and contrast)
2. Imaging time (or more precisely, time spent receiving the signal)
3. Bandwidth – the signal sampling rate
4. Field strength
5. RF coil loading, coupling and sensitivity
6. Voxel volume

EPI carries the advantage (by contrast with the so-called gradient echo methods such as FLASH, GRASS, etc.; Frahm et al. 1986) that the full magnetization is available as signal: In a single shot method, all of the longitudinal magnetization may be used in image formation without a penalty in overall imaging time. The imaging time consideration also works to the advantage of EPI: in a typical EPI sequence, as used in fMRI, signal may be collected for well over 75% of the imaging time, leading to a very high efficiency. EPI pays a penalty in bandwidth, however. The imaging speed in EPI comes from the use of very high amplitude field gradients which, in turn, allow and require very rapid sampling. While conventional MRI may use receiver bandwidths up to about 32 kHz, bandwidths of 300 kHz are typical in EPI and drop the usable SNR by about two thirds. Field strength and RF coil considerations are not pulse sequence-dependent. All told, theoretical analyses and direct measurement have demonstrated a nearly fivefold SNR advantage of EPI over FLASH studies (Cohen and Weisskoff 1991) for comparable voxel volume.

13.4
Bandwidth and Artifacts

The bandwidth of an MR image refers to the difference in MR frequencies between adjacent pixels, as well as to the total range of frequencies that make up an image. In conventional imaging, the bandwidth, per pixel is ordinarily kept comparable to the chemical shift between fat and water. In a 1.5 Tesla instrument, for example, a pixel bandwidth of 125 Hz is typical (the fat-water shift is about 220 Hz). In this case, the fat and water components of a single voxel will be shifted from one another by about one pixel, which is an acceptable imaging artifact. At first, one would expect that the pixel bandwidth in EPI would be very high, due to the rapid sampling rate. This is, in fact, true along the readout axis. The continuous encoding scheme used in EPI, however, results in a relatively low bandwidth along the phase encoding axis; 30 Hz/pixel is typical. This causes several difficult artifacts to occur in EPI.

13.4.1
Chemical Shift

In EPI, the very low bandwidth along the phase encode axis results in substantial chemical shift arti-

facts. At 1.5 Tesla, for example, using a 30 Hz/pixel bandwidth, fat and water are displaced by about eight pixels. Further, the voxel sizes in EPI are usually rather large, for the reasons discussed above. Using a more or less typical 3 mm voxel, fat and water may be displaced from one another by 2.5 cm! This problems scales with field strength, so that in a 3 Tesla scanner the fat water chemical shift approaches 5 cm. Since most body tissues contain at least some water and fat, it is absolutely necessary to correct for the chemical shift problems.

Fortunately, there are a number of good technologies to manage chemical shift (Weiskoff et al. 1989). In the vast majority of cases, only the water component of the MR signal is of clinical interest. This is always the case in functional neuroimaging, where the lipid content of the brain is very low and the dominant source of fat signal is the component found in skin. It is therefore reasonable to simply suppress the fat signal outright. Usually, this is done by applying a fat saturation pulse prior to imaging. Because the chemical shift between fat and water is quite large, one can transmit a 90° pulse at the fat frequency without significantly affecting the water signal. After this pulse the fat signal will be in the transverse plane and it can be dephased easily by applying a gradient pulse. Until the fat signal has had time enough to recover its longitudinal magnetization it will not appear in the images. This so-called chemical shift saturation method does require excellent magnetic field homogeneity so that the frequencies of fat and water are well-resolved. Fortunately, today's imaging instruments easily meet this requirement.

An alternative method of suppression is to use STIR (short TI inversion recovery; Bydder and Young 1985). This approach takes advantage of the T1 difference between fat and other body tissues. An inversion (180°) pulse is applied immediately prior to the EPI sequence, timed such that the magnetization of fat is recovering through zero at the time of the 90° excitation pulse. Because the fat has no magnetization at that time, the 90° pulse does not result in the formation of any signal from fat. While STIR is a very effective method of fat suppression, it has side effects that make it less desirable. First of all, it alters the contrast of the images overall, as it adds T1 contrast. Second, the method works best if the inversion pulse is applied only when the tissue is fully magnetized. The latter requires that inversion recovery be used only with long TR images.

It is possible, also, to use so-called spectral-spatial excitation pulses (Meyer et al. 1990), which excite only the water (or fat) resonance from a well-defined slice. This technology has the advantage that it is temporally efficient, combining both functions, and may avoid certain problems of stimulated echo formation across TR periods. The pulses, however, are typically four or more times as long in duration as the more or less standard spatial only pulses and therefore come at a modest cost to the minimum echo times.

13.4.2
Shape Distortion

The low bandwidth of EPI in the phase direction causes a much less manageable artifact in shape distortion. Even in a well-shimmed magnet, the human head will magnetize unevenly so that the MR frequency may differ from point to point by about 1 part per million (ppm). These small frequency differences result in spatial displacement of the signal in the resulting images. Most investigators simply tolerate the typical one or two pixel distortion as an acceptable artifact. Generally, however, this artifact can be corrected since it is possible to measure the magnetic field in the head and then to apply a correction to the MR image to shift the signal to its correct location (MEYER et al. 1990).

The shape distortions are a frequent cause of concern in functional neuroimaging, as it is often desirable to superimpose regions of brain activation onto higher resolution structural images that are usually acquired conventionally (e.g., with a much higher bandwidth). In this case, the activation maps will not be registered properly with the structural data set.

13.4.3
Ghosting

When the MR field gradients are switched on and off, the time varying magnetic field of the gradients results in current induction (eddy currents) in the various conducting surfaces of the rest of the imaging instrument. These, in turn, set up magnetic field gradients that may persist after the primary gradients are switched off. Such eddy currents are a problem in conventional imaging, but are much more challenging in EPI. The gradient amplitudes, and particularly the gradient switching rates, used in EPI are much greater and induce larger eddy currents. Further, the long readout period in EPI results in more opportunity for image distortion from eddy currents.

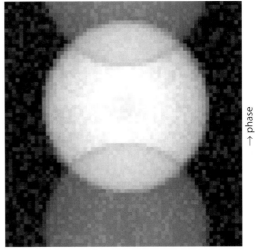

Fig. 13.5. Appearance of a so-called N/2 ghost that occurs frequently in echo-planar imaging. Such ghosts are the result of small line-by-line phase errors that can take place during spatial encoding

A particularly common EPI artifact is so-called "ghosting" from eddy currents. This results from the time-dependent frequency shift created by the time-dependent eddy currents. Because of the back and forth trajectory in k-space used in EPI (Fig. 13.3), the frequency shifts create a phase difference from line to line in the raw data. When the data are Fourier-transformed, the phase shift creates a phase ambiguity in the images, such that part of the signal appears 90° out of phase, or one half image away. This ghosting structure is frequently referred to as an "N/2 ghost." Figure 13.5 shows schematically the appearance of such a ghost image.

The correction of image ghosts may take several forms. Probably the most robust scheme is to design the gradient coils critically such that eddy current induction is minimized. At present the most effective method is to use shielded or "screened" gradient coils, in which a separate set of gradient coils is counterwound around outside the primary coil set to cancel any external magnetic fields. Because gradient efficiency drops as the fifth power of the radius, even a small gap between primary and secondary gradients allows for a non-zero gradient inside the coil and a zero gradient outside (TURNER and BOWLEY 1986).

Elimination of the N/2 ghost also requires critical calibration of the timing between signal digitization and gradient activity. Delays of a few microseconds result in line by line phase discrepancies because of the alternating left-right trajectory along the readout axis in k-space (Fig. 13.3). These errors can be tuned out in hardware by adjusting the sampling clock, and may be adjusted further in software by adding an appropriate phase shift to the raw data. The latter can be performed by an exponential multiplication. An alternative approach to ghost correction is to acquire a reference scan in the absence of phase encoding and to use this as a basis for determination of the time-dependent phase shifts (BRUDER et al. 1989; SCHMITT et al. 1990).

13.5 Resolution

Resolution, or voxel size, depends on the maximum gradient amplitude time product in the raw data. Increases in resolution require either increases in gradient amplitude, increases in gradient duration, or both. Neither is easy to come by. As we will see below, the power requirements for the gradients in EPI can be quite large (DICKINSON et al. 1989; ROHAN 1989). Further, switching gradients rapidly to very high amplitudes may ultimately result in unacceptable safety problems. Increasing the duration of the gradient pulses lowers the effective image bandwidth and increases the sensitivity of the images to shape distortion and other artifacts. At this writing, the highest performance body gradient sets reach amplitudes of up to 3.6 Gauss/cm with a rise time of 179 µs using a sinusoidal waveform. This results in a 3 mm pixel size in the readout axis (COHEN et al. 1996).

Fortunately, a variety of k-space encoding schemes are available to improve spatial resolution. Increases in resolution along the phase encoding axis are available simply by extending the total duration of the echo planar readout (box shown in dotted lines in Fig. 13.4) (COHEN and WEISKOFF 1991). This

increases the total displacement along the ky (phase encoding k axis) at the cost of a decrease in bandwidth and an increase in minimum echo time. Doubling the encoding period, for example, will reduce the pixel size and the bandwidth, per pixel, by a factor of two. Shape distortions from field inhomogeneity will remain constant in distance (as expressed in millimeters), though they will cover double the number of pixels. This tradeoff frequently works well.

A useful way to increase resolution along the readout axis results from the Hermitian symmetry property of k-space (MARGOSIAN 1985; RZEDZIAN 1987). Formally, reflections about the axes in k-space are complex conjugates; a data point at (kx, ky) is equal to the complex conjugate of the data point at (–kx, ky) or at (kx, –ky). This symmetry property implies that it is necessary to acquire only half of the entire MR raw data space to form a complete MR image. A very efficient way to achieve high resolution in a single shot EPI experiment is to use a long readout duration along ky and to acquire only the positive (or negative) values in kx. Prior to image formation, it is a relatively simple matter to calculate the data that make up the uncollected portion of the image and then to Fourier transform the entire raw data set to form a complete image (Fig. 13.6A).

The complex conjugation "trick" outlined above requires a few pre-conditions to work properly. First, it depends on the desired image having no "imaginary" component. What this means in practice is that the user must not be interested in any phase deviations along the image. Such phase difference might result, for example, from local field inhomogeneities or motion and are usually of little concern to the researcher in functional neuroimaging. Second, any phase variations in the image must be relatively small; otherwise, the reconstruction will result in ghost-like artifacts from locations with large phase shifts. Finally, the raw data must be well-centered in k-space for the reflection property to be accurate.

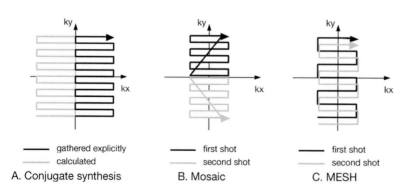

Fig. 13.6A–C. Resolution enhancement approaches for echo-planar imaging (EPI). A The conjugate synthesis method (variously called half-Fourier, half-NEX or partial-k) takes advantage of the conjugate symmetry of k-space so that only half of the raw data need be collected to form a complete MR image. B The Mosaic method collects regions of k-space in tiles. C In MESH, the k-space regions are collected in interleaved fashion, usually with a higher amplitude phase encoding step

A. Conjugate synthesis — gathered explicitly / calculated

B. Mosaic — first shot / second shot

C. MESH — first shot / second shot

Similarly to the process of eddy current correction discussed above, this requirement is achieved by a combination of hardware and software engineering. Figure 13.7 shows example images, each collected in a single shot, using the conjugate synthesis approach. The in-plane resolution is about 1.5 mm.

While true EPI is a single shot experiment (that is, a single excitation pulse results in a complete image), a variety of EPI hybrids, using multiple excitations per image, may be used to increase spatial resolution. The two most often used include the MESH and Mosaic methods (RZEDZIAN 1987). In the Mosaic method (Fig. 13.6B), each excitation is used to cover a different region of k-space and the resulting data are tiled together to form an image of any desired resolution. The MESH technique is slightly subtler. Here, a larger phase encoding step is used so that data collected from separate RF excitations may be interleaved. The important result in MESH imaging is a wider bandwidth in the final image, which may be desirable in reducing imaging artifacts. The multi-shot hybrids have a SNR advantage as well: SNR increases with the square root of the acquisition time, so that the SNR is about 40% better in the two shot than in the single shot scans. The multiple shot and conjugate synthesis methods can be combined over a wide range of variations to produce echo-planar images of very high resolution (COHEN and WEISKOFF 1991).

EPI resolution is limited, ultimately, by the SNR of the images. Since typical EPI data are collected over 40–50 ms or so, as compared to the nearly 1 s of acquisition time spent on a conventional scan, the SNR is down by a factor of more than fourfold at comparable resolution on this basis alone. As shown in Fig. 13.7, single shot images with voxel volumes of $3\times1.5\times1.5$ mm (=6.75 mm^3) offer acceptable SNR at 3 Tesla. In fact, the measured SNR differences between conventional and EPI data in human subjects are much less than predicted on the basis of theory. This is likely due to the fact that tiny motions in the conventional imaging set result in an overall increase in apparent image noise. At the present time, it seems that EPI spatial resolution is largely gradient limited.

13.6
Hardware Requirements

Echo-planar imaging is a demanding sequence for the imaging instrument. Good quality images require high performance gradients with rapid rise times, high peak amplitudes, high accuracy and low eddy currents. The demands on the data acquisition system are considerable as well. Because the data are sampled so rapidly, very fast analog to digital converters (ADCs), up to 2 MHz, are required. The ADC subsystems, however, are becoming more widely available due to advances in semiconductor technology.

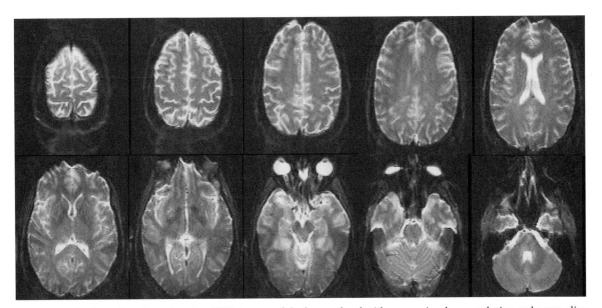

Fig. 13.7. Single-shot echo-planar imaging (EPI) images of the human head with 1.5 mm in-plane resolution and 3 mm slice thickness, collected using the conjugate synthesis method

13.6.1
Gradient Power

A typical body gradient coil in an MR system will have an efficiency of about 1 Gauss/cm per 100 amps. Thus, a current of 250–350 amps is required to produce acceptably high gradient amplitudes for EPI. Further, the inductance of the typical body coil is about 1 milliHenry (mH). The gradient slew rate (the rate of rise) is determined by the rate of change in current (di/dt). This is calculated easily. For example, to achieve a 200 μs rise time to 3.5 Gauss/cm requires that di/dt equal 350 amps/175 μs, or 2×10^6 amps/s. With a coil inductance, L, of 1 mH, the required driving voltage is: V=Ldi/dt=2000 Volts.

A conventional power system would need to deliver 2000 Volts at 350 amps, or 750,000 Watts, to meet this requirement. Most EPI-capable amplifier systems therefore use some form of nonlinear amplification using either inductive or capacitive energy storage devices. These implementations recognize that it is generally not necessary to simultaneously source both high current and high voltage to the highly reactive gradient load.

The required accuracy of the gradient waveforms adds another complicating factor. Any deviations from the ideal waveform could result in phase errors in the images. Such deviations can results from eddy currents, physical instabilities or amplifier distortion. One efficient way to manage this problem is to synchronize the signal digitization to the integral of the measured gradient activity, such that the data are sampled uniformly in k-space.

13.7
dB/dt and Safety and Head Gradients

It has been recognized since the early days of MRI that the rapidly switched magnetic field gradients in imaging instruments result in current induction in the patients. The pioneering work of REILLY (1989a, b, 1990), based on direct modeling using the Hodgkin and Huxley equations for neuronal excitability, suggested operational margins below which gradient switching rate (dB/dt) was not likely to be a cause of concern. At that time, gradient switching rates above the predicted neural firing threshold were not practical to achieve. Once the non-linear amplifier methods became feasible, however, it became possible to routinely exceed the threshold of sensation using imaging gradients (COHEN et al.

1990; BUDINGER et al. 1991; ROHAN and RZEDZIAN 1992; BOURLAND et al. 1990). Most of the present day imaging systems have gradient performance that is limited to just below the typical threshold of sensory stimulation.

There is an alternative, however. The induced current in the patient is proportional not only to the rate of change of the magnetic field, but also to the cross-sectional area of the body exposed to the changing field. For example, it is now well-known that the sensory threshold is higher for gradients that switch along the sagittal axis than for those that switch along the coronal axis, because the cross-sectional area of the typical supine person is much larger in the coronal than in the sagittal plane. Further, the maximum dB/dt occurs at the ends of the imaging coil, where the magnetic fields are at their maximum. A shorter coil, therefore, will have a reduced dB/dt. Probably the best solution in functional neuroimaging is to build head-only gradient coils. Such devices gain safety/sensory threshold margins due both to their reduced length and to the reduced cross-sectional area over which the gradients occur. The cross-sectional area of the human neck is less than one sixth that of the chest. The gradient coil length can be reduced by a factor of at least two, and probably by more than three. Therefore the stimulation threshold, in terms of imaging gradient switching, will be reduced by at least ten-, and probably more than 20-fold.

Shorter and smaller gradients offer another set of advantages: the gradient efficiency scales with fifth power of the radius, so that reducing the diameter twofold can increase the gradient strength by a factor of 32. Thus, the smaller gradients not only enable the use of larger amplitudes with good safety margins, but also make such strong gradients practical to implement. At this writing, the major equipment manufacturers have expressed little interest in special purpose head gradients. In the end, however, it is likely the market will demand such tools for high-performance functional neuroimaging.

13.8
Contrast Variants

Because EPI is fundamentally just a spatial encoding scheme, there are already a wide variety of variants that can be used to offer a correspondingly wide range of contrast behaviors.

13.8.1
Spin Echo

Figure 13.4 (page 137) shows the most common implementation of EPI as used for clinical imaging: the spin echo sequence. Here the spatial encoding "module" is preceded by a 90° excitation pulse and a 180° echo-forming pulse, resulting in the formation of a Hahn echo (HAHN 1950) during the readout period. Such images have a signal intensity (SI) that is well described by the equation:

$$SI = k\varrho(1-e^{-tr/T1})e^{-te/T2}, \tag{13.2}$$

where k represents sequence independent factors such as magnetic field strength and RF coil sensitivity, ρ is the tissue proton density, TR is the repetition time and TE is the echo time or the time from the excitation pulse to the center of the readout period. Such images show relatively little sensitivity to local field inhomogeneities (at least as they relate to contrast) and behave similar to conventional MR images. A key difference, however, is that in a single shot EPI study, the TR is effectively infinite, so that the images are obtained with little or no T1 contrast. This is a decided advantage in clinical T2-weighted studies in which the T1 and T2 contrast mechanisms, when manifest simultaneously, tend to result in an overall reduction in image contrast.

13.8.2
Gradient Echo

The first practical rapid imaging method was arguably the FLASH (fast low angle shot) sequence, developed by FRAHM et al. (1986), which has spawned a large number of variants known collectively as gradient echo techniques. The name refers to the fact that, in these sequences, the 180° echo-forming pulse is omitted, and the signal is refocused solely by the gradients. EPI versions of the FLASH scans are possible and are the most commonly used method for functional neuroimaging today. Figure 13.8 shows the generalized gradient echo EPI sequence.

The gradient echo EPI sequence is used for several reasons. First, and perhaps most importantly for functional imaging, the contrast behavior includes a T2*, as opposed to a T2 component. That is, the SI decays after excitation at a rate determined by local field inhomogeneities. As described in other sections of this book, it is thought that the dominant mechanism in so-called BOLD functional imaging is the

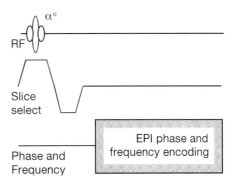

Fig. 13.8. Gradient echo echo-planar imaging (EPI) sequence. In this sequence, the EPI data collection follows a single radiofrequency (RF) pulse, whose flip angle, a, is adjusted to set up the preferred contrast

increased decay rate of the MR signal in the presence of field inhomogeneities produced by deoxyhemoglobin. Thus, an imaging sequence sensitive to such local variations is ideal. In gradient echo EPI it is possible also to use shorter TRs without suffering large signal losses, as the smaller excitation flip angle results in less disturbance from magnetic equilibrium and therefore shorter relaxation recovery times. Gradient echo EPI at frame rates of up to 16 frames/second has been used to produce good quality real-time images of the human heart during the normal contractile cycle (COHEN and WEISKOFF 1991). For non-spin echo scans it is possible to calculate the Ernst angle, α, at which the signal will be maximal for any combination of TR and T1 (ERNST and ANDERSON 1966):

$$\alpha = \cos^{-1}(e^{-tr/T1}), \tag{13.3}$$

Since the ordinary functional imaging application is to acquire a series of EPI scans at a non-infinite TR, the gradient echo methods can confer a slight signal advantage over spin echo studies. This advantage increases at shorter TR.

13.8.3
Offset Spin Echo

By adjusting the relative timing of the Hahn spin echo and the EPI readout module, it is possible to offset the RF echo from the center of k-space. It is by now well-known that the contrast in MR images is dominated by the signal contrast that occurs at the

center of k-space, as this region of the raw data encodes the largest spatial features of the images. In
the offset spin echo method, varying degrees of susceptibility-related contrast are incorporated into the
images. This method has been suggested as an approach to modulating somewhat independently the
signal loss from large and small field perturbers
(BAKER et al. 1992) and as a method for directly
measuring line broadening (HOPPEL et al. 1993). In
the limit, as the Hahn echo is delayed to beyond the
EPI readout, the offset spin echo scan becomes identical to the gradient echo scan. The offset spin echo
method may have increasingly important applications at higher magnetic field strengths where the
inherent functional imaging contrast is greater in
BOLD studies and the artifacts from non-ideal magnetic become more severe. Figure 13.9 shows the offset spin echo sequence.

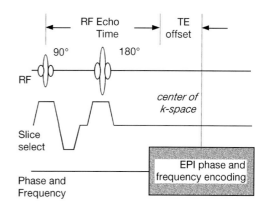

Fig. 13.9. Offset spin echo echo-planar imaging (EPI) sequence. The offset refers to the relative timing of the spin
echo formed by the 90°–180° pulse pair and the center of the
EPI readout period, which ordinarily is the center of k-space

13.8.4
Inversion Preparation

As discussed in the context of fat suppression, the
addition of a 180° inversion pulse prior to the standard spin echo EPI sequence results in an inversion
recovery EPI scan. Such images have easily controlled T1 contrast, according to the equation:

$$SI = k\varrho(1 - e^{-ti/T1} + e^{(te+ti-tr)/T1})e^{-te/T2} \qquad (13.4)$$

where TI is the time between the inversion and excitation pulses. The inversion recovery EPI sequence is
shown in Fig. 13.10.

The inversion recovery method and its several
variants have been used to produced water-sup-
pressed images, similar to the FLAIR method used
conventionally, and have proven useful in the measurement of blood flow and perfusion.

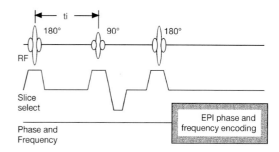

Fig. 13.10. Inversion recovery echo-planar imaging (EPI)
pulse sequence. The addition of a 180° radiofrequency (RF)
pulse at a time, TI, before the standard spin echo EPI scan
results in inversion-recovery contrast behavior

13.9
Volume Echo-Planar Imaging

Echo-planar imaging as typically practiced is a two-
dimensional encoding strategy. In most cases, as
suggested above, the third dimension is provided by
selective excitation. An alternative is to use phase
encoding in the slice selection direction to create a
3D volume image (COHEN et al. 1989, 1991; COHEN
and ROHAN 1989), as shown in Fig. 13.11.

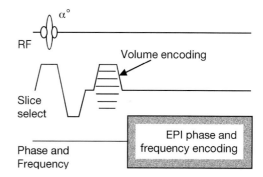

Fig. 13.11. Three-dimensional, or volume echo-planar, scan.
This is a multi-shot echo-planar imaging (EPI) hybrid, in
which an additional phase encoding step is applied along the
slice selection axis with each excitation. After 3D Fourier
transformation, these data yield a contiguous multi-slice image set. The sequence is shown using gradient echo contrast,
though a 180° echo-forming pulse can be added for spin echo
contrast

Volume EPI has theoretical advantages in SNR. Because the same volume is repeatedly sampled, albeit with different phase encoding, the SNR scales with the square root of the number of phase encodes, effectively the number of slices. Thus a 32 slice data set will have nearly sixfold higher SNR than a comparable single slice data set. Using a similar volume sequence, it is possible to collect, for example, a 16 slice volume study of the human heart in only 400 ms (COHEN et al. 1991) This approach should be highly efficient in functional neuroimaging as well, in which contiguous multi-slice image sets are highly desirable. The TR used in the sequence must be reduced by a factor equal to the number of slices to yield the same sampling density. Thus, to acquire an image every 3.2 ms as part of a 32 slice volume, a TR of 100 ms is required. For this reason, shallow flip angle, FLASH-type, imaging is used so that the scanning can be performed at the tissue Ernst angle.

This differs significantly from so-called echo-volumnar imaging (EVI), in which the entire volume is collected following a single excitation pulse (HARVEY and MANSFIELD 1991). As of this writing, EVI is not entirely practical because the extended total readout required greatly exceeds the T2*s of most tissues at clinical field strengths.

13.10
Conclusions

Echo-planar imaging is at this time the fastest and most flexible approach to MRI, offering considerable freedom in the selection of contrast and resolution parameters. It is, however, a technologically challenging method which requires that the imaging system operate at near its performance limits in gradient amplitude and rise times, system stability, and overall noise figure. Further, EPI can suffer from serious artifacts in shape distortion and image ghosts that require extra attention from the researcher. All told, however, the decided advantages of EPI in functional neuroimaging have placed it very much in demand for fMRI applications and have served to drive the technology development both in the academic research laboratory and with major commercial vendors, essentially all of whom now offer EPI products.

Notwithstanding the considerable efforts that have gone into EPI, there are still major advances to be gained. Chief among them will be the practical performance gains that can be achieved with ultra-high performance local gradient coils, which will improve image quality by reducing shape distortions and other bandwidth-related artifacts, while increasing the comfortable operating margin that avoids sensory stimulation.

With the relatively recent dissemination of product level EPI hardware into consumer sites, the future of EPI is rosy indeed and will continue to be driven by the increasingly important clinical applications of functional neuroimaging.

References

Baker J, Cohen MS, Stern C, Kwong K, Belliveau J, Rosen B (1992) The effect of slice thickness and echo time on the detection of signal change during echo-planar functional imaging. In: Society of Magnetic Resonance in Medicine, 11th Annual Meeting, August 8–14, 1992, Berlin, Germany, abstract 1822

Bourland J, Mouchawar G, Nyehuis J, Geddes L, Foster K, Jones J, Graber G (1990) Transchest magnetic (eddy-current) stimulation of the dog heart. Med Biol Eng Comput 28:196–198

Brown T, Kincaid B, Ugurbil K (1982) NMR chemical shift imaging in three dimensions. Proc Natl Acad Sci USA 79:3532–3536

Bruder H, Fischer H, Schmitt F, Reinfelder H-E (1989) Reconstruction procedures for echo planar imaging. In: Society for Magnetic Resonance in Medicine, Eighth Annual Meeting August 8–12, 1989, Amsterdam (abstract 359)

Budinger TF, Fischer H, Hentschel D, Reinfelder HE, Schmitt F (1991) Physiological effects of fast oscillating magnetic field gradients. J Comput Assist Tomogr 15:909–914

Bydder G, Young I (1985) MR imaging: clinical use of the inversion recovery sequence. J Comput Assist Tomogr 9:659–675

Cohen MS Weisskoff RM (1991) Ultra-fast imaging. Magn Reson Imaging 9:1–37

Cohen MS, Rohan M (1989) 3D volume imaging with instant scan. In: Society for Magnetic Resonance in Medicine, Eighth Annual Meeting August 8–12, 1989, Amsterdam (abstract 831)

Cohen MS, Weisskoff RM, Rohan M, Brady T (1991) 400 msec volume imaging of the heart. In: Tenth Annual Meeting of the Society of Magnetic Resonance in Medicine, August 10-16, 1991, abstract 840

Cohen MS, Weisskoff RM, Rzedzian RR, Kantor HL (1990) Sensory stimulation by time-varying magnetic fields. Magn Reson Med 14:409–414

Cohen MS, Weisskoff RM, Kantor H (1989) Evidence of peripheral stimulation by time-varying magnetic fields. In: Radiological Society of North America, Chicago, Illinois (abstract 382)

Cohen MS, Kelley DA, Rohan ML, Roemer PA (1996) An MR instrument optimized for intracranial neuroimaging. Hum Brain Mapping P1A1–007(abstract)

Damadian R, Goldsmith M, Minkoff L (1977) NMR in cancer, FONAR image of the live human body. Physiol Chem Phys 9:97–100

Dickinson R, Goldie F, Firmin D (1989) Gradient power requirements for echo-planar imaging. In: Society for Magnetic Resonance in Medicine, Eighth Annual Meeteing, August 8–12, 1989, Amsterdam, abstract 828

Ernst R, Anderson W (1966) Application of Fourier transform spectroscopy to magnetic resonance. Reviews of Scientific Instruments 37:93–102

Farzaneh F, Riederer SJ, Pelc NJ (1990) Analysis of T2 limitations and off-resonance effects on spatial resolution and artifacts in echo-planar imaging. Magn Reson Med 14:123–139

Frahm J, Haase A, Matthaei D (1986) Rapid NMR imaging of dynamic processes using the FLASH technique. Magn Reson Med 3:):321–327

Hahn E (1950) Spin echoes. Physical Review 80:580–594

Harvey P, Mansfield P (1990) Advances in echo-volumar imaging (EVI). In: European Congress of Radiology (abstract 111)

Hoppel BE, Baker JR, Weisskoff RM, Rosen BR (1993) The dynamic response of DR2 and DR2' during photic activation. In: Society of Magnetic Resonance in Medicine, 12th Annual Meeting, August 14–20, New York, New York, abstract 1384

Ljunggren SA (1983) A simple graphical representation of Fourier-based imaging methods J Magn Reson 54:338–343

Mansfield P (1977) Multi-planar image formation using NMR spin echoes. J Phys C10:L55–L58

Mansfield P Maudsley AA (1977) Medical imaging by NMR. Br J Radiol 50:):188–94

Mansfield P, Pykett IL, Morris PG (1978) Human whole body line-scan imaging by NMR. Br J Radiol 51:921–922

Margosian P (1985) Faster MR imaging – imaging with half the data. In: Society for Magnetic Resonance in Medicine, Fourth Annual Meeting, abstract 1024

Meyer C, Pauly J, Macovski A, Nishimura D (1990) Simultaneous spatial and spectral selective excitation. Magn Reson Med 15:287–304

Pykett IL Mansfield P (1978) A line scan image study of a tumorous rat leg by NMR. Phys Med Biol 23: 961–967

Reilly J (1989a) Peripheral nerve stimulation by induced electric currents: exposure to time-varying magnetic fields. Med Biol Eng Comput 27:101–110

Reilly J (1989b) Cardiac sensitivity to electrical stimulation. Metatec Associates, 10/24/1989, report number MT 89-101

Reilly J (1990) Peripheral nerve stimulation and cardiac excitation by time-varying magnetic fields: a comparison of thresholds. The Office of Science and Technology Center for Devices and Radiological Health, US Food and Drug Administration, Washington DC

Rohan M, Rzedzian R (1992) Stimulation by time-varying magnetic fields. Ann NY Acad Sci 649:118–28

Rohan M (1989) Practical limits to gradient coil design. In: Society of Magnetic Resonance in Medicine, Eighth Annual Meeting, August 8–12, 1989, Amsterdam, abstract 963

Rzedzian R (1987) High speed, high resolution, spin echo imaging by Mosaic scan and MESH. In: Society for Magnetic Resonance in Medicine, Sixth Annual Meeting, abstract 51

Rzedzian R (1988) Method of high speed imaging with improved spatial resolution using partial k-space. US patent number 4,767,991

Schmitt F, Fischer H, Görtler G (1990) Useful filterings and phase corrections for EPI derived from a calibration scan. In: Society for Magnetic Resonance Imaging, works in progress, August 10–16, San Francisco, California, abstract 464

Turner R, Bowley RM (1986) Passive screening of switched magnetic field gradients. J Phys E 19:876–879

Twieg D (1983) The k-trajectory formulation of the NMR imaging process with applications in analysis and synthesis of imaging methods. Medical Physics 10:610–621

Twieg D (1985) Acquisition and accuracy in rapid NMR imaging methods Magn Reson Med 2:437–452

Weisskoff R, Cohen MS, Rzedzian R (1989) Fat suppression techniques: a comparison of results in instant imaging. In: Society for Magnetic Resonance in Medicine, Eighth Annual Meeting, August 8–12, 1989, Amsterdam, abstract 836

14 Spiral Scanning in fMRI

D.C. Noll, V.A. Stenger, A.L. Vazquez, S.J. Peltier

14.1
Introduction

Functional MRI (fMRI) using blood oxygenation level-dependent (BOLD) contrast benefits greatly from high-speed imaging, both for the acquisition of temporal information related to task performance as well as for the reduction of the effects of physiological noise and head movement. The most common imaging methods for MRI involve acquiring data in the two- or three-dimensional Fourier transform space of the object, commonly known as k-space. The spacing of samples in k-space dictates the field of view and the extent of sampling dictates the nominal spatial resolution of the images. The goal of any rapid imaging method, then, is to sample the k-space information with an appropriate spacing and sufficient extent as quickly as possible with a minimum of undesired image artifacts. In this section, we examine the spiral image acquisition method, in which samples are acquired along spiral trajectories

through k-space. Spiral methods have a number of potential advantages over other image acquisition methods, but also some challenges. Spiral acquisitions are generally well-behaved in the presence of motion and flow (Meyer et al. 1992; Nishimura et al. 1995), are very efficient in utilizing available gradient strength, and have multishot variants that can efficiently acquire at high spatial resolution and still provide good temporal information. Many of the potential challenges of using spiral imaging have been addressed by hardware and algorithmic improvements over the last 10 years. For example, eddy current effects have been greatly reduced by the introduction of actively shielded gradient coils (Mansfield and Chapman 1986), high-quality methods for image reconstruction have been developed (O'Sullivan 1985; Jackson et al. 1991), and blur introduced by magnetic susceptibility and field inhomogeneity can be removed by a variety of correction techniques employed in the image reconstruction process. These advantages and improvements have allowed spiral imaging to be used in a variety of applications, including cardiac imaging (Meyer et al. 1992; Brittan et al. 1995) and flow imaging (Nishimura et al. 1995), abdominal imaging (Yacoe et al. 1997), and fMRI (Noll et al. 1995; Glover and Lee 1995). The application of the spiral fMRI technique to the study of basic brain function has been particularly extensive, with numerous high-quality studies conducted using this technique, of which we give a partial listing (Cohen et al. 1994, 1997; Engel et al. 1994; Desmond et al. 1995; Barch et al. 1997; Braver et al. 1997; Gabrieli et al. 1997; Carter et al. 1998; Small et al. 1998; Sobel et al. 1998).

In the following section, the technical considerations for using spiral imaging in fMRI are discussed. This is followed by a description of methods used for correction of physiological noise in spiral fMRI and issues in three-dimensional spiral imaging. Finally, high-spatial resolution and high-temporal resolution acquisition techniques will be demonstrated.

D.C. Noll, PhD; V.A. Stenger, PhD; A.L. Vazquez, PhD; S.J. Peltier, PhD; MR Research Center, Department of Radiology, B-804 PUH, University of Pittsburgh Medical Center, 200 Lothrop St., Pittsburgh, PA 15213, USA
Present address: D.C. Noll, PhD, Department of Biomedical Engineering, University of Michigan, 3304 G. G. Brown, 2350 Hayward, Ann Arbor, Michigan 48109-2125 USA

14.2
Technical Considerations

Spiral imaging typically involves acquisition of samples along an Archimedian spiral path (or trajectory) through k-space. This trajectory was first suggested in a 1981 patent (LIKES 1981). One parameterization of this k-space trajectory for two-dimensional (2D) imaging is:

$$k(t) = \alpha f(t) e^{i2\pi\beta f(t)} \qquad (14.1)$$

where $k(t)=k_x+ik_y(t)$, α and β are scaling factors, and f(t) is a monotonic increasing function of time. The time function, f(t), is typically chosen to satisfy the hardware constraints of a given system. For example, it can be shown that if $f(t)=ct^{1/2}$, then the gradient waveforms that generate the spiral trajectory will have an approximately constant modulus (|G|). An acquisition of this form has several useful benefits. First, for acquisitions in which the peak gradient strength is the limiting factor in gradient design, the sampling pattern will be nearly uniform in density across k-space, which minimizes the noise variance for a given length readout. Since sampling occurs continuously at its maximum rate, a given area in Fourier transform space can be acquired more quickly than other sampling patterns with time- or spatially varying sample densities. Near the center of k-space, the rate of change of the gradients (slew rate) is the hardware constraint that is usually more restrictive than peak gradient strength. This is because the sampling trajectory is tightly coiled requiring the gradient waveforms to change very rapidly. While there are some analytical approximations that can been made (Salustri et al. 1997), the impact of the slew rate hardware limit is generally difficult to quantify. Typically, a numerical solution is required to determine the optimal gradients that satisfy both the peak gradient and slew rate constraints. A graphical design approach is used in most of our studies (Meyer et al. 1996) to insure gradient waveforms that make optimal use of the available gradient hardware.

A spiral trajectory through k-space is smooth, and accordingly time and gradient strength are not consumed in reversing direction of the trajectory. For a desired spatial resolution and a given set of hardware constraints, a spiral acquisition will usually result in a shorter data acquisition period than most other imaging methods, allowing the readout to be shorter than other methods, and thus reducing the effect of magnetic susceptibility and field inho-

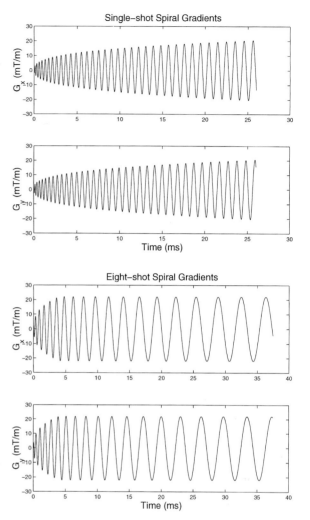

Fig. 14.1a, b. Spiral gradient waveforms optimized for peak amplitude and slew rate gradient constraints of 22 mT/m and 120 mT/m/ms, respectively, for **a** single-shot acquisition and **b** eight-shot acquisition

mogeneity. Moreover, for a desired set of acquisition parameters, a spiral acquisition has reduced hardware requirements when compared to other imaging methods. When comparing different acquisition schemes, it is necessary to make some effort to match spatial resolution. For example, when comparing echo planar imaging (EPI) with spiral imaging, it is necessary to account for the different shapes of the acquisition pattern (EPI is square or rectangular, spiral acquisitions have circular patterns). VAN GELDEREN (1998) found that if k-space area is matched, then the point spread function will have a similar width for square and circular sampling patterns. Table 14.1 contains a comparison of the readout length for EPI and spiral acquisitions for a given set of gradient constraints (peak gradient strength

Table 14.1. Sample gradient designs for spiral and echo planar imaging (EPI) acquisition

Resolution (matrix size)	Acquisition method	Number of shots	Peak gradient strength (mT/m)	Peak slew rate (mT/m/ms)	Readout length (ms)
a. Low (64×64)	EPI	1	22.0	120	30.0
b. Low (72.2 diameter)	Spiral	1	22.0	120	26.0
c. Low (72.2 diameter)	Spiral	1	27.5	120	26.0
d. Low (72.2 diameter)	Spiral	1	22.0	150	23.3
e. High (256×256)	EPI	8	22.0	120	42.3
f. High (288.8 diameter)	Spiral	8	22.0	120	37.5
g. High (288.8 diameter)	Spiral	8	27.5	120	31.2
h. High (288.8 diameter)	Spiral	8	22.0	150	37.1

22 mT/m; peak slew rate=120 mT/m/ms) and a given field of view (24 cm). Rows a. and b. compare these methods for a low resolution, single-shot design (matched for acquisition area) and rows e. and f. compare these methods for a high resolution, eight-shot design. The total acquisition length is reduced by more than 10% for the spiral designs. The gradients that generate spiral acquisitions for high- and low resolution cases are found in Fig. 14.1a and 14.1b, respectively.

While the relationship between hardware limitations and the resultant optimal design of a spiral acquisition is complex, some general concepts can be extracted. For imaging applications that do not require high spatial resolution, the gradient slew rate constraint is more important than the peak gradient strength as a limiting factor for spiral acquisition designs. For high-resolution applications, the peak gradient strength limit is more important. These concepts are also demonstrated in Table 14.1. For the low resolution spiral design (row b.), the effect of increasing the peak gradient strength and peak slew rate by 25% is shown in rows c. and d., respectively. Changing the peak gradient strength had no effect on resultant gradient design since the gradients never reach their peak amplitude (see Fig. 14.1a). Increasing the slew rate constraint did have a substantial effect in reducing the length of the readout. For the high resolution spiral design (row f.), the effects of increasing the peak gradient strength and peak slew rate by 25% are shown in rows h. and i., respectively. For this case, changing the peak gradient strength had a large effect in reducing the length of the readout, but increasing the slew rate constraint had little effect. This is because the waveforms are primarily limited by peak gradient strength for most of the readout as seen in Fig. 14.1b. Finally, the use of multishot acquisition techniques can greatly ease the gradient requirements. For example, if N interleaved

spiral acquisitions are used, then the required peak gradient strength is reduced by a factor of N and the required slew rate is reduced by a factor of N^2. Alternatively, the use of a multishot acquisition can be used for imaging at higher spatial resolution without increasing the hardware requirements or increasing the duration of the acquisition or readout window.

One area in which spiral imaging is more challenging than many other image acquisition techniques is in the reconstruction of images from the set of samples in k-space. For imaging methods in which data are acquired at equally spaced locations along a rectilinear grid, the image reconstruction is simply an inverse 2D fast Fourier transform (FFT). In spiral imaging, the samples, which are located along a spiral trajectory in the Fourier transform space, must first be interpolated to a rectilinear grid prior to performing an inverse 2D FFT. This process is known as "gridding" of the data. While this process is conceptually straight forward, high quality images require attention to the details of the interpolation process. One commonly used and high-quality interpolation method is convolution gridding (O'SULLIVAN 1985; JACKSON et al. 1991), in which the acquired data are spread across the rectilinear grid using a convolution kernel. After performing the inverse 2D FFT, the effects of the convolution process in the Fourier domain can be removed from the image by adjusting the intensity across the image using a function matched to the convolution kernel.

Like all rapid image acquisition methods, spiral imaging is sensitive to the effects of magnetic field nonuniformity. This can arise from inhomogeneity of the main magnetic field or from field distortions related to bulk magnetic susceptibility differences between tissues. This leads to the system center frequency being shifted from the resonant frequency of the tissue of interest, which is known as an off-resonance condition. The impact of field nonuniformity differs by imaging method. In conventional (spin-warp) imaging methods, field nonuniformity results in geometric distortions that are usually very small and are commonly ignored. The sensitivity to magnetic field nonuniformity is much greater in rapid imaging and is due to the long duration of the acquisition readout in these methods. In a manner similar to spin-warp, field nonuniformity in EPI causes geometric distortions, but these are typically larger (several millimeters or more) and, in general, should be corrected. In spiral imaging, field nonuniformity leads to a blurring of the image, which is usually corrected by one of several methods. While there are automatic correction methods that do not require acquisition of a separate map of magnetic field strength, the most commonly applied method makes use of such a map. In fMRI, a magnetic field map can be quickly acquired once per study, minimizing the impact on the overall study duration. Acquisition time for a field map is usually less than 10 s. Once a field map has been acquired, several methods of varying complexity can be used to correct the blur from field inhomogeneity. These range from simple corrections that account for a linear representation of the field map (IRARRAZABAL et al. 1996) to iterative methods (NOLL et al. 1991, 1992) that perform a more complete correction at the expense of computational time in the image reconstruction process. Figure 14.2 contains a demonstration of inhomogeneity corrections applied to a single-shot spiral image. In this example, corrections were required at the front and back of head but not in the center, indicating that the linear correction terms alone would be insufficient to correct for the inhomogeneity-in-

duced blurring and that a full correction (NOLL et al. 1991) of field inhomogeneity is required.

14.3 Physiological Noise Considerations in Multishot Spiral fMRI

With sufficient gradient strength, single-shot spiral imaging can be performed in the same manner as single-shot EPI. One particularly useful form of spiral imaging, however, is the multishot form, which can be used for high spatial resolution imaging or for rapid fMRI using a conventional gradient system. Additionally, the effects of magnetic field nonuniformity can be reduced by increasing the number of acquisitions per image, allowing each to be shorter in duration and thus less influenced by off-resonance effects. Clearly, the use of a multishot technique will come at cost of an increase in scan time, poorer temporal resolution or reduced coverage, but this may be necessary to achieve some other experimental design goal (for example, reduced susceptibility effects). One consequence that is less obvious is the potential increase in image-to-image variation from physiological noise processes, in particular, respiration and cardiac effects. In order for multishot techniques to have a signal-to-noise ratio (SNR) that is equivalent to that found in single-shot imaging, measures must be taken to reduce the effect of the physiological variations.

The presence of signal variations that are linked to the cardiac and respiration cycles is well known

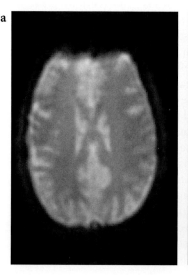 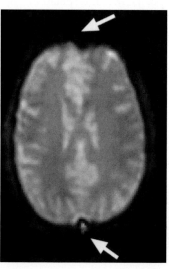

Fig. 14.2a, b. Single-shot spiral, gradient-echo axial slice through the brain **a** before and **b** after correction of susceptibility-induced blurring

(JEZZARD et al. 1993; NOLL et al. 1993; WEISSKOFF et al. 1993), and many techniques have been developed to correct for their effects. In the conventional or spin-warp acquisition technique, these periodic variations lead to a shifting or ghosting of the part of the object that is subject to these variations. In multishot spiral imaging, the manifestation of these variations is inconsistency in the k-space data leading to intensity distortions (for inconsistencies in the low-spatial frequencies) or swirl-like patterns (for inconsistencies in the high-spatial frequencies). In functional MRI, these variations may vary from image-to-image in the time series leading to increased variance and a reduced ability to detect activation signals. For multishot spiral imaging, we have employed several different methods including navigator corrections (HU and KIM 1994; NOLL and SCHNEIDER 1994), oversampling of the low-spatial frequency data in k-space (NOLL et al. 1998), and retrospective estimation and removal from the k-space data (HU et al. 1995; LE and HU 1996). Perhaps the easiest of these techniques to implement is the navigator correction method. In spiral imaging, all of the trajectories begin at the origin in k-space and therefore have the sample of this point in common. Physiological variations that are pervasive across the head will be present and detectable in the samples of the k-space origin. For variations that are nearly constant across the slice of interest, this single sample or "navigator" will be a very good representation of the effect on all spatial frequencies for a given shot in a multishot spiral acquisition. The effect of these variations can then be removed from each acquisition based on the navigator sample. The phase variations associated with the respiration cycle fit this model well, that is, they are nearly constant across each slice, and therefore, navigator correction can provide good correction for this source of variation. Since acquisition of this information requires no modification to the imaging method, we routinely use this correction and have found it to be effective in reducing the time series variance and improving the activation response (NOLL et al. 1998).

Another technique for reducing the effects of physiological noise that can be easily applied to multishot spiral imaging is to provide extra oversampling of the low-spatial frequency data. Since the spiral trajectories begin at the origin in k-space, there is some inherent oversampling that can aid in providing a more accurate measure of the important low-spatial frequencies, which determine the average overall image intensity. By designing spiral trajectories that have a variable sampling density

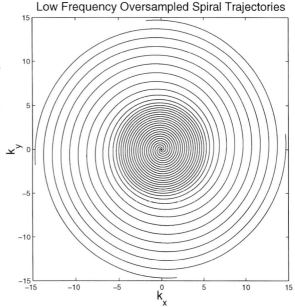

Low Frequency Oversampled Spiral Trajectories

Fig. 14.3. Example of a four-shot spiral k-space trajectory with low-frequency oversampling. The central region (nine samples in diameter) has four times the sampling density as the outer portion of k-space

(MEYER et al. 1993; SPIELMAN et al. 1995; LIAO et al. 1997), additional oversampling can be applied to a broader region of the low spatial frequencies. In Fig. 14.3, we demonstrate a trajectory with extra low-spatial frequency oversampling over a region nine samples in diameter. Use of these oversampled trajectories can be helpful in reducing physiological variation by providing complete sampling of the low-spatial frequency region of k-space with each acquisition of a multishot image. The complete sampling of k-space for each insures that the low-spatial frequency data are fully consistent with each acquisition and therefore, after combining them to make a final image, these data are also fully consistent. Since the low-spatial frequencies contain a dominant part of energy of an image, this technique can have a large effect on reducing image-to-image variations. Use of this technique is relatively simple, requiring only a modification of the design of the spiral waveforms, and comes at the expense of a rather modest increase in readout length (~10%). We have also found this technique to be effective (NOLL et al. 1998) and it is routinely used in our multishot spiral fMRI studies.

The above techniques require no special measures for implementation and use, but may not be able to fully correct for variations that are not manifest in

the central point in k-space or in the low-spatial frequency data. One technique that can be applied to all
spatial frequencies is the retrospective estimation
technique (Hu et al. 1995; Le et al. 1996), in which the
cardiac and respiration variation are estimated for
each k-space point. In its most general form (Hu et
al. 1995), this method requires that the cardiac and
respiration functions be recorded and synchronized
with the scan acquisitions. These waveforms are then
used to evaluate the particular phase of the cardiac
and respiration cycle of each acquisition in a series
of multishot images. For each location in k-space, the
data from each series of images are ordered by phase
of each physiological cycle, and the variation as a
function of position in the cycle is estimated and removed from the data. This is done prior to combining the multishot data together and reconstructing
them into images. For multishot acquisitions, this
must be done prior to image creation, since a reconstructed image will contain data from several different points in the physiological cycles. We have implemented this method for spiral imaging and have
found this to be highly effective in reducing physiological fluctuations in the data (Peltier et al.
1997).

The use of a multishot acquisition technique does
impact the available temporal resolution and the
number of slices that can be acquired, but, in general,
it does not affect the underlying MRI SNR relative to
single-shot methods, provided the image resolution
and readout length are the same. We will look at a
case in which a single-shot and a two-shot acquisition have the same spatial resolution and readout
length. If the TR is held constant, the two-shot acquisition will take twice as long to acquire and therefore
will have one-half the temporal resolution and the
total number of images per slice will be reduced by a
factor of two. The extra acquisition averaged into the
two-shot image will, however, lead to improved image SNR by the square root of two, making the two
single-shot and two-shot acquisitions equivalent in
terms of SNR. Here, the SNR is the same, but temporal resolution has been halved. We now consider a
different case, in which the image-to-image time
(temporal resolution) is held constant, but only one-
half of the number of slices can be acquired in the
two-shot method, but the total number of images for
each slice will be the same. The two-shot method has
a reduced TR and hence signal strength, but if imaging is performed at the optimal flip angle (Ernst
angle), it can be shown that the single-shot and
multishot cases have approximately the same image
SNR (Noll 1995; Noll et al. 1995). In this case, the

number of slices is halved, but the SNR is again unchanged. Therefore, the SNRs of single-shot and
multishot methods are essentially the same. The difference between the methods is primarily a function
of sensitivity to physiological noise. If the physiological noise effects can be eliminated using techniques such as those described above, then costs of
using a multishot technique over a single-shot technique become more clearly defined as a reduction in
volume of coverage or in temporal resolution. The
effects of reduced temporal resolution can be miti-
gated by techniques such as those described below
(Sect. 14.6).

14.4
Three-Dimensional Spiral fMRI

There are several advantages of implementing three-
dimensional (3D) acquisitions in fMRI, including
reduced inter-slice flow (Duyn et al. 1994); higher,
more isotropic resolution (Bomans et al. 1991); and
reduced susceptibility artifacts, resulting from
shorter readouts and thinner slices (Lai and
Glover 1998). Combined with the rapid imaging
characteristics of spiral imaging, 3D spiral fMRI is a
promising technique for acquiring fMRI data. There
are several rapid 3D MRI data acquisition methods
utilizing spiral trajectories (Irarrazabal and
Nishimura 1995). Of these methods, the stacked-
spiral trajectory (Yang et al. 1996), generated from
the 2D spiral pulse sequence by adding phase encoding and rewinding lobes, shows much promise for
fMRI due to its short acquisition time. The following
sections discuss two particularly important applications of 3D stacked-spiral sequence for fMRI data
acquisition: partial k-space acquisitions and physiological view ordering.

14.4.1
Partial k-Space Acquisition

Partial k-space acquisition techniques exploit symmetry properties in the acquired data to reduce imaging time typically by collecting fewer phase encodes (Feinberg et al. 1986; Margosian et al. 1986;
Noll et al. 1991). Reduced imaging time is advantageous for fMRI because of increased temporal resolution. Susceptibility variations, however, destroy the
symmetry properties by introducing imaginary contributions to the imaged object's spin density.

Homodyne detection methods (NOLL et al. 1991) correct for these phase contributions by implementing a phase estimate that is generated from a low resolution image obtained by a slight oversampling (approximately 25% of full k-space) past the zero of k–space. This phase estimate is sufficient only if the true image phase contains predominantly low spatial frequency contributions. This assumption is typically adequate for conventional imaging applications, because these applications normally use either spin echoes or gradient echoes with short TEs (<10 ms). However, optimized sensitivity to the BOLD effect requires gradient echoes with long TEs, which can causes increased phase accumulation and high spatial frequency variations in the phase of the image, particularly for susceptibility variations at tissue boundaries. Therefore, a phase estimate from a low resolution image may be unsatisfactory for accurate image reconstruction. Additionally, there may be time-dependent phase variations making a static high-resolution phase reference impractical. One approach to these challenges is to add static high spatial frequency information to the low resolution phase estimate for each image in the fMRI time-course. By incorporating both time-dependent and high spatial frequency information in the phase estimate, images can be reconstructed from partial k-space fMRI data that are closer to the full k-space images than those reconstructed with standard partial-k techniques (STENGER et al. 1997).

14.4.2
Physiological View Ordering

In a 3D data acquisition, a given image pixel is reconstructed from k-space data which are acquired over a longer period of time compared to a pixel from a multislice 2D data set of identical resolution and field of view (FOV). Therefore, 3D techniques should be more susceptible to physiologically induced motion artifacts than 2D methods. Physiological fluctuations in fMRI are manifested as increased inter-image variation, which could lead to decreased functional sensitivity in the time-course information (JEZZARD et al. 1993; NOLL et al. 1993; WEISSKOFF et al. 1993). Indeed, investigations comparing 2D and 3D spiral acquisitions indicate higher fluctuation noise and decreased functional activity in fMRI data acquired with 3D methods, possibly the result of physiological noise (YANG et al. 1998). Physiological noise minimization, therefore, is an important step required for accurate multishot fMRI acquisitions.

In Sect. 14.3 several strategies are discussed for physiological noise mitigation in multishot spiral fMRI. Another physiological noise compensation method, successfully employed in conventional spin-warp acquisitions, orders the data acquisition such that each view (phase encode or spiral shot) is acquired for only specified values of the physiological phase. In its most common form, this technique is termed respiratory ordering of phase encodes, or ROPE (BAILES et al. 1985). Due to the equivalence between TR and the time between RF pulses, view ordering can easily be extended to 3D. For fMRI applications, the concept of view ordering is simple. The acquisition is ordered such that each view is only acquired during a predetermined value of the physiological phase. As such, in each fMRI image, any ghosting due to physiological noise is placed in the same position with the same amplitude, thereby reducing inter-image variation. The view ordering technique has the advantage that physiological noise reduction is inherent in the data acquisition, requiring no additional assumptions or steps during reconstruction.

To test the efficacy of physiological view ordering, an fMRI experiment was conducted with a 3D spiral sequence for which the spiral interleaves and phase encodes were ordered in real time according to the phase of either the cardiac or respiratory cycle during acquisition (STENGER et al. 1998). The interleaves and phase encodes were distributed linearly across the full range of the physiological period (low frequency sort mode; GLOVER and PELC 1988). It was found that cardiac ordered data acquisitions have a 20% reduction in inter-image variance compared to sequentially ordered acquisitions; equally as effective at mitigating physiological noise as k-space methods (HU et al. 1995). Respiratory ordered data acquisitions show no reduction in variance. The latter is a result of the inefficacy of the view ordering technique due to the close proximity of the respiratory and image acquisition periods for the particular study conducted.

14.5
High Spatial Resolution Spiral fMRI

As described above, one advantage of multishot spiral imaging is the ability to acquire functional images at very high spatial resolution. One example of a high-resolution spiral acquisition is given in Fig. 14.4 in which the motor activation patterns are given

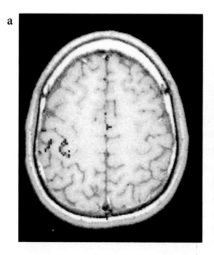
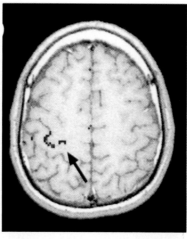

Fig. 14.4a, b. High-resolution (1.6×1.6 ×3.0 mm), four-shot spiral fMRI images at 1.5 T using gradient-echo imaging: **a** finger-thumb sequence task and **b** wrist flexion/extension task. The *arrow* denotes new areas of activation in the wrist flexion/extension task

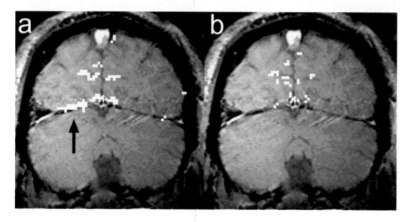

Fig. 14.5a, b. High-resolution (1.5×1.5 ×2.0 mm), eight-shot spiral fMRI images at 3.0 T using a visual checkerboard stimulus: **a** gradient-echo activation map (TE =20 ms) and **b** spin-echo activation map (TE =100 ms). The *arrow* denotes activation signal in the transverse sinus that is removed through use of the spin-echo method

for finger-thumb opposition and wrist flexing movements. This study was conducted at 1.5 T using a four-spiral acquisition with design parameters of peak gradient strength of 16 mT/m, peak slew rate of 120 mT/m per ms, readout length of 28 ms, circular acquisition matrix of diameter 128, and a nominal spatial resolution of 1.6×1.6×3.0 mm. The high-resolution used in this study allows some shifts in the patterns of activation to be visualized.

Because the SNR of MR images is directly proportional to voxel volume, there is a very severe SNR penalty to reducing the linear dimensions of a voxel (volume α cube of the linear dimension). Consequently, improving spatial resolution of fMRI studies may require taking advantage of the improved SNR available from imaging at high magnetic fields (e.g., 3.0 T). Another advantage of imaging at high magnetic fields is that it may allow the use of spin-echo imaging techniques for fMRI, which are potentially advantageous for suppression of vascular signals and reduction of bulk susceptibility dephasing near air/tissue boundaries. Figure 14.5 contains a

demonstration of a high-resolution spiral imaging for both gradient-echo and spin-echo fMRI at 3.0 T for full-field checkerboard stimulation (32 s on/32 s off). This acquisition used an eight-spiral acquisition with design parameters of peak gradient strength of 10 mT/m, peak slew rate of 20 mT/m per ms, readout length of 28 ms, circular acquisition matrix of diameter 135, and a nominal spatial resolution of 1.5×1.5×2.0 mm. The voxel volume in this example is substantially smaller than that commonly used for fMRI studies at 1.5 T (4.5 mm^3 vs the typical 27–60 mm^3). Using a TR of 1 s, the image acquisition time was 8 s for the seven slices studied for both gradient-echo and spin-echo acquisitions. The gradient-echo images used signal averaging over an 8.5 min period and the spin-echo images used signal averaging over a 17 min period. The spin-echo images have reduced SNR overall; however, they exhibit a suppression of vascular signals, both in the transverse between the occipital lobe and the cerebellum and in the smaller vessels in the calcarine fissure.

14.6
High Temporal Resolution Spiral fMRI

Recently, a new class of fMRI studies has been developed based on analysis of data from single-trials or events (BUCKNER et al. 1996; COHEN et al. 1997; COURTNEY et al. 1997; MCCARTHY et al. 1997; ZARAHN et al. 1997). This places demands on the fMRI methods to image with high temporal resolution, which is often in direct conflict with the need to image large parts of the brain at high spatial resolution. One interesting variation on multishot spiral imaging that is helpful for striking a balance between spatial resolution and temporal resolution is the "moving average" reconstruction method. In this method, data are acquired in the usual manner, but during the image reconstruction, a window is used to select the data to be included in the reconstructed image. In the standard multishot image reconstruction, all of the data acquisitions or "shots" necessary for full k-space are acquired before each new image is reconstructed. In other words, for a four-shot acquisition, each new image is generated only after all four-shots are acquired. In the moving average reconstruction, a window surrounding the desired reconstruction time selects the data to be used in the image reconstruction. A different time-point can be gathered by shifting the window to a new reconstruction time. The standard image reconstruction method uses a window to select the data, only that the time-location of the window is set by the location of the first image acquired in a study. These windows can overlap, allowing images to be generated at a finer spacing than in the standard methods. Of course, the additional images generated by overlapping windows do not lead to improved statistical significance because the images are no longer independent samples of the functional activity. Allowing overlapping windows does, however, allow the time-course to be examined on a finer scale without resorting to shifting or jittering the task presentation relative to the image acquisition. The shifting or jittering can all be done in post-processing as part of the image reconstruction.

The standard methods for image reconstruction in multishot imaging equally weight all shots that comprise an image; effectively, this is a rectangular weighting function in time. One possible refinement to the sliding window reconstruction is to interpolate the k-space data to a particular time-point using linear interpolation; effectively, this is a triangular weighting function. Figure 14.6 shows a schematic of the sliding window reconstruction with triangular

weighting function. The rectangular sliding window method has the advantage of having the k-space data used for an image being those data that are closest in time to the "effective time" for an image. The triangular sliding window method, on the other hand, has the advantage that all of the k-space data have an identical "average" acquisition time, the same as the "effective time" for an image. That is, every k-space location is filled with data that are derived by a linear combination of samples acquired before and after the desired time for an image. Additionally, the effective time does not need to fall on a TR interval for the acquisition. This has several potential uses, for example, insuring that all slices in a multislice data set have the same effective time. Typically in a multislice acquisition, different slices are acquired at different times. The moving average reconstruction can shift the effective time for the slices so that they all have the same acquisition time. Another use is aligning data to behavioral effects. Since the effective time can be arbitrarily set, it can be set to external events which could then allow more accurate event-related averaging.

We have used moving window averaging in a study of temporal dynamics in a version of the N-back task using letter stimuli (COHEN et al. 1994; BARCH et al. 1997). In this example, we compare the time-course data for a low-memory load condition (1-back) and a high-memory load condition (3-back). (For a detailed description of the task, see BARCH et al. 1997.) The inter-stimulus interval was 20 s and the imaging was conducted at 1.5 T and used a four-shot spiral acquisition with a 625 ms TR making the image-to-image time 2.5 s. Thus, a total of eight images were acquired over the 20 s period. Figure 14.7a shows a typical time-course for these two

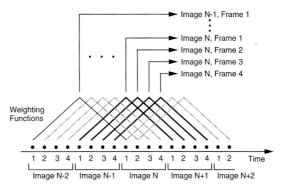

Fig. 14.6. Sliding window reconstruction using a triangular weighting function for a four-shot acquisition. The images from the sliding window data are shown at the *top*, while the images from the standard image reconstruction are denoted at the *bottom* of the figure

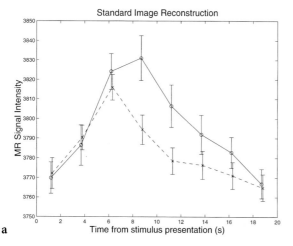

a

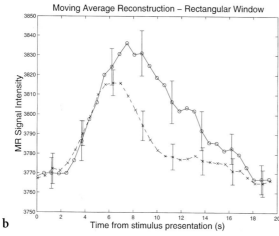

b

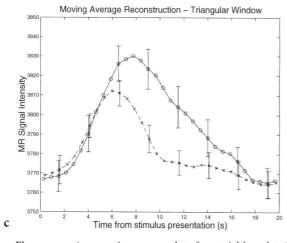

c

Fig. 14.7a–c. Average time-course data for a trial-based task design using the **a** standard image reconstruction, **b** sliding window reconstruction using a rectangular weighting function, and **c** sliding window reconstruction using a triangular weighting function. Task was a 1-back (*dashed line*) and 3-back (*solid line*) verbal working memory task with an intertrial spacing of 20 s

tasks using the standard image reconstruction methods. This time-course is the average signal from a region of interest approximately near Brocca's area. The coarseness of the temporal information makes it difficult to ascertain when, after the stimulus presentation, the fMRI response begins, when the two time-courses deviate in a significant way, when the time-course peaks, and when the time-course returns to baseline. Figure 14.7b and 14.7c demonstrate the time-course data for the same region using the moving average reconstruction method and the rectangular and triangular weighting, respectively. The above features of the time-course can now be much more clearly visualized. The lines between samples in Fig. 14.7a demonstrate linear interpolation performed in the image domain. Clearly, the interpolation performed in the k-space domain (Fig. 14.7c) preserved more detail from the fMRI time-course.

14.7 Summary

Functional MRI using BOLD contrast benefits greatly from high-speed image acquisition. Spiral imaging is a convenient method for rapid fMRI that is applicable to systems with or without high performance gradient subsystems. The methods for image reconstruction and artifact removal have all been refined and are now routine in many laboratories. Multishot methods enable spiral imaging to be used in cases in which gradient performance will not permit single-shot imaging, in which high-resolution is desired, or in which readout lengths must be limited to avoid susceptibility-related distortions. The use of either a single-shot or a multishot method allows for great flexibility in design of the image acquisition. Along with multishot imaging comes challenges related to physiological noise. As discussed above, a variety of methods have been developed that effectively correct for this source of variance. Like EPI, the spiral method can be extended to 3D acquisitions, which opens further schemes for correction of physiological noise. By using a sliding-window image reconstruction, a more detailed presentation of the time-course data can be visualized and more control over the effective time of the imaging data can be achieved. The spiral method is both a flexible and powerful imaging method that is well suited to the study of brain function using MRI.

Acknowledgments. The authors thank Drs. Petr Hlustik, Rao Gullipali, Steven Small, Leigh Nystrom and Jonathan Cohen for use of data presented here. This work was supported by the Whitaker Foundation and U.S. PHS Grant R01-NS32756.

References

Bailes DR, Gilderdate DJ, Bydder GM, Collins AG, Firmin DN (1985) Respiratory ordered phase encoding (ROPE): A method for reducing respiratory motion artefacts in MR imaging. J Comp Assist Tomogr 9:835–838

Barch DM, Braver TS, Nystrom LE, Forman SD, Noll DC, Cohen JD (1997) Dissociating working memory from task difficulty in human prefrontal cortex. Neuropsychologia 35:1373–1380

Bomans M, Hohne K, Laub G, Pommert A, Tiede U (1991) Improvement of 3D acquisition and visualization in MRI. Magn Reson Imaging 9:597–609

Braver TS, Cohen JD, Jonides J, Smith EE, Noll DC (1997) A parametric study of prefrontal cortex involvement in human working memory. NeuroImage 5:49–62

Brittan JH, Hu BS, Wright GA, Meyer CH, Macovski A, Nishimura DG (1995) Coronary angiography with magnetization-prepared T2 contrast. Magn Reson Med 33:689–696

Buckner RL, Bandettini PA, O'Craven KM, Savoy RL, Petersen SE, Raichle ME, Rosen BR (1996) Detection of cortical activation during averaged single trials of a cognitive task using functional magnetic resonance imaging. Proc Natl Acad Sci U S A 93:14878–14883

Carter CS, Braver TS, Barch DM, Botvinick M, Noll DC, Cohen JD (1998) Anterior cingulate cortex, error detection, and the on line monitoring of performance. Science 280:747–749

Cohen JD, Forman SD, Braver TS, Casey BJ, Servan-Scheiber D, Noll DC (1994) Activation of prefrontal cortex in a nonspatial working memory task with functional MRI. Hum Brain Mapping 1:293–304

Cohen JD, Perlstein WM, Braver TS, Nystrom LE, Noll DC, Jonides J, Smith EE (1997) Temporal dynamics of brain activation during a working memory task. Nature 386:604–608

Courtney SM, Ungerleider LG, Keil K, Haxby JV (1997) Hierarchical organization of a distributed extrastiate-prefrontal system for human working memory. Nature 386:608–611

Desmond JE, Sum JM, Wagner AD, Demb JB, Shear PK, Glover GH, Gabrieli JD, Morrel MJ (1995) Functional MRI measurement of language lateralization in Wada-tested patients. Brain 118:1411–1419

Duyn JH, Moonen CTW, van Yperen GH, de Boer RW, Luyten PR (1994) Inflow versus deoxyhemogoblin effects in 'BOLD' functional MRI using gradient echoes at 1.5 T. NMR Biomed 7:83–88

Engel SA, Rumerlhart DE, Wandell BA, Lee AT, Glover GH, Chichilnisky E, Shadlen MN (1994) fMRI of human visual cortex. Nature 369:525

Feinberg DA, Hale JD, Watts JC, Kaufman L, Mark A (1986) Halving MR imaging time by conjugation: Demonstration at 3.5 kG. Radiology 161:527–531.

Gabrieli JD, Brewer JB, Desmond JE, Glover GH (1997) Separate neural bases of two fundamental memory processing in the juman medial temporal lobe. Science 276:264–266

Glover GH, Lee AT (1995) Motion artifacts in fMRI: Comparison of 2DFT with PR and spiral scan methods. Magn Reson Med 33:624–635

Glover GH, Pelc NJ (1988). Method of reducing image artifacts due to periodic signal variations in NMR imaging. U.S. Patent 4,663,591

Hu X, Kim S-G (1994) Reduction of signal fluctuations in functional MRI using navigator echoes. Magn Reson Med 31:495–503

Hu X, Le TH, Parrish T, Erhard P (1995) Retrospective estimation and correction of physiological fluctuation in functional MRI. Magn Reson Med 34:201–212

Irarrazabal P, Nishimura D (1995) Fast three dimensional magnetic resonance imaging. Magn Reson Med 33(5):656–662

Irarrazabal P, Meyer CH, Nishmura DG, Macovski A (1996) Inhomogeneity correction using an estimated linear field map. Magn Reson Med 35:278–282

Jackson J, Meyer C, Nishimura D, Macovski A (1991) Selection of a convolution function for Fourier inversion using gridding. IEEE Trans Med Imaging MI-10(3):473–478

Jezzard P, Le Bihan D, Cuenod C, Pannier L, Prinster A, Turner R (1993) An investigation of the contribution of physiological noise in human functional MRI studies at 1.5 Tesla and 4 Tesla. Proc Soc Magn Reson Med 12th Annu Mtg, pp 1392, New York

Lai S, Glover GH (1998) Three-dimensional spiral fMRI technique: A comparison with 2D spiral acquisition. Magn Reson Med 39:68–78

Le TH, Hu X (1996) Retrospective estimation and correction of physiological artifacts in fMRI by direct extraction of physiological activity from MR data. Magn Reson Med 35:290–298

Liao J-R, Pauly JM, Brosnan TJ, Pelc NJ (1997) Reduction of motion artifacts in cine MRI using variable-density spiral trajectories. Magn Reson Med 37:569–575

Likes RS (1981) Moving gradient zeugmatography. U.S. Patent 4,307,343

Mansfield P, Chapman B (1986) Active magnetic screening of gradient coils in NMR imaging. J Magn Reson 66:573–576

Margosian P, Schmitt F, Purdy D (1986) Faster imaging: Imaging with half the data. Health Care Instrum 1:195

McCarthy G, Luby L, Gore J, Goldman-Rakic P (1997) Infrequent events transiently activate human prefrontal and pariety cortex as measured by functional MRI. J Neurophysiol 77:1630–1634

Meyer C, Hu B, Nishimura D, Macovski A (1992) Fast spiral coronary artery imaging. Magn Reson Med 28:202–213

Meyer CH, Spielman DM, Macovski A (1993). Spiral fluoroscopy. Proc Int Soc Magn Reson Med, 12th Annu Mtg, pp 138, New York

Meyer CH, Pauly JM, Macovski A (1996) A rapid, graphical method for optimal spiral gradient design. Proc Int Soc Magn Reson Med, 4th Annu Mtg, pp 392, New York

Nishimura DG, Irarrazabal P, Meyer CH (1995) A velocity k-space analysis of flow effects in echo-planar and spiral imaging. Magn Reson Med 33:549–556

Noll D, Nishimura DG, Macovksi A (1991) Homodyne detection in magnetic resonance imaging. IEEE Trans Med Imaging 10(2):154–163

Noll D, Pauly J, Meyer C, Nishimura D, Macovski A (1992) Deblurring for Non-2D Fourier transform magnetic resonance imaging. Magn Reson Med 25(2):319–333

Noll DC (1995) Methodologic considerations for spiral k-space functional MRI. Int J Imaging Syst Technol 6:175–183

Noll DC, Schneider W (1994). Theory, simulation, and compensation of physiological motion artifacts in functional MRI. IEEE Int Conf on Image Proc 3, pp 40–44, Austin, Texas

Noll DC, Meyer CH, Pauly JM, Nishimura DG, Macovski A (1991) A homogeneity correction method for magnetic resonance imaging with time-varying gradients. IEEE Trans Med Imaging 10(4):629–637

Noll DC, Schneider W, Cohen JD (1993). Artifacts in functional MRI using conventional scanning. Proc Soc Magn Reson Med, 12th Annu Mtg, pp 1407, New York

Noll DC, Cohen JD, Meyer CH, Schneider W (1995) Spiral K-space MR imaging of cortical activation. J Magn Reson Imaging 5:49–56

Noll DC, Genovese CG, Vazquez AL, O'Brien JL, Eddy WF (1998) Evaluation of respiratory artifact correction techniques in functional MRI using receiver operator characteristic analyses. Magn Reson Med (in press)

O'Sullivan J (1985) A fast sinc function gridding algorithm for Fourier inversion in computer tomography. IEEE Trans Med Imaging 4(4):200–207

Peltier SJ, Vazquez AL, Noll DC (1997) Evaluation of methods of physiological noise correction in spiral fMRI at 1.5 T and 3.0 T. Int Soc Magn Reson Med, 5th Scientific Mtg, pp 1686, Vancouver

Salustri C, Yang Y, Duyn JH, Glover GH (1997). Comparison between analytical and numerical solutions for spiral trajectory in 2D k-space. Proc Int Soc Magn Reson Med, 5th Mtg, pp 1813, Vancouver, BC

Small SL, Flores D, Noll DC (1998) Different neural circuits subservereading before and after therapy for acquired dyslexia. Brain Lang: 62:298–308

Sobel N, Prabhakaran V, Desmond JE, Glover GH, Goode RL, Sullivan EV, Gabrieli JD (1998) Smelling and sniffing: Separate subsystems in the human olfactory cortex. Nature 392:282–286

Spielman DM, Pauly JM, Meyer CH (1995) Magnetic resonance fluoroscopy using spirals with variable sampling densities. Magn Reson Med 34:388–394

Stenger VA, Noll DC, Boada FE (1997) Partial Fourier reconstruction for 3D gradient-echo functional MRI: a comparison of phase correction methods. Magn Reson Med: 40:481–490

Stenger VA, Peltier S, Boada FE, Noll DC (1998) 3D spiral cardiac/respiratory ordered fMRI data acquisition at 3 T. Int Soc Magn Reson Med, 6th Scientific Meeting, pp 297 Sydney, Australia

van Gelderen P (1998) Comparing true resolution in circular versus square sampling. Proc Int Soc Magn Reson Med, 6th Scientific Mtg, pp 424, Sydney

Weisskoff RM, Baker J, Belliveau J, Davis TL, Kwong KK, Cohen MS, Rosen BR (1993) Power spectrum analysis of functionally-weighted MR data: What's in the noise? Proc Soc Magn Reson Med, 12th Annu Mtg, pp 7, New York

Yacoe ME, Li KC, Cheung L, Meyer CH (1997) Spiral spin-echo magnetic resonance imaging of the pelvis with spectally and spatially selective radiofrequency excitation: Comparison with fat-saturated fast spin-echo imaging. Can Assoc Radiol J 48:247–251

Yang Y, Glover GH, Gelderen P, Mattay VS, Santha AKS, Sexton RH, Ramsey NF, Moonen CTW, Weinberger DR, Frank JA, Duyn JH (1996) Fast 3D functional magnetic resonance imaging at 1.5 T with spiral acquisition. Magn Res Med 36:620–626

Yang Y, Glover GH, Gelderen Pv, Patel AC, Mattay VS, Frank JA, Duyn JH (1998) A comparison of fast MR scan techniques for cerebral activation studies at 1.5 tesla. Magn Reson Med 39:61–67

Zarahn E, Aguirre G, D'Esposito M (1997) A trial-based experimental design for fMRI. NeuroImage 6:122–138

15 Optimal Efficiency of 3D and 2D BOLD Gradient Echo fMRI Methods

C.T.W. Moonen, P. Van Gelderen

CONTENTS

15.1 Introduction

Brain stimulation is known to lead to enhanced perfusion which, together with other physiological changes (e.g., blood volume, oxygen consumption)

C. T. W. Moonen, PhD, Résonance Magnétique des Systèmes Biologiques, UMR 5536 CNRS/Université Bordeaux 2, 146 rue Léo Saignat – Case 93, 33076 Bordeaux, France
P. Van Gelderen, PhD NIH In Vivo NMR Research Center, BEIP, NCRR, Building 10, Room B1D-125, Bethesda, MD 20892, USA

results in decreased deoxyhemoglobin levels in the region of neuronal activity (Ogawa et al. 1990a, b). Because deoxyhemoglobin contains a paramagnetic iron, its magnetic susceptibility is high compared to that of oxyhemoglobin, which does not contain a paramagnetic center. Therefore, the magnetic field varies in and around capillaries and veins depending on the local concentration of deoxyhemoglobin and also on the orientation of the vessels with respect to the external magnetic field (Boxerman et al. 1995, Chaps. 9–11, and Chap. 20, this volume). The decreased concentration of deoxyhemoglobin in areas of neuronal activity can be detected by an intensity increase in gradient echo and spin echo functional magnetic resonance imaging (fMRI) methods (Chaps. 11–12, this volume). Because of its high blood oxygen level-dependent (BOLD) sensitivity we will concentrate on gradient echo fMRI methods in this chapter.

Many modern fMRI methods use echo planar imaging (EPI), segmented EPI, or other fast gradient-echo techniques, and repetitively scan multiple 2D slices to achieve a large brain coverage during execution of a specific stimulation paradigm. Several studies have now shown that, because of the small BOLD signal changes upon activation (one to a few percent at 1.5 T), other (non-BOLD and not necessarily local) physiological effects of brain stimulation (enhanced arterial and venous inflow into the observed slice (Duyn et al. 1994, Chap. 7, this volume), enhanced water exchange between capillaries and brain parenchyma (Chaps. 4–6, this volume), stimulus related motion (Hajnal et al. 1994) may also lead to signal changes which may be difficult to interpret unambiguously. Therefore, the sensitivity of BOLD based fMRI techniques should be optimized for blood oxygenation whereas the influence of non-BOLD effects should be minimized. This is especially important when accurate location of brain activity is needed, e.g., for surgical planning (Chap. 44, this volume). In addition, the small changes in BOLD fMRI necessitate careful correction for small rotations and translations between scans and during the scans.

The objective of this chapter is to provide an analysis of the performance of 2D and 3D gradient echo methods for BOLD fMRI. With high performance gradients now available on state-of-the-art clinical 1.5 T scanners and high field research systems, gradient echo EPI methods have become widely available to fMRI researchers. Unfortunately, very fast 3D gradient echo fMRI methods are not yet routinely available, although such methods have potential advantages for fMRI. Central arguments in the discussion are the echo time (TE) dependence of the BOLD effect, maximum available BOLD signal, and signal stability over time due to "physiological noise." Artifacts due to inflow and registration are analyzed for 2D and 3D methods.

15.2
The BOLD Effect as a Function of Echo Time

15.2.1
TE Dependence of BOLD in a Well-Shimmed Magnetic Field

To start with an analysis of optimum BOLD signal, we will first look at the optimum echo time TE of gradient echo fMRI and its consequences for rapid scan fMRI techniques. The phase of the MR signal of water changes with TE under the influence of the local magnetic field. Depending on the amount of deoxyhemoglobin and its distribution in capillaries and veins, the magnetic field varies microscopically within each volume element (voxel). Hence, phase dispersion occurs with increasing TE for the water magnetization arising from different parts of the voxel. When integrating over all water magnetization within one voxel, the MRI signal thus decays with a time constant T_2^*, which is a measure of the extent and distribution of the local variations in the magnetic field over that voxel together with the effect of the transverse relaxation rate T_2. As explained in Chaps. 9–11 the T_2^* value is larger in the activated state than in the rest state because of the decrease in amount of deoxyhemoglobin. In order to determine the TE value at which we will find the maximum BOLD effect we can subtract the T_2^* decay curves in the activated and the rest state. The exact optimum echo time (TE_{opt}) is between the T_2^* value of the resting state (a) and the activated state (b) and can be calculated with Eq. 15.1, in which R_2^* is $1/T_2^*$:

$$TE_{opt} = \frac{\ln(R_2^*(b)) - \ln(R_2^*(a))}{R_2^*(b) - R_2^*(a)} \qquad (15.1)$$

Figure 15.1 shows the T_2^* decay curves of a typical voxel of the human brain at 1.5 T in the activated (T_2^*=75 ms) and resting state (T_2^*=73 ms). The difference between the curves shows that the maximum BOLD amplitude is obtained with a TE of 74 ms. It can also be seen that the difference curve shows a fairly broad maximum. This indicates that the BOLD sensitivity does not critically depend on the exact value of TE. It should be noted that methods with an extended signal acquisition period do not have equal BOLD sensitivity for all acquired data points. In fact, the difference curve of Fig. 15.1 represents a "natural" filter of the data acquired at different echo times and thus influences the actual resolution of BOLD fMRI methods when using extended acquisition periods (such as EPI).

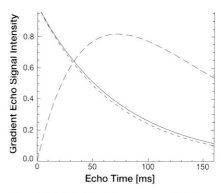

Fig. 15.1. Simulated T_2^* signal decay in a well shimmed voxel during rest (*line with short dashes*, T_2^*=70 ms) and during activation (*solid line*, T_2^*=74 ms). The difference curve is also given (*line with long dashes*), scale ×40, showing a maximum of approximately 2% signal difference at 72 ms

15.2.2
Echo Time Dependence of BOLD for an Inhomogeneous Magnetic Field

The T_2^* value for a voxel is not only determined by the microscopic field heterogeneity due to the presence of deoxyhemoglobin but also by the macroscopic field homogeneity (magnet shimming), and the T_2 relaxation process. We can express the T_2^* process as the sum of those effects:

$$R_2^* = R_2^d + R_{2,mi}' + R_{2,ma}' \qquad (15.2)$$

where R_2^d reflects the T_2 decay including diffusion effects through microscopic field gradients (see

Chap. 11), $R_{2,mi}'$ and $R_{2,ma}'$ the dephasing due microscopic (mi) and macroscopic (ma) effects, respectively. The BOLD effect is predominantly in $R_{2,mi}'$ (decrease upon activation) and, to some extent, in the R_2^d term.

Figure 15.2 shows plots of the magnitude of the BOLD effect as a function of TE for different qualities of field homogeneity. It is evident that not only the magnitude of the BOLD effect depends on the field homogeneity, but also that the optimum TE becomes smaller upon increased field inhomogeneity and that the difference curve narrows significantly upon increased field homogeneity. Therefore, the natural filter for extended acquisition periods changes rather drastically as a function of field homogeneity. Actual resolution in BOLD fMRI methods may thus vary locally as a function of field homogeneity. Since field homogeneity depends on both field strength and resolution, the TE_{opt} should be evaluated for each case specifically.

15.2.3
Typical T_2^* Values for Human Brain at 1.5 T

Figure 15.3 shows histograms of T_2^* values of the human brain at 1.5 T obtained with 3D gradient echo imaging with a range of TE values. The histograms are given for the same brain volume at an isotropic resolution of 1.9 mm, 3.8 mm and 5.7 mm. Only first order gradient adjustment was used for shimming. The distribution of T2* values is rather narrow at high (1.9 mm) resolution, and tends to broaden significantly at low (5.7 mm) resolution. Even at 3.8 mm resolution, many voxels show smaller T_2^* values. At 5.7 mm resolution, 50% of voxels show a T_2^* value below 50 ms, and 20% below 30 ms. Voxels with low T_2^* values are mainly located in cerebellum, frontal and superior cortex, temporal lobes, and near air spaces and irregularly shaped (shimming with higher order gradient shim coils will hardly alter these results). This means that at 1.5 T we have approximately equal sensitivity to BOLD effect (with respect to TE_{opt}) in all voxels when the resolution is 1.9 mm. At 3.8 mm the sensitivity decreases significantly in several brain structures such as cerebellum, frontal and superior cortex and temporal lobe. At 5.7 mm the T_2^* values become much shorter in the majority of voxels. Since macroscopic susceptibility effects scale linearly with magnetic field strength, these results indicate that at 3 T, 4 T, and 8 T, the similar T2* values (due to macroscopic susceptibility effects) will be found at about 3,

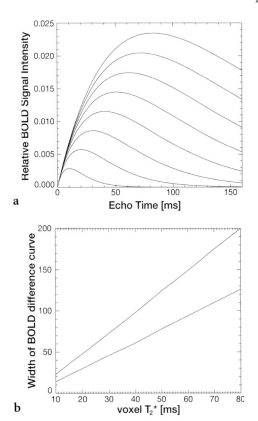

Fig. 15.2. a Magnitude of the BOLD effect as a function of TE for different levels of macroscopic magnetic field inhomogeneity. The graph is obtained with simulations based on Eqs. 15.1 and 15.2. From *top to bottom curve*, T_2^* values for the resting state were 80, 70, 60, 50, 40, 30, 20 ms, and 10 ms, respectively. Note that the optimal echo time and the maximum BOLD effect decrease approximately linearly with decreasing T_2^* values in the resting state. Note also the decreasing width of the curves with decreasing T_2^*, indicated in graph **b** for 75% (*bottom curve*) and 50% (*upper curve*) of the maximum BOLD effect. The decreasing width puts limitations on the duration of the acquisition window of fMRI methods. For example, for a voxel with T_2^*=30 ms, the maximum acquisition period should be approximately 40 ms (range about 15–55 ms) to have at least 75% of the maximum BOLD effects for all data points

2, and 1 mm, respectively for a corresponding decrease in T_2^* values is about 3, 2, and 1 mm, respectively. Note that the slice thickness in many current multi-slice fMRI protocols are often 5–6 mm leading to similar low T_2^* values. For T_2^* values of approximately 20–30 ms, the difference curve in Fig. 15.2 has decreased to such an extent that spin echo methods should become competitive with gradient echo methods.

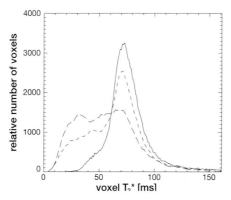

Fig. 15.3. Histograms of the number of voxels with indicated T_2^* obtained from a thick slab through the brain of a volunteer at 1.5 T and comprising the majority of the brain. Histograms are given for the same original data set with isotropic resolution of 1.9 mm (*solid line*), 3.8 mm (*line with short dashes*), and 5.7 mm (*line with long dashes*). Note the strong shift to smaller T_2^* values for lower resolution

15.2.4
Duration of the Acquisition Period in BOLD fMRI

For optimal BOLD effect the TE should be equal to TE_{opt}. How long should the acquisition period be, and what bandwidth should be used? We will later on (Sects. 15.4.4, 15.4.5) come back to the arguments of total imaging time in relation to motion problems, but for the moment we will neglect this problem. Ideally, for maximum signal-to-noise ratio (SNR) in MRI, the acquisition period should be made as long as possible with as low a bandwidth as possible in each repetition time (TR) period. In practical BOLD fMRI, the efficiency and the duration of the acquisition period are limited by the difference curves of Fig. 15.2. In order to have high BOLD sensitivity, while simultaneously reaching high imaging speed, it is advised to limit the acquisition period to the range of TE values for which the BOLD effect is at least 75%. The maximum acquisition period should thus be limited to about 40 ms, 70 ms, and 100 ms for T_2^* values of 30 ms, 50 ms , and 70 ms, respectively. If the signal is acquired at echo times at which the BOLD effect is decreased down to 50%, the duration of the acquisition period can be lengthened. Figure 15.2b shows the maximum duration of the acquisition period for 75% and 50% of the maximum BOLD effect. Long acquisition periods may also lead to image artifacts (distortions) as explained in Sect. 15.3.4 and Chaps. 13 and 14 of this volume.

The difference curves of Fig. 15.2 affect the actual resolution of fMRI images since they form a natural filter over the acquisition window. For extended acquisition periods, the loss in resolution can be analyzed using the point spread function. For example, for a T_2^* period of 30 ms and an acquisition window of 40 ms (see above), 25% loss of image resolution will occur as a result of this T_2^* filter for otherwise unfiltered data, and a 5% additional loss if a cosine window was already used for 25% of the data (leading to a 28% loss in resolution). In practice, this means that identical parameters (matrix size, total duration of acquisition window, bandwidth) for EPI images at 1.5 and 3 T will lead to different BOLD fMRI image resolution in regions where the T_2^* values approach the duration of the acquisition period Unfortunately, resolution in single-shot BOLD fMRI methods at high fields is still mostly (incorrectly) given as the field-of-view divided by the number of encoding steps.

15.2.5
Spatial Variation of Sensitivity to the BOLD Effect

As has been demonstrated previously (BANDETTINI and WONG 1997), the BOLD effect scales with the local blood volume and varies therefore over the brain. Here, we have shown that there is another source of spatial variation of sensitivity to the BOLD effect: the local T_2^* value. Figure 15.3 shows that the effect is noticeable even at 1.5 T at a reasonable resolution of 3.8 mm (slice thickness is generally at least 3 mm, and for whole brain coverage often larger). Please note that the values given in Fig. 15.3 were obtained at 1.5 T. Magnetic susceptibility effects increase linearly with magnetic field strength. Therefore, T_2^* values will decrease significantly at higher field strength. As a result, optimal TE values will decrease accordingly. The maximum BOLD effect will therefore scale less than linearly with field strength (independent of T_1 effects on signal per unit time) for voxels where macroscopic susceptibility effects cannot be neglected.

15.3
Advantages of 3D vs Multi-slice 2D Methods for fMRI

15.3.1
Optimum Signal Amplitude Per Unit Time

In a pure 3D method, the same large volume is excited at the beginning of every TR period by the excitation radiofrequency (RF) pulse, followed by spatial encoding with either one read-out and two phase-encode directions or using spiral or other k-space trajectories. The TR is kept very short for fast imaging, so that TR<<T_1. For multi-slice 2D imaging, the slices are excited sequentially. For typical multi-slice 2D EPI whole brain fMRI protocols, the TR is usually around 3 s for about 20 slices (for spin echo EPI the TR is usually longer). Since TR>>T_1, 90° excitation pulses are used. For 3D MRI and TR<<T_1, the excitation angle is much smaller. For maximum intensity, the optimum flip angle (θ_{opt}) is given as:

$$\cos\theta_{opt} = \exp(-TR/T_1). \qquad (15.3)$$

When comparing the signal intensity per unit time, the 3D methods with small flip angle and short TR show a significant advantage compared to the multi-slice 2D methods with large flip angle and long TR. The theory is identical to that developed by ERNST and ANDERSON (1961). We can express the maximum signal per unit time (S_{max}) as a function of TR/T_1 with Eq. 15.4:

$$S_{max} = \sqrt{\frac{1 - \exp^{-2\,TR/T_1}}{TR}} \qquad (15.4)$$

assuming that the optimum flip angle of Eq. 15.3 has been used. Figure 15.4 shows the maximum signal as a function of TR (for T_1=0.85 s) and demonstrates a significant decrease when TR>T_1 even for optimal flip angle. For the example above, when using multi-slice EPI with a TR of 3 s at 1.5 T (average T_1=0.85 s), the multi-slice method will show about 40% less signal than the 3D method per unit time, of course using otherwise identical parameters such as bandwidth, matrix size and voxel size. In practice, the signal loss is larger since Eq. 15.4 and Fig. 15.4 relate to ideal, rectangular slice profiles. In practice slice profiles have a trapezoidal shape, and therefore overlap of slice profiles will occur to some extent. This

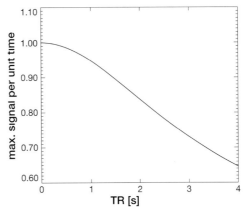

Fig. 15.4. Maximum signal intensity per unit time as a function of TR for T_1=0.85 s when optimal flip angle is used. Short TR periods lead to the highest signal per unit time (intensity 1.0 on the relative intensity scale). Optimal signal decreases significantly for TR>T_1

means that flip angle cannot be optimized for the full slice profile, and signal loss will increase further. For multi-slice spin echo EPI, the losses related to slice profiles are generally larger because saturation effects are related to multiplication of the slice profiles of the excitation and refocusing RF pulses.

Note that 3D methods require spatial encoding in the slab direction. When using phase encoding, the phase of the magnetization in voxels along the slab direction is not coherent, and as a result some signal loss occurs in the imaging experiment along this direction. The amount of signal loss is about 13%. Taken together, the 3D methods have significantly higher signal intensity, in practice about 50% as compared to multi-slice methods with a TR of 3 s at 1.5 T.

15.3.2
Spatial Selectivity: Inflow Artifacts

Because the entire volume is excited in 3D methods by all RF pulses, the saturation level is spatially homogeneous (except for the outer rims of the volume). As a result, changes in inflow of blood will not lead to a different magnetization level. Therefore, 3D fMRI methods generally avoid the confounding inflow effects. Changes in inflow may happen during brain stimulation and may persist in draining veins. For studies requiring accurate localization of the activated areas, such inflow effects should be avoided. Two-dimensional methods, and multi-slice 2D methods show a spatially varying saturation pattern immediately adjacent to the slice. Therefore, inflow effects may occur and investigators should be aware of resulting spatial selectivity problems. Figure 15.5 shows a typical saturation pattern perpendicular to the slice direction in a multi-slice 2D EPI protocol. For comparison the flat saturation profile of 3D methods is also shown in Fig. 15.5. Note that the spatially heterogeneous saturation pattern changes with each RF pulse during every TR period. This changing saturation pattern may also lead to differential sensitivity due to water exchange based on arterial tagging principles (Chaps. 4–6, this volume), independent of the BOLD effect.

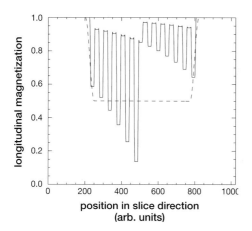

Fig. 15.5. Typical spatially heterogeneous saturation pattern perpendicular to the slice direction in a multi-slice interleaved 2D EPI protocol with 24 slices in 3 s. The longitudinal magnetization is plotted immediately following excitation of slice number 6. The interleaved protocol, consisting of the first 12 even slices followed by the uneven ones, is generally chosen to minimize problems due to slice overlap. For comparison the flat saturation profile of 3D methods obtained with a PRESTO sequence (TR 26 ms, Ernst angle 14°) is also shown (*dashed line*). The spatially heterogeneous pattern of the multi-slice approach changes with every excitation, whereas the homogeneous pattern of the 3D technique remains constant throughout the study

15.3.3
Corrections for Translation and Rotation Between Scans

Small movements of the head inevitably occur during the fMRI study and need to be corrected for (Chap. 26, this volume) as a first step in fMRI data processing. Current correction methods consider the head as a rigid object, necessitating evaluation of six parameters, three translations and three rotations. Three-dimensional images can be easily corrected for such motions. However, multi-slice 2D

scans can give problems for rotations because of the non-rectangular slice profiles. In addition, rotation also leads to modifications of the spatial saturation pattern and thus to modifications in inflow sensitivity.

Since the effects of head motion are often much smaller than the diameter of one voxel, attention must be paid to correct interpolation procedures. Even when this is achieved, interpolation errors may occur, in particular when the image shows high contrast, e.g., between gray, white matter, CSF, skull and "empty" regions. So long as the head can be considered as a rigid body, the six correction parameters can be obtained from the edge of the brain with high accuracy. In order to avoid interpolation errors, it is advantageous to avoid image contrast within the brain. Using $TR \ll T_1$ and scanning with optimal Ernst angle (as used in 3D methods) leads to minimal image contrast since the effects of T_1 and spin density of white, gray matter and cerebrospinal fluid (CSF) on signal intensity are, fortuitously, canceled out. Using long TR periods, image contrast is mainly determined by spin density. Therefore, CSF is hyperintense in such images.

15.3.4
Image Artifacts

With the availability of high quality gradients on state-of-the-art clinical instruments and high field research systems, good quality gradient echo and EPI images can be obtained. Nevertheless, background susceptibility gradients arising from the shape of the object, together with limited gradient ramp times, still lead to some artifacts (Chaps. 12–14, 16, this volume). Such artifacts generally scale with both the duration of the echo train and the magnetic field strength, and can be minimized by using a shortened read-out train. Single-shot methods have limited possibilities to shorten the acquisition period, since all information must be gathered in a single period. Multi-shot methods can limit the duration of the acquisition period, however generally at the cost of total imaging time (except when echo shifting principles are used, see Sect. 15.4.5) and hence increased motion sensitivity (Sect. 15.4.3)

15.4
Signal Stability in 3D and 2D fMRI Methods

The sensitivity of fMRI methods depends not only on the BOLD signal intensity per unit time but also on the signal stability. Usually, "white" noise is not the factor that dominates signal instability, rather fluctuations due to head motion and physiological effects arising from the cardiac and respiratory cycles tend to be major sources of physiological noise. These effects are one of the main drawbacks of 3D methods and need to be carefully corrected for if the inherent advantages of 3D methods are to be realized.

15.4.1
Cardiac and Respiratory Cycle

A typical plot of the phase of the MR signal as a function of time is shown in Fig. 15.6. The results were obtained with a navigated 3D gradient echo MRI sequence (principles of echo shifting with a train of observations, PRESTO, see below). The signal represents an average over the whole brain volume. The cardiac cycle is recognizable as sharp peaks and the breathing as a slow rolling of the baseline. These effects are well above the noise level, and severely affect signal stability. Chapter 16 describes the origin of these instabilities, such as minor head motion, CSF pulsation and distribution of molecular oxygen around the head and in the nasal cavity. Two-dimensional single-shot EPI methods have a total duration that is much below the respiratory cycle. In contrast, even the fastest 3D methods require a total imaging time that is a significant fraction of the respiratory cycle. This the main reason that 3D fMRI methods show less signal stability than 2D single-shot EPI methods. Whereas instabilities due to the cardiac cycle can be easily eliminated by reacquiring data that were obtained during the sharp peaks in Fig. 15.6, corrections for physiological noise during the respiratory cycle are more difficult to accomplish because those effects are rather evenly spread out over the full cycle. What strategies can be followed to correct for such effects? We will look below at the use of navigator echoes, increasing speed, and gating to cardiac and/or respiratory cycle.

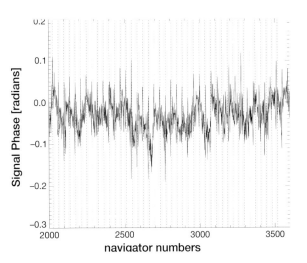

Fig. 15.6. Signal phase of the center of k-space as a function of time during 42 s, with one data point per 26 ms (every fourth point is plotted here for reasons of clarity). The evolution of this zero order navigator signal was measured using the PRESTO method of the full brain with additional gradients in all three principal axes. Note the sharp deviations with the frequency of the cardiac cycle, and the slow rolling evolution with the respiratory cycle

15.4.2
Navigators in 3D and 2D fMRI Methods

The use of navigators for fMRI, and in particular for EPI, is discussed in Chap. 16. Navigator echoes can be very simple, such as a single data point, indicating phase stability of the center of k-space; slightly more complex, such as a read-out gradient without phase encoding; or more complex, such as 2D navigators that describe a circle or spiral in k-space; and even 3D navigators. The use of a single point allows evaluation, and correction, of displacement in the direction of gradients used. The more complex navigator echoes allow evaluation of more than one head motion parameter. Because of the increased instabilities in 3D BOLD methods, the advantages of navigators in 3D methods can be significant. For example, VAN DER VEEN et al. (1997) showed that the use of the simplest navigator in a 3D PRESTO fMRI method (see below) increased the signal stability by about 30%. Total scan duration was 2.5 s per 3D volume. Even after correction, the signal instabilities, as measured by determining the standard deviation, in a series of identical images, was at least twice the white noise in gray and white matter, indicating that the navigator echo allowed only partial correction of physiological noise. More complex navigator echoes may allow further correction. CSF motion is clearly another factor of signal instability. Standard deviation maps obtained from a series of 3D PRESTO volume images clearly show CSF with higher instabilities than gray and white matter. CSF suppression may therefore improve signal stability. However, methods like inversion recovery in 2D methods, or the use of large flip angles in 3D methods (both methods leading to CSF suppression based on its long T_1), cost too much time or lead to other signal instabilities.

15.4.3
Gating in fMRI

The cardiac and/or respiratory cycle can be independently monitored, and fMRI scanning can be started at predetermined time points. However, because of variations in the duration of the cardiac cycle, a varying saturation level will occur leading to variations in the signal intensity which are comparable to, or greater than, those produced by the BOLD effect unless a very long TR is used (at least three times the T_1 of water). Obviously, such a TR is inefficient, and thus gating methods are rarely used in fMRI.

15.4.4
Shortening Total Imaging Time of 3D fMRI

Increasing imaging speed may increase signal stability, in particular when the total imaging time becomes less than the duration of the respiratory cycle. This is evident from Fig. 15.6. For example, when using 3D PRESTO fMRI with total imaging times of 6 s and 2.5 s, by increasing gradient strengths (and read-out bandwidth), white noise was increased but signal instability was virtually unaffected, allowing more time points to be measured during the study and thus increasing statistical power. Unfortunately, gradient performance in current state-of-the-art scanners is limited by safety considerations, in particular avoiding inadvertent nerve stimulation by too high a gradient ramp speed. Therefore, increasing speed (while sampling the same BOLD difference curves of Fig. 15.2) cannot be realistically expected from even faster gradient systems. Instead, a further decrease in total imaging time may come from partial, and/or more efficient, k-space scanning strategies or, alternatively, by the use of echo shifting principles allowing TE>TR in gradient echo imaging.

15.4.5
The Advantage of Echo Shifting in the PRESTO Method

The echo-shifting principle was recently developed to allow fast gradient echo MRI with TE>TR (MOONEN et al. 1992). The gradient echo is shifted in these methods towards the next TR period (or even beyond, LIU et al. 1993a) using gradient pulses that dephase the primary gradient echo, and rephase the shifted echo. In the preferred implementation, two gradient pulses are used with relative intensities –1, and +2 immediately following and immediately prior to the RF pulse, respectively (see VAN GELDEREN et al. 1995 for details). This approach increases the efficiency when a relatively long TE should be used, e.g., for bolus tracking through the brain, for temperature mapping, and also for BOLD fMRI. Note that the method, when used for BOLD fMRI, does not lead to an increase in BOLD signal amplitude per unit time. Rather, the increased speed leads to better signal stability. For example, VAN DER VEEN et al.(1997) compared optimal signal and signal stability of a 3D segmented EPI fMRI of the brain with and without echo shifting (using a total imaging time of 2.5 s and 5.0 s, respectively. Optimal signal strength per unit time was identical, but signal stability was improved by about 25%. Note that the additional gradients used for the echo shifting procedure also lead to some additional signal instability. A single point navigator echo was used to partially correct for this. The segmented (multi-shot) EPI method with echo-shifting principles is called the PRESTO method (principles of echo shifting with a train of observations, LIU et al. 1993b).

The 3D PRESTO has an additional inherent benefit for fMRI, namely, the suppression of signals from within large draining veins, with the principle being similar to the use of "diffusion weighted" gradient echo fMRI methods. As mentioned previously, it is possible that the vein draining a large activated area shows a large BOLD effect extending downstream from the region of neuronal activity. It has been previously demonstrated that a bipolar gradient may eliminate arterial and venous signal because of the phase dispersion resulting from the flow profile in the direction of the gradient. The gradient pulses required by 3D PRESTO for the elimination of the direct gradient echo and the selection of the echo shifted signals will also cause a phase distribution of spins in the vasculature due to the velocity profile of the laminar flow. For example, GRANDIN et al. (1997) measured the average velocity of the large pial veins in the central sulcus using a 2D phase contrast angiographic method. The average velocity was 18 mm/s during rest and 22 mm/s during finger tapping (n=3), corresponding with the known velocity increase during activation (see also Chap. 8, this volume). Based on simulations, it was concluded that the intravascular signals are suppressed in the PRESTO technique on the condition that the average velocity is at least 15 mm/s in the direction of the additional gradients. Indeed, the fMRI signal detected in the voxel containing the pial vein draining the primary sensory motor cortex showed a decrease in difference BOLD signal of 5%–1% when using the additional gradients of the PRESTO method in a 3D fMRI method.

The attenuation of vessel signal due to dephasing resulting from the flow profile has been called, rather unfortunately, diffusion weighting. The term suggests a random incoherent effect. However, the dephasing is in fact coherent and can be reversed. Note that, therefore, dephasing cannot be made direction insensitive by applying consecutive bipolar gradients in the three principal directions. It should also be mentioned that, despite the attenuation of the intravascular draining vein BOLD signals in the PRESTO sequence, the extravascular draining vein BOLD signals still persist when using PRESTO, like any other gradient echo fMRI method.

Figure 15.7 shows an example of a 3D BOLD fMRI experiment during a categorical verbal fluency task

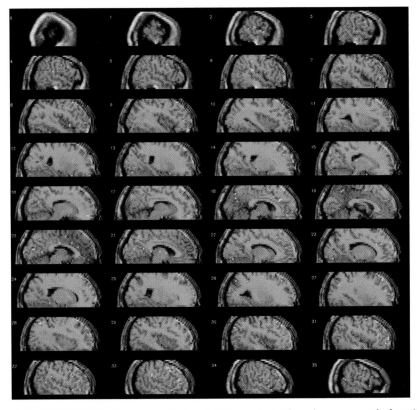

Fig. 15.7. Example of 3D PRESTO fMRI using a categorical verbal fluency task. The volunteer was asked to visualize the objects but to remain silent. Activated voxels are overlaid in color onto anatomical maps. The full 3D volume is represented here as 36 consecutive sagittal slices. Activity can be noticed bilaterally in Broca and Wernicke's area (language), anterior cingulate, dorsolateral frontal cortex bilaterally (working memory), calcarine fissure (visualization). Data were obtained using a Philips 1.5 T scanner with state-of-the-art PowerTrac 6000 gradients (amplitude 23 mTm^{-1} and maximum ramp speed of 115 Tm^{-1}s^{-1}) using the PRESTO method. TR was 26 ms, TE 37 ms. Seventeen echoes per TR period were acquired (maximum difference in TE was 18 ms). Matrix size was 64×51×22. Nominal resolution was 3.75 mm in all directions. Total time was 2 s per 3D volume. Additional gradients were 1.3 and 1.6 s for the first and second additional gradient pulses of each TR with strength 11, 11 and 16 mTm^{-1} for the x, y and z gradient, respectively. Before each echo train, a zero order navigator echo was acquired allowing a correction for translation in the direction of the additional gradients. Total duration of the study was 8 min with 30 s periods of rest and stimulation. All images were registered to the last 3D image. Statistical analysis was performed based on t statistics with a threshold omnibus p value of 0.05. A Bonferroni correction was applied for the total number of voxels in scanned brain tissue

using the PRESTO method, demonstrating activation in areas known to be involved in language, working memory, and visualization tasks.

15.4.6
Spiral, EPI and Other 3D Methods

Image information should be sampled as efficiently as possible during the optimal period in the BOLD difference curves of Fig. 15.2. We have seen in the previous sections that acquisition speed is also of prime importance to achieve signal stability, in particular in 3D methods. Because of the TE dependency of the BOLD effect, scanning should be limited to echo times during which the BOLD effect is larger than 75% (or possibly down to 50%) of the maximum BOLD effect. Several k-space scanning strategies have been suggested for improved efficacy. For example, a spiral scan has the advantage of a continuous acquisition without any time gaps, whereas in blipped EPI (the most used variant, see Chap. 13) the acquisition is interrupted during each blip of the phase encoding gradient (generally even when ramp sampling is used). Unfortunately, the most efficient spirals are rotationally symmetric, and thus lead to square field-of-views. For the average human brain, the length in the posterior-anterior direction is about 20% longer than the left-right direction, and almost double that of the inferior-superior direction. As a result, rectangular field-of-views adjusted to the brain dimensions are more time-efficient. Therefore, the spiral method may not be advantageous compared to a rectangular scanning pattern in this respect. However, the spiral method may have other significant advantages (Chap. 14, this volume). Since each spiral starts at the center of k-space, the first point may be used as a navigator signal. In addition, flow artifacts have a different pattern and are less obvious in the resulting images. When used for 3D fMRI, spiral methods often use a conventional phase encode in the third (slab) direction (YANG et al. 1997; LAI and GLOVER 1997). The volume variant of single-shot EPI, called echo volume imaging (EVI), has also been proposed; however, this is not a practical fMRI method, since the acquisition time becomes much longer than the difference curves of Fig. 15.2. Alternatively, 3D EPI may be accomplished by a volume 2D EPI followed by a conventional phase encode in the third direction. However, the method then loses its speed advantage with respect to the respiratory cycle, and it may then be more advantageous to optimize the ac-

quisition window with respect to the BOLD information, as in Fig. 15.2.

Another significant gain in speed can be obtained by partial k-space scanning and processing the data using the complex conjugate for the remainder of k-space. In principle, a 50% gain in speed can be obtained. Although possible in principle, the method is considerably more complex for gradient echoes with a long acquisition window, since the signal evolution under the influence of the local magnetic field has to be taken into account (contrary to spin echo methods). Thus, field maps might be obtained in order to predict that evolution. Because of the importance of speed, especially in 3D fMRI methods, it is hoped that such partial k-space methods will nevertheless become available for gradient echo fMRI.

15.5
Summary and Discussion

Efficiency of fMRI methods depend strongly on the T_2^* of the voxel. The T_2^*, in turn, strongly depends on both resolution and field strength. In addition, the T_2^* modifies the actual resolution in BOLD fMRI images, when a long acquisition window is used, such as in EPI (in particular in 128+128 matrices or greater at 1.5 T or even 64+64 at 3 T and above). Three-dimensional methods have significant advantages over multi-slice 2D methods: (1) optimum BOLD signal amplitude per unit time; (2) optimal T_2^* weighting over the full k-space; (3) avoidance of confounding inflow effects; (4) straightforward correction for head motions between the scans; (5) improved image quality due to relatively short echo train. The disadvantage of 3D scans is the increased influence of physiological noise, in particular signal instabilities due to the respiratory cycle. Navigator echoes can be used to partially correct for these effects. The echo shifting principle, as employed in the 3D PRESTO methods, leads to a significant increase of imaging speed, and hence to a reduction of signal instabilities, in particular when total imaging time per 3D volume is brought below the duration of the respiratory cycle. With current methods, the stability of 3D PRESTO (comprising 32 slices) with a total imaging time of 2 s is approximately equal to that of multi-slice single-shot EPI.

Because of the recent importance of single event fMRI (Chaps. 21, 36, this volume), it is useful to discuss the relative merits of 2D and 3D methods in this respect. Capturing the hemodynamic response is a crucial element in event-related fMRI. Therefore, two methodological factors need to be considered: temporal resolution and inflow effects. Relatively little work has been presented on the natural variation of latencies in the vascular response. Bandettini (Chap. 19) provides arguments for a range of about 4 s. This would imply that the temporal resolution should be significantly faster than 4 s, say about 2 s. Inflow effects could represent a confounding factor in the experimentally observed range of latencies. Avoiding inflow effects in 3D methods may enhance the precision of the detection of the hemodynamic response (although the extravascular BOLD effect of large draining veins will persist even in 3D gradient echo methods). The temporal resolution of 3D methods is of course inferior to that of 2D methods. Further research in single-event fMRI is needed before the required temporal resolution can be determined, and before the question can be answered whether 3D methods can reach the required temporal resolution. Currently, total imaging times of less than 2 s can be reached for PRESTO 3D fMRI scans using high performance gradients on routine clinical 1.5 T instruments.

Acknowledgments. The authors thank Philipe Thévenaz for making his 3D registration software available to us. We thank Nick Ramsey for Fig. 15.7, Richard Jones and Thomas Loenneker for discussions.

References

Bandettini PA, Wong EC (1997) A hypercapnia based normalization method for improved spatial localization of human brain activation with fMRI. NMR Biomed 10:197–203

Boxerman JR, Hamberg LM, Rosen BR, Weiskoff RM (1995) MR contrast due to intravascular magnetic susceptibility perturbations. Magn Reson Med 34:555

Duyn JH, Moonen CTW, de Boer RW, van Yperen GH, Luyten PR (1994) Inflow versus deoxyhemoglobin effects in "BOLD" functional MRI using gradient echoes at 1.5 T. NMR Biomed 7:83–88

Ernst RR, Anderson WA (1966) Application of Fourier transform spectroscopy to magnetic resonance. Rev Sci Instrum 37:93–102

Grandin CB, Madio DP, Van Gelderen P, Moonen CTW (1997) Reduction of undesirable signal of large veins in functional MRI with PRESTO. Magn Reson Mat Phys Biol Med 5 [Suppl]:14

Hajnal JV, Mayers R, Oatridge A, Schwieso JE, Young IR, Bydder GM (1994) Artifacts due to stimulus correlated motion in functional imaging of the brain. Magn Reson Med 31:289–291

Lai S, Glover GH (1997) Three-dimensional spiral fMRI technique: a comparison with 2D spiral acquisition. Magn Reson Med 39:68–78

Liu G, Sobering G, Olson AW, Van Gelderen P, Moonen CTW (1993a) Fast echo-shifted gradient-recalled MRI: combining a short repetition time with variable T_2^* weighting. Magn Reson Med 30:68

Liu G, Sobering G, Duyn J, Moonen CTW (1993b) A functional MRI technique combining principles of Echo-Shifting with a train of observations (PRESTO). Magn Reson Med 30:764

Moonen CTW, Liu G, van Gelderen, Sobering G (1992) A fast gradient-recalled MRI technique with increased sensitivity to dynamic susceptibility effects. Magn Reson Med 26:184

Ogawa S, Lee TM, Nayak AS, Glynn P (1990a) Oxygenation-sensitive contrast in magnetic resonance imaging of rodent brain at high magnetic fields. Magn Reson Med 14:68

Ogawa S, Lee TM, Ray AR, Tank DW (1990b) Brain magnetic resonance imaging with contrast dependent on blood oxygenation. Proc Natl Acad Sci USA 87:9868

Van der Veen JW, Van Gelderen P, Weinberger DR, Moonen CTW (1997) Characterization of brain motion with a 3D navigator and reduction of motion artifacts in PRESTO. Proc Int Soc Magn Reson Med, 12–18 Apr 1997, Vancouver, Canada, p 466

Van Gelderen P, Ramsey NF, Liu G, Duyn JH, Frank JA, Weinberger DR, Moonen CTW (1995) Three dimensional functional MRI of human brain on a clinical 1.5 T scanner. Proc Natl Acad Sci USA 92:6906

Yang Y, Glover GH, van Gelderen P, Patel AC, Mattay VS, Frank JA, Duyn JH (1997) A comparison of fast MR scan techniques for cerebral activation studies at 1.5 Tesla. Magn Reson Med 39:61–67

16 Physiological Noise: Strategies for Correction

P. Jezzard

CONTENTS

16.1 Introduction

The magnitude of signal changes observed in the various functional MRI methods (BOLD-based contrast, perfusion-based contrast, etc.) is often quite small. Even for functional tasks involving primary sensory or primary motor areas, the fractional change in MRI signal attributable to neuronal activity for most techniques described in this volume is usually less than ≈4%. For more subtle cognitive tasks, for example working memory tasks, or for single event fMRI studies (e.g., Josephs et al. 1997a), the magnitude of the signal changes can be on the order of 1% or less.

Given these small effects, all methods that can improve signal-to-noise ratio or signal-to-artifact ratio ideally should be incorporated into the experiment. Such considerations include the optimization of scanner hardware (such as highly stable radiofrequency amplifiers, state-of-the-art gradient coil amplifiers, and a low noise figure receiver subsystem), careful head immobilizing devices or post-hoc image re-registration (e.g., see Chap. 26), and optimized pulse sequences and perhaps even a specialized magnetic field strength (see Chap. 25, Sect. 25.4).

An additional source of artifact induced in many functional imaging techniques that use MRI is the effect that physiological processes (principally respiration and heart beat) have on the MRI signal (Weisskoff et al. 1993; Jezzard et al. 1993). In fact, respiratory and cardiac motion can induce substantial artifact even in conventional clinical imaging, particularly (and obviously) in imaging of the thorax and abdomen. Hence, a literature has developed to address the problems of these gross physiological artifacts. Simple methods, such as breath holding and respiratory gating, have been implemented. Other more complicated methods include those that order the acquisition of specific phase-encode lines to correspond to particular points in the respiratory cycle (Bailes et al. 1985). Similarly, cardiac gating can be used to correct unwanted cardiac influences in conventional MRI of the heart. In the case of more peripheral imaging, in which cardiac-related pulsatile flow effects cause artifacts (rather than direct bulk motion), gradient moment nulling may be used (for references see, e.g., Ehman and Felmlee 1990).

In fMRI of the brain the artifacts induced by physiological effects are less dramatic than in the thorax. Nevertheless, when all other experimental conditions are optimized it is the physiological processes that dominate the "noise" in the image, or more precisely the temporal stability of the image over repeated acquisitions. With functional imaging techniques that employ FLASH or other two dimensional Fourier transform (2DFT) sequences requiring multiple acquisitions to form an image, ghosting will be induced in the image background along with intensity and phase fluctuations in the image itself. For snapshot techniques, such as snapshot spiral imaging or snapshot echo planar imaging (EPI), more localized intensity variations are induced in the image which are attributable to the physiological processes. For both conventional and snapshot sequences, the physiological processes lead to apparent noise in the time course of the pixels over multiple acquisitions. This is illustrated in Fig. 16.1, which shows power spectra obtained by Fourier transform-

P. Jezzard, PhD, FMRIB Centre, John Radcliffe Hospital, Headington, Oxford OX3 9DU, England

ing the pixel intensity time course taken from small regions of the brain. Fig. 16.1a and 16.1b show the power spectra of the noise for EPI data collected with a scan repeat time of 200 ms at 1.5 Tesla, and Fig. 16.1c and 16.1d show the power spectra of the noise for EPI data collected at 4.0 Tesla. For these data sets the subject was lying still in the magnet and no neurological task was being performed. Significant power in the noise spectra are nevertheless seen at the cardiac frequency ($\approx$0.9 Hz) and its harmonics and at the respiratory frequency ($\approx$0.3 Hz) and its harmonics.

16.2
Theory of Physiological Artifacts in fMRI

16.2.1
Respiratory Effects

Often, the largest source of physiological artifact in fMRI time series is caused by respiration. This is revealed as signal changes which correlate with the breathing cycle. Of particular concern are those blocked fMRI paradigms that have a period which is similar to the respiration period (approx. 4–10 s). Under these conditions it is possible to confound the functional signal of interest with regions of the brain that show strong respiration signal changes.

Experiments which have been performed to determine the origin of respiration-related artifacts have indicated that the effect is largely ascribable to small magnetic field shifts induced in the brain which in turn are caused by gross magnetic susceptibility changes as the lungs in the chest cavity expand and contract. These magnetic field shifts have been measured (NOLL and SCHNEIDER 1994a,b; WOWK et al. 1997a) and have values for maximum inspiration minus maximum expiration of 0.01 ppm at the most superior part of the brain, increasing to 0.03 ppm at the base of the brain (closest to the chest cavity). Figure 16.2 shows the maximum field deviation in the brain over the respiratory cycle in sagittal and coronal views. The figure also shows that the field shifts increase as $1/r^3$ with decreasing distance to the chest (WOWK et al. 1997b), implying that any correction scheme should account for this nonlinear distribution.

Taking some concrete scanning parameters to demonstrate the effect of these field shifts, let us assume a field strength of 2 Tesla and a gradient echo sequence with an echo time (TE) of 40 ms. The field shift at the level of the orbits (roughly 0.015 ppm) will induce phase variations in the received signal of:

$$360 \times \gamma \Delta B_0 TE = 18° \tag{16.1}$$

where γ is in units of Hz/Tesla. Such respiratory-induced phase variations will lead to wave-like ghosting artifacts in conventional imaging sequences, such as FLASH, which require multiple excitations to acquire a complete image, and in interleaved fast imaging sequences, such as interleaved EPI or interleaved spiral sequences. It should also be noted that

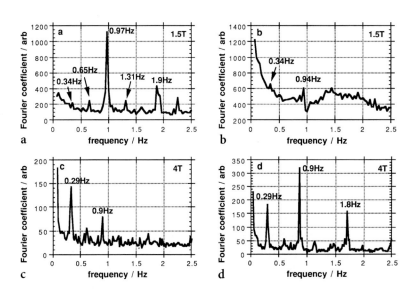

Fig. 16.1a–d. Noise spectra generated by pixel-by-pixel Fourier transformation of 128 single slice echo planar images collected from the brain of a normal volunteer who was lying at rest in the magnet. **a, b** Data obtained at 1.5 Tesla with a TR of 200 ms and a TE of 40 ms. **c, d** Data obtained at 4 Tesla with a TR of 200 ms and a TE of 26 ms. Cardiac and respiratory peaks are evident, along with their harmonics

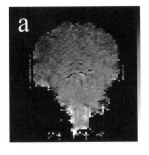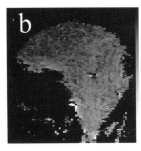

Fig. 16.2a,b. Coronal (**a**) and sagittal (**b**) field maps within the brain generated by subtracting a phase map collected at full expiration from a phase map collected at full inspiration. The magnetic field excursions have values ranging from approx. 0.01 ppm (superior extent) to 0.03 ppm (inferior extent). (Data kindly provided by B. Wowk, M.C. McIntyre and J.K. Saunders, National Research Council Canada)

since the field shifts exhibit a field gradient across the brain (predominantly in the inferior-superior direction) there will also be some fluctuations in signal intensity resulting from intra-voxel dephasing of signal. Experiments by Noll and Schneider (1994a) showed amplitude fluctuations of ±2% for signal collected over an entire slice with a gradient echo time of 40 ms at 1.5 Tesla.

Since, currently, snapshot EPI is the most commonly used pulse sequence for fMRI experiments, it is worth discussing in more detail the effects that field shifts of the sort shown in Fig. 16.2 will have on image quality. Noting that the field shifts vary most in the inferior-superior direction, the effects of respiration will depend partly on the physical axes chosen for the read, slice and phase-encoding directions:

In the axial plane, the collected images will experience small, spatially invariant, zero order phase shifts as the magnetic field changes. The small change in field gradient in the slice direction (≈0.3 Hz/cm over the respiratory cycle) will lead to a small amount of intra-slice dephasing and also to a tiny (<0.02 mm) displacement in the location of the slice, depending on where the slice select radiofrequency pulse falls within the cycle.

In the sagittal and coronal planes, EPI images may be more affected, especially if the phase-encode direction corresponds to the inferior-superior direction. Under these conditions, the respiration-related changes in local magnetic field gradient will cause some (probably nonlinear) scaling of the image (stretching or shrinking) in the phase-encode direction. Towards the edges of the image, this may cause mis-registrations in the images of up to 0.1 pixels.

These effects would be expected to cause respiratory-related artifact most prominently near tissue boundaries (e.g., sulci), which is in agreement with what is observed experimentally.

Finally, the likelihood should be mentioned that bulk motion of the head itself during respiration could be a source of physiological artifact. The most probable manifestation of such movement would be a rotation in the sagittal plane, yielding a flexion/extension cycle as a function of the degree of inspiration (VAN DER VEEN et al. 1997). This would lead to in-plane motions for data taken in the sagittal plane (and consequently to small misregistration artifacts in the image) and to out-of-plane motions for data taken in other orientations. These effects are not straightforward to correct, but may be ameliorated during the process of head motion correction (see Chap. 26).

16.2.2
Cardiac Effects

Whilst it is possible that contraction motions of the heart within the chest cavity could cause susceptibility-induced magnetic field fluctuations at the location of the brain, this would seem to be an unlikely explanation for the cardiac-related noise effects. More likely are, firstly, motions of the brain which are caused by cerebral blood volume and pressure fluctuations and, secondly, the varying effects of inflow of fresh blood spins into the slice of interest over the heart cycle.

In studies unrelated to fMRI, but which lend support to the former proposed mechanism, PONCELET et al. (1992) and ENZMANN and PELC (1992) used motion-sensitive MRI methods with high temporal resolution to characterize the bulk motions of the brain that correlate with the cardiac cycle. They postulated that these motions result from increases in intracranial blood volume following systole (FEINBERG 1992) which, since the skull is a closed cavity, cause the relatively incompressible brain tissue to occupy cerebrospinal fluid (CSF) space (also serving as a pump for CSF circulation). The motions detected using these techniques showed that brain structures close to the brain stem moved with excursions of up to 0.5 mm over the cardiac cycle, whereas cortical regions of the brain moved with excursions that were less than ≈0.05 mm. This implies that bulk motion of the brain caused by cardiac contraction could be a source of artifact particularly in the deeper brain structures. This artifact would most likely reveal itself as image ghosting in conventional or interleaved pulse sequences (through complex phase shifts induced by the nonrigid body motions), and as mis-registration artifacts in the case of snapshot EPI. GLOVER and LEE (1995) have simulated simple forms of pulsatile motion (those which lead to zero order phase shifts) and have shown that conventional 2DFT techniques (such as FLASH) will suffer greater artifact than will sequences such as spiral imaging and projection reconstruction that sample k-space with more frequent collection of the low spatial frequencies.

Pulse sequences that use a short scan repeat (TR) time and a high radiofrequency flip angle may be sensitive to artifacts caused directly by flowing blood itself. The effect results from driving the nuclear spins in a "steady state" condition in which they are unable to relax to their equilibrium magnetization state (fully relaxed along the field direction) before each excitation. Under such conditions fresh nuclear spins in blood that flow into the slice between excitations will in general appear brighter in the image than the stationary (and partially saturated) tissue spins. If the flow increases or decreases (as it does over the cardiac cycle) then pixels containing inflowing blood spins will fluctuate in phase and intensity. This will cause familiar flow artifacts in conventional 2DFT images and punctate increases in temporal variance in the case of snapshot techniques. A further effect that has been proposed is a possible sensitivity of gradient echo imaging techniques to a changing cerebral blood oxygenation level over the cardiac cycle. Though this is feasible (cerebral flow rates will change slightly over the cardiac cycle, which could in turn alter the venous oxygen saturation even with constant metabolism), it would seem unlikely that the arterial oxygen saturation will vary much in normal brain. More probable is that longer time scale breathing depth autoregulations (over many respiratory periods) could lead to CO_2 changes, and hence to flow changes. The associated deoxyhemoglobin changes could explain some of the longer term fluctuations in signal intensity seen in fMRI experiments.

It is worth noting that even when cardiac-related instabilities are present, the frequency spectrum of the cardiac noise may not always show significant peaks (i.e., may not resemble those seen in Fig. 16.1) when the time course of individual pixels are Fourier-transformed. This can occur when the image-to-image acquisition time for snapshot techniques is long compared with the cardiac period (as is invariably the case). This condition can lead to the power

spectrum appearing much more like white noise, a result of random aliasing of the frequencies in the spectrum. It is only when the image-to-image time is brought down to a level comparable to that of the cardiac period that strong peaks in the noise spectrum will be seen. This has implications for correction schemes which use digital filtering to reduce physiological fluctuations, as they can only work properly on raw data which are highly temporally sampled. Otherwise, additional knowledge of the cardiac cycle is required.

16.2.3
Other Effects

Since CSF flows throughout the brain and spinal cord and since CSF has a very long T1 relaxation time (on the order of 4 s.), it is a potential source for signal fluctuation. Several authors have studied the complex motions of CSF as it circulates about the central nervous system (see, for example, SCHROTH and KLOSE 1992a,b; MAIER et al. 1994). They found that the circulation is principally driven by the cardiac pulsations of the brain (mentioned above), with a rhythmic modulation superimposed by breathing. Therefore, it would be expected that regions of CSF in and around the ventricles would show strong cardiac and respiratory frequency fluctuations in signal magnitude and/or phase, with those fluctuations diminishing in the brain with distance away from the ventricles, as the flow effects are diffused. As such, correction for CSF physiological noise will largely be included in the cardiac and respiratory corrections. It is possible, however, to null the CSF signal by inversion nulling (HAJNAL et al. 1992), should this be necessary.

A physiological effect which can easily be overlooked is that of motion of the eyes during the scan. Aside from any neurological processes being engaged during eye movement, it is possible for the eye motion itself to create ghosting effects in the MRI data. CHEN and ZHU (1997) show how eye motion can affect snapshot EPI data by causing increased variance in the region which is displaced field of view (FOV)/2 from the eyes in the phase-encode direction. Clearly, if the phase-encode direction corresponds to anterior-posterior, then eye motion-induced fluctuations can alias into the brain. Similar (although more spatially diffuse) artifacts will be induced in the case of interleaved EPI or 2DFT techniques. CHEN and ZHU (1997) propose using a slab saturation at the location of the eyes to suppress the eye signal, and therefore the ghosted eye signal. Clearly, a judicious choice of phase-encode direction can also ameliorate this problem by making the ghosted fluctuations appear outside the brain region. Particular care in this regard should be taken when there is a possibility of eye motions which correlate with the neurological task, since false activations can result.

Finally, BISWAL et al. (1995) and others have reported very slow fluctuations in the NMR signal intensity of the resting brain (frequencies below 0.1 Hz). These fluctuations are on a time scale similar to that of spontaneous fluctuations in regional cerebral blood flow measured in rats (GOLANOV et al. 1994). Indeed, Biswal and colleagues have cross-correlated these slow signal fluctuations in the primary motor area of one hemisphere and find significant correlations with other motor areas. They propose that these low frequency fluctuations may be explained by correlated neuronal or flow properties which associate areas of the brain with strong axonal connectivity, even when they are at rest.

16.3
Navigator Echo Correction Methods

Navigator echo methods have been used for some years in correcting various effects in MRI data. Ehman and colleagues developed much of the early methods for navigator echo correction of moving structures (e.g., see EHMAN and FELMLEE 1989). The principle is demonstrated in Fig. 16.3, which shows a standard spin-echo pulse sequence to which has been added a second 180° pulse and readout portion, placed before the main readout period. This additional echo is used to monitor any error phases in the main readout echo. Noting that the first (navigator) echo precedes the phase-encoding dephaser gradient, this implies that in the absence of nonsteady state spin excitation or other perturbing influences, the magnitude and phase of the navigator echo should be identical for each phase-encode step. Any changes to the magnitude or phase of the echo may be ascribed to motion of the object or to other artifactual effects which corrupt the signal.
The phase of the navigator echo is more sensitive to motion than its magnitude, and so it is usually the phase of the echo that is used as a monitor of and correction for motion artifacts. For example, a movement of the object in the read-out direction of δx will result in an NMR signal equal to:

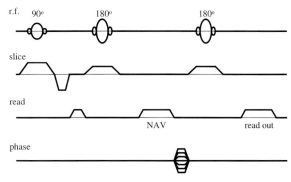

Fig. 16.3. Principle of the navigator echo. A navigator echo is added to an otherwise standard spin echo sequence by preceding the phase encode dephaser with a readout period. Magnitude and phase fluctuations of the navigator echo can be ascribed to nonsteady state behavior of the NMR signal (e.g., motion). The extension of the navigator technique to other pulse sequences is analogous

$$S'(k_x) = \exp(-2\pi i k_x \delta x) \int p(x) \exp(-2\pi i k_x x) dx \qquad (16.2)$$

where $S'(k_x)$ is the k-space navigator signal detected and $\exp(-2\pi i k_x \delta x)$ is the error term induced by the motion, which corresponds to a first order phase shift in k_x. More complicated motions will lead to more complicated phase error terms.

Similarly, motion between the 90° excitation pulse and the readout gradient of the imaging sequence can result in the NMR echo forming slightly later or earlier in the acquisition window. This corresponds to a shift, δk_x, of the signal in k_x, resulting in a linear phase shift within the profile $p(x)$, i.e., analogous to Eq. 16.2 but with k_x and x reversed, and $S'(k_x)$ and $p(x)$ reversed. According to the type of motion being corrected, either the phase of the navigator echo in k-space or the phase of the Fourier-transformed signal, $p(x)$ may be used to rephase the subsequent imaging echo, often resulting in a substantial improvement in image quality.

Navigator echoes can also be used to detect shifts in the static magnetic field which may result from respiration or even MR scanner instabilities (JEZZARD 1996). For a bulk shift of the magnetic field, the NMR signal for a single phase encode step in a conventional 2DFT gradient echo sequence will be zero order phase shifted by an amount $\exp(2\pi i \gamma \Delta B_0 TE)$. This will lead to a displacement of an EPI image in the phase-encode direction by $2\pi \gamma \Delta B_0 N \tau_{pe}$ pixels, where N is the matrix size in the phase encode direction and τ_{pe} is the time between adjacent echoes in the EPI readout train. Monitoring of the phase of a navigator echo can be used to correct these effects.

Navigator echo techniques such as these have been used in functional MRI data to correct for physiologically induced fluctuations in the phase of the NMR signal. NOLL and SCHNEIDER (1994a, b) used a single sampling of the navigator echo phase (in the case of projection reconstruction or spiral imaging one can use the early part of the image data itself) to correct for the effects of respiration. The single point approach presupposes that the respiration artifact is caused by bulk magnetic field shifts which are largely independent of position in the brain, and therefore lead to zero order phase shifts. As was seen in Sect. 16.2.1 this assumption is not strictly true (though it is a close approximation for data taken in the axial plane). Nevertheless, this simple expedient was used to improve the contrast-to-noise ratio substantially. HU and KIM (1994) have also used a single point in a navigator echo collected before a FLASH sequence readout to achieve a 30%–50% reduction in physiologically related artifact. WOWK et al. (1997b) have subsequently used this same form of correction, but have calculated the navigator phase directly from the k-space data contained in the image. This is done by calculating the phase difference between the data collected from each location in k-space collected over time vs the average phase of that location. The error phase is then removed.

A more sophisticated use of navigator echoes in correcting for physiological fluctuations in fMRI data has been proposed by LE and HU (1996). Their approach consists of monitoring the cardiac and respiratory processes using the phase of a navigator echo. This information is then used to construct a "unit cycle" for the respiratory period using the zero order phase of the navigator echo (most likely reflecting respiratory-related field shifts), and a unit cycle for the cardiac period using the magnitude of a point on the navigator profile (most likely reflecting cardiac-related in-flow fluctuations). This is really only possible if the navigator echo is able to subsample both the respiratory and cardiac cycles, since the formation of the cardiac unit cycle (and to a lesser extent the formation of the respiratory unit cycle) rely on digital filtering of the periodic fluctuations to reject random noise. The parameters recommended are as follows: to reject frequencies above 0.5 Hz for construction of the respiratory unit cycle, and to accept frequencies only in the range 0.6–3.0 Hz for construction of the cardiac unit cycle. Once the unit cycles have been generated, a regression is

performed for the time series of each point in k-space vs its respective point in the unit cycle (respiratory or cardiac). This amounts to point-by-point fitting of a Fourier expansion series (to second order) to the scatter plot generated by plotting the k-space phase and magnitude for each image in the time series vs the unit cycle phase, which is defined by:

$$\phi(i) = \frac{T(i) - T_s(j)}{T_s(j+1) - T_s(j)} \qquad (16.3)$$

where $T_s(j)$ is the starting point (relative to some specific point in the respective cycle, e.g., systole) of cycle j, and $T(i)$ is the time of the point in question, which falls within the jth physiological cycle. Once a characteristic fitted curve of this sort is established over a unit cycle, each k-space point in the time series can be phase- and magnitude-corrected according to where it falls in the unit cycle. This process is repeated for all k-space points.

Clearly the above strategy will only be appropriate for imaging sequences which allow a navigator echo to be collected frequently (above the Nyquist frequency threshold for the physiological process being measured). FLASH imaging is easily able to accomplish this, since a typical TR time would be ≈ 50 ms. Most EPI or spiral data collection strategies, though, would not usually satisfy the condition for sampling the cardiac-related fluctuations, although they may be able to sample respiratory fluctuations. Evidence of the ability of this approach to obtain both respiratory and cardiac information is shown in Fig. 16.4. Figure 16.4b shows the time course of the zero order phase of the central k-space point from an EPI time series (Fig. 16.4b, upper plot) vs the abdominal motion recorded using a pressure belt placed around the abdomen. Excellent agreement is seen. Figure 16.4a shows a plot of the magnitude profile of the point picked out by an automatic search algorithm from the navigator profile in a FLASH experiment. This plot shows clearly that the cardiac cycle can be monitored. It is worth noting that, in order to avoid the possibility of confounding any neurological fluctuations of interest with the unwanted physiological processes, one can construct the unit cycle for the respiratory and cardiac cycle from data collected in only a single neurological state (e.g., a rest state). When this physiological information is used to correct for physiological noise a substantial improvement in data fidelity is seen. LE and HU (1996) report a 30%–40% improvement in their ability to detect activated pixels in the images.

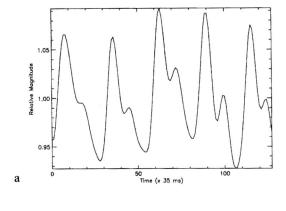

a

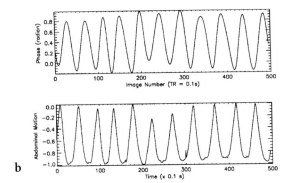

b

Fig. 16.4. a Plot of the magnitude time course (*graph*) of a point on the navigator profile from a FLASH experiment. The point, which clearly shows the cardiac time course, was picked out by an automatic search algorithm. **b** Plot of zero order phase from the central k-space point of an echo planar imaging (EPI) time course (*upper trace*) and the corresponding abdominal movement detected using an external pressure belt (*lower trace*). A TR of 100 ms was used for the EPI data collection. (Data reproduced with permission from LE and HU 1996)

16.4
Non-navigator Echo Correction Methods

HU et al. (1995) had earlier used this same principle for correcting physiological fluctuations using externally collected physiological data. For example, an EKG signal or pulse oximeter signal can be digitized along with the MRI data to give a marker for the cardiac cycle. Similarly, a pressure belt or bellows can be placed around the subject's abdomen to record respiratory motion. The externally collected data can then be used to provide the $T_s(j)$ values in Eq 16.3, and if a temporal marker is recorded each time an image (or phase-encode step) is collected, then all the information required for substitution into Eq 16.3 is available. The advantage of using externally collected physiological information is that one is not constrained to collect navigator echoes (2DFT techniques) or images (EPI, spiral techniques) at a frequency above the Nyquist limit of the cardiac fluctuations. This enables correction of data which have been obtained using a wider range of pulse sequences. An example of the improvement made when this type of physiological noise correction is performed is shown in Fig. 16.5. Figure 16.5a shows the activation area detected without physiological noise correction (*left panel*) and the enlarged area detected with physiological noise correction (*right panel*). Figure 16.5b shows a time course taken from the uncorrected data (*upper trace*) and the corrected data (*lower trace*). The stimulus was present between images 180 and 280.

Less powerful but much simpler methods for partially compensating for physiological effects employ digital filtering at the problematic frequencies. One can accomplish this by external monitoring of respiration and cardiac activity, and then filtering at the frequencies predicted by those external measurements. BISWAL et al. (1996) have shown how one can deal (to first order) with situations in which the cardiac disturbances are aliased in the NMR noise spectrum due to a long TR time. In these instances they suggest decimating a high temporally sampled external signal to match the time points sampled in the NMR experiment. In this way, one can predict where the aliased noise peaks will occur in the NMR data, and one can then digitally filter out signals at these frequencies. Clearly, this approach requires that the cardiac and respiratory cycles are quite constant in length over the course of the experiment. Problems will also occur if an aliased frequency overlaps with the frequency of the neurologic process of interest (when this is run in a cycling block design).

Cardiac gating of the image acquisition itself, either via a peripheral pulse oximeter signal or via an EKG lead, offers a potential method to compensate for cardiac-related artifacts. However, for high flip angle sequences, when the scan TR time is less than 5×T1, cardiac gating is confounded by variability in the cardiac period, leading to NMR relaxation-induced signal fluctuations. Since T1 times in gray matter range between 800 ms and 1500 ms, depending on magnetic field strength, and since the TR times used are typically in the range of 2–5 s for snapshot techniques, the signal intensity changes resulting from the variable T1 recovery can mask the desired fMRI signal changes. Various authors have therefore attempted to compensate for the variable TR signal fluctuations by modeling the T1 recovery

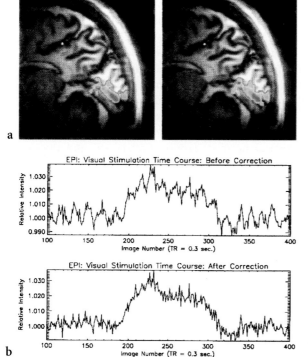

Before correction   **After correction**

a

EPI: Visual Stimulation Time Course: Before Correction

EPI: Visual Stimulation Time Course: After Correction

b

Fig. 16.5. a Functional overlays of a visual stimulus calculated without physiological noise correction (*left panel*) and with physiological noise correction (*right panel*). An enlarged area of activation is detected in the corrected data set. **b** Time course taken from the data shown in (**a**) without physiological noise correction (*upper trace*) and with correction (*lower trace*). An echo planar imaging (EPI) pulse sequence was used with a TR of 300 ms. The stimulus was present during images 180–280. (Data reproduced with permission from Hu et al. 1995)

processes and correcting for them (e.g., see GUIMARAES et al. 1995, 1998; LE and HU 1997).

For a standard snapshot technique, this can be accomplished by noting that the M_z recovery in a given voxel following a 90° pulse excitation is described by:

$$S_i = A[1-\exp(-TR_i/T1)] \qquad (16.4)$$

where S_i is the signal intensity of the voxel following the ith TR interval, and A is the signal intensity for the case of infinite TR. When the radiofrequency flip angle is not 90°, a modified version of Eq. 16.4 must be used which accounts for this.

It would be theoretically possible, although quite time consuming and difficult, to measure voxel-by-voxel the T1 of the brain and then substitute into Eq. 16.4 to correct for changes in cardiac rate. An alternative method is to fit by least squares estimation the

T1 (and, if necessary, the flip angle) value that minimizes the T1-induced signal fluctuations indicated by Eq 16.4. This requires direct measurement of the variable TR times, which is easily accomplished. GUIMARAES et al. (1998) have used this approach to substantially improve the fMRI signal fidelity seen in the colliculi of normal volunteers listening to music. Without cardiac gating (but with constant TR intervals) the significance of the colliculi activation was quite weak, but when the cardiac gating approach described above was used the statistical significance of the activation was greatly enhanced.

ALSOP and DETRE (1997) have used principal component analysis to extract the spatial signature of the physiological fluctuations. Once characterized, the principal components associated with noise are removed by vector subtraction. JOSEPHS et al. (1997b) include physiological noise contributions into the design matrix of their general linear model for signal changes. This, in effect, removes signal fluctuations that match the physiological noise model (constructed using externally collected respiratory and cardiac signals).

16.5 Concluding Remarks

Given the constant struggle to achieve optimal signal-to-noise ratio and contrast-to-noise ratio in fMRI experiments, it seems essential that all efforts should be made to reduce extraneous physiological fluctuations from contaminating the data. In order to realize this, a more complete understanding of those processes is probably needed than is presented here. Once this has been accomplished, it should be possible to minimize physiological fluctuations in fMRI experiments using a combination of optimal pulse sequences, external physiological monitoring, and post-processing techniques of the sort described above. Since the data are acquired in k-space, these corrections will most likely have the best effect when they are applied to the k-space data. Given the current range of correction schemes, it would therefore seem likely that the best are those that combine externally measured physiological information with subsequent k-space data correction. This should enable ever more sensitive fMRI experiments to be conducted.

Acknowledgements. I would like to thank Dr. Peter Robbins at the University of Oxford for helpful discussions regarding this manuscript.

References

Alsop DC, Detre JA (1997) Reduction of excess noise in fMRI using noise image templates. Proceedings of the 5th International Society of Magnetic Resonance in Medicine 3:1687

Bailes DR, Gilderdale DJ, Bydder GM, et al. (1985) Respiratory ordering of phase encoding (ROPE): a method for reducing respiratory motion artifacts in MR imaging. J Comput Assist Tomogr 9:835–838

Biswal B, Yetkin FZ, Haughton VM, et al. (1995) Functional connectivity in the motor cortex of resting human brain using echo-planar MRI. Magn Reson Med 34:537–541

Biswal B et al. (1996) Reduction of physiological fluctuations in fMRI using digital filters. Magn Reson Med 35:107–113

Chen W, Zhu X-H (1997) Suppression of physiological eye movement artifacts in functional MRI using slab presaturation. Magn Reson Med 38:546–550

Ehman RL, Felmlee JP (1989) Adaptive technique for high-definition MR imaging of moving structures. Radiology 173:255–263

Ehman RL, Felmlee JP (1990) Flow artifact reduction in MRI: a review of the roles of gradient moment nulling and spatial presaturation. Magn Reson Med 14:293–307

Enzmann DR, Pelc NJ (1992) Brain motion: measurement with phase-contrast MR imaging. Radiology 185:653–660

Feinberg D (1992) Modern concepts of brain motion and cerebrospinal flow. Radiology 185:630–632

Glover GH, Lee AT (1995) Motion artifacts in fMRI: comparison of 2DFT with PR and spiral scan methods. Magn Reson Med 33:624–635

Golanov EV, Yamamoto S, Reis DJ (1994) Spontaneous waves of cerebral blood flow associated with patterns of electrocortical activity. Am J Physiol 266:R204–214

Guimares AR, Baker JR, Weisskoff RM (1995) Cardiac-gated functional MRI with T1 correction. Proceedings 3rd Society of Magnetic Resonance 2:798

Guimares AR, Melcher JR, Talavage TM, et al. (1998) Imaging subcortical auditory activity in humans. Human Brain Mapping, 6:33–41

Hajnal JV, Bryant DJ, Kasuboski L, et al. (1992) Use of fluid attenuated inversion recovery (FLAIR) pulse sequences in MRI of the brain. J Comput Assist Tomogr 16:841–844

Hu X, Kim S-G (1994) Reduction of signal fluctuation in functional MRI using navigator echoes. Magn Reson Med 31:595–603

Hu X, Le TH, Parrish T, et al. (1995) Retrospective estimation and correction of physiological fluctuation in functional MRI. Magn Reson Med 34:201–212

Jezzard P, LeBihan D, Cuenod C, et al. (1993) An investigation of the contribution of physiological noise in human functional MRI studies at 1.5 Tesla and 4 Tesla. Proceedings of the 12th Society of Magnetic Resonance in Medicine 3:1392

Jezzard P (1996) Effects of B0 magnetic field drift on echo planar functional magnetic resonance imaging. Proceedings of the 4th International Society of Magnetic Resonance in Medicine 3:1817

Josephs O, Turner R, Friston K (1997a) Event related fMRI. Human Brain Mapping, 5:243–248

Josephs O, Howseman AM, Friston K et al. (1997b) Physiological noise modelling for multi-slice EPI fMRI using SPM. Proceedings of the 5th International Society of Magnetic Resonance in Medicine 3:1682

Le TH, Hu X (1996) Retrospective estimation and correction of physiological artifacts in fMRI by direct extraction of physiological activity from MR data. Magn Reson Med 35:290–296

Le TH, Hu X (1997) Reduction in physiological effects using retrospective correction and prospective gating with compensation for TR variation. Proceedings of the 5th International Society of Magnetic Resonance in Medicine 3:1685

Maier SE, Hardy CJ, Jolesz FA (1994) Brain and cerebrospinal fluid motion: real-time quantification with M-mode MR imaging. Radiology 193:477–483

Noll DC, Schneider W (1994a) Respiration artifacts in functional brain imaging: sources of signal variation and compensation strategies. Proceedings of the 2nd Society of Magnetic Resonance 2:647

Noll DC, Schneider W (1994b) Theory, simulation, and compensation strategies of physiological motion artifacts in functional MRI. IEEE International Conference on Imagine Processing 3: 40–44

Poncelet BP, Wedeen VJ, Weisskoff RM,, et al. (1992) Brain parenchyma motion: measurement with cine echo-planar MR imaging. Radiology 185:645–651

Schroth G, Klose U (1992a) Cerebrospinal fluid flow. I. Physiology of cardiac-related pulsation. Neuroradiology 35:1–9

Schroth G, Klose U (1992b) Cerebrospinal fluid flow. I. Physiology of respiration-related pulsations. Neuroradiology 35:10–15

van der Veen JWC, van Gelderen P, Weinberger DR, et al. (1997) Characterization of brain motion with a 3D navigator and reduction of motion artifacts in PRESTO. Proceedings of the 5th International Society of Magnetic Resonance in Medicine 1:466

Weisskoff RM, Baker J, Belliveau, J, et al. (1993) Power spectrum analysis of functionally-weighted MR data: what's in the noise? Proceedings of the 12th Society of Magnetic Resonance in Medicine 1:7

Wowk B, Alexander ME, McIntyre MC, et al. (1997a) Origin and removal of fMRI physiological noise: a multi-modal approach. Proceedings of the 5th International Society of Magnetic Resonance in Medicine 3:1690

Wowk B, McIntyre MC, Saunders JK (1997b) k-space detection and correction of physiological artifacts in fMRI. Magn Reson Med 38:1029–1034

Hu X, Le T-H, Parrish T, Erhard P (1995) Retrospective estimation and correction of physiological fluctuation in functional MRI. Magn Reson Med 34:201–212

17 Simultaneous Acquisition of Multiple Forms of fMRI Contrast

E.C. Wong, P.A. Bandettini

CONTENTS

17.1 Rationales for Embedded Techniques

Functional MRI is a rapidly growing technique for the assessment of neuronal activation locations, timings, and magnitudes. It is also becoming a useful tool for the characterization of cerebral physiology in general. As discussed in several other chapters in this volume, several different types of physiologic information can be mapped using fMRI. These include baseline cerebral blood volume (CBV) (ROSEN et al. 1989; MOONEN et al. 1990); changes in blood volume (BELLIVEAU et al. 1991); baseline and changes in cerebral perfusion (WILLIAMS 1992; DETRE 1992; EDELMAN 1994; KWONG 1994; WONG 1997; WONG 1998; KIM 1995); changes in blood oxygenation (OGAWA et al. 1990; TURNER et al. 1991; KWONG et al. 1992; OGAWA and LEE 1992; BANDETTINI et al. 1992; FRAHM et al. 1992; HAACKE

et al. 1997); and changes in $CMRO_2$ (DAVIS 1998; KIM and UGURBIL et al. 1997; VANZIJL et al. 1998).

Several studies have involved the comparison – using activations or physiologic stresses – of the locations, timings, and magnitudes of fMRI signal changes across different contrast weightings. Information from two or more contrast weightings is extremely helpful in the study of fMRI contrast mechanisms. For example, the ratio of spin-echo to gradient-echo signal changes may reveal the predominant susceptibility perturber size. The dynamics of cerebral blood flow (CBF) changes relative to BOLD changes may reveal details of the underlying changes in CBV and $CMRO_2$.

Comparisons across pulse sequence weightings are typically made by performing separate experiments (collecting separate sets of time series data) for each pulse sequence or test used. The utility of these comparisons is directly related to how accurately they can be made. Hindrances to accurate comparison of these changes include subject motion between separate time series, activation or hemodynamic change non-repeatability (due to changing cognitive or hemodynamic state over time) within and across separate time series, and system instabilities. Simultaneous collection of different contrast weightings is a solution to the these problems. We will refer to this type of strategy as "embedded" contrast weighting, since two or more types of contrast are embedded in a single time series or following a single excitation.

Types of embedded contrast include nearly limitless combinations of the following: (a) TE stepping in a single time series to obtain data on T_2^* (or T_2) and S_0 (the extrapolated signal at TE=0), (b) multiple echoes in a single excitation, (c) gradient-echoes, spin-echoes, and asymmetric spin-echoes, (d) diffusion weighting, (e) arterial spin labeling (ASL) for measurement of CBF, and (f) magnetization transfer contrast. Several combinations of these types of contrast are described in more detail below.

E.C. WONG, PhD, MD; Departments of Radiology and Psychiatry, University of California at San Diego Medical Center, 200 West Arbor Drive, San Diego, CA 92103-8756, USA
P.A. BANDETTINI, PhD; Biophysics Research Institute, Medical College of Wisconsin, 8701 Watertown Plank Rd., Milwaukee, WI 53226, USA

17.2
TE Stepping

Assuming that a gradient-echo sequence is used, the resting and activated MRI signal, S_r and S_a, respectively, can be approximated by:

$$S_r = S_{r0}e^{-R2*rTE}$$
$$S_a = S_{a0}e^{-R2*aTE} \qquad (17.1)$$

The resting and activated signals at TE=0 (S_{r0} and S_{a0}), are modulated by changes in proton density, T_1, or inflow. Transverse relaxation rates, R_2*r ($1/T_2*r$) and R_2*a ($1/T_2*a$) are modulated by changes in the magnetic susceptibility. If TE is systematically modulated during a time series collection of data, temporally and spatially registered measurements of R2* and S_0 during rest and activation are possible, allowing separation of inflow (non-susceptibility) and oxygenation (susceptibility) effects.

An example of this technique is shown in Figs. 17.1 and 17.2, in which a time series of echo planar images was acquired. The TE was stepped between each image; five cycles were acquired. In these data, it appears that a change in S_0 and T_2* takes place in the motor cortex during finger tapping.

Reports describing several different manifestations of TE stepping have appeared in the literature, including multi-echo high-resolution measurements at 4T (MENON et al. 1993), multi-echo low spatial resolution high echo time resolution EPI readout techniques (POSSE et al. 1995 1997; BANDETTINI and WONG 1998a), ; spectroscopic techniques for separating out inflow and susceptibility-related causes for the rapidly occurring pre-undershoot (HENNIG et al. 1994, 1995); double-echo spiral scan (GLOVER

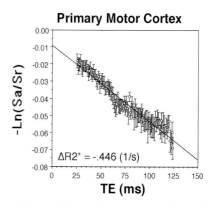

Fig. 17.2. Plot combining the two curves shown in Fig. 17.1

et al. 1996), and single-echo EPI time series, in which the TE was incremented with each successive image (BANDETTINI et al. 1994, 1997).

In addition to the study of contrast mechanisms, the acquisition of two or more gradient echoes allows for B_0 field mapping at every time point. Real time B_0 field mapping may allow correction for dynamic artifacts caused by speaking, swallowing, and breathing (BIRN et al. 1997a,b).

17.3
Combined Gradient-Echo, Spin-Echo, and Asymmetric Spin-Echo Acquisitions

17.3.1
Gradient Echoes with Spin-Echoes

In general, the activation-induced signal changes in spin-echo sequences are thought to arise primarily from blood oxygenation-related field perturbations around red blood cells and capillaries (small compartments). The changes in gradient-echo sequences are thought to arise from field perturbations around red blood cells, capillaries, and larger vessels as well (compartments of all sizes). The ratio of these signal changes, with activation or with the administration of exogenous contrast, may give specific information about the predominant compartment size in each voxel – leading to greater certainty of activation foci (WEISKOFF et al. 1994; OGAWA et al. 1993; BANDETTINI and WONG 1995; KENNAN et al. 1994). Voxel-wise comparisons of these changes require precise registration. A method for precise registration involves the collection of a gradient-echo image, then application of a 180° pulse and subse-

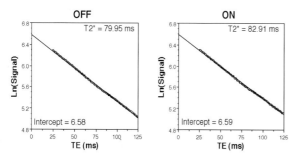

Fig. 17.1. TE dependence of the resting and activated gradient-echo signal. Each point on the decay curve is an average of five echo planar images acquired during a single time series. TR=500 ms. A change in the intercept is likely due to a change in inflow. A change in the slope (R_2*) is due to changes in oxygenation and/or blood volume

Combined Gradient - Echo and Spin - Echo EPI

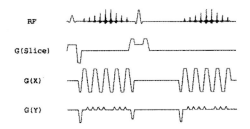

RF

G(Slice)

G(X)

G(Y)

Fig. 17.3. Combined gradient-echo and spin-echo echo planar imaging (EPI), allowing for the collection of spin-echo (T_2^*-weighted) echo planar image pairs within about 50 ms of each other. This sequence is used to obtain spatially and temporally registered gradient-echo and spin-echo time course series for voxel-wise comparison of activation-induced signal change dynamics with different contrast weightings

quent collection of a spin-echo image (BANDETTINI et al. 1993, 1994; BANDETTINI and WONG 1998b; BANDETTINI 1995; PRINSTER 1997). This approach to image acquisition substantially reduces the small amount of systematic error that occurs across separate trials. The pulse sequence is shown in Fig. 17.3.

Typical time series collected using this acquisition strategy are shown in Fig. 17.4. Both time series are from identical voxels in motor cortex. Figure 17.4a is during administration of a bolus of gadolinium during rest. Figure 17.4b is during cyclic on-off finger tapping. Figure 17.5 shows a type of comparison possible with this technique. Changes in R_2^* and R_2, induced by a bolus injection of gadolinium, are compared on a voxel-wise basis.

Image pairs and BOLD contrast functional images created from combined gradient-echo and spin-echo time series are shown in Fig. 17.6. Lastly, systematic incrementation of the two TE values in each sequential time course image also enables the simultaneous mapping of relative transverse relaxation rates (R_2^*, R_2, and R_2') and longitudinal magnetizations (S_0), as well as changes in these values, as shown in Figs. 17.7 and 17.8. Using this method of analysis, a decrease in R_2 is minimally perceptible, and S_0 changes are relatively imperceptible. The reason for this last observation may be that the TR was suboptimal for detection of S_0 changes or that the susceptibility-induced transverse relaxation rate changes do not behave as single exponential functions.

17.3.2
Gradient Echoes with Asymmetric Spin-Echoes

In a variation on the theme described above, one or two asymmetric spin-echoes can be acquired instead of the spin-echo. If the echo planar imaging (EPI) readout window is sufficiently short, then three equally T_2'-weighted images can be obtained within ~150 ms, each having a different T_2 weighting. The first image is collected during the FID, the second prior to the spin-echo (offset by $-\tau$), and the third after the spin-echo (offset by $+\tau$).

Figures 17.9 and 17.10 show an example of this strategy. A time series of 200 axial image triplets was collected: in-plane voxel dimension=3.8×3.8 mm, slice thickness=7 mm, TR=1 ms, gradient echo TE=27.1 ms. The spin-echo occurred at 109.6 ms, and two asymmetric spin-echoes were collected at t offsets of ±27.1 ms. During collection of the time series, self-paced bilateral finger tapping was performed in a cyclic manner (20 s on/20 s off). Figure 17.9 shows the first anatomical images (TR=8) and functional images obtained using this technique. Figure 17.10 shows time series from the same voxels in the motor cortex. Because of T_2 decay, the signal-to-noise ratio in each image decreases, and correspondingly, the contrast-to-noise ratio in the functional images decreases. The functional contrast-to-

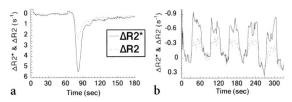

Fig. 17.4a,b. ΔR_2^* and ΔR_2 from identical regions during **a** bolus injection of a susceptibility contrast agent and **b** brain activation. A combined gradient-echo and spin-echo sequence were used

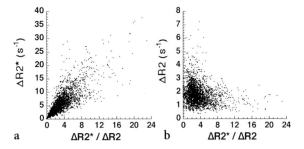

Fig. 17.5a,b. Plots from gray matter of BOLD $\Delta R_2^*/\Delta R_2$ vs **a** ΔR_2^* and **b** ΔR_2. Significantly different correlations are seen

Gradient-Echo TE = 30 ms   Spin Echo TE = 110 ms

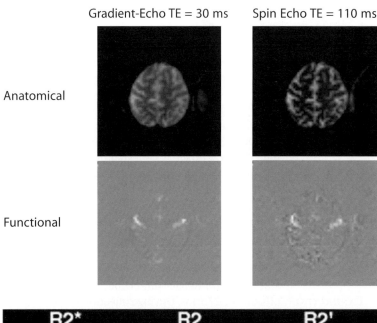

Anatomical

Functional

Fig. 17.6. A pair of anatomical images and the corresponding functional correlation images obtained simultaneously from combined gradient-echo and spin-echo time course series

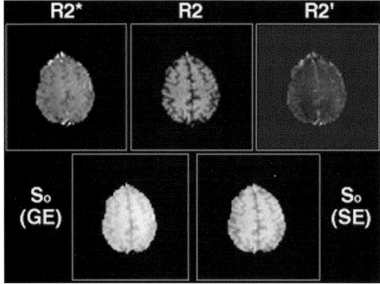

Fig. 17.7. Resting state transverse relaxation rate and S_0 images. The R2' image ($=R_2{}^*-R_2$) is a direct indicator of proton resonance line width

noise ratios in the same motor cortex region were 4.9, 2.0, and 1.6 for the three functional data sets, respectively.

If TE=±τ, then a measure of T_2 can be obtained by fitting the three points to an exponential. In this study, the T_2 from the motor cortex region was 74.2±1 ms. The time series can also be averaged to increase the functional contrast-to-noise ratio.

If at least one of the two t offsets is different from the gradient-echo TE, then T_2 and T_2' measurements may be made at each TR.

17.4
Simultaneous BOLD and Perfusion fMRI

Perfusion fMRI using arterial spin labeling (ASL) (WILLIAMS et al. 1992; DETRE et al. 1995; KWONG et al. 1995; KIM 1995; WONG et al. 1997) is a useful adjunct to conventional BOLD contrast because it provides potentially better spatial localization and absolute quantitation of CBF, but has less sensitivity than BOLD contrast (see Chap. 6, this volume). It is also important for studies of BOLD contrast mechanisms, which involve complex interactions between CBF, $CMRO_2$, and CBV. Techniques for simultaneous acquisition of BOLD and ASL perfusion signals are

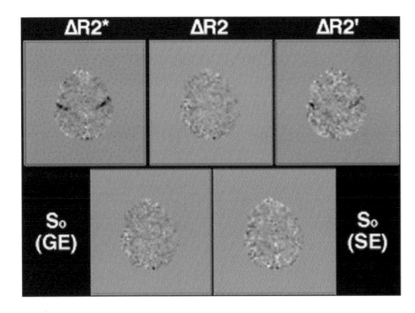

Fig. 17.8. Images of transverse relaxation rate change during bilateral finger tapping. The largest changes are seen in R_2 and almost no change is seen in S_0

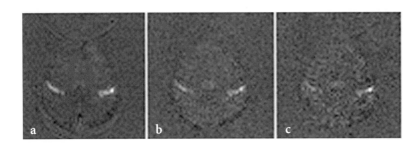

Fig. 17.9a–c. Functional images obtained from a single triple-echo time series. a gradient-recalled echo (GRE; TE=27.1 ms). b Asymmetric spin-echo (ASE); spin-echo occurs at 109.6 ms (t=–27.1 ms). c ASE (t=+27.1 ms)

described below, along with a discussion of the quality of separation between BOLD and perfusion information.

17.4.1
Imaging Techniques

For any imaging technique that is T_2 or T_2^* sensitive, there is some degree of inherent BOLD contrast. Likewise, for all but very specifically designed sequences, there is some degree of inflow weighting, positive or negative. In this section we discuss the factors that affect the separability of flow and BOLD signals.

17.4.1.1
Pulsed ASL

In ASL in general, the magnetization of the static tissue in the imaging slices is immaterial, as long as

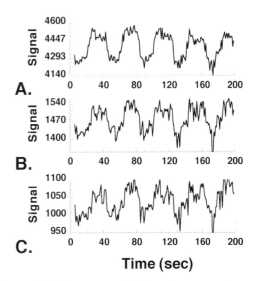

Fig. 17.10A–C. Time course plots from the same motor cortex region as in Fig. 17.9. Plots A, B, C correspond to images A, B, C in Fig. 17.9

it is the same between tag and control conditions (Buxton et al. 1998). For pulsed ASL, it is relatively straightforward to arrange for the magnetization of the imaging planes to be such that both tag and control images can be used for both the ASL and the BOLD signal. This is done in the following manner (Wong et al. 1997; Wong and Bandettini 1996).

The magnetization of the tagged arterial blood follows an inversion recovery curve in the time after the application of the tag, as shown in the bottom curve of Fig. 17.11. In the control state, the arterial magnetization is relaxed, as in the top curve in the figure. If a saturation pulse is applied to the imaging plane immediately prior to the application of the tag pulse, the tissue in the imaging plane undergoes saturation recovery, as in the middle curve of the figure. As usual, the ASL signal is the difference between adjacent tag and control images, irrespective of the static tissue contrast. Under these conditions, the average of adjacent tag/control pairs can be used to construct the BOLD time course. Note that in an average of adjacent images, the time course of the average magnetization of the inflowing arterial blood is the same as the magnetization of the static tissue (i.e., the average of the top and bottom curves in the figure equals the middle curve. Equivalently, the tag condition is negatively flow-weighted (inflow decreases M_z), while the control condition is positively flow-weighted (inflow increases M_z) by the same amount. If the T_1 of arterial blood is identical to that of the static tissue, then these pairwise averaged images are independent of inflow. However, because the T_1 of blood is slightly different from that of brain tissue, there is a very small amount of flow weighting in the BOLD signal, as estimated below.

17.4.1.2
Continuous ASL

For continuous ASL (Williams et al. 1992; Detre et al. 1995), because the inversion of tagged arterial blood is distributed across time, the tagged blood does not follow a simple inversion recovery as in pulsed ASL. For this reason, the scheme outlined above for pulsed ASL does not generate a flow-independent BOLD signal. However, in continuous ASL the control images acquired without perturbation of the inflowing blood are nearly flow independent and can be used as a BOLD time series. There is a very slight positive flow weighting in these images due to the saturation of the imaging slice at the time of image acquisition, and subsequent inflow of relaxed blood, but this effect is small because of the long TR used in continuous ASL.

17.4.2
Separation of BOLD and Perfusion Signals in Pulsed ASL

The raw time course and separated CBF and BOLD components of the signal from a simultaneous pulsed ASL/BOLD finger tapping experiment are shown in Fig. 17.12. In the raw time series, the ASL signal is seen as the rapid image-to-image oscillation, while the BOLD signal is the overall rise and fall of the signal. In the separated time series, the ASL signal is calculated not as a simple pairwise subtraction, but as the difference between each image and the average of the previous and next images. In this manner, the ASL becomes independent of local linear trends in the BOLD signal. Likewise, the BOLD signal is calculated as the average of each image with the average of the previous and next images, providing insensitivity to linear trends in the ASL signal. The residual cross-contamination of the ASL and BOLD signals in the scheme described above is discussed and estimated below.

17.4.2.1
Contamination of the BOLD Signal by Perfusion

Because the T_1 of blood is known to be longer than that of tissue, there is some residual negative flow weighting in the average of tag and control images

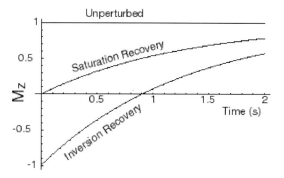

Fig. 17.11. Evolution of magnetization after the time of tag or control application. Arterial blood is unperturbed in the control state and inverted in the tag state. If the imaging plane is saturated at the time of the inversion tag, then static tissue undergoes saturation recovery. Note that at all times, the saturation recovery magnetization equals the average of the unperturbed and the inversion recovery magnetization (see text)

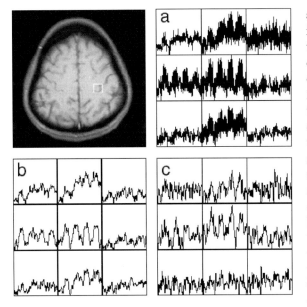

Fig. 17.12a–c. Separation of arterial spin labeling (ASL) and blood oxygen level-dependent (BOLD) components from a raw time series in a combined ASL/BOLD experiment. **a** Raw time series from each of nine pixels shown in the boxed area of the image. **b** BOLD time series; **c** ASL time series (see text)

surements is approximately 20 for 3 min of averaging, so changes on the order of 2%–4% would be at the limit of detectability. Furthermore, functional changes in the flow signal are typically on the order of 50% of the flow signal, and would dominate BOLD-related changes. However, the distributions of tissue that give rise to the flow and BOLD signals are different and may result in a more complex interaction between the flow and BOLD signals. The flow signal arises mostly from small arteries, capillaries, and brain parenchyma. The BOLD signal is primarily from veins and tissue surrounding veins and cannot arise from the arterial side of the circulation because arterial oxygenation is essentially constant. The only overlap between the populations of tissues that give rise to flow and BOLD signals is in brain parenchyma surrounding veins. These extravascular tissues are responsible for only about one third of the BOLD signal, as determined by diffusion-weighted BOLD studies (BOXERMAN et al. 1995, SONG et al. 1996;), and thus produce signal changes that are on the order of 1%. If the BOLD signal only increases the brain tissue signal by 1%, then the tissue component of the ASL signal will be increased by 1%, generating errors in the flow measurement that are typically well within the experimental error.

due to exchange of blood water with tissue water. This residual flow contribution can be estimated by calculating the difference between the magnetization of the tissue compartment in the presence and absence of inflow for a saturation recovery experiment. Using the kinetic inflow model for the ASL signal, in a QUIPSS II experiment with TI_1=700 ms, TI_2=1400 ms, if the transit delay is 1000 ms, the T_1 of blood is 1300 ms, and the T_1 of tissue is 900 ms, the residual flow signal in the average of tag and control images is approximately 18% of the flow signal in the difference signal between tag and control states. This flow contribution has the opposite sign as that of the BOLD signal and thus can only cause underestimation of the BOLD signal.

17.4.2.2
Contamination of the ASL Signal by BOLD

BOLD effects can also contaminate perfusion measurements, but this effect is probably even smaller than the effect of flow on the BOLD signal. To a first approximation, the BOLD effect causes a simple scaling of the MR signal on the order of 2%–4% during activation. If this scaling occurs uniformly throughout the tissue, then this would result in a simple scaling of the flow difference signal. A typical value for the signal-to-noise ratio of the flow mea-

17.5
Embedded Diffusion Weighting

Diffusion weighting (also known in the context of fMRI as flow weighting or velocity nulling) has been shown to reduce fMRI signal changes by removing the intravascular contribution to the signal (BOXERMAN et al. 1995; SONG et al. 1996). To probe the effects of diffusion weighting on a voxel-wise basis, it is useful to embed diffusion weighting within a single time series. Examples are shown of the application of embedded diffusion weighting within time series of interleaved flow and BOLD contrast.

In the example shown here, voxel-wise comparisons are performed on time series containing perfusion, BOLD, and diffusion weighting contrast. All studies were performed on a 1.5 Tesla GE Signa scanner. A balanced torque, three axis gradient coil was used for EPI. Cyclic bilateral finger motion was performed. A single axial imaging plane was obtained using T2*-weighted PICORE (WONG et al. 1997). Selective and nonselective off-resonance inversion was applied for every other image. Diffusion weighting gradients (b=10 s²/mm) were applied for every other pair of images. The in-plane voxel dimension=3.8+3.8 mm, slice thickness=10 mm, TE=40 ms, TR=2 s, TI=1.2 s. A total of 1792 sequential images were obtained, producing four embedded time series of 448 images. Motion correction was performed.

Figure 17.13 shows the anatomical and corresponding functional images created from the four time series. Figure 17.14 shows scatter plots comparing the relative activation induced signal changes (Δ%=percent change, Δ=difference). Two main points can be made: (1) The regions of activation between perfusion and BOLD contrast differ (in Fig. 17.13, compare B,C to D,E). Correspondingly, a small inverse relationship exists between perfusion and BOLD signal change magnitudes (Fig. 17.14 C). Generally, regions of highest perfusion changes correspond to BOLD changes of only about 1%. (2) Dif-

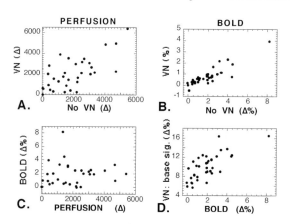

Fig. 17.14A–D. Voxel-wise activation-induced signal change comparisons (Δ%, percent change; Δ, difference). A Perfusion: diffusion weighting (VN; velocity nulling) vs no diffusion weighting; **B** BOLD: diffusion weighting vs no diffusion weighting; **C** BOLD vs perfusion; **D** baseline signal attenuation by diffusion weighting vs BOLD percent change with activation

fusion weighting, while reducing the BOLD fractional signal change (by about one half, as shown in Fig. 17.14B), does not change the location of activation (in Fig. 17.13, compare B to C). Because of extravascular susceptibility effects, the relative signal change magnitudes are still strongly weighted by blood volume, even though the blood signal itself is destroyed by diffusion weighting. Figure 17.14D also demonstrates this by showing that the largest attenuation of baseline signal by diffusion weighting (corresponding to voxels with high blood volume) corresponds to the largest fractional signal change. This largest fractional signal change remains the largest even with diffusion weighting (Fig. 17.14B).

17.6 Conclusions

Embedded contrast is a simple solution to the need for comparisons of different contrast weightings that require a high degree of temporal and spatial registration. These types of comparisons have proven extremely useful for the study of fMRI contrast mechanisms. In this chapter, methods for embedding several types of contrast were discussed. These included combinations of inflow, T_2, T_2^*, and T_2' forms of BOLD contrast, and diffusion weighting.

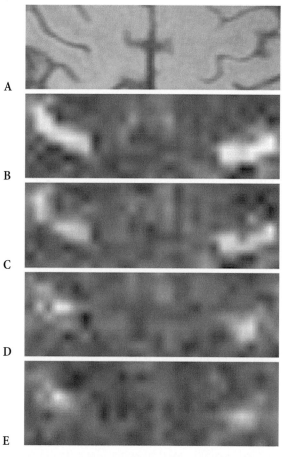

Fig. 17.13. A Anatomical image. The following images are obtained using **B** BOLD and no diffusion weighting; **C** BOLD and diffusion weighting; **D** perfusion and no diffusion weighting; **E** perfusion and diffusion weighting

References

Bandettini PA (1995) PhD dissertation: Magnetic resonance imaging of human brain activation using endogenous susceptibility contrast, Medical College of Wisconsin

Bandettini PA, Kwong KK, Davis TL, Tootell RBH, Wong EC, Fox PT, Belliveau JW, Weiskoff RM (1997) Characterization of cerebral blood oxygenation and flow changes during prolonged brain activation. Human Brain Mapping 5:93–109

Bandettini PA, Wong EC (1995) Effects of biophysical and physiologic parameters on brain activation-induced R2* and R2 changes: simulations using a deterministic diffusion model. Int J Imaging Systems Technology 6:134–152

Bandettini PA, Wong EC (1998a) In: Schmitt F, Stehling M, Turner R (eds) Echo-planar imaging: theory, technique, and application. Springer-Verlag, Berlin, Heidelberg, New York, pp 493–530

Bandettini PA, Wong EC (1998b) Echo time dependence of activation – induced signal change revisited using diced k-space (DK) acquisition. In : Proceedings of the 6th Annual ISMRM Meeting, Sydney, p. 1396

Bandettini PA, Wong EC, Cox RW, Jesmanowicz A, Hinks RS, Hyde JS (1994) Simultaneous assessment of blood oxygenation and flow contributions to activation induced signal changes in the human brain. In: Proceedings of the 2nd Annual SMR Meeting, San Francisco, p. 621

Bandettini PA, Wong EC, Hinks RS, Tikofsky RS, Hyde JS (1992) Time course EPI of human brain function during task activation. Magn Reson Med 25:390–397

Bandettini PA, Wong EC, Jesmanowicz A; Hinks RS, Hyde JS (1993) Simultaneous mapping of activation – induced ΔR2* and ΔR2 in the human brain using a combined gradient-echo and spin-echo EPI pulse sequence. In: Proceedings of the 12th Annual SMRM Meeting, New York

Belliveau JW, Kennedy DN, McKinstry RC, Buchbinder BR, Weiskoff RM, Cohen MS, Vevea JM, Brady TJ, Rosen BR (1991) Functional mapping of the human visual cortex by magnetic resonance imaging. Science 254:716–719

Birn RM, Bandettini PA, Jesmanowicz A, Cox RW (1997a) Bz-Changes in the brain due to speaking and swallowing. In: Proceedings of the 5th Annual Meeting ISMRM, Vancouver, p. 458

Birn RM, Jesmanowicz A, Cox RW (1997b) Correction of dynamic Bz-field artifacts in EPI. In: Proceedings of the 5th Annual Meeting ISMRM, Vancouver, p. 349

Boxerman JL, Bandettini PA, Kwong KK, Baker JR, Davis TL, Rosen BR, Weiskoff RM (1995) The intravascular contribution to fMRI signal change: Monte Carlo modeling and diffusion-weighted studies in vivo. Magn Reson Med 34:4–10

Buxton RB, Frank LR, Wong EC, Siewert B, Warach S, Edelman RR (1998) A general kinetic model for quantitative perfusion imaging with arterial spin labeling. Magn Reson Med 40:383–396

Detre JA, Williams DS, Zhang W, Roberts DA, Leigh JS, Koretsky AP (1995) In: LeBihan D (ed) Diffusion and perfusion: magnetic resonance imaging. Raven, New York, pp 269–305

Davis TL, Kwong KK, Weiskoff RM, Rosen BR (1998) Calibrated functional MRI: mapping the dynamics of oxidative metabolism. Proc Natl Acad Sci USA 95:1834–1839

Frahm J, Bruhn H, Merboldt KD, Hanicke W, Math D (1992) Dynamic MR imaging of human brain oxygenation during rest and photic stimulation. J Magn Reson Imaging 2:501–505

Glover GH, Lemieux SK, Drangova M, Pauly JM (1996) Decomposition of inflow and blood oxygen level-dependent (BOLD) effects with dual-echo spiral gradient-recalled echo (GRE) fMRI. Magn Reson Med 35:299–308

Haacke EM, Al S, Reichenbach JR, Kuppusamy K, Hoogenraad FGC, Takeichi H, Lin W (1997) In vivo measurement of blood oxygen saturation using magnetic resonance imaging: a direct validation of the blood oxygen level-dependent concept in functional brain imaging. Human Brain Mapping 5:341–346

Hennig J, Ernst T, Speck O, Deuschl G, Feifel E (1994) Detection of brain activation using oxygenation sensitive functional spectroscopy. Magn Reson Med 31:85–90

Hennig J, Janz C, Speck O, Ernst T (1995) Functional spectroscopy of brain activation following a single light pulse: examinations of the mechanism of the fast initial response. Int J Imaging Sys Technol 6: 203–208

Kennan RP, Zhong J, Gore JC (1994) Intravascular susceptibility contrast mechanisms in tissues. Magn Reson Med 31:9–21

Kim S-G (1995) Quantification of relative cerebral blood flow change by flow-sensitive alternating inversion recovery (FAIR) technique: application to functional mapping. Magn Reson Med 34:293–301

Kim S-G, Ugurbil K (1997) Comparison of blood oxygenation and cerebral blood flow effects in fMRI: estimation of relative oxygen consumption change. Magn Reson Med 38:59–65

Kwong KK, Belliveau JW, Chesler DA, Goldberg IE, Weiskoff RM, Poncelet BP, Kennedy DN, Hoppel BE, Cohen MS, Turner R, Cheng HM, Brady TJ, Rosen BR (1992) Dynamic magnetic resonance imaging of human brain activity during primary sensory stimulation. Proc Natl Acad Sci USA 89:5675–5679

Kwong KK, Chesler DA, Weiskoff RM, Donahue KM, Davis TL, Ostergaard L, Campbell TA, Rosen BR (1995) MR perfusion studies with T1-weighted echo planar imaging. Magn Reson Med 34:878–887

Menon RS, Ogawa S, Tank DW, Ugurbil K (1993) 4 tesla gradient recalled echo characteristics of photic stimulation-induced signal changes in the human primary visual cortex. Magn Reson Med 30:380–386

Moonen CTW, van Zijl PCM, Frank JA, LeBihan D, Becker ED (1990) Functional magnetic resonance imaging in medicine and physiology. Science 250:53–61

Ogawa S, Lee TM (1992) Functional brain imaging with physiologically sensitive image signals. J Magn Reson Imaging 2(P)-WIP (supplement): S22 (Abstract)

Ogawa S, Lee TM, Kay AR, Tank DW (1990) Brain magnetic resonance imaging with contrast dependent on blood oxygenation. Proc Natl Acad Sci USA 87:9868–9872

Ogawa S, Menon RS, Tank DW, Kim S-G, Merkle H, Ellerman JM, Ugurbil K (1993) Functional brain mapping by blood oxygenation level-dependent contrast magnetic resonance imaging: a comparison of signal characteristics with a biophysical model. Biophy J 64:803–812

Posse S, Olthoff U, Weckesser M, Jancke L, Muller-Gartner HW, Dager SR (1997) Regional dynamic signal changes during controlled hyperventilation assessed with blood oxygen level-dependent functional MR imaging. AJNR 18:1763–1770

Posse S, Tedeschi G, Risinger R, Ogg R, LeBihan D (1995) High speed 1H spectroscopic imaging in human brain by echo planar spatial-spectral encoding. Magn Reson Med 33:34–40

Prinster A, Pierpaoli C, Turner R, Jezzard P (1997) Simultaneous measurement of $\Delta R2$ and $\Delta R2^*$ in cat brain during hypoxia and hypercapnia. NeuroImage 6:191–200

Rosen BR, Belliveau JW, Chien D (1989) Perfusion imaging by nuclear magnetic resonance. Magn Reson Q 5:263–281

Song AW, Wong EC, Tan SG, Hyde JS (1996) Diffusion weighted fMRI at 1.5 T. Magn Reson Med 35:155–158

Turner R, LeBihan D, Moonen CTW, Despres D, Frank J (1991) Echo-planar time course MRI of cat brain oxygenation changes. Magn Reson Med 22:159–166

van Zijl PCM, Eleff SM, Ulatowski JA, Oja JME, Ulug AM, Traystman RJ, Kauppinen RA (1998) Quantitative assessment of blood flow, blood volume, and blood oxygenatoin effects in functional magnetic resonance imaging. Nature Med 4:159–167

Weiskoff RM, Zuo CS, Boxerman JL, Rosen BR (1994) Microscopic susceptibility variation and transverse relaxation: theory and experiment. Magn Reson Med 31:601–610

Williams DS, Detre JA, Leigh JS, Koretsky AP (1992) Magnetic resonance imaging of perfusion using spin-inversion of arterial water. Proc Natl Acad Sci USA 89:212–216

Wong EC, Bandettini PA (1996) Two embedded techniques for simultaneous acquisition of flow and BOLD signals in functional MRI. In: Fourth Meeting, International Society for Magnetic Resonance in Medicine, New York, p. 1816

Wong EC, Buxton RB, Frank LR (1997) Implementation of quantitative perfusion imaging techniques for functional brain mapping using pulsed arterial spin labeling. NMR Biomed 10:237–249

Spatial and Temporal Resolution of BOLD

18 Spatial Resolution of BOLD and Other fMRI Techniques

S.-G. Kim, S.P. Lee, B. Goodyear, A.C. Silva

CONTENTS

18.1 Introduction

Functional magnetic resonance imaging (fMRI) has been used for visualization of the human brain function with relatively high spatial resolution. In most human fMRI studies, typical spatial resolution is between 3 and 5 mm in-plane with 3–10 mm slice thickness, which is still better than other noninvasive functional mapping techniques such as positron emission tomography (PET) and single photon emission computerized tomography (SPECT). Since MRI can, in principle, be acquired with very high spatial resolution, high resolution fMRI imaging is feasible. Many groups have obtained high spatial resolution fMRI; for example, Frahm et al. (1993) obtained a voxel volume of 2.5 µl, and Menon et al. (1997) achieved 1.2 µl resolution during visual stimulation.

S.-G. Kim, PhD; S.P. Lee, MS; A.C. Silva, PhD
Center for Magnetic Resonance Research, University of Minnesota Medical School, Minneapolis, MN 55455, USA
B. Goodyear, MS
Laboratory for Functional Magnetic Resonance Research, University of Western Ontario, London, Ontario N6A 5K8, Canada

Three spatial resolution groups are classified; one is on the order of a few millimeters to a centimeter scale (referred to as a macroscale), the second is a column scale, a few hundred micrometers to a millimeter, and the last is a single capillary scale, less than 50 µm. Higher spatial resolution in fMRI means that voxels with signal changes are closer to neuronally active areas. To obtain high spatial resolution, the following issues should be considered: (1) improvement of task-induced signal change to signal fluctuation ratio (contrast-to-noise ratio, CNR), (2) minimization of large vascular contributions, and (3) spatial limitations of hemodynamic responses. To achieve high spatial resolution in fMRI, both the signal-to-noise ratio (SNR) and the CNR should be adequate enough to detect regional signal changes induced by hemodynamic alterations during the performance of a task. Further, since the origin of the fMRI signal is the hemodynamic/vascular response, signal changes should be detected at tissue level, not in large vessels for high resolution fMRI. The ultimate limitation of hemodynamic-based mapping techniques including fMRI is localization of the hemodynamic response during increased neural activity. These issues will be discussed in this chapter.

18.2 Technical Considerations

18.2.1 Contrast-to-Noise Ratio

To achieve high spatial resolution in fMRI, the task-induced signal change should be maximized and the noise should be minimized. Task-induced signal change is dependent on both image contrast, i.e., blood oxygen level-dependent (BOLD) and cerebral blood flow (CBF) methods and imaging techniques (gradient echo and spin echo) used for fMRI. In the most commonly used gradient echo-based BOLD technique, the signal change induced by neural activity (ΔS) can be described by:

$$\Delta S = \rho \times S_{cont} \times (e^{-TE \times \Delta R_2^*} - 1)$$

where ρ is the fraction of total voxel volume that is active in a single voxel, S_{cont} is the signal intensity during the resting (control) period, TE is the echo time, and ΔR_2^* is the change in the apparent transverse relaxation rate in the active partial volume. When spin echo imaging techniques are used, ΔR_2^* is replaced by ΔR_2. In perfusion-based techniques, $TE\Delta R_2^*$ is substituted by $TI\Delta R_1^*$ where TI is the spin tagging time (i.e., the inversion time for pulsed tagging methods), and ΔR_1^* is the change in the apparent longitudinal relaxation rate in the active partial volume.

Since S_{cont} decreases linearly with the voxel volume, higher spatial resolution means less ΔS. If the signal change area is smaller than a pixel ($\rho < 1.0$), higher spatial resolution will increase ρ until ρ reaches 1.0, resulting in an increase of ΔS. One practical approach to improve S_{cont} is to use a high quality receiver coil such as a small surface coil with high sensitivity. The more expensive method is to use higher magnetic fields. Theoretical modeling (OGAWA et al. 1993; WEISSKOFF et al. 1994; BANDETTINI and WONG 1995) and preliminary data (TURNER et al. 1993; SONG et al. 1995; GATI et al. 1997) in BOLD images suggest strongly that higher magnetic fields provide stronger task-induced signal changes. Higher magnetic fields will provide higher CNR provided that instrumental problems do not dominate the signal fluctuations. Recent studies by GATI et al. (1997) show that a CNR of tissue at 4 T is higher than that at 1.5 T and 0.5 T.

Sources of signal fluctuations include random white noise, physiological fluctuations, bulk head motion, and system instability, if it exists. Random noise is independent between voxels, while other noise sources may be coherent among voxels, resulting in spatial and temporal correlation. In fMRI, coherent noises are the major source of signal fluctuation. Bulk head motion can be reduced by head restraints and further minimized by motion correction algorithms (see Chap. 26). However, the rigid-body registration algorithms may not be effective when motion is sufficiently large so that, coupled with image distortions dependent on magnetic field inhomogeneities and/or gradient nonlinearity, it induces a transformation that is no longer a rigid body motion. When voxel dimension decreases, image quality is more sensitive to bulk head motion. An-

other coherent noise is physiological motion, which is mainly due to respiration and cardiac pulsation and can be reduced by post-processing (see Chap. 16). After minimizing coherent noise components, random incoherent noise is left. The simple, effective approach to minimize the noise is to use a high quality preamplifier with a low noise figure. A typical noise figure is >1.5 dB in a wide-band bipolar-based preamplifier used in MRI systems, and can be reduced significantly using a narrow frequency GaAs-based preamplifier.

18.2.2
Imaging Techniques

Technically, high spatial resolution can be obtained easily by conventional imaging techniques such as FLASH. Using these conventional techniques, high spatial resolution in BOLD-based fMRI has been achieved (FRAHM et al. 1993; KIM et al. 1994; MENON et al. 1997). These techniques have poor temporal resolution because the data collection time of a single image is: (number of phase encoding steps)×(repetition time). To use statistical analyses for determining active voxels in fMRI, many images are needed and thus it is important to have adequate temporal resolution. To acquire an image faster, the segmented, interleaved fast imaging techniques described in Chaps. 13–15 can be used for high resolution studies. An example of the use of segmented echo planar imaging (EPI) techniques for fMRI studies is shown in Fig. 18.1 (see also Fig. 18.4). A BOLD-based functional map of somatosensory stimulation with 150×150 μm^2 in-plane resolution is overlaid on an original EPI image at 9.4 T. Two-shot EPI with a gradient echo time of 10 ms was used. Coronal brain images of an α-chloralose-anesthetized rat were obtained every two respiratory cycles (about 0.8 s per ventilator pumping cycle) during stimulation with repeated electric pulses (1.5 mA amplitude, 3 Hz frequency, and 0.3 ms duration) for a total of 2 min. The activation site is localized to the contralateral forelimb somatosensory area. Note that since a surface coil is used for data detection, high sensitivity can be obtained with a narrow field of view. A similar segmented approach can be used for high resolution CBF-based fMRI (KWONG et al. 1992; EDELMAN et al. 1994; KIM 1995), in which multiple segments are acquired sequentially without any additional delay after a single spin tagging pulse (KIM et al. 1996).

High Resolution fMRI

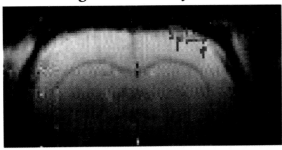

Fig. 18.1. High resolution blood oxygen level-dependent (BOLD)-based functional map of rat brain during electric forepaw stimulation overlaid on an original echo planar imaging (EPI) image. Spatial resolution is 150×150×2000 μm³. Coronal two-shot, segmented gradient echo EPI images were acquired at 9.4 T with gradient echo time of 10 ms. A 1.5 mA current was applied to a forepaw in a rat for 2 min. Box-car cross correlation was used to calculate a statistical map and a correlation value of 0.6 was applied for threshold. Activation is located at the contralateral somatosensory area, which is consistent with stereotaxic coordinates of forelimb S1. (From PAXINOS and WATSON 1986)

18.3
Vasculature Considerations

If the observed image intensity changes can only be detected in large (macroscopic) vessels which drain/supply the functionally involved gray matter regions (see Chaps. 7, 8 for large vessel inflow effect and Chap. 20 for draining veins), then fMRI will be somewhat spatially nonspecific for the functionally activated areas. Therefore, the ability to distinguish the macro- vs the microvascular effects is of particular importance, whether they are based on CBF changes only or on the BOLD phenomenon. Since large size vessels can run several centimeters in length, it becomes difficult to discern the actual gray matter region of increased neuronal activity. Hence, effective spatial resolution is degraded. However, there is considerable dilution of deoxyhemoglobin changes downstream from the neuronally active region by blood draining from inactive areas. This reduces the probability of significant contributions from large vessels in BOLD fMRI. In the macroscale spatial resolution, this may not be a major problem. However, in column level spatial resolution, large vessel contributions in both BOLD and CBF-based fMRI should be avoided. Here it is defined that the microvasculature is arterioles, capillaries and venules which cannot be spatially resolved in high resolution MR images, while the macrovasculature consists of large arteries and veins.

18.3.1
Separation of Macrovascular Inflow Effects in fMRI

In T1-based fMRI techniques, macro- and microvascular effects can be differentiated by adjusting the delay time between spin tagging pulse(s) and data collection (i.e., inversion time) (KIM and TSEKOS 1997). Radiofrequency (RF)-tagged blood proton spins move into the imaging slice through large arterial vessels. Then, they are delivered into capillaries and exchange with tissue water proton spins (perfusion). Depending on the travel distance and inversion time, contributions from macro- and microvessels will be different. Complete refreshment of tagged spins occurs when the inversion time is greater than or equal to travel distance/velocity. For example, with a travel distance of 10 mm and flow velocities of >5 cm/sec, fresh blood spins will be completely replenished during the inversion time of >0.2 s, regardless of control or stimulation periods. Thus, increases in these flows do not induce significant task-related signal changes. In human studies, when inversion time was 0.4 s, large arterial vessels had significant signal changes during finger opposition, while tissue areas were dominant when inversion time was set to 1.4 s (KIM and TSEKOS 1997). In order to reduce the macrovascular contributions in the functional images, a thinner inversion slab and/or a longer inversion time can be used.

BOLD contrast images obtained under rapid RF pulsing conditions can have an "inflow" component from large vessels (LAI et al. 1993; MENON et al. 1993; DUYN et al. 1994; FRAHM et al. 1994; KIM et al. 1994; SEGEBARTH et al. 1994) that is dominated by fast flowing macrovascular blood in arteries and large veins. This macrovascular inflow effect has probably been the major source of "activation" in numerous early functional imaging studies conducted with conventional techniques (e.g., FLASH) which used large tip angles and rapid pulsing in order to have adequate SNR. Especially in high resolution fMRI using multiple RF pulses, regardless of conventional imaging or multi-segmented fast imaging, the inflow area may have a high CNR because the velocity increase in large vessels changes the magnitude of replenishment of "fresh" spins. This effect, however, can be easily eliminated by allowing full relaxation between sequential RF pulses, or minimized by pulsing slowly relative to excitation flip angles with a consequent loss of SNR. Alternatively, spin echo-based techniques can be used in which signals from stationary tissues will refocus at the spin echo time, while spins of fast moving components dephase, resulting in loss of signal intensity.

18.3.2
Separation of Micro- and Macrovascular BOLD Effects

When the inflow component is suppressed, it is possible to specifically examine the vascular origin of the BOLD phenomenon. The BOLD phenomenon has two components (Ogawa et al. 1993; Weisskoff et al. 1994); one is due to dephasing of the magnetization in the presence of susceptibility-induced gradients of relatively large venous vessels, and the other is due to diffusion within the steep, susceptibility-induced gradients from small vessels (capillaries and venules). The first component induces high percentage signal changes. Generally, areas with some of the most intense stimulation-related signal change lie over large venous vessels. This component may have contributed predominantly to the fMRI maps acquired at short TE and/or at low magnetic fields (Lai et al. 1993; Menon et al. 1993;

Frahm et al. 1994; Kim et al. 1994). The second component induces small signal changes in diffuse areas which are not associated with any detectable large venous vessels. The BOLD effect in these areas presumably arises from tissues around and inside small vessels (sub-millimeter diameter). Spin echo images are less sensitive to susceptibility effects in large vessels than gradient echo images (Ogawa et al. 1993; Weisskoff et al. 1994). However, the T2 of blood in large venous vessels is changed during specific tasks (Thulborn et al. 1982; Ogawa et al. 1993; Bandettini and Wong 1995). Therefore, spin echo or asymmetric spin echo techniques are not immune to large vessel BOLD contributions.

Large venous vessel contribution to BOLD can be examined by comparing BOLD maps with CBF-based fMRI maps; because CBF technique is sensitive to microvessels (Bandettini and Wong 1997; Kim and Tsekos 1997). Figure 18.2 shows a comparison of fMRI maps measured by BOLD and CBF-based techniques. The flow-sensitive alternating inversion recovery (FAIR) technique was used during left thumb-finger opposition (Kim et al. 1997); the BOLD map was obtained from non-slice selective in-

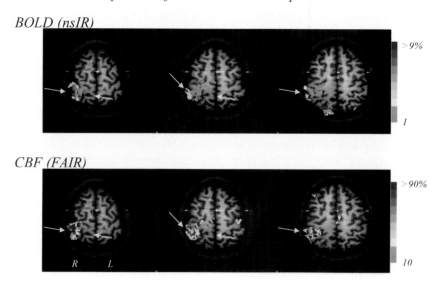

Comparison of BOLD and CBF maps

BOLD (nsIR)

CBF (FAIR)

Fig. 18.2. Representative three-slice relative percent change maps overlaid on T1-weighted echo planar imaging (EPI) during left hand finger opposition. The flow-sensitive alternating inversion recovery (FAIR) technique was used to acquire blood oxygen level-dependent (BOLD; *top*) and cerebral blood flow (CBF; *bottom*) contrast simultaneously. BOLD maps were obtained from non-slice selective IR (nsIR) images and CBF maps were calculated from differences between slice-selective and non-slice selective inversion (IR) images. A cross-correlation value of 0.3 was used for threshold. For BOLD images, each color increment represents a 1% increment starting from the bottom 1%, while for CBF images, each color increment represents a 10% increment starting from the bottom 10%. *Arrows* indicate the right (contralateral) central sulcus; *R* and *L* refer to right and left hemispheres, respectively. The *oblique arrow* at the middle slice shows no activation in the CBF map, but a large signal increase in the BOLD map, suggesting BOLD is sensitive to large draining veins

version recovery images and the CBF map from subtraction of non-slice selective from slice selective inversion recovery images. Since the inversion time was 1.4 s, only microvascular components will contribute to the CBF-based map. In macroscale spatial resolution, activation areas are consistent between the maps measured by both techniques. However, pixel-by-pixel comparison shows discrepancies between the two maps. Large signal changes in BOLD are located at draining veins, indicated by arrows in the middle slice, while no signal change was observed in CBF. Tissue areas with high percent CBF changes have low BOLD signal changes. When higher spatial resolution is obtained with lower SNR and CNR, only areas with large percent change are more likely to be active, which means large vessels in BOLD. This large vascular contribution should be minimized for high resolution studies.

One approach to minimize macrovascular components is to use bipolar gradients (as employed in diffusion-weighted images), which, with a b value of ~30 s/mm^2, are expected to leave only the microvascular/extravascular contribution (LE BIHAN et al. 1986; NEIL et al. 1991). At 1.5 T, SONG et al. (1994)

showed that task-related BOLD signal changes were eliminated at a b value of 42 s/mm^2, suggesting that the macrovascular component dominates the BOLD effect. A further study at 1.5 T showed that 60% of BOLD signals in visual stimulation were lost with a b value of 600 s/mm^2 (BOXERMAN et al. 1995). At high magnetic fields (3 and 4 Tesla), signal changes induced by visual and motor activation persisted significantly even at b values of >400 s/mm^2 (MENON et al. 1994; SONG et al. 1995), suggesting that extravascular and intravascular components coexist at high fields. Thus, to increase BOLD effects at the microvascular (including intra- and extravascular) level, higher magnetic fields can be used. To further examine microvascular contributions of BOLD at ultra-high magnetic field, a spin echo imaging technique with bipolar diffusion gradients was used at 9.4 T in rats during electric forepaw stimulation. Figure 18.3 shows functional maps with b values of 6.1 and 438 s/mm^2, an anatomic image with region of interest (ROI), and time courses in ROI. Since SNR is higher in images with low gradient strength than those with high b value, different thresholds were used; cross-correlation values were 0.8 for images

Diffusion-weighted Spin Echo BOLD fMRI

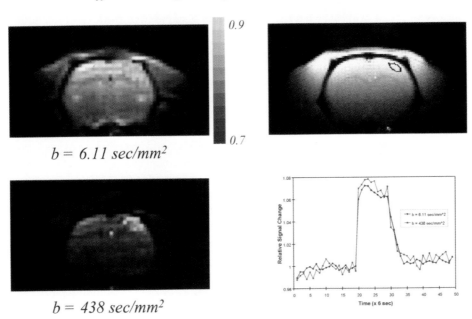

Fig. 18.3. Representative diffusion-weighted fMRI of rat brain during electric forepaw stimulation. A single-shot spin echo echo planar imaging (EPI) technique with bipolar diffusion-weighted gradient was used at 9.4 T. Spatial resolution is 470×470×2000 μm^2. Two fMRI maps with b values of 6.1 (*left top*) and 438 s/mm^2 (*left bottom*) were calculated using cross-correlation values of 0.8 and 0.7, respectively. A TurboFLASH image with region of interest (ROI) is shown in the *right upper corner*; time courses of diffusion-weighted images within ROI are shown in the *right bottom corner*. Clearly, relative signal changes are the same in both images with different b values, suggesting that only microvascular/extravascular components contribute to BOLD at 9.4 T

with b of 6.1 s/mm^2 and 0.7 for images with b of 438 s/mm^2. The activation area was located at the forepaw somatosensory area in both fMRI maps. If large vascular components contribute, it is expected to decrease relative signal changes when higher b value is used. Interestingly, relative signal changes in the somatosensory area marked in the anatomic image are the same, 7%, suggesting that the microvascular component is dominant. This indicates that high spatial resolution can be obtained with spin echo techniques with bipolar gradients at high magnetic fields.

18.4
Physiological Considerations

To obtain the spatial resolution of the column or on a higher scale, large vessel components should be minimized. Thus, in this section, no macrovascular component contribution is assumed.

It is generally thought that the spatial extent of alterations in glucose metabolism, oxygen consumption, and CBF is consistent with the location of increased neuronal activity (RAICHLE 1987).

To investigate the spatial extent of metabolic and hemodynamic responses, a whisker/barrel model has been used (WOOLSEY and VAN DER LOOS 1970). In rats and mice, layer IV of the somatosensory area contains discrete cytoarchitectonic units which are called barrels and which receive a one-to-one projection from the whiskers on the contralateral face (WOOLSEY and VAN DER LOOS 1970; SIMON and WOOLSEY 1979; YANG et al. 1996). The larger whiskers on the upper lip, organized in a neat and predictable order, are "whiskered" (to and from movements of the whisker pad) in exploratory behaviors. A single barrel in the rat cortex (300–500 μm in diameter) can be found by stereotaxis without functional assays (CHAPIN 1986). This widely accepted and well documented whisker/barrel model serves as an important model to study the relationship between cortical organization and function (JONES and DIAMOND 1995). According to CBF and glucose metabolism studies in animals using invasive 2-deoxyglucose (2DG) and ^{14}C-iodoantipyrine (IAP) autoradiographic methods (KENNEDY et al. 1976; HUBEL and WIESEL 1977; LEVAY et al. 1985), corresponding neuronally active columns/barrels show specific increases of CBF and glucose consumption rate. Recently, YANG et al. (1996, 1997) studied whisker stimulation using the BOLD fMRI technique and

found that this technique detects activation of a single barrel at 7 T. Spatial distribution of BOLD fMRI signal change is consistent with that of neuronal activity (YANG et al. 1997). This study suggests that the BOLD technique provides column level spatial resolution. However, some may argue that a whisker/barrel vascular structure is unique and findings based on this model may not be generalized.

Recently, Grinvald and coworkers have raised fundamental questions about the specificity of CBF/CBV (cerebral blood volume) response to elevated neuronal activity based on intrinsic optical imaging studies of ocular dominance columns in monkeys and cats (MALONEK and GRINVALD 1996). They found that an increase of deoxyhemoglobin concentration within 3 s (early time point) after onset of stimulation was observed at both active, although a little more, and inactive columns due both to an early increase of oxygen consumption rate and a late CBV response. This suggests that the area with a metabolic response is larger than the area of electrical activity. At a later time point, CBV increased more than elevation of oxygen consumption, resulting in decrease of deoxyhemoglobin. This increase of CBV (sum of oxy- and deoxyhemoglobin) was observed at both active, again a little more, and inactive columns. Compared to the area of metabolic response, spatial correspondence of CBV with the actual site of electrical activity is poor because, in the terminology of these authors, the cerebral vasculature "waters the whole garden for the sake of one thirsty flower." Although the area with later deoxyhemoglobin decrease is less specific than that with earlier deoxyhemoglobin increase, both hemodynamic (CBF/CBV) and metabolic (oxygen consumption) responses are more widespread than electric activity, which may be due to increased synaptic activity including excitatory activity in the active column and inhibitory activity in the inactive column. This argument was supported by NUDO and MASTERSON (1986); they studied the glucose consumption in the auditory system of cats and found that glucose consumption increased during synaptic activity whether excitatory or inhibitory without the necessity of electric discharge. This indicates that if the area of synaptic activity is larger than that of electrical activity, the "active area," as determined by metabolic- and hemodynamic-based techniques, is larger than the area of electrical activity.

To improve spatial resolution in the column resolution, the initial period of deoxyhemoglobin changes (FROSTIG et al. 1990; GRINVALD et al. 1991;

MALONEK and GRINVALD 1996) was used in optical images, suggesting that higher spatial resolution may be obtained when BOLD effects are observed within 2–3 s following stimulation. This initial period is assumed to be related to oxygen consumption (metabolism) rather than CBF change and its area to be more spatially specific to increased neuronal activity. Similar to optical imaging studies, negative initial BOLD signal change has been used during visual stimulation in humans (MENON et al. 1995; HU et al. 1997) (see Chap. 22). The area with the initial negative change is smaller than that with a later positive BOLD change. The negative BOLD signal is small and requires high temporal resolution and a long inter-task interval. To get column level spatial resolution, high spatial resolution is needed in addition to high temporal resolution (see Chaps. 19, 22).

An alternative approach to obtain high spatial resolution is to compare (initial negative or later positive) signal changes induced by one and the other tasks. This approach was used by MENON et al. (1997) to map ocular dominance columns in humans. Right and left eye stimulation was alternated. By comparing the images of two tasks, the pixels only related to the right or the left eye response were found to be interleaved, perpendicular to the cortical ribbon. In this study, conventional FLASH technique was used. To improve SNR with high temporal resolution, a segmented EPI technique was employed to map ocular dominance columns in humans at 4 T (Fig. 18.4). The slice thickness was 4 mm with an inplane resolution of 0.55 mm (256×256, 14 cm FOV). Blue indicates pixels more highly activated during left eye stimulation, while red represents those during right eye stimulation. Right and left eye dominance columns are interleaved, as expected from optical imaging and single neuron recording in animals. This study shows that fMRI can be used to map functional activation with a column level spatial resolution. This method is extremely valuable for finding functional organizations at the column level in humans and animals. One potential problem arises, since we do not whether the areas activated by the two tasks are distinct. In this case, the areas active in common to both tasks can be canceled out by comparing fMRI images during the two tasks.

The above-mentioned high resolution studies, including whisker/barrel and ocular dominance columns, are based on BOLD contrast. Since the BOLD effect is based on complete or partial uncoupling between CBF and oxygen consumption, an interplay between CBF and oxygen consumption changes will be important for determining spatial resolution. Let us examine one hypothetical condition assuming that metabolic change is localized to the neuronally active area, while hemodynamic response is more spread out (MALONEK and GRINVALD 1996). Figure 18.5 shows an example of spatial extents and relative changes of various physiological parameters. As we assumed, the metabolic change (oxygen consumption) will give the best localization. Since degree of CBF modulation correlates well with metabolic activity, CBF techniques with thresholding would provide a reasonably accurate localization of neuronal activity. However, in BOLD, the neuronally active area has a lower percent change than the nonactive area. If an fMRI map is generated using a certain threshold, less metabolically active areas are likely seen, rather than the areas of high neuronal activity (see also Fig. 18.2). Furthermore, if CBF and oxygen consumption are coupled completely, BOLD-based techniques cannot provide high spatial resolution because the most neuronally active spot will not be detected. At column level spatial resolution, this will

fMRI of Ocular Dominance Columns in Humans

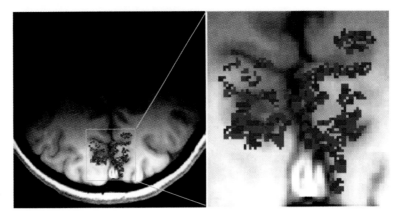

Fig. 18.4. Activation map of pixels exhibiting significant ocular dominance (p<0.001). Blue (red) indicates pixels more highly activated during stimulation of the left (right) eye. Functional images were collected using an 8-shot, interleaved echo planar imaging (EPI) imaging sequence with centric ordering of k-space and navigator echo correction. The slice thickness was 4 mm with an in-plane resolution of 0.55 mm (256×256, 14 cm FOV)

Spatial Distribution and Relative Changes of Signals

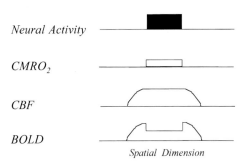

Fig. 18.5. Relative changes and spatial extents of neural activity, oxygen consumption (CMRO$_2$), cerebral blood flow (CBF), and blood oxygen level dependence (BOLD). In this model, we assumed that metabolic response is well-localized to neuronally active area, while CBF response is spread out widely. The BOLD signal is calculated by difference between oxygen consumption and CBF increase

be an obvious concern. Especially at the capillary level, further compounding effects will be contributed since the BOLD effect is dependent on vessel orientation and size. It is imperative to understand BOLD phenomena in order to obtain high spatial resolution using BOLD contrast.

18.5
Conclusion

A few millimeters to centimeter spatial resolution can be easily obtained using current fMRI imaging approaches. To obtain higher spatial resolution such as at column level, large vascular contributions should be minimized. In addition, higher magnetic fields and high sensitivity surface detection coils are desirable to obtain adequate CNR. By comparing fMRI signals obtained during two or more tasks, column level spatial resolution can be obtained.

Acknowledgments. We thank all colleagues in the CMRR at the University of Minnesota and the Imaging Center at the John Robarts Institute for helpful discussion and providing figures. This work is supported by NIH (MH57180 and RR08079) and the Whitaker Biomedical Foundation.

References

Bandettini PA, Wong EC (1995) Effects of biophysical and physiologic parameters on brain activation-induced R2* and R2 changes: Simulations using a deterministic diffusion model. Int J Imaging Syst Technol 6:133–152

Bandettini PA, Wong EC (1997) Analysis of embedded-contrast fMRI: Interleaved perfusion, BOLD and velocity nulling. 5th Sci Mtg Int Soc Magn Reson Med, Vancouver, Canada, pp 157

Boxerman JL, Bandettini PA, Kwong KK, Baker JR, Davis TL, Rosen BR, Weisskoff, RM (1995) The intravascular contribution to fMRI signal change: Monte Carlo modeling and diffusion-weighted studies in vivo. Magn Reson Med 34:4–10

Chapin JK (1986) Laminar differences in sizes, shapes, and response profiles of cutaneous receptive fields in the rat SI cortex. Exp Brain Res 62:549–559

Duyn JH, Moonen CTW, Van Yperen GH, De Boer RW, Luyten PR (1994) Inflow versus deoxyhemoglobin effects in BOLD functional MRI using gradient echoes at 1.5 T. NMR Biomed 7 (1/2) :83–88

Edelman RR, Siewert B, Darby DG, Thangaraj V, Nobre AC, Mesulam MM, Warach S (1994) Qualitative mapping of cerebral blood flow and functional localization with echo-planar MR imaging and signal targeting with alternating radio frequency. Radiology 192:513–520

Frahm J, Merboldt KD, Henicke W (1993) Functional MRI of human brain activation at high spatial resolution. Magn Reson Med 29:139–144

Frahm J, Merboldt K-D, Hanicke W, Kleinschmidt A, Boecker H (1994) Brain or vein-oxygenation or flow? On signal physiology in functional MRI of human brain activation. NMR Biomed 7 (1/2) :45–53

Frostig RD, Lieke EE, Ts'o DY, Grinvald A (1990) Cortical functional architecture and local coupling between neuronal activity and the microcirculation revealed by in vivo high-resolution optical imaging of intrinsic signals. Proc Natl Acad Sci USA 87:6082–6086

Gati JS, RS M, Ugurbil K, Rutt BK (1997) Experimental determination of the BOLD field strength dependence in vessels and tissue. Magn Reson Med 38:296–302

Grinvald A, Frostig RD, Siegel RM, Bartfeld RM (1991) High-resolution optical imaging of functional brain architecture in the awake monkey. Proc Natl Acad Sci USA 88:11559–11563

Hu X, Le TH, Ugurbil K (1997) Evaluation of the early response in fMRI in individual subjects using short stimulus duration. Magn Reson Med 37:877–884

Hubel DH, Wiesel TN (1977) Functional architecture of macaque monkey visual cortex. Proc R Soc Lond B198 (1–59)

Jones EG, Diamond IT (eds) (1995) Cerebral cortex. The barrel cortex of rodents. Plenum, New York

Kennedy C, Des Rosiers MH, Sakurada O (1976) Metabolic maps of the primary visual system of the monkey by means of autoradiographic 14C-deoxyglucose technique. Proc Natl Acad Sci USA 73:4230–4234

Kim S-G (1995) Quantification of relative cerebral blood flow change by flow-sensitive alternating inversion recovery (FAIR) technique: application to functional mapping. Magn Reson Med 34:293–301

Kim S-G, Tsekos NV (1997) Perfusion imaging by a flow-sensitive alternating inversion recovery (FAIR) technique: Application to functional mapping. Magn Reson Med 37:425–435

Kim S-G, Hendrich K, Hu X, Merkle H, Ugurbil K (1994a) Potential pitfalls of functional MRI using conventional gradient-recalled echo techniques. NMR Biomed 7 (1/2) :69–74

Kim S-G, Ugurbil K, Strick PL (1994b) Activation of cerebellar output nucleus during cognitive processing. Science 265:949–951

Kim S-G, Hu X, Adriany G, Ugurbil K (1996) Fast interleaved echo-planar imaging with navigator: High resolution anatomic and functional images at 4 Tesla. Magn Reson Med 35:895–902

Kim S-G, Tsekos NV, Ashe J (1997) Multi-slice perfusion-based functional MRI using the FAIR technique: Comparison of CBF and BOLD effects. NMR Biomed 10:191–196

Kwong KK, Belliveau JW, Chesler DA, et al. (1992) Dynamic magnetic resonance imaging of human brain activity during primary sensory stimulation. Proc Natl Acad Sci USA 89:5675–5679

Lai S, Hopkins AL, Haacke EM, et al. (1993) Identification of vascular structures as a major source of signal contrast in high resolution 2D and 3D functional activation imaging of the motor cortex at 1.5 T: preliminary results. Magn Reson Med 30:387–392

Le Bihan D, Breton E, Lallemand D, Grenier P, Cabanis E, Laval-Jeantet M (1986) MR imaging of intravoxel incoherent motions: Application to diffusion and perfusion in nerologic disorders. Radiology 161:401–407

LeVay S, Connolly M, Houde J (1985) The complete pattern of ocular dominance stripes in the striate cortex and visual field of the macaque monkey. J Neurosci 5:486–501

Malonek D, Grinvald A (1996) Interactions between electrical activity and cortical microcirculation revealed by imaging spectroscopy: Implication for functional brain mapping. Science 272:551–554

Menon RS, Ogawa S, Tank DW, Ugurbil K (1993) 4 Tesla gradient recalled echo characteristics of photic stimulation-induced signal changes in the human primary visual cortex. Magn Reson Med 30:380–386

Menon RS, Hu X, Adriany G, Andersen P, Ogawa S, Ugurbil K (1994) Comparison of SE-EPI, ASE-EPI and conventional EPI applied to functional neuroimaging: The effect of flow crushing gradients on the BOLD signal. Proc Soc Magn Reson 2:622

Menon RS, Ogawa S, Hu X, Strupp JP, Anderson P, Ugurbil K (1995) BOLD based functional MRI at 4 Tesla includes a capillary bed contribution: Echo planar imaging correlates with previous optical imaging using intrinsic signals. Magn Reson Med 33:453–459

Menon RS, Ogawa S, Strupp JP, Ugurbil K (1997) Mapping ocular dominance columns in human V1 using fMRI. J Neurophysiol 77:2780–2787

Neil JJ, Scherrer LA, Ackerman JJH (1991) An approach to solving the dynamic range problem in measurement of the pseudodiffusion coefficient in vivo with spin echoes. J Magn Reson 95:607–614

Nudo RJ, Masterson RB (1986) Stimulation-induced 14C-2-deoxyglucose labeling of synaptic activity in the central auditory system. J Comp Neurol 245:553–565

Ogawa S, Menon RS, Tank DW, Kim S-G, Merkle H, Ellermann JM, Ugurbil K (1993a) Functional brain mapping by blood oxygenation level-dependent contrast magnetic resonance imaging. Biophys J 64:800–812

Ogawa S, Lee TM, Barrere B (1993b) Sensitivity of magnetic resonance image signals of a rat brain to changes in the cerebral venous blood oxygenation. Magn Reson Med 29:205–210

Paxinos G, Watson C (1986) The rat brain in stereotaxic coordinates. Academic, San Diego

Raichle ME (1987) Circulatory and metabolic correlates of brain function in normal humans. Handbook of physiology-The nervous system, vol V, American Physiological Society, Bethesda, MD, pp 643–674

Segebarth C, Belle V, Delon C, Massarelli R, Decety J, Le Bas JF, Décorps M, Benabid AL (1994) Functional MRI of the human brain. Predominance of signals from extracerebral veins. Neuro Report 5(7):813–816

Simon DJ, Woolsey TA (1979) Functional organization in mouse barrel cortex. Brain Res 165:327–332

Song AW, Wong EC, Bandettini PA, Hyde JS (1994) The effect of diffusion weighting on task-induced functional MRI. Proc Soc Magn Reson 2:643

Song AW, Wong EC, Jezmanowicz A, Tan SG, Hyde JS (1995) Diffusion weighted fMRI at 1.5 T and 3 T. 3rd Sci Mtg Soc Magn Reson Med, Nice, France, pp 457

Thulborn KR, Waterton JC, Mattews PM, Radda GK (1982) Oxygenation dependence of the transverse relaxation time of water protons in whole blood at high field. Biochem Biophys Acta 714:265–270

Turner R, Jezzard P, Wen H, Kwong KK, Le Bihan D, Zeffiro T, Balaban RS (1993) Functional mapping of the human visual cortex at 4 and 1.5 Tesla using deoxygenation contrast EPI. Magn Reson Med 29:277–279

Weisskoff RM, Zuo CS, Boxerman JL, Rosen BR (1994) Microscopic susceptibility variation and transverse relaxation: Theory and experiment. Magn Reson Med 31:601–610

Woolsey TA, Van der Loos H (1970) The structural organization of layer IV in the somatosensory region (SI) of mouse cerebral cortex: The description of a cortical field composed of discrete cytoarchitectonic units. Brain Res 17:205–242

Yang X, Hyder F, Shulman RG (1996) Activation of single whisker barrel in rat brain localized by functional magnetic resonance imaging. Proc Natl Acad Sci USA 93:475–478

Yang X, Hyder F, Shulman RG (1997) Functional MRI BOLD signal coincides with electrical activity in the rat whisker barrels. Magn Reson Med 38:874–877

19 The Temporal Resolution of Functional MRI

P.A. Bandettini

CONTENTS

19.1
Introduction

Since its inception (Bandettini et al. 1992; Frahm et al. 1992; Kwong et al. 1992; Ogawa and Lee 1992), functional MRI (fMRI) has been steadily advancing from a brain activation mapping tool to a means for dynamically assessing brain activation characteristics across time scales ranging from days, to minutes, to tens of milliseconds. Changes in neuronally modulated hemodynamic states across seconds is routinely used to map brain function with fMRI. Changes in the magnitudes and locations of these activated regions over minutes to days with priming, learning, habituation, and reorganization have been studied (Breiter et al. 1996; Buckner et al. 1998a; Buckner and Koutstaal 1998; Cao et al. 1994; Cohen et al. 1997; Karni et al. 1995; Sakai et al. 1998; Schacter and Buckner 1998).

P. A. Bandettini, PhD, Biophysics Research Institute, Medical College of Wisconsin, 8701 Watertown Plank Rd., Milwaukee, WI 53226, USA

Since fMRI contrast is based on hemodynamic changes, the limits of interpretability over any time scale are dependent on the differentiability of neuronally independent hemodynamic changes from neuronally transduced hemodynamic changes. Particularly on the very rapid time scale (milliseconds to seconds), hemodynamic timing variability plays a central role in the limits of fMRI interpretability. It is argued in this chapter that the practical upper limit on functional temporal resolution is determined primarily by the variation of the hemodynamic response latencies in space and in time. To increase the temporal resolution, these variations first need to be better understood.

This chapter is an overview of fMRI temporal resolution. First, the basics of fMRI contrast, as they relate to temporal resolution, are reviewed. Second, fMRI temporal resolution issues are described, and high temporal resolution fMRI strategies are discussed.

19.1.1
Basics of fMRI Contrast

Several types of physiologic information can be mapped using fMRI, including baseline cerebral blood volume (Moonen et al. 1990; Rosen et al. 1989), changes in blood volume (Belliveau et al. 1991), baseline and changes in cerebral perfusion (Detre et al. 1992; Edelman et al. 1994; Kim 1995; Kwong et al. 1994; Williams et al. 1992; Wong et al. 1997, 1998), and changes in blood oxygenation (Bandettini et al. 1992; Frahm et al. 1992; Haacke et al. 1997; Kwong et al. 1992; Ogawa and Lee 1992; Ogawa et al. 1990; Turner et al. 1991). Recently, quantitative measures of the cerebral metabolic rate of oxygen ($CMRO_2$) changes with activation have been derived from fMRI data (Davis et al. 1998; Kim and Ugurbil 1997; van Zijl et al. 1998).

Because of its sensitivity and ease of implementation, the contrast used to observe susceptibility changes with changes in blood oxygenation, coined blood oxygenation level-dependent (BOLD) contrast by OGAWA et al. (1990), is the most commonly used functional brain imaging contrast used and is the technique that will be primarily discussed in this chapter.

With each of the above-mentioned techniques, the precise type of observable cerebrovascular information can be more finely delineated. Regarding susceptibility contrast imaging, spin-echo sequences are more sensitive to small susceptibility compartments (capillaries and red blood cells) and gradient-echo sequences are sensitive to susceptibility compartments of all sizes (BANDETTINI and WONG 1995; BOXERMAN et al. 1995b; KENNAN et al. 1994; OGAWA et al. 1993). Outer volume radiofrequency (RF) saturation removes inflowing spins (DUYN et al. 1994), therefore reducing non-susceptibility-related inflow changes when using short TR sequences. Diffusion weighting or "velocity nulling," involving the use of b>50 s²/mm-reduces the intravascular signal (BOXERMAN et al. 1995a; SONG et al. 1996) therefore reducing, but not eliminating, large vessel effects (intravascular effects are removed but extravascular effects remain) in gradient-echo fMRI and all large vessel effects in spin-echo fMRI. Going to higher field strengths has the same effect as diffusion weighting in the context of susceptibility-based contrast because the T2* and T2 of venous blood become increasingly shorter than the T2* and T2 of gray matter as field strength increases, therefore less signal will arise from within venous blood vessels, at higher field strengths, in sequences having TE=T2 and T2* of gray matter (MENON et al. 1993).

Regarding arterial spin labeling techniques that image perfusion, the time between the inversion "tag" and the image acquisition, the inversion time (TI) roughly determines the predominant vasculature being imaged. A short TI selects rapidly flowing spins (protons in arteries). A long TI selects spins that take longer to reach the imaging plane (protons that are either in capillaries or have exchanged with tissue). Again, as with susceptibility contrast, diffusion weighting gradients reduce or remove intravascular signal in perfusion imaging, allowing the creation of maps that exclusively delineate intravascular capillary and exchanged protons (WONG et al. 1997; YE et al. 1997). The issues of hemodynamic specificity, in the context of improving temporal resolution, will be discussed in detail in Sect. 19.3.1.

19.1.2
Neuronal-Hemodynamic Cascade of Events

Since fMRI contrast is based on cerebral hemodynamics, to begin to understand the issues in fMRI temporal resolution it is important to have a clear understanding of the cascade of hemodynamic events that follow neuronal activation. After the onset of activation, or rather, after the neuronal firing rate has passed an integrated temporal-spatial threshold, either neuronal, metabolic, or neurotransmitter-mediated signals reach arterial sphincters, causing vessel dilatation. The time for this initial process to occur is likely to be on the order of 100 ms. After vessel dilatation, the blood flow rate increases by 10%–200%, depending on the location and spatial scale of the measurement. The time for blood to travel from arterial sphincters, through the capillary bed to pial veins is thought to be about 2–3 s. This transit time determines when the blood oxygenation saturation increases in each part of the vascular tree.

19.1.2.1
Draining Vein Effects

In the resting state, hemoglobin oxygen saturation is about 95% in arteries and 60% in veins. The increase in hemoglobin saturation with activation is largest in veins, changing in saturation from about 60% to 90%. Likewise, capillary blood oxygen saturation changes from about 80% to 90%. Arterial blood, already saturated, shows practically no change in hemoglobin oxygen saturation. The fact that the largest oxygen saturation change is in veins is one reason why the strongest BOLD effect is usually seen in this part of the vasculature.

The second reason why the strongest BOLD effect is seen in draining veins is that activation-induced BOLD contrast is highly weighted by blood volume in each voxel (BANDETTINI and WONG 1997b; BOXERMAN et al. 1995a; HAACKE et al. 1995; JESMANOWICZ et al., 1998; KENNAN et al. 1994; OGAWA et al. 1993; VAN ZIJL et al. 1998). Since capillaries are much smaller than a typical imaging voxel, an extremely large range of voxel volumes in gray matter will likely have a constant 2%–4% capillary blood volume. In contrast, since the size and spacing of draining veins is on the same scale as most imaging voxels, it is likely that veins dominate the relative blood volume in any voxel that they happen to pass through. Voxels that pial veins pass through can have 100% blood volume while voxels that contain no pial veins may have only 2% blood volume. This stratification in blood volume distribution strongly determines the magnitude stratification of the BOLD signal.

One of the first observations made regarding fMRI signal changes is that after activation, the BOLD signal takes about 2–3 s to begin to deviate from baseline. The time for venous oxygenation to begin to increase appears to be directly correlated to the time that it takes blood to travel from arteries to capillaries and draining veins – about 2–3 s.

19.1.2.2
Blood Volume Change and CMRO$_2$ Change Effects

Other changes, including blood volume dynamics and CMRO$_2$ dynamics relative to flow and oxygenation dynamics, are less well characterized. These relative dynamics are typically invoked to explain other aspects of the BOLD signal change such as the occasionally observed pre-undershoot and the more frequently observed post-undershoot, which represent are essentially decreases in the BOLD signal observed prior to and after the activation-induced signal increase. Evidence exists that blood volume changes are slower than blood flow changes (MANDEVILLE et al. 1998), providing a compelling explanation for the post-undershoot signal. Models constructed to explain the pre-undershoot by blood volume dynamics require a rapid increase of capillary and venous volume (BUXTON et al. 1998a, b).

Although no direct measures of rapid CMRO$_2$ changes have been published, the dynamics of CMRO$_2$ changes relative to flow changes have been invoked in the same manner as blood volume dynamics to explain the pre- and post-undershoot in the BOLD contrast signal. The basic hypothesis is that CMRO$_2$ changes happen more rapidly than subsequent flow increases, therefore immediately reducing the saturation of hemoglobin prior to the flow increase that subsequently overcompensates for this effect (HENNIG et al. 1995; HU et al. 1997; MENON et al. 1995a). This hypothesis has been most strongly advocated by laboratories performing optical imaging (GRINVALD et al. 1991), since the maps created using this effect show extremely fine detail – suggesting a close proximity to direct metabolic changes and not to secondary hemodynamic effects. The post-undershoot has been explained in a similar manner. Again, the hypothesis is that activation-induced increase in CMRO$_2$ lingers on longer than time for flow to return to a baseline state, therefore

reducing the oxygen saturation of hemoglobin until CMRO$_2$ returns to baseline (FRAHM et al. 1996).

What matters in the context of temporal resolution is not the time constants or the rapidity of the various activation-induced signal increases and decreases, but the temporal variability of these changes and how accurately these changes can be measured. Figure 19.1 is a representation of the hypothesized approximate onset latency (x axis) and variability (width of shaded regions in x direction) of the cascade of hemodynamic changes that occur following neuronal activation. Also shown are the approximate distance from the neuronal activation source (y axis) and the variability in the distance (width of shaded regions in y direction). The area of the shaded regions give an approximate measure of the spatial and temporal variability. If these areas were reduced to points on a line (i.e., no spatial or temporal variability), then, regardless of the temporal offset and spatial proximity of the hemodynamic event, neuronal activation time and place (the zero intercept) could be precisely determined.

19.2
Temporal Resolution Issues

The temporal resolution of fMRI has been variably defined in the literature. These definitions include the image acquisition rate, the time it takes for the activation-induced response to rise or fall a given

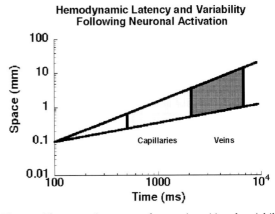

Fig. 19.1. The approximate onset latency (*x axis*) and variability (*width of shaded regions in x direction*) of the hemodynamic changes within capillaries or veins that occur following neuronal activation. Also shown are the approximate distances from the neuronal activation source (*y axis*) and the variability in the distance (*width of shaded regions in y direction*)

amount – otherwise phrased as the time constant of the measured changes, the maximum rate at which activation can be turned on and off and still generate a detectable response, the smallest detectable activation duration, the smallest detectable difference in latency (between two identical activations that have different onset times) in an individual voxel or region of interest (ROI), and the smallest detectable difference in latency across separate voxels or ROIs. Each of these aspects of fMRI temporal resolution are discussed below.

19.2.1
Image Acquisition Rate

The rate at which images are acquired is determined by the choice of pulse sequence. Multi-shot functional imaging techniques, while generally not needing specialized gradient hardware, usually require at least 3 s for image acquisition (FRAHM et al. 1993; GLOVER and LEE 1995; KIM et al. 1993; NOLL 1995; OGAWA et al. 1992). A faster technique, single shot echo planar imaging (EPI) (COHEN and WEISSKOFF 1991; SCHMITT et al. 1998; STEHLING et al. 1991), generally requires specialized gradients or gradient-switching hardware. The readout window width of an echo planar image is about 20–40 ms. Hybrid techniques such as multi-shot EPI (BUTTS et al. 1994; MCKINNON 1993) provide a good compromise in spatial resolution and time, but suffer from the same shot-to-shot instability as other multi-shot techniques. These instabilities in multi-shot techniques, primarily caused by respiration and cardiac cycle effects, are reduced by spiral scanning strategies (GLOVER and LEE 1995; NOLL 1995), retrospective k-space realignment techniques (LE and HU 1996), and navigator pulses (HU and KIM 1994).

In the context of fMRI, a TE in the range of 30–60 ms is optimum ($\approx$T2* of gray matter from 4 T to 1.5 T, respectively), and the minimum time between successive image acquisitions (TR) is typically about 100 ms. With the use of partial k-space acquisition techniques and a shorter and therefore nonoptimal TE, image acquisition rates as high as 60 images per second have been reported (BISWAL et al. 1997). Issues regarding the tradeoffs between image acquisition rate and functional contrast have not yet been fully resolved. From a practical standpoint, collection of a multi-slice, whole-brain, volumetric EPI data set requires a TR of about 2 s. The limit of a long TR can be overcome in the context of the cyclic on-off activation time series. Finer temporal sampling of cyclic on-off activation cycle is achievable using a TR that is not an even multiple of the on-off cycle time (BUXTON et al. 1998a).

19.2.2
Basic Dynamic Characteristics of the BOLD Signal

Figure 19.2 shows a typical BOLD contrast response from an ROI in motor cortex during repeated cycles of 20 s on, 20 s off finger tapping. Figure 19.2b is the average of the 12 on-off cycles shown in Fig. 19.2a. Several aspects of the BOLD contrast are illustrated here. First, the signal is generally stable over time, although FRAHM and colleagues have observed a small drift downward of the baseline and the activation-induced signal change magnitude within the first minutes of either continuous or cyclic on-off visual stimulation (FRAHM et al. 1996; FRANSSON et al. 1998).

With activation, the time for the BOLD response to first significantly increase from baseline is approximately 2 s (DEYOE et al. 1994; FRANSSON et al. 1998; KWONG et al. 1992). The time to plateau in the on state is approximately 6–9 s (DEYOE et al. 1994). With cessation of activation, the time to return to baseline is longer than the rise time by about 1 or 2 s (BANDETTINI et al. 1995). As mentioned, several

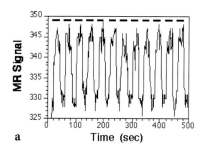

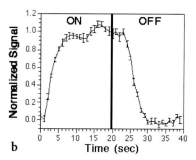

Fig. 19.2. a Typical blood oxygen level-dependent (BOLD) response from a region of interest (ROI) in motor cortex during repeated cycles of 20 s on, 20 s off finger tapping. The time series of echo planar images (EPIs) of the motor cortex were obtained using EPI at 1.5 T. TR=2 s; TE=40 ms. **b** The average of the 12 on-off cycles shown in **a**

groups have reported a pre-undershoot or initial dip during the first 500 ms (HENNIG et al. 1995) to 2 s of the signal (HU et al. 1997; MENON et al. 1995a). More commonly observed is a post-undershoot, which is observed more in visual cortex than in motor cortex and has an amplitude that is dependent on stimulus duration (DAVIS et al. 1994). On cessation of activation, the post-undershoot signal can take up to a minute to return to baseline (BANDETTINI et al. 1997; FRANSSON et al. 1998).

The hemodynamic response can be thought of as a low-pass filter (FRISTON et al. 1994). A straightforward method to determine the filter characteristics is to modulate the input and observe the output. Figure 19.3 demonstrates the effect of modulating the on-off motor cortex activation rate from 24 s on, 24 s off to 1 s on, 1 s off. Because the time to reach a baseline after cessation of activity is slightly longer than the time to plateau in an on state, the signal becomes saturated in the on state with the faster on-off frequencies. The relative activation-induced signal amplitude in motor cortex does not show a significant decrease until the switching frequency is higher than 0.06 Hz (8 s on, 8 s off), and does not follow the activation timing above 0.13 Hz. Other work has shown that with sufficient averaging a constant on-off rate of 2 s on, 2 s off is able to induce a measurable hemodynamic response (BANDETTINI and COX 1998). Also, the time to reach the saturated on state decreases as the on-off rate increases.

19.2.3
The Hemodynamic Response to Transient Activation

Linear deconvolution of a neuronal input function from the measured hemodynamic response gives a hemodynamic "impulse response" that resembles the type of response that is induced by a brief stimulus – modeled as a Poisson function (FRISTON et al. 1994) and a γ function (COHEN 1997) among others. The implicit assumption in this analysis is that the hemodynamic response is linear and that the neuronal input is a binary box-car function. Issues related to the linearity of the hemodynamic response become important when considering experimental design and signal interpretability issues and are discussed later in this chapter. Regardless, a brief impulse of activation elicits a response that quite closely resembles the shape of a deconvolved neuronal impulse response. The first "event-related" fMRI experiments were performed using primary

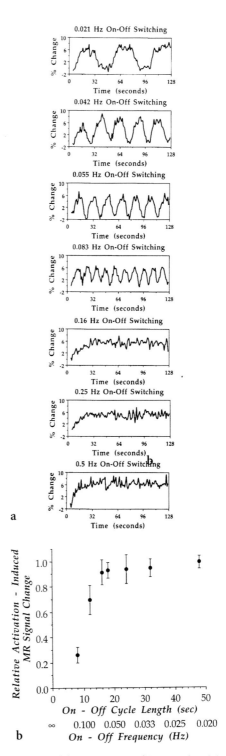

Fig. 19.3. a Signal from a region of interest (ROI) in motor cortex obtained during cyclic on/off finger movement. As the on-off frequency is increased from 0.024 Hz to 0.5 Hz, the activation-induced amplitude becomes decreased and the signal becomes saturated in the on state. b Summary of the dependence of the relative amplitudes of the activation-induced signal on switching frequency shown in a. The relative signal change amplitude is reduced at on-off rates above 0.06 Hz

visual and motor activation (BANDETTINI et al. 1993, 1995; BLAMIRE et al. 1992; SAVOY et al. 1994, 1995), demonstrating the critical fact that a single transient activation (2 s or less) can induce a measurable hemodynamic response. The general response was shown to peak at about 4–6 s following activation, then return to baseline at about 10 s following activation. Details of this transient activation-induced hemodynamic response are discussed below.

19.2.3.1
The Minimum Detectable Stimulus Duration

One of the first questions asked after fMRI was discovered was: What is the shortest stimulus duration necessary to elicit a measurable response? First, BLAMIRE et al. (1992) reduced a visual stimulus duration to 2 s, successfully showing a response. Then, BANDETTINI et al. (1993, 1995) demonstrated a response to 500-ms duration finger tapping. Figure 19.4 shows these early results obtained from a region in motor cortex. The time series consist of two finger tapping durations of 500 ms, 1 s, 2 s, 3s, and 5 s. The responses czn be clearly delineated from each other based on the finger tapping duration. The amplitude and time to peak systematically shift with stimulus duration. Also, even after waiting 20 s between stimuli, the baseline has shifted to a lower level, due to the time it takes for the post-undershoot to dissipate.

SAVOY et al. (1994, 1995) reduced the stimulus duration further, performing a study in which the fMRI response to stimulus durations of 1000 ms, 100 ms, and 34 ms were compared. A measurable response was obtained using all stimulus durations. The re-

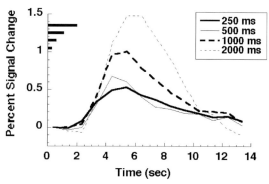

Fig. 19.5. Averaged signal from a region of interest (ROI) in visual cortex across four separate runs during which the subject was given a full field black and white alternating checkerboard stimulus for 250, 500, 1000, and 2000 ms. The total on-off cycle time was 14 s for each stimulus duration. The amplitude and peak time of the response decreases only until 500 ms. The responses to 500 ms and 250 ms stimuli are not significantly different, suggesting a minimum neuronal or hemodynamic activity time of at least 250 ms regardless of the briefness of the input stimulus. TR=1 s

sponses to the 100 ms and 34 ms stimuli were considerably smaller than the response to the 1000 ms stimulus and were similar in shape and amplitude to each other. These results suggest that the minimum stimulus duration has not yet been determined, but that below a specific stimulus duration, the hemodynamic response remains constant.

Figure 19.5 demonstrates a similar basic effect as shown by SAVOY et al. (1994, 1995), but at longer stimulus durations. Stimulus durations of 250 ms, 500 ms, 1 s, and 2 s were compared. The amplitude and peak time of the response decrease only until 500 ms. The responses to 500 ms and 250 ms stimuli are not significantly different. These data suggest a minimum neuronal or hemodynamic activity time of at least 500 ms regardless of the briefness of the input stimulus.

19.2.3.2
A Paradigm Shift in Experimental Design: Event-Related fMRI

A critical question in event-related fMRI was whether a transient cognitive activation could elicit a significant and usable fMRI signal change. In 1996, BUCKNER et al. demonstrated that in fact, event-related fMRI lent itself quite well to cognitive activation questions. In their study, a word stem completion task was performed using a "block-design" strategy and an event-related strategy. Robust activation in the regions involved with word generation was observed in both cases.

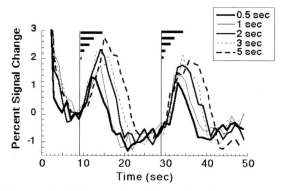

Fig. 19.4. Signal from a region of interest (ROI) in motor cortex across five separate runs during which the subject was cued to perform finger tapping for 0.5, 1, 2, 3, and 5 s twice during the time series. The time between the two finger tapping periods was 20 s; TR=1 s

Given the substantial number of recent publications that use event-related fMRI (BANDETTINI and COX, submitted; BIRN et al., 1999; BOYNTON et al. 1996; BUCKNER et al. 1998a, b; BUCKNER and KOUTSTAAL 1998; BUROCK et al. 1998; CLARK et al., 1998; DALE and BUCKNER 1997; FRISTON et al. 1998a, b; HENNIG et al. 1995; HICKOK et al. 1997; JOSEPHS et al. 1997; KONISHI et al. 1996; LUKNOWSKY et al. 1998; MCCARTHY et al. 1997; ROSEN et al. 1998; SCHACTER et al. 1997; ZARAHN et al. 1997), it is clearly an exciting recent development in fMRI. Several papers describing event-related signal change characteristics and analysis techniques have been recently published (BOYNTON et al. 1996; COHEN 1997; DALE and BUCKNER 1997; FRISTON et al. 1998a; JOSEPHS et al. 1997; VASQUEZ and NOLL 1998).

The advantages of event-related activation strategies are many (ZARAHN et al. 1997). These include the ability to more completely randomize task types in a time series, the ability to selectively analyze fMRI response data based on measured behavioral responses to individual trials, and the option to incorporate overt responses into a time series. Separation of motion artifact from BOLD changes is possible by the use of the temporal response differences between motion effects and the BOLD contrast-based changes (BIRN et al. 1998).

19.2.3.3
Experimental Design Issues in Event-Related fMRI

Experimental design and interpretation depend on whether the activation-induced hemodynamic response behaves like a linear system. Evidence is currently somewhat conflicting. BOYNTON et al. (1996) demonstrated that under most circumstances, the hemodynamic response behaves in a linear manner. Nevertheless, they also observed that the amplitude of the response to brief stimuli is larger than a linear system would predict.

This non-linear system observation is supported by BANDETTINI and COX (1998). In that study, the optimal interstimulus interval (ISI) was determined and the functional contrast in single event paradigms (2 s stimulus duration) was compared with the contrast of a blocked design (20 s on, 20 s off) paradigm. For comparison, a series of simulated responses were created by linear convolution of the hemodynamic impulse response (COHEN 1997) with a box-car function representing hypothesized underlying neuronal activity. Figure 19.6 shows the ex-

perimental and simulated linear system contrast (blocked design contrast=1) of a 2 s stimuli as the ISI is varied. The functional contrast is maximized at ISIs in the range of 10–12 s for both the experimental and simulated responses. The experimentally derived contrast, relative to blocked design contrast, is significantly higher than the simulated contrast. This suggests that the amplitude of the response with brief stimuli is greater than that which would be predicted by a linear system.

It is important to note that these results are from averaged ROIs in visual and motor cortex and may vary significantly across voxels within and between activated brain regions. Preliminary data also suggest differences in the event-related response with different types of stimuli (JANZ et al. 1998).

Reasons for nonlinearities in the event-related response can be neuronal, hemodynamic, and/or metabolic in nature. The neuronal input may not be a simple box-car function. Instead, an increased neuronal firing rate at the onset of stimulation (neuronal "bursting") may cause a slightly larger amount of vasodilatation that later plateaus at a lower steady-state level. The amount of neuronal bursting necessary to significantly change the hemodynamic response, assuming a linear neuronal-hemodynamic coupling, is quite large. For example, to account for the almost double functional contrast for the experimental relative to the linear convolution-derived single-event responses, the integrated neuronal response over 2 s must double. Assuming that neuronal

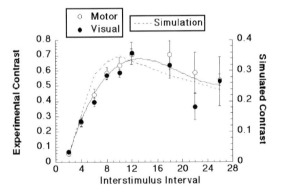

Fig. 19.6. Synthesized and experimental single-event contrast per unit time vs interstimulus interval (ISI). Contrast is normalized to the contrast obtained during the block design time series (blocked design contrast=1). The experimental optimal ISI for a 2 s stimulus duration is shown to be about 12 s. At the optimal ISI, the experimental contrast per unit time is only 35% lower than that of a blocked design paradigm. The synthesized optimal ISI is shown to be about 10 s. At the optimal ISI, the synthesized contrast per unit time is 65% lower than that of a blocked design paradigm

firing is only at a higher rate for about the first 50 ms of brain activation, the neuronal firing rate must be 40 times greater than steady state for this duration.

As is well known, BOLD contrast is highly sensitive to the interplay of blood flow, blood volume, and oxidative metabolic rate. If, with activation, any one of these variables changes with a different time constant, the fMRI signal can show fluctuations until a steady state is reached (BUXTON et al. 1998b; FRAHM et al. 1996; MENON et al. 1995b). For instance, an activation-induced increase in blood volume would slightly reduce the fMRI signal since more deoxyhemoglobin would be present in the voxel. If the time constant for blood volume changes were slightly longer than that of flow changes, then the activation-induced fMRI signal would first increase then be reduced as blood volume later increased. The same could apply if the time constant of oxidative metabolic rate were slightly slower than that of flow and volume changes. Evidence for increased oxidative metabolic rate after 2 min of activation is given by FRAHM et al. (1996), but no evidence suggests that the time constant of the increase in oxidative metabolic rate is only seconds longer than the flow increase time constant – as would be required to be applicable only to relatively high amplitude single- event responses. These hemodynamics, which may also differ on a voxel-wise basis, remain to be characterized fully.

From the above information, it is clear that when using a constant ISI, the optimal ISI is about 10–12 s, and that the response is nonlinear. Nonlinearities have also been shown demonstrated by other studies (FRISTON et al. 1998b; VASQUEZ and NOLL 1998). DALE and BUCKNER (1997) have nevertheless shown that responses to visual stimuli, presented as rapidly as once every 1 s, can be adequately separated using overlap correction or deconvolution methods. These methods are possible if the ISI is varied during the time series. BUROCK et al. (1998) demonstrated that remarkably clean activation maps can be created using an average ISI of 500 ms and deconvolution methods to extract overlapping responses. Assuming the hemodynamic response is essentially a linear system, there is no obvious minimum ISI. Rather, there exists an optimal ISI distribution. As suggested by Dale, an exponential distribution of ISIs, having a mean as short as psychophysically possible, is optimal from a statistical standpoint. Of course the speed with which stimuli can be presented ultimately depends on the study being performed. Many cognitive tasks may require a lower presentation rate. Several cognitive studies have been successfully performed using intermixed, rapidly presented trials (BUCKNER et al. 1998a; CLARK et al., 1998).

While excellent activation maps can be created using rapidly presented stimuli and deconvolution methods, interpretation of details of the deconvolved responses depends on the linearity of the system. Future work in event-related experimental optimization lies in what further information can be derived from these responses. Between-region, between-voxel, between-subject, and stimulus-dependent variations in amplitude, latency, shape, and responsiveness of the event-related fMRI responses are still relatively uncharacterized. The reasons for these differences are also still unclear.

19.2.3.4
Single-Event fMRI: Single Thought Measurement

It should be noted that while individual responses to individual events are easily detectable at low field strengths, the studies described in previous sections involved relatively long time series and considerable averaging or binning of the individual responses into specific categories. These approaches are extremely powerful, but repeatability of individual activation patterns is likely to be somewhat imperfect, especially across trials spaced several minutes apart.

Several recently published studies have demonstrated the ability to create functional maps and to derive useful information using only a single response to a single input. RICHTER and colleagues have been able to derive the relative onset of activation of supplementary motor cortex relative to primary motor cortex using a delayed motor task following a readiness cue (KIM et al. 1997; RICHTER et al. 1997a). Also, RICHTER et al. (1997b) have demonstrated the ability to correlate individual response widths to the duration of a mental rotation task. The larger the angle that an object was mentally rotated the longer the task took and the wider was the event-related parietal region response.

These types of studies represent yet another exciting new direction in fMRI paradigm design. It is imagined that measurement of complex responses from large arrays of cognitive manipulations are achievable in a single time series using this approach. This approach may represent a large jump in one aspect of fMRI temporal resolution – that of usable information per unit time. The combination of single-event fMRI paradigm design with analysis techniques that involve linear regression of multiple expected responses in a single time series (COURTNEY et al. 1997) may improve even further the utility of fMRI.

19.2.4
Latency Discernment Within a Voxel or Region of Interest

If a task onset or duration is modulated, such as in the above-mentioned motor cortex tasks or mental rotation studies (KIM et al. 1997; RICHTER et al. 1997a, b), the accuracy with which one can temporally correlate the modulated input parameters to the measured output signal depends on the variability of the signal within a voxel or region of interest.

SAVOY and colleagues (1995) have begun to address this issue of latency estimation accuracy. The variability of several temporal components of an activation-induced response function was determined. Six subjects were studied, and for each subject ten activation-induced response curves were analyzed. The relative onsets were determined by finding the latency with which each of the temporal components was maximized with each of three reference functions, representing three components of the response curve: the entire curve, the rising section, and the falling section. The standard deviations of the entire curve, rising phase, and falling phase were found to be 650 ms, 450 ms, and 1250 ms, respectively. The reasons for the differences between the rising phase and falling phase variability remain unclaer.

19.2.5
Latency Discernment Across Voxels or Regions of Interest

Researchers have reported observing across-region differences in the onset and return to baseline of the BOLD signal during cognitive tasks (BINDER et al. 1993; BUCKNER et al. 1996). For example, during a visually presented, event-related word stem completion task BUCKNER et al. (1996) reported that the signal in visual cortex increased about 1 s before the signal in the left anterior prefrontal cortex. One might argue that this is expected since the subject first observes the word stem then, after about a second, generates a word to complete this task. Others would argue that the neuronal onset latencies should not be more than about 200 ms. Can inferences of the spatial-temporal cascade characteristics of networked brain activation be made on this time scale from fMRI data? Without controlling for the intrin-

sic temporal variability of the BOLD signal over space, such inferences cannot be easily made for temporal latency differences below about 4 s. If appropriate controls are performed, then the variability approaches that of a single response in an individual voxel – described in Sect. 19.2.4.

LEE et al. (1995) were the first to observe that the fMRI signal change onset within visual cortex during simple visual stimulation varied from 6 s to 12 s. These latencies were also shown to roughly correlate somewhat with the underlying vascular structure. The earliest onset of the signal change appeared to be in gray matter and the latest onset appeared to occur in the largest draining veins. This basic observation was also made in the motor cortex (BANDETTINI 1995; BANDETTINI and WONG 1997c). In one study, latency differences did not show a clear correlation of latency with location of draining veins (SAAD et al. 1996).

Figure 19.7 demonstrates three sources of temporal variability. Figure 19.7a is a plot of the average time course from the motor cortex resulting from 2 s finger tapping. The first source of variability is the intrinsic noise in the time series signal. The standard deviation of the signal is on the order of 1%. The second source of variability is that of the hemodynamic response. As mentioned, this ranges from 450 ms to 1250 ms depending on whether one is observing the rising phase of the signal or the falling phase. The third source of variability is the latency spread over space.

The plot in Fig. 19.7a was used as a reference function for correlation analysis and was allowed to shift ±2 s. Figure 19.7b is a histogram of the number of voxels in an activated region that demonstrated a maximum correlation with the reference function at each latency (relative to the average latency) to which the reference function was shifted. As can be seen, the spread in latencies is over 4 s. Figure 19.7c includes a map of the dot product (measure of signal change magnitude) and latency, demonstrating that the regions showing the longest latency roughly correspond to the regions that show the largest signal changes. These largest signal changes are likely to arise from downstream draining veins.

To obtain information about relative onsets of cascaded neuronal activity from latency maps, it is important to characterize the underlying vasculature-related latency distribution at which one is looking. SAVOY et al. (1994; ROSEN et al. 1998) demonstrated that activation onset latencies of 500 ms were discernible using a visual stimulation timing described as follows. First, the subject viewed a fixa-

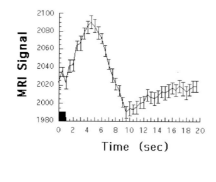

a

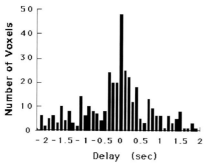

b

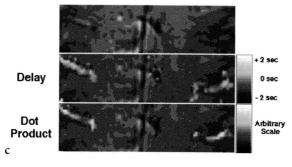

Delay

Dot
Product

c

+2 sec

0 sec

-2 sec

Arbitrary
Scale

Fig. 19.7a–c. Demonstration of several of the limits of fMRI temporal resolution. Echo planar imaging was performed at 3 Tesla using a Bruker Biospec 3 T/60 equipped with a local head gradient coil. An time course series of axial images (matrix size=96×96, FOV=20 cm, TE=40 ms, TR=500 ms, flip angle=80°) through motor cortex was obtained. Bilateral finger tapping was performed for 2 s, alternating with 18 s rest. The figures demonstrate that the upper temporal resolution is determined by the variability of the signal change in time and space. a Time course of the signal elicited by tapping fingers for 2 s. The standard deviation at each point was in the range of 1%–2%. The standard deviation of the hemodynamic change, in time, is in the range of 450–650 ms. b Map of the dot product (a measure of the activation-induced signal change magnitude) and the relative latencies or delays of the reference function (the plot in a was used as the reference function) at which the correlation coefficient was maximized. The spatial distribution of hemodynamic delays has a standard deviation of about 900 ms. The longest delays approximately match the regions that show the highest dot product and the area where veins are shown as dark lines in the T2*-weighted anatomical image. c Histogram of relative hemodynamic latencies. This was created from the latency map in b

tion point for 10 s. Then, the subject's left visual hemifield was activated 500 ms before the right. Both hemifields were activated for 9 s, then the left hemifield stimulus was turned off 500 ms before the right.

While these onset differences can be shown in a time series derived from an ROI, maps of latency cannot reveal the onset differences because the 4-s variability over space dominates the experimentally inserted 500 ms variability from left to right hemifield. In addition, the onset latency, as derived from a time course obtained from a ROI, is extremely sensitive to the choice in ROI, since the spatial variability is so extreme.

Modulation of the stimulation timing has allowed relative latency differences to be mapped. In the following study, the left-right onset order was switched so that in the first run, the left hemifield was activated and turned off 500 ms and 250 ms prior to the right, and in the second run the right hemifield was activated and turned off 500 ms and 250 ms prior to the left. Latency maps were made for each onset order and subtracted from each other to reveal clear delineations between right and left hemifield that were not apparent in each of the individual maps. This operation is shown in Fig. 19.8. It should be noted that the maps are of the change in onset of one area relative to another and not of absolute latency. Maps such as these may be extremely useful in determining which regions of activation are modulated relative to other areas, given a specific and measurable task timing or response variation.

A similar study by LUKNOWSKI et al. (1998) has shown that the mean accuracy of latency measures from multi-voxel ROIs is ±27 ms, which is comparable to that of electrophysiological experiments.

19.3
Increasing the Temporal Resolution

The current upper temporal resolutions of fMRI, and some variables that determine these resolution, as described above, are summarized in Table 19.1. The last estimate in Table 19.1 – that of the range of latencies over space – can be reduced to the standard deviation of the onset time per voxel if the appropriate normalization procedure is performed (as in Sect. 19.2.5) and if only relative latency is desired.

Methods discussed below have potential for increasing the temporal resolution even further. These

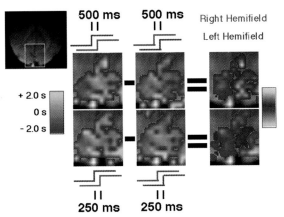

Right Hemifield

Left Hemifield

Fig. 19.8. Activation within a region of visual cortex is shown for two separate conditions. In one condition (*left*), the right visual hemifield stimulation precedes the left by 500 ms (*top*) and 250 ms (*bottom*). In the other condition (*middle*), the left precedes the right by 500 ms and 250 ms. Latency maps from both of these conditions show an intrinsic spread of ±2.5 s, which is too large to clearly identify the relative latencies across hemifields. However, once the data are normalized for this intrinsic variance by directly comparing the hemodynamic response from the two different lags within individual voxels, the offset between left and right hemifield can be observed (*right*). This is a demonstration that suggests that normalization of the hemodynamic lag can allow small relative temporal offsets to be identified. These normalized offsets can then be compared across regions to make inferences about neuronal delay. For this experiment the TR was 400 ms

Table 19.1. Functional fMRI temporal resolution factors

Temporal resolution factors	Values for each factor
Fastest image acquisition rate	≈64 images/s
Minimum time for signal to significantly deviate from baseline	≈3 s
Fastest on-off rate in which amplitude-is not compromised	≈8 s on, 8 s off
Fastest on-off rate in which hemodynamic response keeps up	≈2 s on, 2 s off
Minimum activation duration	≈30 ms (no limit determined yet, but the response behaves similarly below 500 ms)
Standard deviation of baseline signal	≈1% (less if physiological fluctuations and system instabilities are filtered out)
Standard deviation of onset time estimation	≈450 ms
Standard deviation of return to baseline time estimation	≈1250 ms
Standard deviation of entire on-off response time estimation	≈650 ms
Range of latencies over space	± 2.5 s

include increasing the hemodynamic specificity and the possibility of observation of a non-hemodynamic phenomenon with MRI.

19.3.1
Hemodynamic Specificity

Figure 19.9 shows a stylized depiction of the vascular tree and the corresponding blood transit delay associated with it. Pulse sequence sensitivity is also indicated. As is shown, the hemodynamic sensitivity can be improved by choosing the pulse sequence that is sensitive to the vasculature having the smallest spatial and temporal spread. As suggested by Fig. 19.9, arterial spin labeling (ASL) techniques allow exquisite control over the vasculature that is observed. If the appropriate TI and diffusion weighting are applied, capillary perfusion effects may be selectively observed. Several studies have compared regions of activation between perfusion based sequences and BOLD-based sequences (BANDETTINI and WONG 1997a, c; KIM and UGURBIL 1997), but

none to date have compared the latency ranges in regions demonstrating perfusion changes with voxels showing only BOLD changes. It is hypothesized that such a study would reveal that the distribution of latencies across voxels showing perfusion changes (because of the capillary specificity) would be smaller than the distribution of latencies across voxels showing BOLD changes.

A practical issue is that ASL techniques, while having more selective sensitivity to capillary effects, have about two to four times less sensitivity. Also, because of the long TI necessary and because pairs of sequentially obtained images are collected, the time between acquisition of each image is long (≈4 s), making any temporal sampling prohibitively coarse. One way around this temporal sampling problem is by having the on-off cycle rate not be divided evenly by the image acquisition rate, therefore each on-off cycle will be sampled at a slightly different time.

Alternatively, if high contrast to noise and short temporal spacing are necessary, perhaps ASL may be used in the identification of voxels showing only

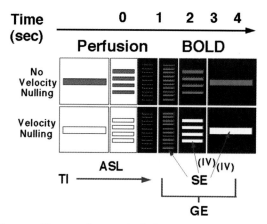

Fig. 19.9. The vascular tree, including arteries (*left*), arterioles, capillaries, and veins (*right*). If the inside of the vessel is filled in, the signal is arising from intravascular spins. Arterial spin labeling (*ASL*) is differentially sensitive to the arterial-capillary region of the vasculature, depending on the TI used and whether or not velocity nulling (diffusion weighting) gradients are used. A small amount of velocity nulling and a TI of about 1 s makes ASL techniques selectively sensitive to capillaries. Susceptibility-based techniques, including gradient-echo (*GE*) and spin-echo (*SE*), are also differentially sensitive to specific aspects of the vasculature. GE techniques are sensitive to susceptibility perturbers of all sizes, therefore they are sensitive to all intravascular and extravascular effects. SE techniques are sensitive to susceptibility perturbers about the size of a red blood cell or capillary, making them sensitive to intravascular (*IV*) effects in vessels of all sizes and to extravascular capillary effects. Velocity nulling makes GE sequences sensitive to extravascular capillary to vein effects, and makes SE sequences selectively sensitive to only capillary effects

capillary effects; then gradient-echo sequences with shorter TR values may be used to observe the signal change dynamics from these voxels.

Susceptibility-based techniques have different vascular sensitivities and therefore different temporal accuracy, depending on the vasculature. Gradient-echo techniques are sensitive to susceptibility perturbers of all sizes, and therefore sensitive to all intravascular and extravascular effects. Interestingly, (multi-shot) gradient-echo techniques that use short TR may be more sensitive to inflow effects which mostly happen upstream in arteries. The onset of these effects may be earlier than those observed using capillary-based contrast. Spin-echo techniques are sensitive to susceptibility perturbers about the size of a red blood cell or capillary, causing them to be sensitive to intravascular effects in vessels of all sizes and to extravascular capillary effects. Velocity nulling causes gradient-echo sequences to be sensitive to only extravascular effects (from capillaries to veins), and causes spin-echo sequences to be selec-

tively sensitive only to capillary effects. As with ASL techniques, spin-echo sequences have two to four times less functional contrast than gradient-echo sequences, and the addition of velocity nulling reduces this contrast further. Again, it might be useful to select the specific regions using a spin-echo velocity nulled sequence, then use the higher contrast to noise gradient-echo imaging to more accurately characterize the dynamics.

19.3.2
Neuronal Current Mapping Using NMR Phase Maps?

As discussed extensively in this chapter, the temporal resolution of fMRI is limited by the variability of the hemodynamic response. A question that most fMRI developers have probably asked themselves is: Are there any other MRI-measurable signatures of brain activation that allow more precise temporal and spatial accuracy? One phenomenon that is, by most calculations, likely to be too small by at least an order of magnitude is magnetic field changes caused by coherent neuronal currents in the brain. These electrical currents and magnetic fields are measured at the scalp using electroencephalography (EEG) and magnetoencelography (MEG), respectively. The hypothesis is that these currents may be measurable at their source, using changes in NMR phase-sensitive to subtle coherent B_0 shifts. A recent abstract has demonstrated that currents on the order of 10 µA are detectable (Li et al. 1998). A useable map of brain function using this technique remains to be seen. Nevertheless, the hope of obtaining images of the brain having the spatial resolution of MRI and the temporal resolution of MEG is extremely motivating.

19.4
Conclusions

As of June 1998, fMRI temporal resolution remains a moving target as it is changing at a rate that is so fast that any characterization becomes obsolete within a short time. New results, providing new hopes or new reasons for caution, are being rapidly published. It has hopefully been made clear in the chapter that the upper temporal resolution of fMRI depends not only on how well we understand neuronal-hemodynamic coupling, but also on how robustly the spatially dependent variables that affect neuronal-hemodynamic coupling and underlying temporal variability can be characterized or controlled on a voxel-wise basis during each experiment.

The temporal resolution of fMRI also strongly depends on the question being asked, as illustrated in Table 19.1. For specific questions, it compares well with the fastest techniques. For others, it is extremely coarse. Synergistic use of fMRI with other techniques may precipitate significant improvements as well. In general, robust characterization of individual and cascaded neuronal events remains a realistic goal with fMRI.

Acknowledgments. This work was supported by the National Institute of Mental Health grant MH51358. Ted DeYoe, Ph.D. and Ziad Saad were critical in obtaining the results shown in Fig. 19.5. Many of the elements of this chapter were brought together as a result of an ongoing lecture given by the author at the MGH visiting fellowship fMRI course, organized by Robert Savoy, Ph.D.

References

Bandettini PA (1995) Magnetic resonance imaging of human brain activation using endogenous susceptibility contrast. PhD dissertation, Biophysics Research Institute, Medical College of Wisconsin, Milwaukee

Bandettini PA, Cox RW (1998) Contrast in single-trial fMRI: interstimulus interval dependency and comparison with blocked strategies. In: Proc ISMRM 6th Annu Meeting, Sydney, p.161

Bandettini PA, Cox RW Functional contrast in event-related fMRI: theory and experiment. Hum Brain Mapp (submitted)

Bandettini PA, Wong EC (1995) Effects of biophysical and physiologic parameters on brain activation-induced R2* and R2 changes: simulations using a deterministic diffusion model. Int J Imag Syst Technol 6:134–152

Bandettini PA, Wong EC (1997a) Analysis of embedded-contrast fMRI: interleaved perfusion, BOLD, and velocity nulling. In: Proc ISMRM 5th Annu Meeting, Vancouver, p.156

Bandettini PA, Wong EC (1997b) A hypercapnia-based normalization method for improved spatial localization of human brain activation with fMRI. NMR Biomed 10:197–203

Bandettini PA, Wong EC (1997c) Magnetic resonance imaging of human brain function: principles, practicalities, and possibilities. Neurosurg Clin North Am 8:345–371

Bandettini PA, Wong EC, Hinks RS, Tikofsky RS, Hyde JS (1992) Time course EPI of human brain function during task activation. Magn Reson Med 25:390–397

Bandettini PA, Wong EC, DeYoe EA, Binder JR, Rao SM, Birzer D et al. (1993) The functional dynamics of blood oxygenlevel dependent contrast in the motor cortex. In: Proc SMRM 12th Annu Meeting. New York, p.1382

Bandettini PA, Wong EC, Binder JR, Rao SM, Jesmanowicz A, Aaron EA et al. (1995) Functional MRI using the BOLD approach: dynamic characteristics and data analysis methods. In: LeBihan D (ed) Diffusion and perfusion: magnetic resonance imaging. Raven, New York, pp 335–349

Bandettini PA, Kwong KK, Davis TL, Tootell RBH, Wong EC, Fox PT et al. (1997) Characterization of cerebral blood oxygenation and flow changes during prolonged brain activation. Hum Brain Mapp 5:93–109

Belliveau JW, Kennedy DN, McKinstry RC, Buchbinder BR, Weisskoff RM, Cohen MS et al. (1991) Functional mapping of the human visual cortex by magnetic resonance imaging. Science 254:716–719

Binder JR, Jesmanowicz A, Rao SM, Bandettini PA, Hammeke TA, Hyde JS (1993) Analysis of phase differences in periodic functional MRI activation data. In: Proc SMRM 12th Annu Meeting, New York, p.1383

Birn RM, Bandettini PA, Cox RW, Shaker R (1998) FMRI during stimulus correlated motion and overt subject responses using a single trial paradigm. In: Proc ISMRM 6th Annu Meeting, Sydney, p.159

Birn RM, Bandettini PA, Cox RW, Shaker R (1999) Event-related fMRI of tasks involving brief motion. Hum Brain Mapp 7:106-114

Biswal B, Jesmanowicz A, Hyde JS (1997) High temporal resolution FMRI. In: Proc ISMRM 5th Annu Meeting, Vancouver, p. 1629

Blamire AM, Ogawa S, Ugurbil K, Baker JR, Davis TL, Rosen BR, Rothman D, McCarthy G, Ellermann JM et al. (1992) Dynamic mapping of the human visual cortex by high-speed magnetic resonance imaging. Proc Natl Acad Sci USA 89:11069–11073

Boxerman JL, Bandettini PA, Kwong KK, Baker JR, Davis TL, Rosen BR et al. (1995a) The intravascular contribution to fMRI signal change: Monte Carlo modeling and diffusion-weighted studies in vivo. Magn Reson Med 34:4–10

Boxerman JL, Hamberg LM, Rosen BR, Weisskoff RM (1995b) MR contrast due to intravascular magnetic susceptibility perturbations. Magn Reson Med 34:555–566

Boynton GM, Engel SA, Glover GH, Heeger DJ (1996) Linear systems analysis of functional magnetic resonance imaging in human V1. J Neurosci 16:4207–4221

Breiter HC, Etcoff NL, Whalen PJ, Kennedy WA, Rauch SL, Buckner RL et al. (1996) Response and habituation of the human amygdala during visual processing of facial expression. Neuron 17:875–887

Buckner RL, Koutstaal W (1998) Functional neuroimaging studies of encoding, priming, and explicit memory retrieval. Proc Natl Acad Sci USA 95:891–898

Buckner RL, Bandettini PA, O'Craven KM, Savoy RL, Peterson SE, Raichle ME et al. (1996) Detection of cortical activation during averaged single trials of a cognitive task using functional magnetic resonance imaging. Proc Natl Acad Sci USA 93:14878–14883

Buckner RL, Goodman J, Burock M, Rotte M, Koutstaal W, Schacter D et al. (1998a) Functional-anatomic correlates of object priming in humans revealed by rapid presentation event-related fMRI. Neuron 20:285–296

Buckner RL, Koutstaal W, Schacter DL, Wagner AD, Rosen BR (1998b) Functional-anatomic study of episodic retrieval using fMRI. Neuroimage 7:151–162

Burock MA, Buckner RL, Dale AM (1998) Understanding differential responses in event related fMRI through linear simulation. In: Proc ISMRM 6th Annu Meeting, Sydney, p. 245

Butts K, Riederer SJ, Ehman RL, Thompson RM, Jack CR (1994) Interleaved echo planar imaging on a standard MRI system. Magn Reson Med 31:67–72

Buxton RB, Luh WM, Wong EC, Frank LR, Bandettini PA (1998a) Diffusion-weighting attenuates the BOLD signal change but not the post-stimulus undershoot. In: Proc ISMRM 6th Annu Meeting, Sydney, p. 7

Buxton RB, Wong EC, Frank LR (1998b) Dynamics of blood flow and oxygenation changes during brain activation: the balloon model. Magn Reson Med 39:855–864

Cao Y, Vikingstad EM, Huttenlocher PR, Levin DN (1994) Functional magnetic resonance studies of the reorganization of the human hand sensorimotor area after unilateral brain injury in the perinatal period. Proc Natl Acad Sci USA 91:9612–9616

Clark VP, Maisog JM, Haxby JV (1998) fMRI study of face perception and memory using random stimulus sequences. J Neurophys 79:3257–3265

Cohen JD, Perlstein WM, Braver TS, Nystrom LE, Noll DC, Jonides J et al. (1997) Temporal dynamics of brain activation during a working memory task. Nature 386:604–607

Cohen MS (1997) Parametric analysis of fMRI data using linear systems methods. Neuroimage 6:93–103

Cohen MS, Weisskoff RM (1991) Ultra-fast imaging. Magn Reson Imaging 9:1–37

Courtney SM, Ungerleider LG, Keil K, Haxby JV (1997) Transient and sustained activity in a distributed neural system for human working memory. Nature 386:608–611

Dale AM, Buckner RL (1997) Selective averaging of rapidly presented individual trials using fMRI. Hum Brain Mapp 5:329–340

Davis TL, Weisskoff RM, Kwong KK, Savoy R, Rosen BR (1994) Susceptibility contrast undershoot is not matched by inflow contrast undershoot. In: Proc SMR 2nd Annu Meeting, San Francisco

Davis TL, Kwong KK, Weisskoff RM, Rosen BR (1998) Calibrated functional MRI: mpping the dynamics of oxidative metabolism. Proc Natl Acad Sci USA 95:1834–1839

Detre JA, Leigh JS, WIlliams DS, Koretsky AP (1992) Perfusion imaging. Magn Reson Med 23:37–45

DeYoe EA, Bandettini P, Neitz J, Miller D, Winans P (1994) Functional magnetic resonance imaging (FMRI) of the human brain. J Neurosci Methods 54:171–187

Duyn JH, Moonen CTW, vanYperen GH, de Boer RW, Luyten PR (1994) Inflow versus deoxyhemoglobin effects in BOLD functional MRI using gradient-echoes at 1.5 T. NMR Biomed 7:83–88

Edelman RR, Sievert B, Wielopolski P, Pearlman J, Warach S (1994) Noninvasive mapping of cerebral perfusion by using EPISTAR MR angiography. J Magn Reson Imaging 4(P):68 (abstract)

Frahm J, Bruhn H, Merboldt K-D, Hanicke W, Math D (1992) Dynamic MR imaging of human brain oxygenation during rest and photic stimulation. J Magn Reson Imaging 2:501–505

Frahm J, Merboldt K-D, Hanicke W (1993) Functional MRI of human brain activation at high spatial resolution. Magn Reson Med 29:139–144

Frahm J, Krüger G, Merboldt K-D, Kleinschmidt A (1996) Dynamic uncoupling and recoupling of perfusion and oxidative metabolism during focal activaiton in man. Magn Reson Med 35:143–148

Fransson P, Krüger G, Merboldt K-D, Frahm J (1998) Temporal characteristics of oxygenation-sensitive responses to visual activation in humans. Magn Reson Med 39:912–919

Friston KJ, Jezzard P, Turner R (1994) Analysis of functional MRI time-series. Hum Brain Mapp 2:69–78

Friston KJ, Fletcher P, Josephs O, Holmes A, Rugg MD, Turner R (1998a) Event-related fMRI: characterizing differential responses. Neuroimage 7:30–40

Friston KJ, Josephs O, Rees G, Turner R (1998b) Nonlinear event-related responses in fMRI. Magn Reson Med 39:41–52

Glover GH, Lee AT (1995) Motion artifacts in fMRI: comparison of 2DFT with PR and spiral scan methods. Magn Reson Med 33:624–635

Grinvald A, Frostig RD, Siegel RM, Bratfeld E (1991) High-resolution optical imaging of functional brain architecture in the awake monkey. Proc Natl Acad Sci USA 88:11559–11563

Haacke EM, Lai S, Yablonski DA, Lin W (1995) In vivo validation of the BOLD mechanism: a review of signal changes in gradient-echo functional MRI in the presence of flow. Int J Imag Syst Technol 6:153–163

Haacke EM, Lai S, Reichenbach JR, Kuppusamy K, Hoogenraad FGC, Takeichi H et al. (1997) In vivo measurement of blood oxygen saturation using magnetic resonance imaging: a direct validation of the blood oxygen level-dependent concept in functional brain imaging. Hum Brain Mapp 5:341–346

Hennig J, Janz C, Speck O, Ernst T (1995) Functional spectroscopy of brain activation following a single light pulse: examinations of the mechanism of the fast initial response. Int J Imag Syst Technol 6:203–208

Hickok G, Love T, Swinney D, Wong EC, Buxton RB (1997) Functional MR imaging during auditory word perception: a single-trial presentation paradigm. Brain Language 58:197–201

Hu X, Kim S-G (1994) Reduction of signal fluctuations in functional MRI using navigator echoes. Magn Reson Med 31:495–503

Hu X, Le TH, Ugurbil K (1997) Evaluation of the early response in fMRI in individual subjects using short stimulus duration. Magn Reson Med 37:877–884

Janz C, Schmitt C, Fischer H, Speck O, Hennig J (1998) Variability of the hemodynamic response to different stimuli in single event paradigms. In: Proc ISMRM 6th Annu Meeting, Sydney

Jesmanowicz A, Bandettini PA, Hyde JS (1998) Single-shot half k-space high-resolution gradient-recalled EPI for fMRI at 3 tesla. Magn Reson Med 40:754–762

Josephs O, Turner R, Friston K (1997) Event-related fMRI. Hum Brain Mapp 5:243–248

Karni A, Meyer G, Jezzard P, Adams MM, Turner R, Ungerleider LG (1995) Functional MRI evidence for adult motor cortex plasticity during motor skill learning. Nature 377:155–158

Kennan RP, Zhong J, Gore JC (1994) Intravascular susceptibility contrast mechanisms in tissues. Magn Reson Med 31:9–21

Kim S-G (1995) Quantification of relative cerebral blood flow change by flow-sensitive alternating inversion recovery

(FAIR) technique: application to functional mapping. Magn Reson Med 34:293–301

Kim S-G, Ugurbil K (1997) Comparison of blood oxygenation and cerebral blood flow effects in fMRI: estimation of relative oxygen consumption change. Magn Reson Med 38:59–65

Kim S-G, Ashe J, Georgopoulos AP, Merkle H, Ellermann JM, Menon RS (1993) Functional imaging of human motor cortex at high magnetic field. J Neurophysiol 69:297–302

Kim S-G, Richter W, Ugurbil K (1997) Limitations of temporal resolution in fucntional MRI. Magn Reson Med 37:631–636

Konishi S, Yoneyama R, Itagaki H, Uchida I, Nakajima K, Kato H et al. (1996) Transient brain activity used in magnetic resonance imaging to detect functional areas. Neuroreport 8: 19–23

Kwong KK, Belliveau JW, Chesler DA, Goldberg IE, Weisskoff RM, Poncelet BP et al. (1992) Dynamic magnetic resonance imaging of human brain activity during primary sensory stimulation. Proc Natl Acad Sci USA 89:5675–5679

Kwong KK, Chesler DA, Weisskoff RM, Rosen BR (1994) Perfusion MR imaging. In: Proc SMR 2nd Annu Meeting, San Francisco

Le TH, Hu X (1996) Retrospective estimation and correction of physiological artifacts in fMRI by direct extraction of physiological activity form MR data. Magn Reson Med 35:290–298

Lee AT, Glover GH, Meyer CH (1995) Discrimination of large venous vessels in time-course spiral blood-oxygen-level-dependent magnetic-resonance functional neuroimaging. Magn Reson Med 33:745–754

Li S-J, Jesmanowicz A, Bodurka J, Hyde J (1998) Current-induced magnetic resonance phase imaging. In: Proc ISMRM 6th Annu Meeting, Sydney, p.1495

Luknowsky DC, Gati JS, Menon RS (1998a) Mental chronometry using single trials and EPI at 4 T. In: Proc ISMRM 6th Annu Meeting, Sydney, p.167

Mandeville JB, Marota JJA, Kosofky BE, Keltner JR, Weissleder R, Rosen BR et al. (1998) Dynamic functional imaging of relative cerebral blood volume during rat forepaw stimulation. Magn Reson Med 39:615–624

McCarthy G, Luby M, Gore J, Goldman-Rakic P (1997) Infrequent events transiently activate human prefrontal and parietal cortex as measured by functional MRI. J Neurophysiol 77:1630–1634

McKinnon GC (1993) Ultrafast interleaved gradient-echo-planar imaging on a standard scanner. Magn Reson Med 30:609–616

Menon RS, Ogawa S, Tank DW, Ugurbil K (1993) 4 Tesla gradient recalled echo characteristics of photic stimulation-induced signal changes in the human primary visual cortex. Magn Reson Med 30:380–386

Menon RS, Ogawa S, Strupp JP, Anderson P, Ugurbil K (1995a) BOLD based functional MRI at 4 tesla includes a capillary bed contribution: echo-planar imaging correlates with previous optical imaging using intrinsic signals. Magn Reson Med 33:453–459

Menon RS, Ogawa S, Ugurbil K (1995b) High-temporal-resolution studies of the human primary visual cortex at 4 T: teasing out the oxygenation contribution in FMRI. Int J Imag Syst Technol 6:209–215

Moonen CTW, van Zijl PCM, Frank JA, LeBihan D, Becker ED (1990) Functional magnetic resonance imaging in medicine and physiology. Science 250:53–61

Noll DC (1995) Methodologic considerations for spiral k-space functional MRI. Int J Imag Syst Technol 6:175–183

Ogawa S, Lee TM (1992) Functional brain imaging with physiologically sensitive image signals. J Magn Reson Imaging 2(P)-WIP (Suppl):S22 (abstract)

Ogawa S, Lee TM, Kay AR, Tank DW (1990) Brain magnetic resonance imaging with contrast dependent on blood oxygenation. Proc Natl Acad Sci USA 87:9868–9872

Ogawa S, Tank DW, Menon R, Ellermann JM, Kim S-G, Merkle H et al. (1992) Intrinsic signal changes accompanying sensory stimulation: functional brain mapping with magnetic resonance imaging. Proc Natl Acad Sci USA 89:5951–5955

Ogawa S, Menon RS, Tank DW, Kim S-G, Merkle H, Ellerman JM et al. (1993) Functional brain mapping by blood oxygenation level-dependent contrast magnetic resonance imaging: a comparison of signal characteristics with a biophysical model. Biophys J 64:803–812

Richter W, Andersen PM, Georgopolous AP, Kim S-G (1997a) Sequential activity in human motor areas during a delayed cued finger movement task studied by time-resolved fMRI. Neuroreport 8:1257–1261

Richter W, Ugurbil K, Georgopouloos A, Kim S-G (1997b) Time-resolved fMRI of mental rotation. Neuroreport 8:3697–3702

Rosen BR, Belliveau JW, Chien D (1989) Perfusion imaging by nuclear magnetic resonance. Magn Reson Q 5:263–281

Rosen BR, Buckner RL, Dale AM (1998) Event-related functional MRI: past, present, future. Proc Natl Acad Sci USA 95:773–780

Saad ZS, Ropella KM, Carman GJ, DeYoe EA (1996) Temporal phase variation of FMR signals in vasculature versus parenchyma. In: Proc ISMRM 4th Annu Meeting, New York

Sakai K, Hikosaka O, Miyauchi S, Takino R, Sasaki Y, Putz B (1998) Transition of brain activation from frontal to parietal areas in visuomotor sequence learning. J Neurosci 18:1827–1840

Savoy RL, O'Craven KM, Weisskoff RM, Davis TL, Baker J, Rosen B (1994) Exploring the temporal bourdaries of fMRI: measuring responses to very brief visual stimuli. In: Book of Abstracts, Soc Neurosci 24th Annu Meeting, Miami

Savoy RL, Bandettini PA, Weisskoff RM, Kwong KK, Davis TL, Baker JR et al. (1995) Pushing the temporal resolution of fMRI: studies of very brief visual stimuli, onset variablity and asynchrony, and stimulus-correlated changes in noise. In: Proc SMR 3rd Annu Meeting, Nice, p.450

Schacter DL, Buckner RL (1998) Priming and the brain. Neuron 20:185–195

Schacter DL, Buckner RL, Koutstaal W, Dale AM, Rosen BR (1997) Late onset of anterior prefrontal activity during true and false recognition: an event related fMRI study. Neuroimage 6:259–269

Schmitt F, Stehling MK, Turner R (1998) Echo-planar imaging: theory, technique, and application. Springer, Berlin Heidelberg New York

Song AW, Wong EC, Tan SG, Hyde JS (1996) Diffusion weighted fMRI at 1.5 T. Magn Reson Med 35:155–158

Stehling MK, Turner R, Mansfield P (1991) Echo-planar imaging: magnetic resonance imaging in a fraction of a second. Science 254:43–50

Turner R, LeBihan D, Moonen CTW, Despres D, Frank J (1991) Echo-planar time course MRI of cat brain oxygenation changes. Magn Reson Med 22:159–166

van Zijl PCM, Eleff SM, Ulatowski JA, Oja JME, Ulug AM, Traystman RJ, Kauppinen RA (1998) Quantitative assessment of blood flow, blood volume and blood oxygenation effects in functional magnetic resonance imagning. Nature Med 4:159–167

Vasquez A, Noll D (1998) Nonlinear aspects of the BOLD response in functional MRI. Neuroimage 7:108–118

Williams DS, Detre JA, Leigh JS, Koretsky AS (1992) Magnetic resonance imaging of perfuusion using spin-inversion of arterial water. Proc Natl Acad Sci USA 89:212–216

Wong EC, Buxton RB, Frank LR (1997) Implementation of quantitative perfusion imaging techniques for functional brain mapping using pulsed arterial spin labeling. NMR Biomed 10:237–249

Wong EC, Buxton RB, Frank LR (1998) Quantitative imaging of perfusion using a single subtraction (QUIPSS and QUIPSSII). Magn Reson Med 39:702–708

Ye FQ, Smith AM, Yang Y, Duyn J, Mattay VS, Ruttimann UE et al. (1997) Quantitation of regional cerebral blood flow increases during motor activation: a steady-state arterial spin tagging study. Neuroimage 6:104–112

Zarahn E, Aguirre G, D'Esposito M (1997) A trial-based experimental design for fMRI. Neuroimage 6:122–138

20 Spatial Selectivity of BOLD Contrast: Effects In and Around Draining Veins

S. Lai, G.H. Glover, E.M. Haacke

CONTENTS

20.1 Introduction

Building on the foundation laid with other neurofunctional imaging modalities, i.e., positron emission tomography (PET) and single photon emission computerized tomography (SPECT), functional MRI (fMRI) has, since its inception in the early 1990s, revolutionized the field of neurofunctio-nal imaging. The major advantage of fMRI is that, in addition to its high spatial and temporal resolution, it noninvasively depicts brain function by using blood as an endogenous contrast agent to image hemodynamics accompanying neuronal activation. Two signal contrast mechanisms have been identified to have functional sensitivity in MRI. The first mechanism is based on the shortening of effective longitudinal relaxation times in tissues due to increased perfusive inflow of unsaturated blood into the imaging volume (KWONG et al. 1992). The other mechanism, dubbed blood oxygenation level-dependent (BOLD) contrast (OGAWA et al. 1990a), depends on the fact that deoxyhemoglobin is paramagnetic (PAULING and CORYELL 1936) and that there is a change in blood oxygenation as a consequence of uncoupling between focal changes in blood flow and oxygen consumption, as originally suggested by PET data (FOX and RAICHLE 1986) and recently validated by optical imaging of intrinsic signals (FROSTIG et al. 1990) and by using MRI (LAI et al. 1996a; HAACKE et al. 1997). Among the two fMRI approaches, BOLD imaging has been the mainstay of brain fMRI studies because of its wide accessibility and relatively higher functional sensitivity.

The BOLD technique exploits the so-called susceptibility effects resulting from the magnetic susceptibility difference between the venous vasculature and the surroundings. Changes in the susceptibility of blood cause alterations in the magnetic field microgradients established in and near the capillaries, venules, and veins. Alterations in the field heterogeneity in turn affect the local transverse relaxation time, T2*. Gradient echo (GE) sequences have been shown to be sensitive to both small and large vessels (WEISSKOFF et al. 1994). With high enough signal-to-noise ratio, signal changes originating from the capillary bed are observable, although these signals are only a fraction of the signal change at 1.5 T (OGAWA et al. 1992; BOXERMAN et al. 1995). However, signals from large vessels are much stronger and often dominate the fMRI signals (LAI et al. 1993; MENON et al. 1993). The extravascular diffusion-in-

S. LAI, PhD, Department of Diagnostic Imaging and Therapeutics, University of Connecticut School of Medicine, 263 Farmington Avenue, Farmington, CT 06030-2017, USA
G.H. GLOVER, PhD, Lucas MR Center, Department of Radiology, Stanford University Stanford, CA 94305-5488, USA
E.M. HAACKE, PhD, Mallinckrodt Institute of Radiology, Washington University, St. Louis, MO 63110, USA

duced signal change in a spin echo (SE) acquisition has been theoretically predicted to be more sensitive to capillary-sized vessels (on the order of a few microns; Fisel et al. 1991; Muller et al. 1991; Weisskoff et al. 1994); nevertheless, due to the strong dependence of blood T2 on oxygenation (Thulborn et al. 1982), SE fMRI signals can also be dominated by large vessels (Bandettini et al. 1994). Furthermore, very large inflow effects can be seen with large vessels (Duyn et al. 1994; Frahm et al. 1994; Kim et al. 1994; Segebarth et al. 1994; Gao et al. 1996) and can be important in GE acquisitions with short repetition times (TR; Glover and Lee 1995; Haacke et al. 1995).

Because the BOLD signal from larger vessels can dominate the weaker signals from the capillary bed, there is a potential for spatial mismapping of the site of activation because the flowing blood can cause contrast downstream from the actual site of metabolic activity. Accordingly, the ultimate spatial resolution of a BOLD experiment may be limited by these flow effects. Engel et al. (1997) have measured the modulation transfer function (MTF) in the visual cortex using neural traveling-wave fMRI experiments and found localization precision within about 1.1 mm, but Gaussian-equivalent spatial resolution of only about 3.5 mm. In such studies, therefore, blurring of the boundaries among the different visual areas may arise due to the temporal effects from large vessels. It is not known if these results can be generalized to other cortical regions, since the visual cortex has relatively dense vascularization, and the signals in sensory cortex are in general much stronger than elsewhere.

For these reasons, a comprehensive understanding of the BOLD signal associated with large vessels is important for the assessment of the spatial selectivity of BOLD techniques. In this chapter, we are primarily concerned with the BOLD signals from large veins. We present simulations for the roles of both intravascular and extravascular signals and discuss methods for the visualization and discrimination of large vessels. This work represents a portion of the doctoral dissertation of one of the authors (Lai 1996).

20.2
Field Inhomogeneity
In and Around a Vein

To understand the signal behavior in and around a vein, it is imperative to have a quantitative view of the field inhomogeneity associated with the vein. Paramagnetic deoxyhemoglobin in blood induces a magnetic susceptibility difference, $\Delta\chi$, between the blood vessel and its surrounding. Because of its large ratio of length to diameter, a vein (pial vein or venule) can be reasonably modeled as an infinitely long cylinder (Fig. 20.1). Equations 20.1 and 20.2 describe the change in the magnetic field inside and outside the vein:

$$\Delta B_{in}(\theta)=2\pi\Delta\chi B\hat{0}(\cos^2\theta-1/3), \; r\leq R_o \tag{20.1}$$

$$\Delta B_{ex}(r,\theta,\psi)=2\pi\Delta\chi B_0\sin^2\theta\cos(2\psi)(R_0/r)^2, \; r>R_o \tag{20.2}$$

where r is the radial distance from the observation point to the axis of the cylinder, R_0 is the radius of the cylinder, θ is the angle between the axis of the cylinder and the static field, and ψ is the angle between the projections of the position vector of this point and B_0 into the plane perpendicular to the axis of the cylinder. Figure 20.2 gives an example of the field inhomogeneity profile in and around a vein that is perpendicular to B_0. As may be seen, strong field gradients are established in the perivascular space by the paramagnetic deoxyhemoglobin. These microgradients in turn induce significant signal loss in a T2*-weighted image, so that venous blood vessels often appear as dark structures, a phenomenon Ogawa originally observed at high fields (Ogawa et al. 1990b). The change of $\Delta\chi$ is associated with neuronal activity-induced blood flow change accompanied by a nearly constant oxygen consumption rate. The resulting intravascular and extravascular changes in local field inhomogeneity lead to the observed fMRI signals.

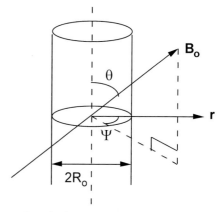

Fig. 20.1. The cylinder model

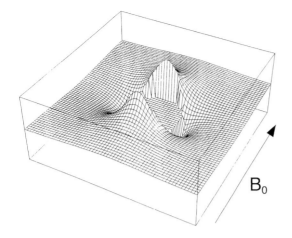

B_0

Fig. 20.2. Field inhomogeneities in and around a cylindrical vein. The vessel has a bulk susceptibility difference from the outside medium. The bulk field offset is homogeneous inside the cylinder while it is strongly position-dependent outside the cylinder

20.3
Mechanisms of BOLD Signals
In and Around a Vein

As suggested by the above discussion, the BOLD mechanism can be subdivided into intravascular and extravascular components. The importance of these two components depends on the imaging methods (GE or SE), imaging parameters and vascular geometry. A comprehensive understanding of the relative importance of these different components is paramount to the assessment of the spatial selectivity of BOLD imaging. In the following, we assess the relative contribution of each of the following BOLD mechanisms for a large vein:

1. Intravascular: change of blood T2/T2* due to the relaxation dependence on oxygenation (Thulborn et al. 1982). This effect is presumably due to the secular diffusion of protons through the microgradients near blood cells (Gillies and Koenig 1987). Furthermore, in a GE acquisition, the change of intravascular coherent frequency results in an altered NMR phase shift of blood signal relative to the tissue signal which alters the intravoxel spin dephasing in a voxel not fully occupied by blood (Haacke et al. 1994).

2. Extravascular: T2* change of the perivascular surroundings due to the change of the field inhomogeneity resulting from altered susceptibility

difference between the blood and surroundings. The extravascular diffusion effect is small for large vessels (Weisskoff et al. 1994) and will be ignored here.

20.3.1
Intravascular Effects: Blood T2/T2* Dependence on Oxygen Saturation

The transverse relaxation time, T2, of blood has a strong dependence on blood oxygenation, Y (Thulborn et al. 1982). Based on the Luz-Meiboom model of magnetization relaxation in the presence of exchange (Luz and Meiboom 1963), it was found empirically that the blood T2 has the following dependence on Y:

$$R2(Y)=R2_0+k(1-Y)^2 \qquad (20.3)$$

where $R2_0$ is the relaxation rate of fully oxygenated blood (i.e., Y=100%), and k is a constant that depends on field strength. For 1.5 T, Wright and co-workers (1991) found $R2_0$=4.02 s^{-1}, k=41.5 s^{-1}.

More recently, Li et al. (1998) have shown that the T2* of blood *in vivo* can be written approximately as:

$$R2^*(Y)=R2_0^*+k^*(1-Y) \qquad (20.4)$$

for 0.5≤Y≤1.0, where $R2_0^*$=5 s^{-1} and k*=14 s^{-1}. For a change in Y of 0.15, R2* changes by 2.5 s^{-1}, which, if blood is the only source of the fMRI signal, would lead to a change of roughly 8% for TE=40 ms.

The dependence of blood T2 on oxygenation indicates that SE fMRI signals can also be dominated by large vessels, despite the fact that extravascular diffusion effect is more sensitive to small vessels (Weisskoff et al. 1994). Apparently, the relative contribution from this mechanism increases with blood volume fraction in the imaging voxels of interest. Distinct from other BOLD components as detailed in the following, the fMRI signal due to blood T2/T2* dependence on Y does not change with the orientation of the vessel. For a voxel completely occupied with blood, the signal change due to the blood T2/T2* change constitutes the only mechanism of BOLD signal.

20.3.2
Coherent Intravascular NMR Phase Effects: Cancellation of Blood Signal with Surrounding Brain Parenchyma

20.3.2.1
Intravoxel Dephasing

In a GE image, the blood signal develops a phase shift relative to the surrounding tissue according to Eq. 20.1:

$$\phi_b = 2\pi\gamma\Delta\chi\hat{B0}(cos^2\theta - 1/3)TE \qquad (20.5)$$

where $\gamma = 2.68 \times 10^8$ rad/Tesla per second is the gyromagnetic ratio for protons.

This intravascular NMR phase will contribute to fMRI signals in a voxel not completely occupied by blood, since the change of Dc will result in a change of ϕ_b, and consequently a change in fMRI signal through intravoxel dephasing. The relative contribution of this mechanism to the fMRI signal has a strong dependence on the orientation of the vessel; particularly, maximal contribution is expected when the vessel is parallel to B_0. It also depends on the size of the vessel through the partial volume effects.

20.3.2.2
Measuring Blood Oxygenation by Measuring Intravascular NMR Phase

This intravascular phase shift can be invoked for the measurement of blood oxygenation (HAACKE et al. 1995, 1997; LAI et al. 1996a), since $\Delta\chi$ is linearly proportional to the oxygenation level of blood via $\Delta\chi = 0.072(1-Y)$ (WEISSKOFF and KIIHNE 1992). Using high resolution GE imaging and measuring the phase angle in a large pial vein found to have significant signal enhancement with a finger tapping task, the oxygenation levels in this vessel were calculated to be 0.54 and 0.70 for the resting and the activation states, respectively (LAI et al. 1996a; HAACKE et al. 1997). Significantly, the resting state oxygenation was found to be similar in many other large veins in other brain areas and in different subjects. Furthermore, similar results were obtained at both lower (HOOGENRAAD et al. 1998) and higher (LIU et al. 1998) field strengths. Moreover, these results are consistent with findings using near infrared optical techniques (MALONEK and GRINVALD 1996).

20.3.3
Extravascular Spin Dephasing

As a result of the extravascular field offset (Eq. 20.2), spins at different locations precess at different rates, thus causing intravoxel spin dephasing. During brain activation, the susceptibility difference $\Delta\chi$ between blood and tissue changes, which results in changes in the perivascular gradients. This in turn alters the degree of spin dephasing in a GE acquisition which is manifested as an fMRI signal change. For a long echo time GE acquisition, the extravascular diffusion effect is found to be negligible for large vessels at 1.5 T (WEISSKOFF et al. 1994). Diffusion effect is the only extravascular signal mechanism in a SE acquisition and is maximal for vessels of a few microns (i.e., capillaries). However, for larger vessels this extravascular diffusion effect is small and negligible relative to the intravascular fMRI signal due to the blood T2 change.

20.4
Relative Contributions of Different BOLD Mechanisms for a Large Vessel

Computer simulations can be used to predict the fMRI signal from a large vein. A key issue of great concern and controversy is the relative importance of the intravascular vs the extravascular contribution to the fMRI signal. The answer will offer some insight into the issue of the spatial selectivity of BOLD contrast. By including or excluding blood signal in the simulations, it is relatively easier to investigate this important issue than in experiments (LAI et al. 1995; BOXERMAN et al. 1995).

A two-component model is used in the following, with gray matter (GM) filling the whole imaging slice except for the space occupied by blood vessels. The vessels are modeled as infinitely long cylinders with appropriate in vivo oxygenation levels. Because we consider the case of relatively large vessels, the results are displayed as a function of vessel orientation relative to the magnetic field rather than averaging over a random orientation as might be appropriate for modeling the microvasculature.

20.4.1
Functional MRI Signal Dependence on Vessel Orientation

Equations 20.1 and 20.2 assert that the BOLD signal from a vein has a strong dependence on the vessel orientation. Figure 20.3 shows the fMRI signal dependence on the vessel orientation for a vessel which occupies a 4% volume fraction in the array of voxels containing the vessel (e.g., a vessel with diameter of 225 µm in a 1 mm^3 voxel). Specifically, three different BOLD effects are taken into account one by one: (1) extravascular signal only (i.e., blood signal nulled); (2) extravascular effect and blood T2 dependence on oxygenation; (3) further adding the effect of a coherent intravascular phase.

We draw the following points from this figure: (1) The extravascular signal change monotonically increases with the angle between the vessel and the static field. This is due to the linear dependence of the extravascular field offset on $\sin^2\theta$ (Eq. 20.2). (2) The blood T2 dependence on oxygenation leads to a signal increase which is independent of vessel orientation. (3) However, when the effect of coherent intravascular phase is added, the fMRI signal shows a minimum around $\theta \approx 40°$. This is because, in each state (resting or activation), the intravascular signal vector makes a phase angle, ϕ_b (Eq. 20.5) with the extravascular signal, and $\phi_b=0°$ at $\theta \approx 55°$. Because of this, the total fMRI signal has a minimum around $\theta \approx 40°$. (4) Even with only 4% blood volume fraction, the intravascular signal (IV) is already at least as im-

portant as the extravascular (EV) signal. Figure 20.4 elucidates the relative contribution of the IV term to the total fMRI signal change. With a large angle between the vessel and the static field ($\theta=50°\sim90°$), the IV contribution is about 25% of the total fMRI signal. The IV contribution increases very rapidly with decreasing θ. Averaging over θ ("θ-averaging"), the fractional contribution of the IV term to the total fMRI signal is about 60%, while the total signal change is about 2.8%. These results are similar to the results for a network of small vessels (BOXERMAN et al. 1995). Worth noting is that, when the vessel is parallel to the static field, all the signal is from the IV contribution and is already larger than 2% even for a nominal blood volume fraction of 4%. As we will demonstrate in the next subsection, the IV contribution to the fMRI signal becomes increasingly larger relative to the EV signal when the blood volume fraction increases.

20.4.2
Functional MRI Signal Dependence on Blood Volume Fraction

In the last section, it was shown that, even with a minimal 4% blood volume fraction, the IV signal provides the major component of the fMRI signal. In this subsection, we investigate the effect of blood volume fraction on fMRI signal change. The blood volume fraction is altered by varying the vessel size.

As an example, Fig. 20.5 shows the results when the vessels are perpendicular to B_0. Several important points are demonstrated in this figure. First, even in this extreme case, in which the largest EV

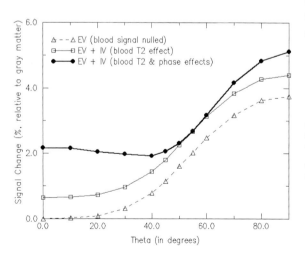

Fig. 20.3. Functional MRI (fMRI) signal dependence on vessel orientation. Blood volume fraction = 4%, TE = 40 ms, Y(rest) = 0.55, Y(act.) = 0.70. The signal change was normalized to a voxel containing 100% gray matter and far away from the vessel

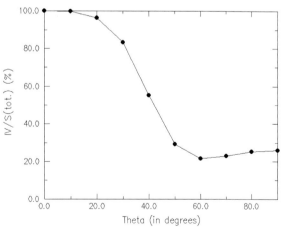

Fig. 20.4. Relative contribution of the intravascular component to the total fMRI signal as a function of the angle between the vessel and the static field

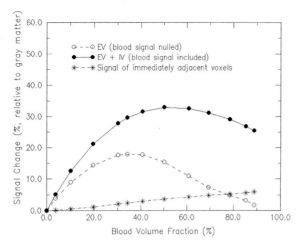

Fig. 20.5. Blood oxygen level-dependent (BOLD) functional MRI (fMRI) signal dependence on blood volume fraction. The vessels are perpendicular to the static field. TE=40 ms, Y(rest)=0.55, Y(act.)=0.70. The data for the immediately adjacent voxels were from the simulations when the blood signal was not included. Simulations with blood signal included gave the same results except for the last points for which larger signals were seen when blood signal was included

signal occurs (θ=90°), the IV contribution to the fMRI signal change becomes increasingly dominant when the blood volume fraction increases. As we have seen in the last section, the EV signal will diminish rapidly when the vessel is tilted away from being perpendicular to the static field, due to the dependence of EV gradients on $\sin^2\theta$ (Eq. 20.2). In fact, as $\theta\rightarrow0$, the EV component approaches zero quadratically. Second, the EV signal change for a voxel containing a vessel initially increases with the increased vessel size (i.e., blood volume fraction). After this signal change passes a peak at about 38% blood volume (e.g., a vessel with diameter of 700 μm in a 1 mm³ voxel), it decreases with increased blood volume fraction and becomes zero when the voxel is fully occupied with blood. This can be understood from the cos(2ψ) dependence of the EV field offset (Eq. 20.2, and Fig. 20.2), because with increasing blood volume fraction, a cubic voxel contains a larger and larger proportion of EV spins with ψ close to 45° (the angle with no resonance frequency shift, thus no signal change). The peak reveals that vessels occupying 30%–80% voxel volume (e.g., diameter of 500 μm to 800 μm in a 1 mm³ voxel) are the most efficient source to induce EV signal change. The signal change in the adjacent voxels (labeled in Fig. 20.5 with filled stars) shows continued increase with increased vessel size, i.e., the conventional T2* behavior. This is easy to understand from the R_0^2 dependence of the EV field offset (Eq. 20.2). It is worth not-

ing that a large vessel induces a few percent signal enhancement in the immediately adjacent voxels. In fact, quite large signal enhancement can often be observed in areas with no visible vessels (HAACKE et al. 1994). From the results here, we see that such signals can be due to the long-range effect from the adjacent slices containing large vessels.

20.4.3
Functional MRI Signal Dependence on Echo Time

There has been great interest in investigating the relationship between the fMRI signal and echo time. Experimentally, the linear dependence of the fMRI signal on TE has been largely used as the main criterion by which to judge whether the observed signal is based on the susceptibility effect from blood or not. Therefore, in this section, the effect of echo time is examined using simulations. Of special interest is the partial volume effect present with voxels containing both blood and tissue. To elucidate this effect, we consider three cases with different angles between the vessel and the static field: θ=0, 45°, 90°.

20.4.3.1
Signal Oscillation Phenomenon Due to Intravascular NMR Phase: Case of θ=0

As illustrated in Sect. 20.4.1, when a vessel is parallel to the static field there is no EV dephasing, and the IV mechanism is the only one contributing to the BOLD signal. Figure 20.6 shows the fMRI signal dependence on TE for a vessel parallel to $\mathbf{B}_0$, with blood volume fraction of 4%. The results for other blood volume fractions are characteristically similar, but the signal amplitudes scale according to blood volume fraction. The various signals in the figure are defined as following (a bold letter indicates a complex signal, i.e., the signal has a magnitude and phase):

Contrast (rest)=[S(rest)–S(GM)]/S(GM) (20.6)

Contrast (act.)=[S(act)–S(GM)]/S(GM) (20.7)

Magnitude subtraction=[S(act)–S(rest)]/S(GM) (20.8)

Complex subtraction=|$\mathbf{S}$(act)–$\mathbf{S}$(rest)|/S(GM) (20.9)

In each state (resting or activated), the blood signal develops a phase angle, given by ϕ_b=4$\pi\gamma\Delta\chi\hat{B_0}$TE/3,

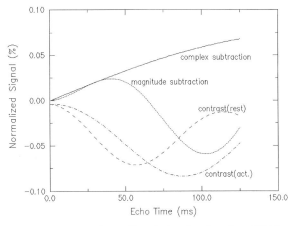

Fig. 20.6. Functional MRI (fMRI) signal as function of TE for a vessel parallel to B_0. The blood volume fraction was 4%. Y(rest)=0.55, Y(act.)=0.70. Complex subtraction avoids the difficulty of negative signal change with TE longer than 60 ms seen with magnitude subtraction

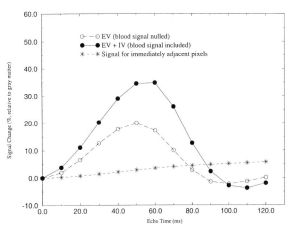

Fig. 20.7. Functional MRI (fMRI) signal dependence on echo time (TE). The vessel makes an angle of 90° with the static field, and the blood volume fraction is 34%

relative to the gray matter signal, thus the contrast in each state shows a periodic oscillation with TE. The period is:

$$(TE)period=1.5/(\gamma\Delta\chi B_0)\propto(1-Y)^{-1} \qquad (20.10)$$

Consequently, the oscillation period is shorter in the resting state than in the activation state (about 120 ms vs 180 ms). Therefore, the magnitude subtraction also shows an oscillation behavior with a period of about 360 ms. Such signal oscillation leads to negative signal change when TE is longer than about 60 ms. To avoid this difficulty, complex subtraction should be used. As seen in the figure, upon complex subtraction, the fMRI signal monotonically increases with TE. Clearly, both the contrast and the magnitude of the fMRI signal do not follow the conventional, near-exponential behavior.

20.4.3.2
Signal Oscillation Phenomenon Due to Extravascular Effect: Case of θ=90°

Figure 20.7 shows the TE dependence of GE fMRI signal for a vessel perpendicular to the static field. A blood volume fraction of 34% is considered because it induces the maximal EV contribution to the fMRI signal (Fig. 20.5). We note that: (1) For voxels containing the vessel, both EV and EV+IV signals oscillate with TE, with maximum signals occurring around TE=50~60 ms, and minimum signals occurring around TE=100~110 ms. This may explain the experimental results (MENON et al. 1993; DUYN et al. 1995) that fMRI signals associated with a large vessel

initially increased with TE, then decreased with TE after reaching a peak around TE~50 ms. Importantly, this oscillation phenomenon asserts that the T2* concept or near-exponential nature of the signal loss is not valid for voxels containing large vessels when TE>50 ms, as supported by recent experimental results (ANDERSON et al. 1994; CHEN et al. 1996). (2) The EV+IV signal peaks at TE slightly longer than that for the EV signal, reflecting the role of the IV oscillation mechanism. (3) With long enough TE (~100 ms), negative signal change is possible. This might be explained by the fact that the intravoxel dephasing is actually larger in the activation state than in the resting state at such long echo times. (4) For voxels immediately adjacent to those containing the vessel, the fMRI signal is essentially linearly dependent on TE, demonstrating conventional T2* signal behavior, but at low amplitude.

20.4.3.3
Minimal Effect from Intravascular NMR Phase: Case of θ=45°

Figure 20.8 shows the TE dependence of the GE fMRI signal when a vessel makes an angle of 45° with the static field. This angle is of interest because it is the median angle between a vessel and the static field and close to the point at which the IV contribution is minimal (see Sect. 20.4.1). For voxels immediately adjacent to those voxels containing the blood vessel, the fMRI signal increases linearly with TE as expected from the T2* theory. For voxels containing the vessel, within the most often used range of TE (between 20 ms and 80 ms) in experiments at 1.5

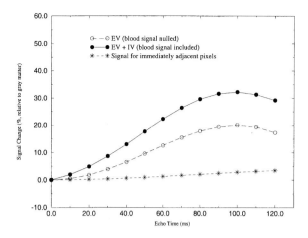

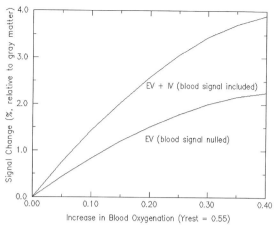

Fig. 20.8. Functional MRI (fMRI) signal dependence on echo time (TE). The vessel makes an angle of 45° with the static field, and the blood volume fraction is 34%

Fig. 20.9. Functional MRI (fMRI) signal dependence on oxygenation change. Blood volume fraction is 4%, TE=40 ms, θ=45°

Tesla, the signal changes (EV and EV+IV) are roughly linearly dependent on TE. However, with TE longer than 80 ms, this quasi-linearity breaks down, and the fMRI signals (EV and EV+IV) show peaks at about 100 ms. Compared with the case of θ=90° (Fig. 20.7), the maximum signal is obtained when TE is roughly two times longer, at the same amplitude. This can be readily explained by the fact that the product $TE\sin^2\theta$ remains invariant. For the EV+IV signal, according to Eq. 20.5, modulation from the coherent intravascular NMR phase is expected to be significantly reduced relative to the case of θ=90°, i.e., the echo time of the peak EV+IV signal is mainly determined by the extravascular mechanism. Consequently, the EV+IV signal reaches a maximum at the same TE as the EV signal.

20.4.4
Functional MRI Signal Dependence on Oxygenation Change

In the previous sections, we have used the oxygenation levels measured in a motor cortex study (HAACKE et al. 1997), i.e., Y(rest)=0.55, Y(act.)=0.70. In practice, of course, other values of oxygenation level change can be expected depending on the neuronal activity. Therefore, we investigate the dependence of the fMRI signal change on blood oxygenation change. Figure 20.9 shows simulations for a 4% blood volume fraction with TE=40 ms and θ=45°. The results demonstrate that, in this case, the fMRI signal increases monotonically with ΔY. However, this may not be the case for larger vessels based on our observation of the complicated signal behavior discussed above. Following the argument about the

extravascular mechanism, the EV phase can be generalized to $\phi_{ex}(r,\theta,\psi)=F(\Delta\chi,\theta,R_0,TE)2\pi\gamma B_0\cos(2\psi)(1/r)^2$ with $F(\Delta\chi,\theta,R_0,TE)=\Delta\chi R_0^2 TE\sin^2\theta$. We expect to see the fMRI signal oscillating with ΔY if a large vessel is involved. The oscillation period will be dependent on vessel size, orientation, echo time, and ΔY.

In summary, when a voxel contains a large vessel, the fMRI signal behavior depends on the vessel size, orientation, echo time, and the change of oxygenation. Generally speaking, the concept of T2* (signified by linear signal dependence on TE) is not valid for a voxel containing a large vessel, except for short enough TE.

20.5
Discrimination of Large Vessels

It is generally believed that signals arising in microvasculature regions are more specific to the underlying neuronal activation, whereas signals from draining veins may be distal to the activated areas, although the issue of vessel size and functional vascular territory is still poorly understood. Various methods have been proposed for the discrimination of large vessels.

The first method is the use of MR angiography (MRA) (LAI et al. 1993; SEGEBATH et al. 1994; KIM et al. 1994). By collecting MRA images at the same location as the BOLD images, activated pixels from large vessels visible in the MRA images can be excluded. Unfortunately, difficulties may arise with this approach. For example, even a 200 μm diameter vein may be too small to be seen with MRA, but as seen from the previous analysis, it can nevertheless induce a several percent signal change with typical fMRI imaging parameters. In addition, misregistration due to scan-to-scan motion may also occur (HAJNAL et al. 1994), which leads to imprecision in generating the mask.

Another method is based on the paramagnetic property of deoxyhemoglobin. In the typical long TE gradient echo fMRI images, large veins often appear as dark structures, especially in the low-oxygenation state, i.e., the resting state, thus providing a way to localize large veins. Since this comes from the fMRI scan itself, this method does not have the same problem of possible scan-to-scan motion as the MRA approach. With high resolution, quite small venous vessels can be seen since the susceptibility effects of a vessel extend into the extravascular space roughly one diameter from the vessel. This intravoxel signal loss phenomenon has been explored to obtain high resolution venograms (REICHENBACH et al. 1997) and highly localized fMRI results (LAI et al. 1996b). An example minimum-intensity-projection (mIP) image is shown in Fig. 20.10, where the dark structures represent the veins.

The third approach uses temporal phase of the fMRI signal time course. In a visual stimulation study, LEE and GLOVER (1995) demonstrated that the activated voxels can be divided into two groups that have distinctive temporal phases. The voxels having the normal 6–8 s temporal delay are believed to originate from parenchyma, whereas the voxels showing much larger time delay are believed to be associated with large draining veins. This is based on the understanding that there is a transit time for the blood to traverse the brain parenchyma and be swept into the draining veins. Therefore, keeping only the voxels with shortest time lags relative to the stimulus cycle may exclude the venous signals.

The fourth method is the application of velocity dephasing gradients to dephase flowing spins (BOXERMAN et al. 1995; SONG et al. 1996). With increased diffusion gradients (or b-value), the number of activated voxels decreases, especially those voxels associated with large vessels. Elegant as it seems, this method suffers the problem that there is a global decrease in signal-to-noise ratio, leading to reduced detectability of fMRI signals. Furthermore, even when the blood signals from large vessels are dephased, the extravascular effects remain. More investigation is needed to assess the applicability of this method in fMRI.

One promising approach is the use of NMR phase images. As addressed in Sect. 20.3.2, in addition to magnitude changes, blood oxygenation elevation upon activation also results in observable MR phase changes in voxels containing large vessels (HAACKE et al. 1994; LEE and GLOVER 1995). Therefore, a product image of the magnitude activation map and its corresponding MR phase activation map can be used to single out those voxels containing significant venous blood volume, most likely associated with large veins (LAI and GLOVER 1997).

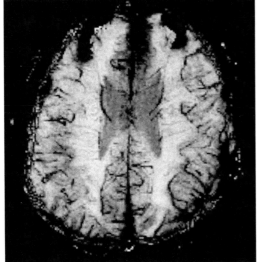

Fig. 20.10. A minimum-intensity-projection (mIP) image from eight contiguous axial slices acquired with a 3D gradient-echo (GE) sequence (TE=50 ms, in-plane resolution 1 mm×1 mm, slice thickness 1 mm). The *dark structures* represent veins

20.6
Significance of BOLD Signals Associated with Large Veins in fMRI Studies

A primary concern with BOLD signals emanating from venous structures is that the apparent location of activation may be propagated from the cortical bed because of the blood flow. However, the geometry of the venous circulation tends to suggest that the oxygenation change originating in the activation site will be rapidly attenuated as one travels downstream because of dilution by venous blood branches from nonactivated regions. In the bat wing, capillary flow is diluted approximately 70 times in traversing the post-capillary venules (7.3 μm diameter, length 210 μm), venules (21 μm diameter, length 1 mm) and small veins (37 μm diameter, length 3.4 mm; WIEDEMAN 1963). Thus, the signal changes may not propagate more than ~3 mm before being lost to dilution. This is consistent with the ~3.5 mm spatial resolution observed in mapping the retinotopy of human visual cortex (ENGEL et al. 1997). In practice, single-shot echo planar imaging (EPI) or spiral techniques have been widely used, and their resolution is typically 2–4 mm. Therefore, signals from large veins are most likely within one pixel from the activation site. Indeed, it is comforting that the activation maps of various human brain functions obtained by the current BOLD techniques generally conform with the known brain functional anatomy.

20.7
Summary

This chapter addresses one aspect of the spatial selectivity of the BOLD contrast mechanism by investigating the signal behavior associated with large veins. It has been shown that the signals from large veins can be quite large in the typical fMRI imaging setting, often dominating the signals from smaller vessels and the capillary bed. Although the spatial selectivity of BOLD is still poorly understood, it is clear that these venous signals can provide rich information about brain function. The effects from draining veins clearly play a key role in much of the observed effects in functional brain MR imaging as it is practiced today.

References

Anderson A, Kirsch JE, Chen Q, Avison MJ (1994) Data analysis for multi-echo acquisition in fMRI. In: Proc ISMRM 2nd Annu Meeting, San Francisco, p 639

Bandettini PA, Wong EC, Jesmanowicz A, Hinks RS, Hyde JS (1994) Spin-echo and gradient-echo EPI of human brain activation using BOLD contrast: a comparative study at 1.5 T. NMR Biomed 7:12–20

Boxerman JL, Bandettini PA, Kwong KK, Baker JR, Davis TL, Rosen BR, Weisskoff RM (1995) The intravascular contribution to fMRI signal changes: Monte Carlo modeling and diffusion-weighted studies in vivo. Magn Reson Med 34:4–10

Chen Q, Andersen AH, Avison MJ (1996) TE-dependence of gradient echo signal decay. In: Proc ISMRM, 4th Annu Meeting, New York, p 290

Duyn JH, Moonen CTW, Van Yperen GH, De Boer RW, Luyten PR (1994) Inflow versus deoxyhemoglobin effects in BOLD functional MRI using gradient echoes at 1.5 T. NMR Biomed 7:83–88

Duyn JH, Frank JA, Ramsey NR et al. (1995) Effects of large vessels in functional magnetic resonance imaging at 1.5 T. Int J Imag Syst Technol 6:245–252

Engel SA, Glover GH, Wandell BA (1997) Retinotopic organization in human visual cortex and the spatial precision of functional MRI. Cereb Cortex 7:181–192

Fisel CR, Ackerman, Buxton RB, Garrido L, Belliveau JW, Rosen BR, Brady T (1991) MR contrast due to microscopically heterogeneous magnetic susceptibility: numerical simulations and applications to cerebral physiology. Magn Reson Med 17:336–347

Fox PT, Raichle ME (1986) Focal physiological uncoupling of cerebral blood flow and oxidative metabolism during somatosensory stimulation in human subjects. Proc Natl Acad Sci USA 83:1140–1144

Frahm J, Merboldt DK, Hänicke W, Kleinschmidt A, Boecker H (1994) Brain or vein – oxygenation or flow? On signal physiology of functional MRI of human brain activation. NMR Biomed 7:45–53

Frostig RD, Lieke EE, Ts'o DY, Grinvald A (1990) Cortical functional architecture and local coupling between neuronal activity and the microcirculation revealed by in vivo high resolution optical imaging of intrinsic signals. Proc Natl Acad Sci USA 87:6082–6086

Gao JH, Miller I, Lai S, Xiong J, Fox PT (1996) Quantitative assessment of blood inflow effects in functional MRI signals. Magn Reson Med 36:314–319

Gillis P, Koenig S (1987) Transverse relaxation of solvent protons induced by magnetized spheres: application to ferritin, erythrocytes, and magnetite. Magn Reson Med 5:323–345

Glover GH, Lee AT (1995) Motion artifacts in fMRI: comparison of 2DFT with PR and spiral scan methods. Magn Reson Med 33:624–635

Haacke EM, Hopkins AL, Lai S et al. (1994) 2D and 3D high resolution gradient echo functional imaging of the brain: venous contributions to signal in motor cortex studies. NMR Biomed 7:54–62

Haacke EM, Lai S, Yablonskiy DA, Lin W (1995) In vivo validation of the BOLD mechanism: a review of signal changes in gradient echo functional MRI in the presence of flow. Int J Imag Syst Technol 6:153–163

Haacke EM, Lai S, Reichenbach JR et al. (1997) In vivo measurement of blood oxygen saturation using magnetic resonance imaging: a direct validation of the blood oxygen level-dependent concept in functional brain imaging. Hum Brain Mapping 5:341–346

Hajnal JV, Myers R, Oatridge A, Schwieso JE, Young IR, Bydder GM (1994) Artifacts due to stimulus correlated motion in functional imaging of the brain. Magn Reson Med 31:283–291

Hoogenraad FGC, Reichenbach JR, Haacke EM, Lai S, Kuppusamy K, Sprenger M (1998) In vivo measurement of changes in venous blood-oxygenation with high resolution functional MRI at 0.95 Tesla by measuring changes in susceptibility and velocity. Magn Reson Med 39:97–107

Kim SG, Hendrich K, Hu X, Merkle H, Ugurbil K (1994) Potential pitfalls of functional MRI using conventional gradient-recalled echo techniques. NMR Biomed 7:69–74

Kwong KK, Belliveau JW, Chesler DA et al. (1992) Dynamic magnetic resonance imaging of human brain activity during primary sensory stimulation. Proc Natl Acad Sci USA 89:5675–5679

Lai S (1996) Brain functional magnetic resonance imaging using blood as an endogenous susceptibilty contrast agent. PhD thesis, Case Western Reserve University, Cleveland

Lai S, Glover GH (1997) Detection of BOLD fMRI signals using complex data. In: Proc ISMRM 5th Annu Meeting, Vancouver, p 1671

Lai S, Hopkins AL, Haacke EM et al. (1993) Identification of vascular structures as a major source of signal contrast in high resolution 2D and 3D functional activation imaging of motor cortex at 1.5 T: preliminary results. Magn Reson Med 30:387–392

Lai S, Haacke EM, Yablonskiy D (1995) Heterogeneous susceptibility-induced MR contrast: time domain computer simulations and applications to fMRI. In: Proc ISMRM, 3rd Annu Meeting, Nice, p 826

Lai S, Haacke EM, Reichenbach JR, Kuppusamy K, Hoogenraad F, Takeichi H, Lin W (1996a) In vivo quantification of brain activation-induced change in cerebral blood oxygen saturation using MRI. In: Proc ISMRM 4th Annu Meeting, New York, p 1756

Lai S, Reichenbach JR, Haacke EM (1996b) Commutator filter: a novel technique for the identification of structures producing significant susceptibility inhomogeneities and its application to functional MRI. Magn Reson Med 36:781–787

Lee AT, Glover GH (1995) Discrimination of large venous vessels in time-course spiral blood oxygen dependent magnetic resonance functional neuroimaging. Magn Reson Med 33:745–754

Li D, Wang Y, Waight DJ (1998) Blood oxygen saturation assessment *in vivo* using T2* estimation. Magn Reson Med 39:685–690

Liu YJ, Fox PT, Gao JH (1998) Quantification of dynamic changes in cerebral venous oxygenation with MR phase imaging. Magn Reson Med (to be published)

Luz Z, Meiboom S (1963) Nuclear magnetic resonance study of the protolysis of trimethylammonium ion in aqueous solution: order of the reaction with respect to the solvent. J Chem Phys 39:366–370

Malonek D, Grinvald A (1996) Interactions between electrical activity and cortical microcirculation revealed by imaging spectroscopy: implications for functional brain mapping. Science 272:551–554

Menon RS, Ogawa S, Tank DW, Ugurbil K (1993) 4 Tesla gradient recalled echo characteristics of photic stimulation-induced signal changes in the human primary visual cortex. Magn Reson Med 30:380–386

Muller R, Gillis P, Moiny F, Roch A (1991) Transverse relaxivity of particulate MRI contrast media: from theories to experiments. Magn Reson Med 22:178–182

Ogawa S, Lee TM, Kay AR, Tank DW (1990a) Brain magnetic resonance imaging with contrast dependence on blood oxygenation. Proc Natl Acad Sci USA 87:9868–9872

Ogawa S, Lee TM, Nayak AS, Glynn P (1990b) Oxygenation-sensitive contrast in magnetic resonance image in rodent brain at high magnetic fields. Magn Reson Med 14:68–78

Ogawa S, Tank DW, Menon RS, Ellerman JM, Kim SG, Merkle H, Ugurbil K (1992) Intrinsic signal changes accompanying sensory stimulation: functional brain mapping using MRI. Proc Natl Acad Sci USA 89:5951–5955

Pauling L, Coryell CD (1936) The magnetic properties and structure of hemoglobin, oxyhemoglobin and carbonmonooxyhemoglobin. Proc Natl Acad Sci USA 22:210–216

Reichenbach JR, Venkatesan R, Schillinger DJ, Kido DK, Haacke EM (1997) Small vessels in the human brain: MR venography with deoxyhemoglobin as an intrinsic contrast agent. Radiology 204:272–277

Segebarth C, Belle Y, Delon C et al. (1994) Functional MRI of the human brain: predominance of signals from extracerebral veins. Neuroreport 5:813–816

Song AW, Wong EC, Tan SG, Hyde JS (1996) Diffusion weighted fMRI at 1.5 T. Magn Reson Med 35:155–158

Thulborn KR, Waterton JC, Matthews PM, Radda GK (1982) Oxygenation dependence of the transverse relaxation time of water protons in whole blood at high field. Biochem Biophys Acta 714:263–270

Weisskoff RM, Kiihne S (1992) MRI susceptometry: image-based measurement of absolute susceptibility of MR contrast agents and human blood. Magn Reson Med 24:375–383

Weisskoff RM, Zuo CS, Boxerman JL, Rosen BR (1994) Microscopic susceptibility variation and transverse relaxation: theory and experiment. Magn Reson Med 31:601–610

Wiederman MP (1963) Dimensions of blood vessels from distributing artery to collecting vein. Circ Res 12:375–378

Wright G, Hu B, Macovsky A (1991) Estimating oxygen saturation of blood in vivo with MR Imaging at 1.5 T. J Magn Reson Imaging 1:275–283

21 Functional MR Bold Spectroscopy

J. Hennig, C. Janz

CONTENTS

21.1
Introduction

The possibility to use methods of localized proton spectroscopy as a means to measure BOLD-related changes (functional magnetic resonance spectroscopy, fMRS) in the observed water signal was proposed in 1993 (Hennig et al. 1993). There are several reasons to exploit this experimental approach, which differs radically from the imaging techniques commonly used in functional magnetic resonance imaging (fMRI). At least potentially, single voxel techniques offer a number of attractive features compared to methods such as echo planar imaging (EPI) and long-TE fast gradient echo imaging (FLASH): (1) increased signal-to-noise ratio (S/N), (2) increased signal stability, and (3) the possibility to characterize the signal changes during activation not just by a single value (the signal intensity in an observed pixel) but by a free induction decay which allows characterization of the mechanism behind the observed signal changes.

In the beginning, the higher S/N and greater stability were the driving forces behind the use of BOLD-based spectroscopy. With further improvements in scanner soft- and hardware, which led to better imaging results, the possibility to monitor the

J. Hennig, PhD; C. Janz, PhD; Professor, Uniklinik Freiburg, Radiologische Klinik, Abteilung Kernspintomographie, Hugstetterstrasse 55, 79106 Freiburg, Germany

exact nature of the activation-dependent signal changes increasingly became the focus of spectroscopy studies.

The disadvantage of the application of single-voxel techniques to fMRI is, of course, the limitation of the observation to one (or a few) voxels. The area of activation must therefore be known beforehand. By contrast, fMRS has been used more or less exclusively in mechanistic studies to examine the time course of signal changes after activation, and not for localization studies.

21.2
Methodology

Experiments using BOLD-based functional spectroscopy have so far been performed using a PRESS (point resolved spectroscopy) technique identical to the one applied in "real" 1H-MRS to observe metabolites in the brain (Fig. 21.1). Since water resonance is the target of observation, water suppression is deleted from the sequence. A more subtle difference compared to 1H-MRS is the less stringent re-

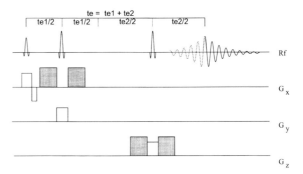

Fig. 21.1. The point resolved spectroscopy (PRESS) sequence. *Rf*, radiofrequency pulses consecutively applied under three orthogonal gradients *Gx*, *Gy*, and *Gz* and the echo generated by them at the time TE=TE₁+TE₂. The *shaded gradients* are used as spoilers to destroy unwanted signals from outside the voxel of interest generated by any single Rf pulse or combinations thereof

quirement to include spoiler gradients in the sequence in order to block unwanted tissue from outside the voxel. This is afforded by the fact that the intensity of the water signal is 5000–10 000 higher than that of the commonly observed metabolites; therefore much higher residual signals can be tolerated while observing water resonance without any measurable artifact. The echo time can thus be considerably reduced compared to 1H-MRS without appreciable disadvantage.

21.2.1
Signal-to-Noise

In a normal clinical setup, imaging techniques and spectroscopy are applied in different contexts (although increasingly within the same examination). Therefore, there is some misconception that the techniques are in some way fundamentally different. This is of course not the case. Imaging as well as spectroscopy use the same signal. The observed spins have no way of "knowing" whether a given experiment is meant to acquire an image or to measure a spectrum. The difference lies more in the practical implementation than in any fundamentally different method of signal generation.

For a comparison let us thus start by considering two complementary experiments: The first one is a single voxel, non-water suppressed PRESS experiment (Fig. 21.1) with an acquisition time of T_{aq} for the observation of the free-induction decay generated by the three pulses acting on three orthogonal slices. The spectral bandwidth for signal observation is typically on the order of 2 kHz, which, according to the Nyquist theorem, corresponds to a sampling time of 0.5 ms per (complex) data point. With 256 acquired data points, this leads to an acquisition time of 128 ms and a spectral resolution of roughly 8 Hz.

The second experiment uses an EPI sequence with the same acquisition time. The image matrix of the EPI experiment is chosen such that one image voxel has the same size as the voxel measured by the spectroscopic sequence. For an image matrix of 64×64, the sampling time will be 31.25 ms in the read direction and 2 ms in the phase-encoding direction.

In an ideal experiment, both sequences are first applied to a probe with a spin distribution given by a δ-function at the center of the gradient system. In that case the observed spins will not see any effect from any of the gradients used for imaging. The resulting signal will be fundamentally the same in both experiments (Fig. 21.2a), the only difference be-

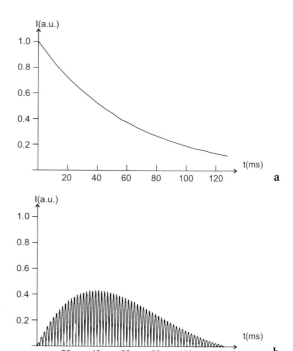

Fig. 21.2a,b. Simulated signals from functional magnetic resonance imaging (fMRI) and functional magnetic resonance spectroscopy (fMRS). If the spin distribution is assumed to be a δ-function at the center of the magnet, imaging and spectroscopy will produce an identical signal characterized by an exponential decay with the time constant T2*(=60 ms) **a**. For a homogeneous distribution within one single voxel at the center of a 64×64 image matrix, the signal measured by fMRI will be attenuated by dephasing across the voxel **b**, whereas the signal measured by fMRS will remain unchanged

ing that the sampling rate of data acquisition in EPI is much higher. It is a basic fact of signal theory that increasing the sampling rate at a constant acquisition time does not alter the S/N of a given observed signal. (This is the basis of oversampling, which is commonly used in most imaging experiments in order to avoid fold-over of signals from outside of the field-of-view.) Since the observed signal intensity of the voxel at the center can be shown to be equal to the integral over the corresponding signal, the signal intensities measured by both techniques will be identical if T2 relaxation during voxel selection is neglected as well as any saturation effects and a flip angle of 90° is used for EPI.

A first step from this ideal experiment towards reality is to change the spin distribution from a δ-function to a continuous distribution filling exactly the same voxel. For the fMRS experiment this does not change anything. For EPI, however, intravoxel dephasing must now be taken into account. According to the basic theory of two-dimensional image formation, signal dephasing will lead to sinusoidal signal attenuation along both imaging directions. The integral over the resulting signal and thus the signal intensity will be reduced to about 37% of that of the fMRS experiment for $T2^* = 60$ ms (Fig. 21.2b). This is the inherent penalty paid by any imaging experiment for the signal dephasing caused by the fact that a continuous distribution of spins is measured by a discrete sampling strategy.

A further important issue for consideration is the fact that, for fMRS, one normally uses voxels which are much larger than the typical resolution of an imaging experiment. In order to make sure that the activated area under study is contained within the selected voxel, typically a voxel size of $1 \times 1 \times 1 - 2 \times 2 \times 2$ ml is chosen. As long as there are no confounding effects from the nonactivated tissue within this voxel, and if the activation-dependent signal change is assumed to be homogeneous over the activated part of the cortex, the observed signal change will linearly scale with the size of the activated area.

For measurement with an imaging technique, the total effect-to-noise is measured as the average signal change over the activated area. Averaging improves the measured S/N only with the square-root of the number of voxels. For activation in an area covered by n voxels in an imaging experiment but all contained within the voxel selected by fMRS, this leads to a further volume-dependent increase in the effect-to-noise measured by fMRS compared to imaging by a factor of $\sqrt{n}$.

Taking these two sources of improved S/N together gives fMRS an advantage of a factor of ten or more, dependent on the volume of activation. This advantage, based on ideal conditions, can, however, not be carried over to a practical experiment. The most important confounding factor is that the S/N along the time axis of a repetitive experiment is not limited by the S/N of a single acquisition, but by physiological and technical signal fluctuations. For a PRESS spectrum from a $2 \times 2 \times 2$ ml voxel and a repetition time of 400 ms, we have measured signal fluctuations of 0.07%, whereas the stability of a single pixel in a typical EPI experiment was 0.4%. With averaging over several pixels a maximum stability of 0.13% can be achieved with EPI for averaging over about 10 pixels. For larger regions-of-interest no further increase in the stability is achieved, indicating that this value represents the true scanner stability for this particular experiment (WEISSKOPF 1996).

For a state-of-the art scanner it can be shown that the signal fluctuations in repetitive scans on volun-

teers are considerably higher than those on phantoms. Therefore, the reproducibility of the experiment can be assumed to be mainly determined by physiological factors. Typical values range in the order of 1%–2% on a pixel-by-pixel basis in an imaging experiment. Consequently, observation of activation by fMRS will not automatically lead to improved effect-to-noise as compared to fMRI. The in-plane S/N of an EPI-based fMRI experiment easily exceeds the S/N along the time axis. Observation of the same stimulation paradigm with fMRS will consequently lead to improved S/N in each single measurement but not necessarily to an improvement along the time series. The improved S/N of fMRS can therefore only be played out for those experiments in which the low amplitude of the effect and a low basic signal amplitude lead to severe limitations of fMRI examinations. In our institute, we have thus used this technique predominantly for examinations of the time course after brief and weak visual stimuli, which lead to only small stimulation effects in the visual cortex and for which we were able to observe subtle effects such as the initial undershoot.

21.2.2
Signal Processing

A few words should be said about the signal processing of fMRS data. First it should be noted that the observed signal nearly always consists of a superposition of the signal from brain parenchyma with a T2 of about 50–60 ms (at 2 T) and cerebrospinal fluid (CSF) with a T2 in the order of 1–3 s. It has been shown that a corresponding biexponential fit is in excellent agreement with the observed data. Such a fit is in fact used in quantitative 1H-MRS for measuring the partial volume effect of CSF (ERNST et al. 1993). In order to avoid the errors inherent in fitting a function as a superposition of multiple exponentials, we have found it advisable to fit the difference signals between the two states (normally on-off). These can be shown to be nicely represented by a difference of two mono-exponentials, since the CSF signals remain unchanged upon stimulation and are canceled out. Data evaluation is performed on the time domain signals rather than on the Fourier-transformed spectra, since time domain fitting allows better treatment of effects including frequency drifts and baseline shifts.

Given the fact that the change in $T2^*$ upon stimulation is small, it can be easily shown that the difference signal shows a maximum at a time corresponding to the averaged observed T2* (Fig. 21.3). For experiments aimed at the observation of T2* effects alone, the first few points of the signal can be used as a navigator signal, which is used to normalize all observed signals in a time series. This leads to a further improvement of the scan-to-scan reproducibility at the cost of information about possible changes in signal intensity.

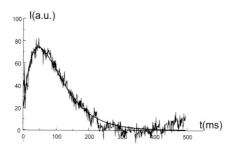

Fig. 21.3. Difference of the signal with and without activation as measured by functional magnetic resonance spectroscopy (fMRS). The curve is characterized by a maximum at a time corresponding to the approximate average of the signal decay constants T2* as long as the change in T2* upon activation is small

21.3
Applications

As already mentioned, the fMRS experiment is mainly used for mechanistic studies to examine the time course of signal changes after stimulation. The main result of these experiments is the notorious and elusive initial fast response, whose existence was first reported in 1994 (ERNST and HENNIG 1994) and which has meanwhile been confirmed by fMRI experiments at high field strengths (MENON et al. 1995; HU et al. 1997; see also Chap. 22). The experiment used in this study was performed with a very long recovery time of 15 s and a brief stimulus of 1 s duration consisting of a flicker display provided by stimulation goggles. The effect, as observed immediately (100–500 ms) after onset of the stimulus, was a small (–0.25%) but significant dip in the observed BOLD signal. In a second study, experiments were performed with much better temporal resolution (TR=400 ms) and by varying the stimulus application time and the echo readout time (HENNIG et al. 1995). These studies clearly established a triphasic response with a small negative effect immediately after onset of the stimulus (Fig. 21.4, top), a BOLD difference signal as shown in Fig. 21.3 (Fig. 21.4,

middle) and a negative BOLD effect (Fig. 21.4, bottom) about 10 s after the onset of stimulation (and long after the stimulus was switched off again), which had already been reported in one of the initial fMRI papers by KWONG et al. (1992). The most remarkable result of our study was that the main contribution to the observed negative BOLD effect is an amplitude change by –0.44%±0.15% at TE=30 ms and 1 s stimulus time, whereas the T2* change was determined to be 0.09%±0.08%.

A summary of the result of varying the stimulus length is seen in Fig. 21.5. The diagrams display the integrated intensities over the length of the observed signals and thus do not allow a distinction between T2* effects and effects of the initial signal amplitude. A rather surprising result of this study was the observation that the initial dip vanished for the longest stimulus with TS=2 s (Fig. 21.5, bottom). The observation of an effect 400 ms after the onset of the stimulus at TS=1 s, but no such effect at TS=2 s looks puzzling at first. How does the parenchyma know at 400 ms that the stimulus would be switched off 600 ms later, and why should there be any signal change in one condition, but not the other? This seemingly paradoxical result was resolved in a fur-

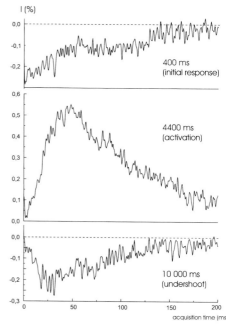

Fig. 21.4. Triphasic response after activation with a short (1 s) light flash. The initial response (400 ms after the onset of the stimulus) is characterized by a negative change in the initial amplitude of the signal difference as well as a change in T2* followed by a BOLD-type response, as shown in Fig. 21.3 and a negative undershoot at 8–50 s after the onset of the stimulus, which corresponds also to a pure (but negative) T2* effect. (From HENNIG et al. 1995)

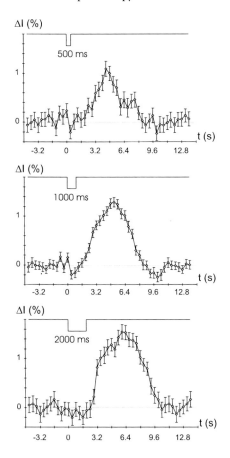

Fig. 21.5. Response vs time for three durations of the stimulus. The diagrams show the integral over the observed difference signals; changes in T2* are therefore not distinguished from changes in the initial amplitude of the signal. Note that both the initial as well as the final undershoot have vanished at 2 s stimulus duration compared to the experiments with shorter stimuli. (From Hennig et al. 1995)

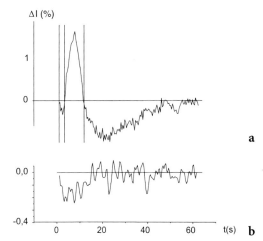

Fig. 21.6. Change in initial signal amplitude (**b**) vs total signal change (**a**) for an experiment using four stimuli of 2 s duration applied at 6 s intervals. The repetition time for the activation sequence was 60 s. It is demonstrated that the negative effect in the initial signal amplitude persists throughout the BOLD phase of the response. (From Janz et al. 1997)

mental series we were also able to show that the time course of the response very nicely fits a linear response model with respect to the first two phases (but not with respect to the late undershoot). This demonstrates that the experiments are performed under conditions well below arterial saturation, which leads to strongly nonlinear effects produced by block paradigms commonly used in fMRI localization studies (Janz et al. 1998b).

From the results of these experiments, together with literature data from optical and near-infrared experiments (Frostig et al. 1990, 1995; Obrig and Villringer 1996; Malonek and Grinvald 1996), we were able to derive a refined model for the events

ther study aimed at determining the inherent time constants of the various events that are triggered by the stimulus.

It was demonstrated that the negative undershoot occurring in the third phase after the BOLD effect returns to baseline only after nearly 60 s (Janz et al. 1997). This confirmed the hypothesis that the negative dip at 2 s stimulus time was quenched by the negative undershoot, which still existed at the 15 s stimulus repetition time TP in the previous study. At TP=30 and 60 s the negative dip reappeared for the 2 s stimulus.

These experiments further revealed that the initial negative change in the signal amplitude persists all through the positive BOLD phase. As shown in Fig. 21.6, the dip in the initial amplitude reaches the baseline only after about 20 s. In the same experi-

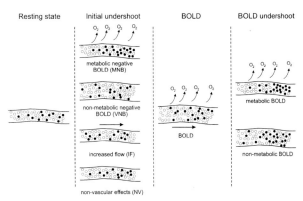

Fig. 21.7. The events occurring during and after stimulation in accordance with the triphasic response demonstrated in Figs. 21.4–21.6. For explanation, see text. (From Janz et al. 1997)

occurring after cortical activation. This is demonstrated in Fig. 21.7, where it is shown that several mechanisms each contribute to explaining the observed effects.

The T2* drop during the initial undershoot can be due to a combination of two mechanisms: A metabolic negative undershoot (MNB) caused by the immediate onset of oxygen consumption, in accordance with the results of MALONEK and GRINVALD (1996), and/or a nonmetabolic negative undershoot (VNB) caused by the fast vasodilation known to follow after the onset of activation (MALONEK and GRINVALD 1996; KUSCHINSKY and PAULSON 1992). Possible sources for the amplitude change are either an intravoxel incoherent motion (IVIM) effect caused by the increased flow (IF), or any of the known nonvascular effects such as changes in neuronal cell size or rearrangements in the membrane bound water which occur as a consequence of membrane depolarization (NV) (COHEN 1973; ANDREW and MacVICAR 1994).

The current understanding of the late undershoot tends to be that a nonmetabolic BOLD effect caused by increased volume of the post-capillary veins is a more likely candidate than a metabolic effect driven by prolonged oxygen consumption. It remains in fact something of a mystery why the hemodynamic response should be driven by the increased energy demand of the activated neurons given the fact that the oxygen extraction is only about 20% (and glucose consumption less than 2%), which means that the perfusion in the unstimulated condition would be by far sufficient to cope with the increased energy demand during and after activation. It has indeed been demonstrated that immediate regulation of the hemodynamic response after activation is independent of the local oxygen concentration and that, therefore, the increased oxygen supply delivered by the increased perfusion is a beneficial side effect, but not the cause of the hemodynamic response (JANZ et al. 1998a). The question of the uncoupling of the hemodynamic response after extended stimulation (FOX and RAICHLE 1986) has also been examined by fMRS (FRAHM et al. 1996).

The fact that the observation of a negative response is not an artifact of an fMRS experiment has been confirmed by fMRI studies performed at 4 T. The EPI technique used therein does not allow to distinguish amplitude effects from T2* effects, but the initial dip was nevertheless clearly demonstrated. A comparison with our results reveals similar findings, but also some differences in the timing and amplitude of the triphasic effect.

EPI experiments performed on our scanner at 2 T confirm the fMRS observations. As shown in Fig. 21.8, the area activated by these simple activation paradigms leads to activation within area V1 of the visual cortex (Fig. 21.8a) (for a discussion of the activation pattern, see JANZ et al. 1998b). The signal time course over the activated voxels (Fig. 21.8b) for brief stimuli is practically identical to the one shown in Fig. 21.6. It is demonstrated that the response after a brief stimulus is largely independent of the type of stimulus at least for different visual stimuli (JANZ et al. 1998c). Figure 21.8b shows the remarkable uniformity of the response curves in marked contrast to the different response curves measured with a block paradigm for stimulus presentation.

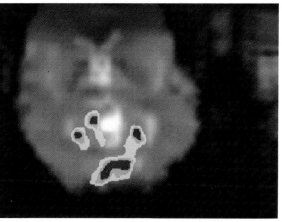

a

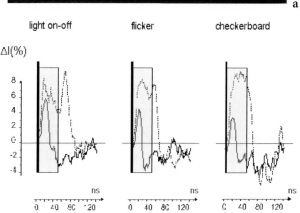

b

Fig. 21.8. a Activation map after stimulation with a checkerboard stimulus of duration 2 s. b Signal time courses averaged over the pixels with positive activation after 4 s for brief (2 s, full line) and extended (20 s, dotted line) application of the stimulus. The results correspond to a single-subject measurement. Note that the different stimuli produce nearly identical response curves for brief presentation of the stimulus, but show significant differences for longer stimulation times. The horizontal axes represents the scan number, the repetition time of the paradigm was 60 s (=150 scans at a scan repetition time of 400 ms)

21.4
Conclusion

Functional magnetic resonance spectroscopy has been very successfully used over the last few years to elucidate the neurophysiological events during and after stimulation. It has been the "motor" for several studies revealing very subtle effects way below the 1% range. With improvements of scanner hardware and the development of new imaging sequences, these applications might, in the future, be replaced by more sophisticated experiments combining the spatial resolution of fMRI with the parametric information gained by fMRS. Very encouraging results have already been demonstrated with multi-image EPI experiments, in which several EPI images with different echo times are acquired with each excitation of the spin system. This allows a parametric signal analysis comparable to the one used in fMRS, but with the benefit of the additional spatial information.

The higher reproducibility and the possibility of more sophisticated signal analysis of the observed time-variant signal time course obtained by the presentation of brief stimuli have meanwhile also been exploited for fMRI localization studies. Such "event-related paradigms" (SCHAD et al. 1995; FRISTON et al. 1998) have been introduced into fMRI only recently, but have already found a number of interesting and important applications.

References

Andrew RD, MacVicar BA (1994) Imaging cell volume changes and neuronal excitation in the hippocampal slice Neuroscience 62:371–383

Cohen LB (1973) Changes in neuron structures during action potential propagation and synaptic transmission. Physiol Rev 53:373–418

Ernst TH, Hennig J (1994) Observation of a fast response in functional MR. Magn Reson Med 32:146–149

Ernst TH, Kreis R, Ross BD (1993) Absolute quantitation of water and metabolites in the human brain. I. Compartments and water. J Magn Reson 102:1–8

Fox PT, Raichle ME (1986) Focal physiological uncoupling of cerebral blood flow and oxidative metabolism during somatosensory stimulation in human subjects. Proc Natl Acad Sci USA 83:1140–1144

Frahm J, Krüger G, Merboldt KD, Kleinschmidt A (1996) Dynamic uncoupling and recoupling of perfusion and oxidative metabolism during focal brain activation in man. Magn Reson Med 35:143–148

Friston KJ, Fletcher P, Josephs O, Holmes A, Rugg MD, Turner R (1998) Event-related fMRI: characterizing differential responses. Neuroimage 7(1):30–40

Frostig RD, Lieke, EE, Ts'o DY, Grinvald A (1990) Cortical functional architecture and local coupling between neuronal activity and the microcirculation revealed by in vivo high resolution optical imaging of intrinsic signals. Proc Natl Acad Sci USA 87:6082–6086

Frostig RD, Masino SA, Kwon MC, Chen CH (1995) Using light to probe the brain: intrinsic signal optical imaging. Int J Syst Tech 6:216–224

Hennig J, Ernst TH, Speck O, Laubenberger J (1993) Functional spectroscopy: a new tool for the observation of brain activation. Proc XIIth Annu Meeting SMRM, p 12

Hennig J, Janz C, Speck O, Ernst TH (1995) Functional spectroscopy of brain activation following a single light pulse: examinations of the mechanism of the fast initial response. Int J Imag Sci Technol 6:203–208

Hu X, Le TH, Ugurbil K (1997) Evaluation of the early response in fMRI in individual subjects using short stimulus duration. Magn Reson Med 37(6):877–884

Janz C, Speck O, Hennig J (1997) Time-resolved measurements of brain activation after a short visual stimulus: new results on the physiological mechanisms of the cortical response. NMR Biomed 10:222–229

Janz C, Schmitt C, Speck O, Fischer H, Hennig J (1998a) Decoupling of the hemodynamic response and the blood oxygen concentration: direct demonstration using an event-related disactivation paradigm. Proc 6th Annu Meeting ISMRM, p. 4

Janz C, Schmitt C, Speck O, Hennig J (1998b) Regional differences in the hemodynamic response to different visual stimuli observed with block paradigms vs. single event observations. Proc 6th Annu Meeting ISMRM, p 1544

Janz C, Schmitt C, Speck O, Fischer H, Hennig J (1998c) Variability of the hemodynamic response to different stimuli in single event paradigms. Proc 6th Annu Meeting ISMRM, p. 165

Kuschinsky W, Paulson O (1992) Capillary circulation in the brain. Cerebrovasc Brain Metab Rev 4:261–268

Kwong KK, Belliveau JW, Chesler DA et al (1992) Dynamic magnetic resonance imaging of human brain activity during primary sensory stimulation. Proc Natl Acad Sci USA 89:5675–5679

Malonek D, Grinvald A (1996) The imaging spectroscope reveals the interaction between electrical activity and cortical microcirculation: implication for optical, PET, and MR functional brain imaging. Science 272:551–554

Menon RS, Ogawa S, Hu X et al (1995) BOLD based functional MRI at 4 Tesla includes a capillary bed contribution: echo-planar imaging correlates with previous optical imaging using intrinsic signals. Magn Reson Med 33(3):453–459

Obrig H, Villringer A (1996) What is the typical NIRS-response to functional brain activation? Adv Exp Med Biol 388:219–224

Schad LR, Wiener E, Baudendistel KT, Muller E, Lorenz WJ (1995) Event-related functional MR imaging of visual cortex stimulation at high temporal resolution using a standard 1.5 T imager. Magn Reson Imaging 13(6):899–901

Weisskoff RM (1996) Simple measurement of scanner stability for functional NMR imaging of activation in the brain. Magn Reson Med 36(4):643–645

Incompletely Understood BOLD Contrast Observations

22 Functional MRI Signal Decrease at the Onset of Stimulation

X. Hu, E. Yacoub, T.H. Le, E.R. Cohen, K. Ugurbil

CONTENTS

22.1 Introduction

Over the past several years, functional magnetic resonance imaging (fMRI) based on endogenous contrast has evolved into a widely used methodology for examining the function of both normal and diseased brains. The majority of the fMRI studies are based on the blood oxygenation level-dependent (BOLD) contrast (OGAWA and LEE 1990; OGAWA et al. 1990a, b), which is derived from the paramagnetic property of deoxyhemoglobin in the blood (THULBORN et al. 1982), and the fact that neuronal activation within the cerebral cortex leads to a localized increase in blood flow without a commensurate increase in oxygen extraction (Fox and RAICHLE 1986). As a result of neuronal activity, capillary and venous deoxyhemoglobin concentrations decrease in relevant brain regions, leading to an increase in $T2^*$ and $T2$ and thereby an elevation of intensity in $T2^*$- and $T2$-weighted MR images.

X. Hu, PhD; E. Yacoub, BS; T.H. Le, MD, PhD; E.R. Cohen, BS; K. Ugurbil, PhD; Center for Magnetic Resonance Research, 385 East River Road, Minneapolis, MN 55455, USA
T.H. Le, MD, PhD; E.R. Cohen, BS; K. Ugurbil, PhD; Department of Radiology, University of Minnesota Medical School, Minneapolis, MN 55455, USA

Although BOLD-based fMRI has been extensively used for mapping various neuronal functions to date (KIM and UGURBIL 1997), the exact nature of its underlying mechanism is not yet fully elucidated. In particular, the correspondence between the location of the MR signal change and the site of neuronal activity has not been fully established. This lack of spatial correspondence may be a result of inflow effects in large veins, and/or BOLD contrast in and surrounding large draining veins (DUYN et al. 1994; FRAHM et al. 1994; KIM et al. 1994; LAI et al. 1993; LEE et al. 1995; MENON et al. 1993; SEGEBARTH et al. 1994). A number of experimental studies have revealed that activation maps were dominated by large vessel contributions (KIM et al. 1994; LAI et al. 1993; MENON et al. 1993; SEGEBARTH et al. 1994), although small but detectable contributions from gray matter areas devoid of large vessels were present (KIM et al. 1994; LEE et al. 1995; MENON et al. 1993). Large vessel contributions can be distinguished, to a large extent, from parenchymal contributions or reduced using an assortment of approaches (BOXERMAN et al. 1995; FRAHM et al. 1994; KIM et al. 1994; LEE et al. 1995; MENON et al. 1994; MENON et al. 1993; SONG et al. 1996).

The lack of spatial specificity of fMRI may also arise from the notion that the hemodynamic response is somewhat distant from the actual site of neuronal activity. This view is supported by intrinsic signal optical imaging studies (FROSTIG et al. 1990; GRINVALD et al. 1991; MALONEK and GRINVALD 1996), which have the ability to achieve high spatial and temporal resolutions and assess the oxygenation state of hemoglobin. Optical imaging studies have revealed that the deoxyhemoglobin concentration following the onset of neuronal stimulation/activation is biphasic, consisting of a small rise, peaking at 2 s and lasting approximately 4 s, and a subsequent decrease that persisted until several seconds after the cessation of the stimulation. In a recent optical imaging study examining cortical columns in the visual cortex in cats, MALONEK and GRINVALD (1996) have reported that the delayed response extended beyond the true area of activation, thereby suggesting that the fundamental spatial resolution limitation of current fMRI technique is approximately 2–3 mm. However, they also demonstrated that, when the initial deoxyhemoglobin increase is selectively mapped, the differential optical imaging signal provided column-specific changes, indicating that the mapping of the early response can potentially overcome the spatial limitation of the current fMRI methodology. These results suggest that the majority of fMRI studies, which are based on the mapping of the delayed response, may be inherently limited in spatial specificity or resolution, and a more specific alternation may be the mapping of the early increase in deoxyhemoglobin concentration, which is reflected as a decrease in fMRI signal. The questions are whether this early response can be reliably detected with MR methods, and whether it is spatially more specific as suggested by the optical imaging studies. A number of MR studies which focused on answering these question are summarized in this chapter.

22.2
Detection of the Early Response with Functional Spectroscopy

Functional spectroscopy is a technique introduced by Hennig and his colleagues for detecting neuronal activation-related MR signal in a localized volume of interest (VOI) (Hennig et al. 1994). The technique is based on the principle of single voxel spectroscopy. The idea is to acquire signal from a region of interest defined by selective excitation using a combination of radiofrequency (RF) pulses and gradients. When implemented as a tool for observing neuronal function, localized spectroscopy is used to detect the water signal in a user-specified VOI and to examine possible changes in this signal arising from neuronal activity.

With the high speed afforded by the spectroscopic data acquisition, functional spectroscopy provides a convenient vehicle for investigating the temporal response of the MR signal following a sensory stimulation/neuronal task. In a study performed at 2 Tesla by Ernst and Hennig (1994), free induction decays (FIDs) from a VOI ($2\times2\times2$ cm^3) localized to the visual cortex were collected using a stimulus-gated PRESS sequence (Bottomley 1987). Visual stimulation consisted of 0.5 s or 1 s nonflickering light generated by a pair of goggles that were controlled by

the MR scanner. In the study, baseline FIDs were acquired just before the goggles were turned on whereas delayed FIDs were collected 0, 100, 500, 1500, or 5000 ms after the stimulus onset. The baseline acquisition and delayed acquisition were interleaved and repeated. The average of the subtraction of the baseline data from those acquired with one of the delays showed a –0.25% signal change at the 500 ms delay and a subsequent signal increase (0.59%) which occurred at 1.5–5 s. This MRS study suggested a possible early negative change in the MR signal in response to visual stimulation.

In a subsequent study, performed also at 2 Tesla, the same group examined the early fast response with functional spectroscopy more thoroughly by studying the echo time dependence and stimulus duration dependence (Hennig et al. 1995). Using a TR of 400 ms and a voxel of $2\times2\times2$ cm^3, FIDs were collected consecutively prior to, during and after visual stimulation. The visual stimulus was again nonflickering light presented by goggles controlled by the MR scanner. In this study, three echo times (TEs) were used for the stimulus duration of 1 s. For the TE of 60 ms, the stimulus duration varied between 0.5 s and 3 s. The experimental data from this study suggested a decrease in the amplitude of the early response with increasing TE as well as with stimulus duration. This observation seemed to contradict the BOLD nature of the early response. The authors proposed several hypotheses, including that of a change in the ionic environment of neurons caused by the influx of Na$^+$, to account for this behavior. However, an exact explanation of this data is not yet available.

The initial negative response observed using the spectroscopic study is only qualitatively in agreement with the optical imaging study. The amplitude and the duration of the negative response, however, are not in agreement with those revealed by optical imaging data. In addition, the echo time dependence is somewhat puzzling. One explanation of this discrepancy may be the partial voluming effect that is substantial for the spectroscopic study. This explanation is indirectly supported by the imaging studies described below.

22.3
Observation of the Early Response with MRI

22.3.1
The Initial Study

The first MR imaging study of the initial response, which occurred shortly after the functional spectroscopy study, was performed on a 4 Tesla whole body system using a head-gradient insert and surface RF coil (MENON et al. 1995). Photic stimulation consisted of red light flickering at 8 Hz generated with light emitting diode (LED) goggles (Grass instruments, Quincy, MA) controlled by the MR scanner. A blipped echo planar imaging (EPI) sequence (TR/TE: 100/30 ms) was used for the study. Imaging parameters were: 5° flip angle, 20×20 cm FOV, 64×64 matrix and 5–8 slice. A total of 500 images were acquired, with 100 images collected during a 10 s baseline period, followed by 100 images acquired during the visual stimulation (10 s) and finally 300 images made during the recovery (30 s). Activation maps were made by subtracting the average of the control period images from average images acquired during one of two phases of the 10 s photic stimulation period. The first phase consisted of images acquired between 0.5 and 2.5 s after the onset of visual stimulation and the second included all images between 5 s and 15 s after the beginning of the visual stimulation. The difference maps were subsequently thresholded with a Student's t test ($p<0.01$).

Maps were generated from a single trial on a single subject for both the initial signal decrease phase and subsequent hyperemic response phase. The map of pixels exhibiting the negative response contained more focal areas which, on comparison with a high resolution FLASH image, were identified as cortical gray matter above and below the calcarine fissure. In contrast, the map corresponding to all pixels possessing a significant positive response is more widespread spatially, including some large veins. Time-courses from pixels displaying the positive response or the negative response, respectively, were averaged over all subjects. The time course for pixels exhibiting the early negative response shown in Fig. 22.1b indicates that the negative response reached a maximum at 2 s after stimulus onset and had a peak amplitude of approximately 1% of the baseline signal intensity. A positive response followed and reached a maximum of 2%. The time course for pixels exhibiting only the positive response (Fig. 22.1a) rose monotonically until a peak of 6% was reached.

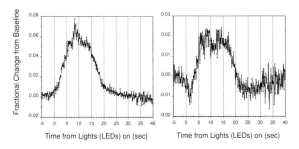

Fig. 22.1a, b. Averaged echo planar imaging (EPI) time courses from 13 trials in five subjects for two different regions. a Time course data from regions exhibiting only the positive response. b Time course data from regions that displayed the initial negative response (Adapted from MENON et al 1995)

This initial study demonstrates that some focal areas of gray matter display an initial negative change in signal intensity after the onset of photic stimulation, while other areas, including those where draining veins are visible, show only a positive signal change. This result is in very good agreement with published optical imaging data, in which a deoxygenation phase has been shown to occur in specific cortical columns (MALONEK and GRINVALD 1996). Along with the optical imaging data, the initial MRI result lends support to the current view of the BOLD phenomena. The initial activity of the neurons draws oxygen out of the local capillary network, resulting in a local increase in paramagnetic deoxyhemoglobin and hence a decrease in MR image intensity. The hemodynamic response eventually overcompensates for this initial oxygen demand, resulting in a net decrease in local deoxyhemoglobin concentration, and thereby an increase in the MR signal.

22.3.2
Study in Individual Subjects and with Variable Stimulus Duration

The first MRI study of the early response (MENON et al. 1995) relied on subject breathhold, prohibiting the use of multiple epochs in each run. Thus, intersubject averaging was utilized in obtaining the temporal characteristics of the early response, making the result sensitive to intersubject variation. In addition, with a single stimulus duration of 10 s, that study did not examine the stimulus duration of the early response. In view of the recent optical imaging study which examined visual stimuli of various duration between 2 and 4 s and that the early response was independent of the stimulus durations used, a more thorough investigation of the early response was carried out to: (1) demonstrate the early response in individual subjects, and (2) to examine the stimulus duration dependence of the early response. This extensive study was made possible by taking advantage of a technique for removing physiological fluctuations (Hu et al. 1995; Le and Hu 1996) so that experiments were performed without breathhold to acquire multiple epochs in individual runs.

In this imaging study conducted at 4 Tesla(Hu et al. 1997), functional MRI experiments were conducted on 14 normal volunteers using a head gradient insert and a quadrature surface coil designed to maximize sensitivity in the occipital cortex (Merkle et al. 1993). In each study, a sagittal slice approximately 6 mm off the midline was selected based on anatomic images obtained with inversion-recovery-prepared ultrafast gradient echo imaging (Haase 1990). Binocular stimulation was achieved with LED goggles (Grass Instruments, Quincy, MA) flashing at a frequency of 8.6 Hz. The switching of the goggles was synchronized with the MR scanner. Functional MRI experiments were performed with either a 4-segment EPI sequence (Kim et al. 1996) (matrix: 128×128, slide: 5 mm, TR/TE: 600/30 ms, FOV: 20×20 cm², and seven subjects) or a single-shot EPI sequence (matrix: 64×64, slide: 5 mm, TR/TE: 300/30 ms, and FOV: 20×20 cm², and seven subjects). The segmented EPI sequence employed a variable flip angle approach (Frahm et al. 1985). The flip angle for the single-shot EPI was approximately 20°. In each experimental run, T2*-weighted images of the sagittal slide were acquired consecutively while epochs of stimulus OFF and stimulus ON were repeated. On each subject, several runs were executed, each using one of the durations for stimulus ON. With the four-segment EPI sequence, stimulus durations of 4.8, 3.6, 2.4 s were employed, and each run contained 500 images for eight ON/OFF epochs with each OFF period lasting 25–30 s. For studies using the single shot EPI, three durations, 6, 3, and 1.5 s, were used, and each run consisted of 1200 images acquired during six ON/OFF epochs, each with a 34–40 s OFF period. To reduce the physiological fluctuation, respiratory and cardiac activities were monitored concurrently with the MR data acquisition. Using the physiological data, respiratory and cardiac fluctuations in the MR data were removed with a retrospective approach described previously (Hu et al. 1995; Le and Hu 1996). In addition to removing physiological fluctuations, N/2 ghosts in EPI images were minimized by using phase-encoded reference calibration (Hu and Le 1996).

Epochs in each experimental run were averaged to generate a single epoch for further analysis. Functional MRI maps were generated corresponding to two types of responses, one for those voxels that displayed the early response (signal decrease or the dip) and the other for those voxels that exhibited the delayed positive response (signal increase). Both types of maps were generated using a cross-correlation technique (Bandettini et al. 1993) with correlation templates chosen to reflect the early negative response or the positive response accordingly and a threshold corresponding to $p<0.01$. To account for possible stimulus duration dependence of the dip, a family of templates that varied in width were initially applied and the template that had the largest correlation in the occipital cortex was chosen in the final analysis. Subtraction images were also generated to visualize the spatio-temporal characteristics of the competing responses. Time courses of regions exhibiting the early response were subsequently examined and compared.

In studies performed with the segmented EPI sequence, the early signal decrease was statistically significant in the primary visual area (V1) with all three stimulus durations (2.4, 3.6, and 4.8 s) in four out of the seven subjects. In the other three subjects, the early response was significant in only one or two of the three durations. Functional maps corresponding to the early and delayed responses in a subject are shown in Figs. 22.2a and 22.2b, respectively. As depicted in these maps, the areas exhibiting the initial signal decrease are focused along the primary visual area and more localized than the pixels that displayed the delayed positive response. The spatio-temporal dynamics of the signal change for a 4.8 s stimulus is portrayed with subtracted images shown in Fig. 22.3. These subtraction images vividly depict the localized negative response at the onset of the stimulus, the subsequent positive response which is more widespread, and the post-stimulus undershoot which usually correlates spatially with the delayed positive response. The negative change starts in V1 shortly after the stimulus onset, remains in V1 and lasts 4 s until the positive response begins. The positive change starts in V1 and spreads to other areas, presumably those containing large veins. Upon cessation of the stimulus, the positive change sustains for approximately 5 s and an undershoot follows in areas that exhibited the positive signal change. For the three stimulus durations used (2.4 s, 3.6 s and 4.8 s), the initial signal decrease peaked at 2–3 s and 1%–2%, depending on the subject. In each subject, the magnitude of this signal decrease varied only slightly with the stimulus duration, especially for stimuli with 3.6 s or longer, and the time at which the

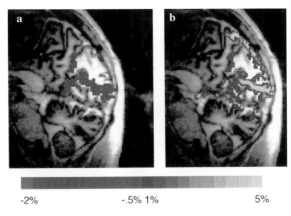

Fig. 22.2. a Functional map corresponding to pixels exhibiting the early response and b that corresponding to pixels displaying only the positive response. (Adapted from Hu et al. 1997)

early response reached its maximum was also independent of stimulus duration. A plot showing the effect of stimulus duration on the different temporal components of the fMRI time course is shown in Fig. 22.4 for a single subject. The early response remained relatively constant, particularly for stimuli of 3.6 s and 4.8 s, while both the delayed positive response and the post-stimulus undershoot increased with stimulus duration. Comparison of the response in different subjects revealed that the characteristics of the early response varied substantially from subject to subject.

Similar early response maps were obtained from the single-shot EPI studies. Interestingly, the early response was found to be reduced for the shortest duration used in this study. For stimuli of 1.5 s, the magnitude of the early response was reduced and statistically significant only in four of the seven subjects. This reduction of the early response is clearly seen in Fig. 22.5, which illustrates the time courses for the three stimulus durations used in this study. Further quantitative measurements of the temporal characteristics also confirmed that the early response becomes dependent on the stimulus duration when it is short. In addition, for short stimulus duration, the post-stimulus undershoot is diminished.

This study further demonstrated the early negative response in individual subjects and systematically revealed the temporal characteristics of the fMRI time course. The experimental results confirmed the existence of this initial negative change in the MR signal. The ability to map the negative signal change in individual subjects makes it possible to study human brain function using the initial deoxygenation phase which is believed to be more specific. Despite the large disparity in spatial resolution, the fMRI time courses experimentally observed mirror those detected with intrinsic signal optical imaging (FROSTIG et al. 1990; GRINVALD et al. 1991; MALONEK and GRINVALD 1996) in three aspects. First, the duration and the peak location of the early response are identical to those revealed by the opti-

Fig. 22.3. A sequence of images derived from the original images subtracted by the average baseline image, overlaid on the T1-weighted anatomic image; the subtraction images were masked by the delayed response map and colored with purple and blue for negative value and red and yellow for positive. The spatiotemporal dynamics of the fMRI response is clearly depicted in this figure. (Adapted from Hu et al. 1997)

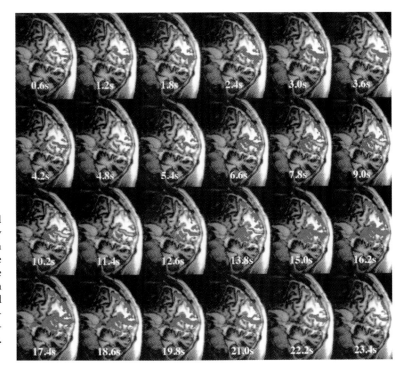

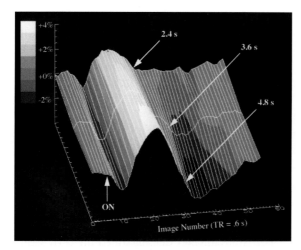

Fig. 22.4. Time courses for stimulus durations of 2.4, 3.6, and 4.8 s in the V1 region of an individual subject studied with segmented echo planar imaging (EPI). The *gray scale bar* indicates the percentage signal change from baseline. For three stimulus durations used, the initial negative response is approximately constant. (Adapted from Hu et al. 1997)

cal imaging studies. Second, the stimulus duration dependence observed is consistent with the optical imaging data in that the early response in the MR signal is independent of the stimulus duration above 2 s. Third, the ratio of the peak positive signal change to the peak negative signal change is in accordance with the optical imaging observation, which indicated that the initial increase in deoxyhemoglobin is about one third of the subsequent decrease in deoxyhemoglobin arising from the over compensation. As expected from the optical imaging result (FROSTIG et al. 1990; GRINVALD et al. 1991; MALONEK and GRINVALD 1996), the maps from the early response are more focal than the maps obtained from the hyperemic positive response. Although maps based on detecting the early response may include veins directly draining the active cortex, these veins are expected to be very close to the area of activation. Therefore, early response mapping may be more desirable for high resolution fMRI studies.

The stimulus duration dependence of the fMRI early response is concordant with the current hypothesis about the underlying mechanism of functional imaging and has provided additional insight into the temporal characteristics of the related events. The onset of stimulus leads to a local increase in oxygen consumption and thereby an increase in deoxyhemoglobin which is reflected in a decrease of the MR signal. The subsequent increase in cerebral blood flow (CBF) eventually overcompensates the

increased oxygen utilization, leading to a net decrease in deoxyhemoglobin and hence an elevation of the MR signal. The temporal behavior of the early MR response reflects the combination of these two competing mechanisms. The observed stimulus duration independence indicates that the CBF increase occurs before the complete rise of the deoxygenation phase. The observation that the negative response decreases, in both magnitude and temporal span, with stimulus shorter than 2 s in duration indicates that the rise time of the early response is approximately 2 s. Based on this observation, the optimal stimulus duration for selectively detecting the early response is between 2–3 s.

A significant amount of variability among subjects was observed in the fMRI response. This variability may arise from a number of factors including the slice position variation and subject dependence of the hemodynamic response and arousal. It should be noted that, due to this variability, averaging data between subjects may blur the time course and should be avoided.

The temporal characteristics of the early response observed with imaging differs from that revealed with the spectroscopic studies. The smaller and shorter early response reported by the fMRS study may be due to the shorter stimulus used in the study as well as the partial volume effect arising from the large voxel size in the fMRS study.

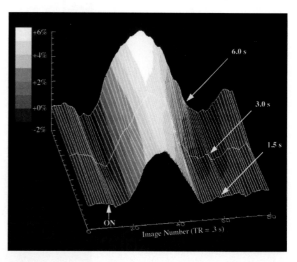

Fig. 22.5. Time courses for stimulus durations of 1.5, 3.0, and 6.0 s in the V1 region of a subject studied with single shot echo planar imaging (EPI). The *gray scale bar* indicates the percentage signal change from baseline. The initial negative response for the 1.5 s stimulus is substantially reduced. (Adapted from Hu et al. 1997)

22.3.3
Echo-Time Dependence

Despite its remarkable agreement with the optical imaging data, the physiological origin of the early response observed in MR studies is still under debate. For example, the echo time dependence observed with the functional spectroscopy study (HENNIG et al. 1995) did not find a significant T2* dependence of the early response, suggesting mechanisms other than BOLD. To probe the early response further, the echo time dependence of the early response has been examined in two imaging studies which revealed a T2* nature of the early response.

A preliminary study was conducted on a 4.1 T system using a six-segment spiral imaging sequence (McINTOSH et al. 1996). Stimulus presentation consisted of 20 s epochs of alternating darkness and flashing checkerboard that were repeated six times in each run. In each epoch, one of the six spiral segments was acquired with a TR of 200 ms. Upon combining data from all epochs, the effective temporal resolution was 200 ms. The images were acquired with a 64×64 matrix over a 22 cm FOV and a slice thickness of 5 mm. Three echo times, 10, 20, and 25 ms, were used to investigate the echo time dependence. Pixels corresponding to the early response were detected using a *t* test. The amplitude of the negative response at three echo times was calculated. The data showed that there is a log-linear dependence on the echo time, consistent with a T2* dependence. However, due to the use of a brief interstimulus delay and short echo times, the result of this study is somewhat controversial.

In another study conducted by our group (YACOUB et al. 1997), the TE dependence was examined more rigorously. This study was performed on our 4 Tesla whole body system. Images were acquired using a T2*-weighted single-shot EPI sequence at echo times of 21, 30, and 45 ms (matrix: 64×64, slice thickness: 5 mm, TR: 300 ms, FOV: 20cm×20 cm). Each run, at one of the echo times, consisted of 550 images of a sagittal slice a few millimeters to the left or right of the mid-line. During each run, flashing lights (8 Hz) were presented to the subjects three times via LED goggles, each lasting 3.6 s and 45 s apart. Two runs were conducted for each echo time. Cardiac pulsations and respiratory pressure data were acquired for physiological fluctuation corrections. The data were corrected using a retrospective technique (HU et al. 1995; LE and HU 1996), averaged over the three stimulus presentations in

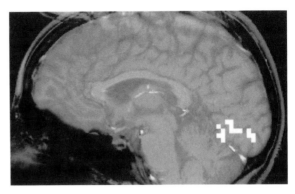

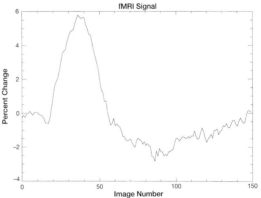

Fig. 22.7a, b. Result of an early response study using visual stimulation performed at 1.5 T. a The functional map of pixels exhibiting the early response. b The time course of the activated pixels shown in (a) The image TR is 300 ms and the visual stimulus was on from images 10–30

each run as well as the two runs for each echo time. The pixel time courses were correlated with an early response model to identify those pixels having a correlation threshold of at least 0.5. The map generated from the data acquired with a TE of 30 ms was used to define an ROI for comparing the amplitude of the dip at the three echo times. The early response was found significant at all three each times in four out of the five subjects studied. Data from one subject is shown in Fig. 22.6. The amplitude of the response increases linearly with increasing echo time. This result confirms a T2* nature of the early response, which is in agreement with the BOLD model and consistent with an initial increase in oxygen consumption not matched by the hemodynamic response. This suggests a closer spatial correspondence between the early response and the site of neuronal activation.

The discrepancy in TE dependence between the spectroscopy data and the imaging data may be attributed to partial volume effect. The fMRS study (HENNIG et al. 1995) reported that the amplitude of the early response decreases with increasing TE and subsequently attributed the early response to changes in T1 and proton density. While changes in T1 and proton density are possible sources of the early response, the fMRS observation is consistent with the BOLD contrast if the partial volume effect is taken into consideration. When the TE is increased, the contribution from the functionally active area is relatively reduced in the total MRS signal because these areas, consisting of gray matter and veins, have a shorter T2* relative to the rest of the VOI such as the white matter. As a result, the relative change in the total signal is diminished with increasing echo time. This interpretation is also consistent with the spectroscopic observation of a decrease in the delayed response with increasing echo time.

22.3.4
Study at Other Field Strengths

While most imaging experiments demonstrating the early response have been conducted at 4 Tesla, experimental studies at other field strengths have also been performed, demonstrating that the early response can be detected at lower field strength and providing an assessment of the field strength dependence of the early response.

In a study performed at 3 Tesla with a spiral imaging sequence, a visual paradigm consisting of a whole-field 8 Hz inverting checkerboard was studied (VAZQUEZ et al. 1997). The imaging sequence employed TR/TE of 75/35 ms, four spiral interleaves (300 ms per image), and a flip angle of 10°. The visual stimulation paradigm, which consisted of 28 s of fixation and 2 s of visual stimulation, was repeated 30 times in each subject. Upon data averaging, z statistic for the early response and the hyperemic response was calculated and thresholded to generate corresponding functional maps. Spatial characteristics of the maps were comparable to those observed at 4 T. Interestingly, the amplitude of the early response relative to the amplitude of the late response is about 1:5, smaller than that reported at 4 T.

We have recently performed a study at 1.5 Tesla (Siemens Medical Systems, Iselin, NJ) examining the early response. Physiological noise reduction was used in this study. A T2*-weighted single shot EPI sequence (matrix: 64×64, FOV: 20×20 cm, TE: 60 ms, TR: 300 ms, flip angle: 55°) was used to acquire 600 images of a sagittal slice 6 mm off the mid-line while LED goggles flashing at 8 Hz were turned on for 3.6 s at intervals of 45 s. Each run consisted of three re-

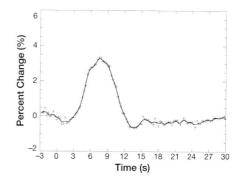

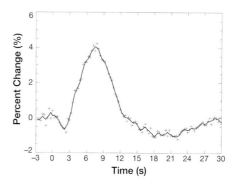

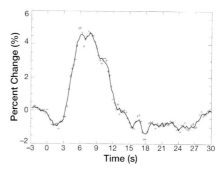

Fig. 22.6a–c. Early response time course for TEs of **a** 21, **b** 30 and **c** 45 ms from a visual stimulation study conducted at 4 T

peats of the visual stimulus. In each subject, four runs were performed. The pixel time courses were averaged over all repeats and runs in each subject, correlated with an early response model, and thresholded at a level of 0.5 for identifying pixels exhibiting a significant early response. A statistically significant early negative response was detected in three out of four subjects. As shown in Fig. 22.7a, the map generated from the early response is well localized to the calcarine fissure. The average time course of pixels displaying the negative response (Fig. 22.7b) indicates that the peak of the negative change is about one tenth of the peak positive response.

The results from these studies, when compared to those obtained at 4 T, indicate that the relative amplitude of the early response scales more rapidly with the field strength than the positive response. This observation is concordant with the view that the early response may predominantly reflect changes in the microvascular circulation, whose BOLD contrast is expected to scale quadratically with the field while the positive response may scale less than quadratically.

22.4 Discussion

This chapter provides an overview of MR studies aimed at demonstrating and characterizing the early response at the onset of neuronal stimulation. The existence of an early negative response in the MR signal is confirmed. The temporal characteristics of the early MR response, especially that revealed by the imaging studies, is in good agreement with that of the optical imaging data. In addition, despite the discrepancy in spatial resolution between the MR study and the optical experiments, the spatial characteristics of the early response relative to the late positive response is consistent with the prediction of the optical data, suggesting that the early response may arise from the microvasculature, which is more specific to the site of neuronal activation.

The echo time dependence and field strength dependence of the early response have provided some insights into the origin of the early response. While the exact physiological origin is not known at this point, the echo time dependence as observed by the MR imaging studies indicate that the dip is likely of a BOLD contrast, consistent with an initial increase in deoxyhemoglobin concentration as shown more directly with optical imaging. Furthermore, the field strength dependence, albeit preliminary, suggests that the early response is mostly of microvascular origin. While the deoxygenation model is rather compelling, alternative hypotheses regarding the origin of the early response cannot be ruled out at this point. One interesting model that is also consistent with BOLD is the balloon model based on a hypothesis of mechanical response of the vessel (Buxton et al. 1997).

It is worth noting that the functional spectroscopy data are not in full agreement with the imaging results. This discrepancy most likely arises from the difference in the stimuli used and the severe partial volume effect associated with the spectroscopic studies.

22.5 Summary

The early increase in deoxyhemoglobin concentration reported by optical imaging studies is investigated by a number of MR experiments that are summarized in this chapter. Experimental data have demonstrated that the early response is clearly detectable with various functional MR approaches. The characteristics of the early response were found to be in agreement with previous optical imaging results (Frostig et al. 1990; Grinvald et al. 1991; Malonek and Grinvald 1996). Additional studies examining the echo time dependence and the field strength dependence are consistent with the view that the early response reflects BOLD contrast and is possibly of microvasculature origin. These studies also suggest that the early response may be used for more specific functional mapping. Of course, further experimental studies are still needed to evaluate the early response in fMRI.

Acknowledgements. This work is supported by the National Center for Research Resources at the National Institutes of Health (grants RR08079 and R01MH55346). Helpful discussions with Drs. Amiram Grinvald, Seiji Ogawa, Seong-Gi Kim, and Ravi Menon are greatly appreciated. We thank Drs. Peter Andersen and Gregor Adriany for technical assistance.

References

Bandettini PA, Jesmanowicz A, Wong EC, Hyde JS (1993) Processing strategies for time-course data sets in functional MRI of the human brain. Magn. Reson. Med. 30: 161–173

Bottomley PA (1987) Spatial localization in NMR spectroscopy in vivo. Ann NY Acad Sci 508: 333–348

Boxerman JL, Bandettini PA, Kwong KK, Baker JR, Davis TJ, Rosen BR, Weisskoff RM (1995) The intravascular contribution to fMRI signal changes: Monte Carlo modeling and diffusion-weighted studies in vivo. Magn Reson Med 34: 4–10

Buxton RB, Wong EC, Frank LR (1997) A biomechanical interpretation of the BOLD signal time course: the balloon model. Fifth Annual Meeting of the International Society of Magnetic Resonance in Medicine, Vancouer, Canada, 2: 743

Duyn JH, Moonen CTW, Yperen GH, Boer RW, Luyten PR (1994) Inflow versus deoxyhemoglobin effects in BOLD functional MRI using gradient echoes at 1.5 T. NMR Biomed 7: 83–88

Ernst T, Hennig J (1994) Observation of a fast response in functional MR. Magn Reson Med 32: 146–149

Fox PT, Raichle ME (1986) Focal physiological uncoupling of cerebral blood flow and oxidative metabolism during somatosensory stimulation in human subjects. Proc Natl Acad Sci USA 83: 1140–1144

Frahm J, Haase A, Matthaei D, Merboldt KD, Hanicke W (1985) Rapid NMR imaging using stimulated echoes. J Magn Reson 65: 130–135

Frahm J, Merboldt KD, Hanicke W, Kleinschmidt A, Boecker H (1994) Brain or vein-oxygenation or flow? On signal physiology in functional MRI of human brain activation. NMR Biomed 7: 45–53

Frostig RD, Lieke EE, Ts'o DY, Grinvald A (1990) Cortical functional architecture and local coupling between neuronal activity and the microcirculation revealed by in vivo high-resolution optical imaging of intrinsic signals. Proc Natl Acad Sci USA 87: 6082–6086

Grinvald A, Frostig RD, Siegel RM, Bartfeld RM (1991) High-resolution optical imaging of functional brain architecture in the awake monkey. Proc Natl Acad Sci USA 88: 11559–11563

Haase A (1990) Snapshot FLASH MRI: Application to T_1, T_2, and Chemical Shift Imaging. Magn Reson Med 13: 77–89

Hennig J, Ernst T, Speck O, Deuschl G, Feifel E (1994) Detection of brain activation using oxygenation sensitive functional spectroscopy. Magn Reson Med 31: 85–90

Hennig J, Janz C, Speck O, Ernst T (1995) Functional spectroscopy of brain activation following a single light pulse: examination of the mechanism of the fast initial response. Int J Imag Sys Tech. 6: 203–208

Hu X, Le TH (1996) Artifact reduction in EPI with phase-encoded reference scan. Magn Reson Med 36: 166–171

Hu X, Le TH, Parrish T, Erhard P (1995) Retrospective estimation and correction of physiological fluctuation in functional MRI. Magn Reson Med 34: 201–212

Hu X, Le TH, Ugurbil K (1997) Evaluation of the early response in fMRI in individual subjects using short stimulus duration. Magn Reson Med 37: 877–884

Kim S-G, Hendrich K, Hu X, Merkle H, Ugurbil K (1994) Potential pitfalls of functional MRI using conventional gradient-recalled echo techniques. NMR in Biomed 7: 69–74

Kim S-G, Hu X, Adriany G, Ugurbil K (1996) Fast interleaved echo-planar imaging with navigator: High resolution anatomic and functional images at 4 Tesla. Magn Reson Med 35: 895–902

Kim SG, Ugurbil K (1997) Functional magnetic resonance imaging of the human brain. J Neurosci Methods 74: 229–243

Lai S, Hopkins AL, Haacke EM, Li D, Wasserman BA, Buckley P, Friedman L, Meltzer H, Hedera P, Friedland R (1993) Identification of vascular structures as a major source of signal contrast in high resolution 2D and 3D functional activation imaging of the motor cortex at 1.5 T: Preliminary results. Magn Reson Med 30: 387–392

Le TH, Hu X (1996) Retrospective estimation and correction of physiological artifacts in fMRI by direct extraction of physiological activity from MR data. Magn Reson Med 35: 290–298

Lee AT, Glover GH, Meyer GH (1995) Discrimination of large venous vessels in time-course spiral blood-oxygen-level-dependent magnetic resonance functional neuroimaging. Magn Reson Med 33: 745–754

Malonek D, Grinvald A (1996) The imaging spectroscope reveals the interaction between electrical activity and cortical microcirculation: Implication for optical, PET, and MR functional brain imaging. Science 272: 551–554

McIntosh J, Zhang Y, Kidambi S, Harshbarger T, Mason G, Prohost GM, Twieg D (1996) Echo-time dependence of the functional MRI 'fast response'. Soc Magn Reson Med, 4th Scientific Meeting, New York, NY, 1: 284

Menon RS, Hu X, Adriany G, Andersen P, Ogawa S, Ugurbil K (1994) Comparison of spin-echo EPI, asymmetric spin-echo EPI and conventional EPI applied to functional neuroimaging: The effect of flow crushing gradients on the BOLD signal. Second Conference of Society of Magnetic Resonance, San Francisco, 2:622

Menon RS, Ogawa S, Hu X, Strupp JS, Andersen P, Ugurbil K (1995) Bold based functional MRI at 4 Tesla includes a capillary bed contribution: Echo-planar imaging mirrors previous optical imaging using intrinsic signals. Magn Reson Med 33: 453–459

Menon RS, Ogawa S, Tank DW, Ugurbil K (1993) 4 Tesla gradient recalled echo characteristics of photic stimulation-induced signal changes in the human primary visual cortex. Magn Reson Med 30: 380–386

Merkle H, Garwood M, Ugurbil K (1993) Dedicated circularly polarized surface coil assemblies for brain studies at 4 T. Soc Magn Reson Med, 12th Annual Meeting, New York, 3: 1358

Ogawa S, Lee T-M (1990) Magnetic resonance imaging of blood vessels at high fields: In vivo and in vitro measurements and image simulation. Magn Reson Med 16: 9–18

Ogawa S, Lee T-M, Kay AR, Tank DW (1990a) Brain magnetic resonance imaging with contrast dependent on blood oxygenation. Proc Natl Acad Sci USA 87: 9868–9872

Ogawa S, Lee T-M, Nayak AS, Glynn P (1990b) Oxygenation-sensitive contrast in magnetic resonance image of rodent brain at high magnetic fields. Magn Reson Med 14: 68–78

Segebarth C, Belle V, Delon C, Massarelli R, Decety J, Le Bas J-F, Decorps M, Benabied AL (1994) Functional MRI of the human brain: Predominance of signals from extracerebral veins. NeuroReport 5: 813–816

Song AW, Wong EC, Tan SG, Hyde JS (1996) Diffusion weighted fMRI at 1.5 T. Magn Reson Med 35: 155–158

Thulborn KR, Waterton JC, Mattews PM, Radda GK (1982) Oxygenation dependence of the transverse relaxation time of water protons in whole blood at high field. Biochem Biophys Acta 714: 265–270

Vazquez A, Peltier S, Davis D, Noll D (1997) Evidence of the fast response at 3.0 T. Fifth Annual Meeting of the International Society of Magnetic Resonance in Medicine, Vancouer, Canada, 2: 726

Yacoub E, Cohen ER, Hu X (1997) Echo-time dependence of the early negative response in functional MRI. 27th Annual Meeting of the Society for Neuroscience, New Orleans, 23: 1576

23 The Post-Stimulus Undershoot of the Functional MRI Signal

R.B. Buxton, E.C. Wong, L.R. Frank

CONTENTS

23.1
The Mystery of the Post-Stimulus Undershoot

In 1992, Kwong and coworkers published a seminal paper in functional neuroimaging, in which they demonstrated that the magnetic resonance (MR) signal increases by a few percent in activated areas of the brain associated with performance of sensory and motor tasks (Kwong et al. 1992). The source of the effect is an alteration of the local concentration of deoxyhemoglobin, and this blood oxygenation level-dependent (BOLD) effect is the basis of functional MR imaging (fMRI) for mapping patterns of activation in the working human brain. But even in this early paper, the authors noted a curious feature of the BOLD signal response to activation. At the end of the stimulus the signal dipped below the baseline level, and remained depressed for a considerable

time (tens of seconds). Figure 23.1 shows their original data measured at 1.5 T from the visual cortex in response to a flashing grid of red lights. In Fig. 23.1 this post-stimulus undershoot appears as a lowering of the baseline after the first stimulus, and this pattern is often seen when the stimulus and the control periods are the same.

Figure 23.2 shows a more recent example of the BOLD response, measured at 3 T in the visual cortex in response to a similar flashing light stimulus lasting 20 s, and with the off period increased to 40 s for better visualization of the undershoot (Buxton et al. 1998a). This curve illustrates the general features of the BOLD response. The BOLD signal ramps up to its peak value over several seconds after the beginning of the stimulus, ramps down again after the end of the stimulus, and then undershoots the baseline. The post-stimulus undershoot in these data has about half the magnitude of the peak itself, and the undershoot takes about 20 s to resolve. Although the post-stimulus undershoot is not always evident, numerous examples can be found in the fMRI literature (Ogawa et al. 1992; Turner et al. 1993; Menon et al. 1995; Merboldt et al. 1995; Hu et al. 1997). In particular, Frahm and coworkers have reported ex-

R.B. Buxton, PhD; Department of Radiology, University of California at San Diego, 200 West Arbor Drive, San Diego, CA 92103-8756, USA
L.R. Frank, PhD; Department of Radiology, VA Medical Center 9114/MRI, 3350 La Jolla Village Drive, San Diego, CA 92161, USA
E.C. Wong, MD, PhD; Department of Radiology and Psychiatry, University of California at San Diego, 200 West Arbor Drive, San Diego, CA 92103-8756, USA

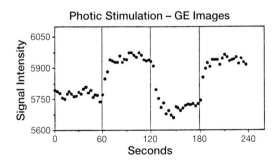

Fig. 23.1. Original demonstration of functional MRI (fMRI) based on the blood oxygen level-dependent (BOLD) effect (reproduced from Kwong et al. 1992; with permission of the author). The plot shows signal intensity changes within the visual cortex during darkness and 8 Hz photic stimulation, measured at 1.5 T. The post-stimulus undershoot is evident as an apparent lowering of the baseline after the first stimulus period

amples of pronounced undershoots that take more than a minute to resolve (see Fig. 23.3) (FRAHM et al. 1996; KRUGER et al. 1996).

The cause and significance of the post-stimulus undershoot have been sources of speculation since the beginning of fMRI. From the basic theory of the BOLD effect, a signal change is observed when the local deoxyhemoglobin content is altered. During activation the cerebral blood flow (CBF) increases much more than the cerebral metabolic rate of oxygen (CMRO$_2$), and as a result the venous blood is more oxygenated and the decrease in deoxyhemoglobin leads to an increase of the BOLD signal. But in addition to the changes in CBF and CMRO$_2$, a change in the cerebral blood volume (CBV) will also produce a change in the local deoxyhemoglobin content. All three of these physiological quantities increase with activation, but the effects of these changes on deoxyhemoglobin content are opposite. The large CBF change compared to the CMRO$_2$ change tends to decrease local deoxyhemoglobin content, but the CBV change tends to increase it. The net BOLD signal change thus depends in a somewhat complex way on the combined changes in several physiological parameters. The post-stimulus undershoot is a transient effect and clearly suggests that some physiological quantity is slow to return to baseline at the end of the stimulus. Because the BOLD signal depends on changes in CBF, CMRO$_2$ and CBV, all three of these are potential sources of the undershoot.

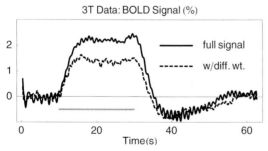

Fig. 23.2. The blood oxygen level-dependent (BOLD) response in the visual cortex, measured at 3 T (BUXTON et al. 1998a). The plot shows the average response of three subjects to 20 s of 8 Hz photic stimulation alternated with 40 s of darkness. In this example the transient post-stimulus undershoot is pronounced and requires about 20 s to fully resolve. Also plotted is the BOLD response when bipolar gradient pulses (diffusion weighting) are added to the pulse sequence to spoil the intravascular component of the BOLD signal. The peak BOLD signal is reduced, consistent with approximately one third of the BOLD signal change being intravascular, but the post-stimulus undershoot is unchanged, consistent with the undershoot being a purely extravascular signal change

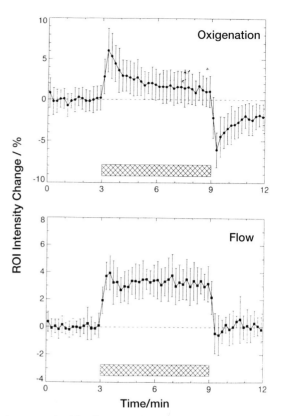

Fig. 23.3. The blood oxygen level-dependent (BOLD) and flow-sensitive response measured in the visual cortex with sustained stimulation (reproduced from KRUGER et al. 1996 with permission of the publisher). The plot shows a more extreme example of the post-stimulus undershoot, which has a magnitude larger than the plateau BOLD signal itself and requires several minutes to resolve. Note also that in this example there is a pronounced overshoot at the beginning of the stimulus. When the experiment was performed using an imaging pulse sequence directly sensitive to inflow effects, rather than the BOLD effect, the transients are not present. This indicates that the post-stimulus undershoot is not a flow undershoot. This pattern has been interpreted as evidence of an initial uncoupling of cerebral blood flow (CBF) and cerebral metabolic rate of oxygen (CMRO$_2$), a recoupling during the plateau portion, and uncoupling again after the end of the stimulus (FRAHM et al. 1996; KRUGER et al. 1996)

Perhaps the simplest explanation for the post-stimulus undershoot would be that CBF itself dips below baseline. That is, a naive interpretation of the BOLD signal would be that it simply reflects the flow change. If CBF and CMRO$_2$ are uncoupled, perhaps CMRO$_2$ stays approximately constant, but flow fluctuates more strongly. Then if flow dipped below baseline while CMRO$_2$ remained at baseline, more oxygen would be extracted, the deoxyhemoglobin content would increase, and the BOLD signal would decrease, thus producing the undershoot. However, there is substantial evidence that this explanation is incorrect. In the original paper of Kwong et al. (1992) and in later work (Davis et al. 1994b), when the same experiment was performed with an inversion recovery (IR) pulse sequence, there was no post-stimulus undershoot. An IR image is more directly sensitive to inflow of blood and when collected with a spin-echo acquisition the signal is only weakly sensitive to the BOLD effect. Kruger et al. (1996) also showed that a pronounced and long lasting undershoot of the BOLD signal was not present when the experiment was repeated with a flow-sensitive pulse sequence (Fig. 23.3). Figure 23.4 shows an example from a more recent motor activation study we performed using an arterial spin labeling technique that allows simultaneous measurement of both the quantitative flow change and the BOLD change (Buxton et al. 1998c). There is a clear divergence of the data in the post-stimulus period, with the flow change returning smoothly to baseline after the end of the stimulus while the BOLD signal shows a distinct undershoot.

The post-stimulus undershoot is thus a potent reminder that the BOLD signal change depends on the combined changes in several physiological parameters and cannot be interpreted as a simple reflection of CBF. And although this complicates the quantitative interpretation of the BOLD signal change, it also provides a window for investigating the physiological changes that form the basis of fMRI. In particular, study of the transient aspects of the BOLD signal, such as the post-stimulus undershoot, may help to clarify the nature of the physiological changes that accompany brain activation.

23.2
What Happens During Brain Activation?

The post-stimulus undershoot has been a continuing subject of discussion and debate because it was felt that this simple piece of observable data might shed light on the basic metabolic changes that follow brain activation. Despite the widespread use of fMRI for mapping brain activation, a quantitative understanding of the physiological changes that underlie the BOLD signal is still lacking. In broad terms, the basic picture is believed to be that increased neural activity leads to increased local consumption of adenosine triphosphate (ATP), which in turn triggers an increase of local energy metabolism. This involves an increase in CBF, the cerebral metabolic rate of glucose (CMRGlc), $CMRO_2$, and also CBV. As

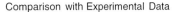

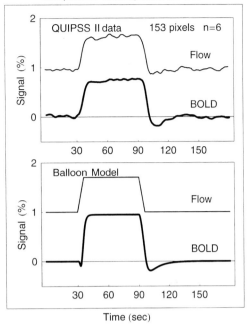

Fig. 23.4. Simultaneous measurement of the flow and blood oxygen level-dependent (BOLD) response in the motor cortex (*upper panel*) compared with theoretical calculations based on the balloon model (reproduced from Buxton et al. 1998c with permission from the publisher). Measurements were done at 1.5 T using an arterial spin labeling technique (QUIPSS II) which allows simultaneous measurement of both the change in cerebral blood flow (CBF) and the BOLD signal. The data are an average response of all voxels exhibiting a flow change of greater than 40% in six subjects performing a simple bilateral finger tapping task. A modest post-stimulus undershoot is apparent in the BOLD signal but not the flow signal. Theoretical curves calculated with the balloon model are able to reproduce the data reasonably well. In the balloon model, CBF and cerebral metabolic rate of oxygen ($CMRO_2$) are tightly coupled throughout, and the undershoot arises because the CBV is slow to return to baseline

noted above, the essential problem is that the BOLD signal is not a simple reflection of any one of these physiological parameters.

The imbalance in the changes of CBF and $CMRO_2$ during activation is the primary physiological phenomenon that creates the BOLD signal change and makes possible fMRI. When first reported based on positron emission tomography (PET) measurements (Fox and Raichle 1986; Fox et al. 1988), this imbalance was termed an "uncoupling" of flow and oxygen metabolism, in the sense that the flow appeared to increase much more than was necessary to support the small increase in oxygen metabolism. This PET result was particularly unexpected because virtually all of the energy metabolism of the brain is derived from the oxidative metabolism of glucose, and the glucose metabolic rate showed similar large changes to those of CBF. This clearly suggested that a significant amount of anaerobic metabolism was associated with brain activation. With the advent of fMRI it has become clear that this imbalance of the changes in flow and oxygen metabolism is not an artifact of the PET techniques but instead is a real and widespread physiological phenomenon. But if CBF and $CMRO_2$ changes are truly uncoupled, we are left with a fundamental unanswered question: Why does flow increase so much? Furthermore, if CBF and $CMRO_2$ changes are unrelated, and the BOLD signal depends on both, is it possible to develop any quantitative interpretation of the BOLD signal changes in terms of the underlying physiological changes?

The large change in CBF with activation is even more puzzling because it should not be required to support the change in CMRGlc. The brain extraction fraction of glucose from the blood is relatively low (OLDENDORF 1971), suggesting that glucose delivery to brain cells is not flow-limited, and even at rest only about half of the glucose that leaves the capillary and becomes available for metabolism is actually metabolized (GJEDDE 1987). In short, it seems that glucose is delivered in substantial excess of what is required at rest, so the increases associated with activation should be met easily without any increase in flow (BUXTON and FRANK 1997).

In trying to interpret BOLD changes in terms of CBF changes, a common working assumption has been that $CMRO_2$ does not change. This allows one to eliminate one of the physiological variables that affects the deoxyhemoglobin content and develop quantitative relationships between BOLD changes and CBF changes. Physiologically, this amounts to an assumption that all of the additional energy metabolism associated with activation is met by anaerobic glycolysis. But there is now substantial evidence that the change in $CMRO_2$, although smaller than the change in CBF, is not zero. In their original work, Fox and RAICHLE (1986) found that a 30% flow increase was accompanied by a 5% increase in oxygen metabolism, and in earlier work an increase of 13% in $CMRO_2$ was measured (SEITZ and ROLAND 1992). More recently, strong evidence for an increase in $CMRO_2$ with activation was reported based on using MRI techniques for direct measurement of perfusion in conjunction with BOLD signal measurements (DAVIS et al. 1998). In these experiments flow and BOLD signal changes were compared between an activation paradigm and a paradigm which altered the CO_2 content of the subject's inspired air. Both activation and increased CO_2 are expected to alter CBF, but altered CO_2

has been found to have no effect on $CMRO_2$. The experimental result was that, for the same change in flow, the activation experiment showed a smaller BOLD change, consistent with larger oxygen extraction and $CMRO_2$ during activation. Thus, any quantitative interpretation of BOLD changes must include $CMRO_2$ as well as CBF changes.

Furthermore, even a small change in $CMRO_2$ compared to the change in CMRGlc is not negligible in terms of the metabolic energy budget. Comparing aerobic and anaerobic metabolism, for each molecule of glucose that is fully oxidatively metabolized, approximately 16 times as many ATP molecules are generated as in glycolysis alone (SIESJO 1978). Then, for example, if $CMRO_2$ increases by 5% while CMRGlc increases by 30%, the change in ATP production is only about 6.6%, but 75% of this change comes from oxidative metabolism (BUXTON and FRANK 1997).

23.3
Are Flow and Oxygen Metabolism Coupled During Activation?

A simple proposed explanation for the observed imbalance of flow and oxygen metabolism changes during activation is that the $CMRO_2$ increase occurs on a fine spatial scale, but that CBF is only controlled on a coarser scale (TURNER and GRINVALD 1994; MALONEK and GRINVALD 1996). In this context CBF and $CMRO_2$ changes are indeed coupled and of similar magnitude over a small spatial region, but the focal $CMRO_2$ change is diluted in the measurements of larger tissue volumes, creating a small average increase in $CMRO_2$. The flow change is more spatially widespread and so is not diluted, producing the apparent imbalance of CBF and $CMRO_2$ changes. This has been described as "watering the garden for the sake of one thirsty flower" (TURNER and GRINVALD 1994; MALONEK and GRINVALD 1996). However, this explanation does not address the observed large increase in CMRGlc, which would suggest that glucose metabolism is increased over a much wider area than that of increased $CMRO_2$. This hypothesis also suggests that the magnitude of the observed imbalance between CBF and $CMRO_2$ may vary substantially between brain regions, and perhaps even within the same region in response to different stimuli that activate different neuronal populations.

Recently, we proposed a different interpretation for the imbalance of CBF and $CMRO_2$ changes, arguing that this imbalance is required to support the small change in $CMRO_2$ (BUXTON and FRANK 1997). The idea behind this oxygen limitation model is that the brain metabolizes virtually all of the oxygen that leaves the capillary and becomes available for metabolism, so that the observed net oxygen extraction fractions of about 40% are also the unidirectional extraction fractions. In other words, only a fraction of the oxygen delivered by blood flow actually leaves the capillary and enters the extravascular space (KASSISSIA et al. 1995). If oxygen delivery is limited at rest and the flow change is accomplished by increased blood velocity rather than capillary recruitment, then the decreased capillary transit time associated with increased flow leads to a reduced extraction of oxygen. The result is that, although the delivery of oxygen to the capillary bed increases dramatically, the fraction of the oxygen which leaves the capillary and becomes available for metabolism is reduced. In the context of this oxygen limitation model, flow and oxygen metabolism are tightly coupled, but in a nonlinear way that requires a large change in flow to support a small increase in oxygen delivery to the tissue. When this idea is developed in a quantitative model, the prediction is that an increase of 5% in $CMRO_2$ requires a 30% increase in flow when the resting oxygen extraction fraction is 40%, in good agreement with the PET results. This model also does not directly address why the increase in CMRGlc is so large, and suggests that CMRGlc is uncoupled from CBF and $CMRO_2$.

The two proposals above both argue for a coupling of flow and oxygen metabolism. In the model of coarse spatial control of CBF, the $CMRO_2$ changes are as large as the flow changes but occur in a smaller volume than the flow changes, and so in effect are artifactually smaller. In the oxygen limitation model, the $CMRO_2$ change is indeed smaller, but is as large as can be supported by the flow change. In principle, these two hypotheses are not incompatible. One can imagine that both effects may contribute to the observations, and further experiments, particularly those that push the current limits of spatial resolution, will be required to test these hypotheses.

23.4
Is the Post-Stimulus Undershoot Evidence for Uncoupling of Flow and Oxygen Metabolism?

An alternative picture of brain activation has been proposed, largely based on fMRI observations of the post-stimulus undershoot. This explanation invokes an uncoupling of flow and metabolism with CBF returning to baseline while $CMRO_2$ remains elevated during the undershoot. This basic explanation of the undershoot has been suggested by a number of investigators (TURNER et al. 1993; DAVIS et al. 1994a) and has been most clearly developed in the works of Frahm and colleagues (FRAHM et al. 1996; KRUGER et al. 1996). Figure 23.3 shows a striking example from their data, with a substantial post-stimulus undershoot that takes more than a minute to resolve. The data also show an initial overshoot of the BOLD signal relative to the steady state plateau signal. These investigators proposed that this pattern could be evidence that $CMRO_2$ changes more slowly than CBF. The picture of brain activation is then, initially, CBF increases without much change in $CMRO_2$, producing a large decrease in deoxyhemoglobin and a resulting strong BOLD signal increase. As $CMRO_2$ slowly increases to its new level, more deoxyhemoglobin is created and the BOLD signal is reduced to the plateau level. At the end of the stimulus, CBF returns to baseline more quickly than $CMRO_2$, and so deoxyhemoglobin content is increased above baseline, producing the post-stimulus undershoot. This picture is then one of an initial uncoupling of flow and oxygen metabolism, a recoupling during the plateau phase, and a transient uncoupling again at the end of the stimulus.

This model has at its heart the idea that flow and oxygen metabolism can be fundamentally uncoupled, and in a rather broader way than what was originally proposed by Fox and RAICHLE (1986). Based on their observation that CBF increased more than $CMRO_2$, Fox and Raichle argued for uncoupling in the sense that the CBF increase appeared to serve some need other than support of a $CMRO_2$ increase, implying that the increased $CMRO_2$ requirements could have been met with a smaller increase in flow. But the interpretation of Frahm and colleagues appears to go further and suggest that a flow increase is not even necessary in order to increase $CMRO_2$, because, at least transiently, $CMRO_2$ can remain elevated after CBF has returned to baseline. This view is directly opposed to the hypothesis of tight coupling of CBF and $CMRO_2$, as developed in the oxygen limitation model. If this view is correct, and the post-stimulus undershoot represents an uncoupling of flow and oxygen metabolism, then the fundamental questions remain: Why does CBF increase so much, and is there any relationship between CBF and $CMRO_2$ changes?

23.5
Or, Is the Post-Stimulus Undershoot a Blood Volume Effect?

More recently, MANDEVILLE et al. (1998) have reported evidence for another possible explanation, that the elevated blood volume associated with activation is slow to resolve after the end of the stimulus. In rat studies with forepaw stimulation they found strong BOLD signals with a pronounced post-stimulus undershoot. By using an intravascular contrast agent, they were also able to show that the blood volume recovered very slowly, requiring more than 30 s to reach baseline, in good agreement with the observed BOLD undershoot (see Fig. 23.5). Note that the explanation of the undershoot as a blood volume effect does not require invoking an uncoupling of flow and oxygen metabolism. If both CBF and $CMRO_2$ have returned to baseline shortly after the end of the stimulus, then the blood oxygenation would also return to baseline, but the total deoxyhemoglobin would remain elevated above baseline simply because the blood volume remains elevated.

Thus, the two leading theories for the source of the undershoot are that either $CMRO_2$ or CBV remains elevated after CBF has returned to the resting level. The initial experimental evidence from animal studies supports the volume theory, but more experimental data, particularly in human subjects, is required. Another approach to testing these theories is to exploit the fact that the MR signal has both intra- and extravascular contributions (BOXERMAN et al. 1995). The extravascular signal change depends primarily on the total amount of deoxyhemoglobin within a voxel, and both hypotheses predict an increase in the total. In the elevated $CMRO_2$ theory this is due to an elevated blood *concentration* of deoxyhemoglobin, rather than an elevated blood *volume*, but both predict an undershoot of the extravascular BOLD signal. But the two theories differ in their predictions of the intravascular signal change. With the elevated $CMRO_2$ hypothesis the blood oxygenation is reduced, so the undershoot should also be present in the intravascular signal because the blood oxygenation is altered, but the elevated CBV hypothesis suggests that the intrinsic intravascular signal should have returned to baseline, so there should be no undershoot in the intravascular signal. Experimentally, the intravascular signal can be suppressed by applying bipolar gradient pulses (diffusion weighting) to spoil the signal of moving blood. Figure 23.2 shows the results of our

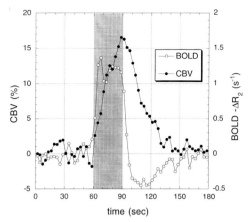

Fig. 23.5. Blood oxygen level-dependent (BOLD) and cerebral blood volume (CBV) response to rat forepaw stimulation, measured at 4.7 T (MANDEVILLE et al. 1998, reprinted with permission of the publisher). In this study animals (7 forepaws, 5 rats) were injected with an intravascular contrast agent in order to directly monitor changes in CBV during activation. After the end of the stimulus, CBV returns slowly to baseline, requiring more than 30 s to normalize. During this period the BOLD signal exhibits a post-stimulus undershoot. These data are consistent with the undershoot being a blood volume effect, rather than an uncoupling of cerebral blood flow (CBF) and cerebral metabolic rate of oxygen ($CMRO_2$)

initial studies based on this approach using a visual stimulation paradigm (BUXTON et al. 1998a). With added spoiler pulses the peak BOLD signal is reduced by about one third, but the undershoot is unaffected. This result, although preliminary, is consistent with the post-stimulus undershoot being a purely extravascular effect and supports the elevated CBV hypothesis.

23.6
The Balloon Model

In addition to the experimental work described above, we recently proposed a mathematical model, called the balloon model, which illustrates in a quantitative way how the post-stimulus undershoot can arise from a blood volume effect (BUXTON et al. 1998c). In an initial comparison with experimental data measured in the motor cortex, the model was able to reproduce the data reasonably well (see Fig. 23.4). Furthermore, the balloon model incorporates the oxygen limitation model for the coupling of flow and oxygen metabolism and demonstrates that transients similar to those observed experimentally are entirely consistent with tight coupling throughout the activation and recovery period.

The balloon model is based on a few simple assumptions. These assumptions are undoubtedly overly simplistic, but they serve to illustrate that pronounced transient features, such as the post-stimulus undershoot, can arise in a natural way from the dynamics of the physiological changes during activation. The mathematical details of the model can be found in BUXTON et al. (1998c), but the basic physical picture represented by the balloon model is as follows: The capillary bed is treated as a fixed set of pipes (i.e., there is no capillary recruitment). The small, post-capillary veins, however, are distensible, and the changes in blood volume all occur on the venous side (the arteriolar dilatation that produces a flow increase is assumed to be a negligible change in blood volume). The vascular bed within a small volume of tissue is then modeled as an expandable venous compartment (a balloon) that is fed by the output of the capillary bed. The volume flow rate (ml/s) into the tissue, $F_{in}(t)$, is an assumed function of time that drives the system. The volume flow out of the system, $F_{out}(t)$, is assumed to depend primarily on the pressure in the venous compartment. And this pressure, in turn, is assumed to depend on the volume of the balloon. Then outflow is modeled as a function of volume, with the curve $F_{out}(v)$ playing a role analogous to a stress/strain curve for the venous balloon.

The physical picture of activation is that after the arteriolar resistance is decreased, producing an increase in F_{in}, the venous balloon swells and the pressure increases until F_{out} matches F_{in} (a new steady state). The amount of swelling that occurs will depend on the biomechanical properties of the vessel as reflected in the pressure/volume curve of the venous balloon. The rate of change of the volume of the balloon is the difference between F_{in} and F_{out}. Applying mass balance for deoxyhemoglobin and blood leads to two coupled equations for the total deoxyhemoglobin content of the voxel and the volume of the balloon. From these two quantities, the dynamic BOLD signal change is calculated, taking into account the changes in both the extravascular (OGAWA et al. 1993) and intravascular (BOXERMAN et al. 1995) signals.

Because the dynamical equations of the balloon model are based on mass balance for deoxyhemoglobin, a critical ingredient is an expression for the oxygen extraction fraction over time, $E(t)$, which governs the rate at which deoxyhemoglobin is delivered to the balloon. If flow and oxygen metabolism are uncoupled, then this is an unknown function. But if instead they are coupled according to the oxygen limitation model (BUXTON and FRANK 1997), this unknown function of time can be replaced by a known function of flow. That is, a central assumption of the balloon model is that flow and oxygen metabolism are tightly coupled throughout the stimulus and recovery period, so that $CMRO_2$ increases by as much as can be supported by the current value of the inflow.

The final ingredient of the balloon model is the form of the curve of $F_{out}(v)$, the rate of outflow from the balloon as a function of the volume of the balloon. As noted above, this curve is analogous to the stress/strain curve of the balloon wall and so is dependent on the mechanical properties of the vessels. Different forms of $F_{out}(v)$ will yield different BOLD response curves. The shape of this curve for the small post-capillary vessels of the brain is unknown, but with the balloon model we can explore the effects of different mechanical properties. For example, if the vessel becomes stiffer as it inflates, this would correspond to a steepening of the curve of $F_{out}(v)$ as v increases. Figure 23.6 shows an example of how this shape of the curve introduces transients into the BOLD response. A strong post-stimulus undershoot occurs because the volume is slow to return to baseline, and this shape for $F_{out}(v)$ also produces an initial dip in the BOLD signal. An initial dip has been reported in several high field fMRI studies (ERNST and HENNIG 1994; MENON et al. 1995: HU et al. 1997), and MENON et al. (1995) observed that, when the initial dip was detected, it was usually accompanied by a post-stimulus undershoot. An initial overshoot of the deoxyhemoglobin content, corresponding to this initial dip, has been observed in optical experiments and attributed to an initial increase of $CMRO_2$ prior to the increase of CBF (MALONEK and GRINVALD 1996). But in the context of the balloon model, any increase of $CMRO_2$ must be supported by an increase of CBF, and in these calculations the dip occurs because of an early increase of blood volume due to the shallow initial slope of the curve $F_{out}(v)$.

However, the initial dip is more rarely seen than the post-stimulus undershoot, and the data in Fig. 23.3 show an initial overshoot, rather than a dip. This type of behavior can result if the curve of $F_{out}(v)$ exhibits hysteresis, such that the curve differs during inflation and deflation of the balloon. This effect can be incorporated into the balloon model equations in a simple way by introducing a viscosity parameter (BUXTON et al. 1998b). The goal is to mimic viscoelastic effects, in which rapid changes in volume are resisted. Figure 23.7 shows examples of the type of BOLD response curves which result. With a mod-

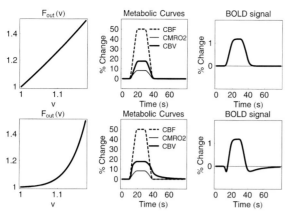

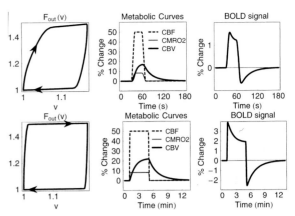

Fig. 23.6. Balloon model calculations illustrating how a non-linear form of the outflow curve as a function of balloon volume leads to transients in the deoxyhemoglobin content and the blood oxygen level-dependent (BOLD) signal (Buxton et al. 1998c). The panels in each row show F_{out} (v) (*left*), the physiological curves (*middle*), and the resulting BOLD signal (*right*). For all of these calculations the steady state volume change was taken to be of the form f^a (where f is the maximum flow change) with a=0.4 (Grubb et al. 1974); a resting blood volume of 2% and a resting oxygen extraction of 40% were assumed; and the inflow curve was assumed to be a trapezoid with 8 s ramps and a 50% flow increase. In the *first row* F_{out} (v) simply follows the power law with exponent 0.4, and there are no transients in the BOLD signal. In the *second row* F_{out} (v) steepens as v increases (but with the same steady state endpoint), representing an initially distensible balloon that stiffens as it inflates. The initial shallow slope of this curve leads to an initial rapid filling of the balloon, which produces an initial dip in the BOLD signal, and a slow drainage of the balloon after the end of the stimulus, producing a post-stimulus undershoot. Cerebral blood flow (CBF) and cerebral metabolic rate of oxygen (CMRO$_2$) are tightly coupled throughout according to the oxygen limitation model (Buxton and Frank 1997)

Fig. 23.7. Balloon model calculations illustrating the effect of hysteresis. For these calculations the effects of viscoelastic behavior were approximated by allowing the curve F_{out} (v) to be different during inflation and deflation of the balloon by introducing a viscosity parameter into the balloon model (Buxton et al. 1998b) so that rapid volume changes are resisted. With moderate viscous effects and a short 30 s stimulus, the curves are similar to those in Fig. 23.5. With larger viscous effects, a larger resting blood volume of 4%, a larger maximum volume change corresponding to a=0.5, and a longer 4 min stimulus the curves are similar to those in Fig. 23.3

23.7
The Significance of the Post-Stimulus Undershoot

The animal experiments of Mandeville et al. (1998) showing that blood volume changes resolve slowly suggest that the post-stimulus undershoot may simply be a secondary effect and does not reflect the more basic physiological changes in flow and oxygen metabolism. This is supported by theoretical calculations based on the balloon model, which show that a wide range of transient phenomena in the BOLD response can be produced when blood volume changes resolve at a different rate than do the flow and metabolism changes, and indeed such transients can arise in the presence of tight coupling of flow and oxygen metabolism. In the context of this model the volume change passively follows the flow change, and so does not reflect directly on energy metabolism. But further studies are required to confirm this view. The development of techniques for dynamic assessment of blood volume changes in humans will greatly expand the range of stimuli which can be investigated (Wong et al. 1997). And more sophisticated models of the viscoelastic behavior of small blood vessels are required to refine the predictions of the balloon model and quantitatively compare theoretical curves with experimental data.

erate viscous effect (upper row), the shape of the CBV and BOLD curves are similar to those found experimentally by Mandeville et al (1998; compare with Fig. 23.5). With a larger viscous effect (lower row), the shape of the BOLD curve is similar to that reported by Kruger et al. (1996; compare with Fig. 23. 3), showing an initial overshoot and a strong post-stimulus undershoot with a long time constant. Again, in the context of the balloon model these transient features are entirely due to blood volume effects.

In short, blood volume effects are sufficient to account for the observed transients in the BOLD signal, but a definitive confirmation requires more work. But whatever the source of the undershoot phenomenon, an intriguing question that remains to be answered is why it varies so much in different experiments. It is not always present, and when it is, its quantitative features, such as magnitude and duration, vary over a wide range from subject to subject. In some cases the undershoot was found to vary depending on the nature of the stimulus itself. In an experiment alternating low spatial frequency color stimuli and high spatial frequency black and white stimuli, the undershoot was only found with the black and white stimuli (BANDETTINI et al. 1997). These stimuli are thought to activate different subcompartments of the imaging voxel (blobs and interblobs, respectively), suggesting that the BOLD response varies on a fine spatial scale. The source of the different responses is unknown, but these data suggest that the undershoot may provide a way to probe events on a sub-voxel spatial scale.

In addition to its significance as a physiological phenomenon, the existence of the post-stimulus undershoot has consequences for the practical analysis of fMRI data. The broadening effect of the hemodynamic response places limits on the detection of responses to stimuli that are close together, and so fundamentally affects the temporal resolution of fMRI. The presence of an undershoot with a long recovery time suggests that the response to even a short stimulus may influence the BOLD signal tens of seconds after the stimulus was applied. In practice, analysis of a measured fMRI time series usually involves correlation with an assumed hemodynamic response function, and in many applications this function should include an undershoot.

Furthermore, such a response function often is calculated as a convolution of the stimulus pattern with an assumed "impulse response." This is essentially an assumption of linearity, that the hemodynamic response to an extended stimulus is simply a sum of shifted versions of the response to a single, short stimulus. Experimental approaches testing the linearity of the BOLD response have found that while it is approximately linear, there are measurable nonlinear effects (BOYNTON et al. 1996; DALE and BUCKNER 1997). In particular, it appears that the post-stimulus undershoot for a very short stimulus is weaker than that for a longer stimulus. At least qualitatively, this type of nonlinearity is consistent with the balloon model. For short stimuli the full blood volume change does not develop and so the peak BOLD signal is stronger and the undershoot is reduced. For longer stimuli the larger volume change reduces the plateau BOLD signal and deepens the undershoot. Further studies of the post-stimulus undershoot are thus important for understanding the ultimate limits on the linearity and temporal resolution of fMRI.

Acknowledgments. This work was supported by grant NS36722 from the National Institutes of Health.

References

Bandettini PA, Kwong KK, Davis TL, Tootell RBH, Wong EC, Fox PT, Belliveau JW, Weisskoff RM, Rosen BR (1997) Characterization of cerebral blood oxygenation and flow changes during prolonged brain activation. Hum Brain Mapping 5:93–109

Boxerman JL, Bandettini PA, Kwong KK, Baker JR, Davis TL, Rosen BR, Weisskoff RM (1995) The intravascular contribution to fMRI signal change: Monte Carlo modeling and diffusion-weighted studies in vivo. Magn Reson Med 34:4–10

Boynton GM, Engel SA, Glover GH, Heeger DJ (1996) Linear systems analysis of functional magnetic resonance imaging in human V1. J Neurosci 16:4207–4221

Buxton RB, Frank LR (1997) A model for the coupling between cerebral blood flow and oxygen metabolism during neural stimulation. J Cereb Blood Flow Metab 17:64–72

Buxton RB, Luh W-M, Wong EC, Frank LR, Bandettini PA (1998a) Diffusion weighting attenuates the BOLD peak signal change but not the post-stimulus undershoot. 6th Mtg Int Soc Magn Reson Med, Sydney, Australia, pp 7

Buxton RB, Miller K, Frank LR, Wong EC (1998b) BOLD signal dynamics: the balloon model with viscoelastic effects. 6th Mtg, Int Soc Magn Reson Med, Sydney, Australia, pp 1401

Buxton RB, Wong EC, Frank LR (1998c) Dynamics of blood flow and oxygenation changes during brain activation: the balloon model. Magn Reson Med 39:855–864

Dale AM, Buckner RL (1997) Selective averaging of rapidly presented individual trials using fMRI. Hum Brain Mapping 5:329–340

Davis TL, Weisskoff RM, Kwong KK, Boxerman JL, Rosen BR (1994a) Temporal aspects of fMRI task activation: Dynamic modeling of oxygen delivery. Int Soc Magn Reson, 2nd Annu Mtg, San Francisco, pp 69

Davis TL, Weisskoff RM, Kwong KK, Savoy R, Rosen BR (1994b) Susceptibility contrast undershoot is not matched by inflow contrast undershoot. Int Soc Magn Reson, 2nd Annu Mtg, San Francisco, pp 435

Davis TL, Kwong KK, Weisskoff RM, Rosen BR (1998) Calibrated functional MRI: mapping the dynamics of oxidative metabolism. Proc Natl Acad Sci U S A 95:1834–1839

Ernst T, Hennig J (1994) Observation of a fast response in functional MR. Magn Reson Med:146–149

Fox PT, Raichle ME (1986) Focal physiological uncoupling of cerebral blood flow and oxidative metabolism during somatosensory stimulation in human subjects. Proc Natl Acad Sci U S A 83:1140–1144

Fox PT, Raichle ME, Mintun MA, Dence C (1988) Nonoxidative glucose consumption during focal physiologic neural activity. Science 241:462–464

Frahm J, Krüger G, Merboldt K-D, Kleinschmidt A (1996) Dynamic uncoupling and recoupling of perfusion and oxidative metabolism during focal activaiton in man. Magn Reson Med 35:143–148

Gjedde A (1987) Does deoxyglucose uptake in the brain reflect energy metabolism? Biochem Pharmacol 36:1853–1861

Grubb RL, Raichle ME, Eichling JO, Ter-Pogossian MM (1974) The effects of changes in PCO_2 on cerebral blood volume, blood flow, and vascular mean transit time. Stroke 5:630–639

Hu X, Le TH, Ugurbil K (1997) Evaluation of the early response in fMRI in individual subjects using short stimulus duration. Magn Reson Med 37:877–884

Kassissia IG, Goresky CA, Rose CP, Schwab AJ, Simard A, Huet PM, Bach GG (1995) Tracer oxygen distribution is barrier-limited in the cerebral microcirculation. Circ Res 77:1201–1211

Kruger G, Kleinschmidt A, Frahm J (1996) Dynamic MRI sensitized to cerebral blood oxygenation and flow during sustained activation of human visual cortex. Magn Reson Med 35:797–800

Kwong KK, Belliveau JW, Chesler DA, Goldberg IE, Weisskoff RM, Poncelet BP, Kennedy DN, Hoppel BE, Cohen MS, Turner R, Cheng H-M, Brady TJ, Rosen BR (1992) Dynamic magnetic resonance imaging of human brain activity during primary sensory stimulation. Proc Natl Acad Sci U S A 89: 5675–5679

Malonek D, Grinvald A (1996) Interactions between electrical activity and cortical microcirculation revealed by imaging spectroscopy: implications for functional brain mapping. Science 272:551–554

Mandeville JB, Marota JJA, Kosofsky BE, Keltner JR, Weissleder R, Rosen BR, Weisskoff RM (1998) Dynamic functional imaging of relative cerebral blood volume during rat forepaw stimulation. Magn Reson Med 39:615–624

Menon RS, Ogawa S, Strupp JP, Anderson P, Ugurbil K (1995) BOLD based functional MRI at 4 tesla includes a capillary bed contribution: echo-planar imaging correlates with previous optical imaging using intrinsic signals. Magn Reson Med 33:453–459

Merboldt KD, Kruger G, Hanicke W, Kleinschmidt A, Frahm J (1995) Functional MRI of human brain activation combining high spatial and temporal resolution by a CINE FLASH technique. Magn Reson Med 34:639–644

Ogawa S, Tank DW, Menon R, Ellermann JM, Kim S-G, Merkle H, Ugurbil K (1992) Intrinsic signal changes accompanying sensory stimulation: functional brain mapping with magnetic resonance imaging. Proc Natl Acad Sci USA 89:5951–5955

Ogawa S, Menon RS, Tank DW, Kim S-G, Merkle H, Ellerman JM, Ugurbil K (1993) Functional brain mapping by blood oxygenation level – dependent contrast magnetic resonance imaging: a comparison of signal characteristics with a biophysical model. Biophys J 64:803–812

Oldendorf WH (1971) Brain uptake of radiolabeled amino acids, amines, and hexoses after arterial injection. Am J Physiol 221:1629–1639

Seitz RJ, Roland PE (1992) Vibratory stimulation increases and decreases the regional cerebral blood flow and oxidative metabolism: a positron emission tomography (PET) study. Acta Neurol Scand 86:60–67

Siesjo BK (1978) Brain energy metabolism. Wiley, New York

Turner R, Grinvald A (1994) Direct visualization of patterns of deoxygenation and reoxygenation in monkey cortical vasculature during functional brain activation. Int Soc Magn Reson, 2nd Annu Mtg, San Francisco, pp 430

Turner R, Jezzard P, Wen H, Kwong KK, Bihan DL, Zeffiro T, Balaban RS (1993) Functional mapping of the human visual cortex at 4 and 1.5 tesla using deoxygenation contrast EPI. Magn Reson Med 29:277–279

Wong EC, Buxton RB, Frank LR (1997) A method for dynamic imaging of blood volume. 5th Mtg, Int Soc Magn Reson Med, Vancouver, pp 372

24 Functionally Related Correlation in the Noise

J.S. Hyde and B.B. Biswal

24.1 Introduction

Low-frequency spontaneous oscillations of regional cerebral blood flow and oxygenation have been observed by several investigators in animal models using a variety of measurement techniques, including laser Doppler flowmetry (LDF) (Golanov et al. 1994; Hudetz et al. 1992, 1995), fluororeflectometry (Dora and Kovach 1980; Vern et al. 1988), fluorescence video microscopy (Biswal and Hudetz 1996), and polarographic measurement of brain tissue PO_2 with microelectrodes (Moskalenko 1980; Cooper et al. 1966; Halsey and McFarland 1974).

Several early reports of similar phenomena in humans appeared shortly after the initial discovery of fMRI (Ogawa et al. 1992; Jezzard et al. 1993; Biswal et al. 1993; Weisskoff et al. 1993). Of these, the abstract by Weisskoff et al. (1993) is particularly instructive. They show Fourier transforms of pixel time courses in visual area V1, white matter, CSF, sagittal sinus, and background. Several bands of

J.S. Hyde, PhD; B.B. Biswal, PhD; Biophysics Research Institute, Medical College of Wisconsin, 8701 Watertown Plank Road, Milwaukee, WI 53226, USA

signals were observed, including peaks at the cardiac rate as well as harmonics of this rate, a peak at the respiratory rate, and an intense peak at very low frequencies of the order of 0.1 Hz in the gray matter V1 time course. This low-frequency peak is the subject of the present chapter.

Although the literature on the low-frequency peak has become extensive, no full papers have appeared that address in detail the nature of the other bands. Nevertheless, some information has been accumulating. For example, the cardiac peak and its harmonics arise from several superimposed biophysical processes including modulation of the static magnetic field by the beating heart, physical displacement of the brain, CSF pulsatility, vessel wall displacement, and blood flow and oxygenation pulsatility. In addition, the heart rate changes during the respiratory cycle, resulting in the generation of respiratory "sidebands" on either side of the cardiac peak in the Fourier transform display. Biswal and Hyde (1997a) studied the effect of the concentration of oxygen in the breathing gas mixture on the respiratory and cardiac peaks. Biswal et al. (1997g), using a half k-space echo planar imaging (EPI) pulse sequence that had been developed by Jesmanowicz et al. (1998), studied the harmonic content of CSF to frequencies as high as 15 Hz. In subsequent unpublished work, this was extended to 30 Hz. Fluctuations in CSF exist above thermal noise to the highest frequency observed thus far. It is apparent that the further study of these various effects will yield useful physiological information. These other bands will not be considered further in this chapter.

Work is currently in progress to determine the relationships between the animal literature on low-frequency spontaneous oscillations and the human fMRI literature on low-frequency physiological fluctuations. Much of the animal literature involves pathophysiological preparations that may not be relevant. However, two recent reports on normal rat cortex support the hypothesis that in normal brain the underlying biophysics of the observed fluctuations are the same in rats and in humans. The key observation in humans, as discussed in the next section, is the existence of a temporal correlation of fluctuations between well-separated focal regions. Abstracts by VERN et al. (1997) and BISWAL et al. (1997b), presented at the meeting of the International Society of Oxygen Transport in Tissues in 1997 as part of a general symposium, demonstrated for the first time interhemispheric synchrony of spontaneous oscillations in focal regions. Parallel human and animal studies on physiological fluctuations are a promising direction for future research.

24.2
Functional Connectivity

In 1995 the authors together with their colleagues YETKIN and HAUGHTON reported correlation of low-frequency fluctuations between time courses acquired during rest from pixels that were known from fMRI to have a commonality of response to a finger tapping paradigm (HYDE et al. 1995; BISWAL et al. 1995b, c). FRISTON et al. (1993) had previously defined functional connectivity as the temporal correlation of a neurophysiological index measured in different brain areas. These studies supported the hypothesis that low-frequency physiological fluctuations constituted such a neurophysiological index.

The experimental protocol was designed to avoid rehearsing or imagining motor activity during acquisition from resting brain.
1. Subjects were biomedical research and MRI naive.
2. Subjects were recruited for an unrelated MRI project.
3. There was no initial mention of finger motion or hand motion studies.
4. Resting state multislice data were the first to be acquired.
5. Subjects were told that they would be asked to perform an auditory task. The task was performed, but multislice data were collected in the motor cortex region.
6. A task-induced finger tapping multislice study was performed at the end of the exam to define the motor cortex region. Cross-correlation with a boxcar waveform was used.

Step 6 permits labeling of every pixel in a slice as being in the left motor cortex (L), the right motor cortex (R), or in other brain regions (O). This step serves only to permit labeling of pixel time courses

acquired in either step 4 or step 5 by subscripts L, R, or O. These three indices, taken together, enumerate all pixel time courses in a slice. Data acquired in step 6 are not otherwise used. Signal processing proceeded as follows.

Each pixel time course in the left motor cortex, there being n_R such time courses, is cross-correlated with all other pixel time courses in a slice, and resulting cross-correlation coefficients (CCCs) are divided into three groups: CCC_{RR}, CCC_{RL}, and CCC_{RO}. Cross-correlation coefficients between all possible pairs in the left motor region carry the index RR, between all intrahemisphere motor pairs the index RL, and between the right motor area and all other areas RO. For example, if there are 30 pixel time courses in the left motor cortex, 30 in the right, and 1000 other time courses, corresponding to $n_L=n_R=30$, $n_O=1000$, there are 30×29 entries in the CCC_{RR} category (noting the deletion of the entry corresponding to self-correlation), 30×30 entries in CCC_{RL}, and 30×1000 in CCC_{RO}. In a similar manner CCC_{LL} and CCC_{LO} are formed. Necessarily, $CCC_{RL} \equiv CCC_{LR}$.

Figure 24.1 shows histograms of CCC values from BISWAL et al. (1995c), pooling data across seven subjects. Resting state CCC distributions are compared with task activation data that were acquired in step 6 of the protocol and processed in the manner described above (i.e., cross correlation between pairs of task-activated time courses rather than the more customary use of a reference waveform). It is apparent that there is a considerable amount of synchrony of low-frequency physiological fluctuations during rest and that performance of the task increases the overall synchrony.

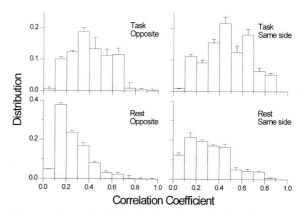

Fig. 24.1. Normalized distribution of magnitudes of correlation coefficients for all entries in regions L and R of the correlation-coefficient matrix for two experiments: resting (*lower*) and task activation (*upper*). Pixel pairs for opposite sides are at the left and for the same side at the right. (From BISWAL et al. 1995c)

Images can be formed from resting state data. BISWAL et al. (1995c) used a resting state correlation coefficient of 0.35, corresponding to a significance $P<10^{-3}$, and a single color was assigned to all CCCs above this value. Since there are n_R+n_L activated pixels, n_R+n_L separate independent maps can be produced in this manner from a single subject. Figure 24.2 shows one such map, which is compared with the original task activation map produced according to step 6 above. The general similarity is apparent. (The yellow regions in the figure represent significant *negative* correlations, an observation not yet pursued in the literature to date.)

Table 24.1 shows data on the degree of congruency of task-defined motor areas using a CCC of 0.5 with areas defined by analysis of physiological fluctuations with a CCC of 0.35. Variation of TR in the data of this table was carried out in order to test possible effects of aliasing of the heart rate into the low-frequency region.

Table 24.1. Correlation coefficient data from resting brain

Subject	TR (ms)	$\bar{n}_{LL}/n_L$ (%)	$\bar{n}_{LR}/n_L$ (%)	$\bar{n}_{RR}/n_R$ (%)	Mean	$\bar{n}_{OL}+\bar{n}_{OR}/n_O$ (%)
1	250	88±8	65±11	74±9	73±10	1.8
2	250	84±9	63±13	75±10	71±11	2.2
3	250	93±5	77±12	85±9	83±12	2.4
4	250	83±11	66±17	74±12	72±15	1.6
5	500	71±14	56±19	62±9	61±16	1.7
6	400	79±12	61±17	67±14	67±15	0.9
7	1000	79±9	67±13	74±10	72±11	1.6
8	1000	73±7	53±9	70±8	65±8	3.5
9	1000	69±11	42±9	71±12	60±11	1.9
10	1000	82±9	69±10	79±8	76±9	3.5
11	1000	77±9	59±12	65±11	67±11	4.3

The resting state data may be even better than Fig. 24.2 and Table 24.1 would suggest. Region c of Fig. 24.2 was not considered in the analysis but lies in Broadman's area 6 and can probably be assigned to the supplementary motor area (SMA). The area labeled d may be an extension of the primary sensorimotor area into the inner hemispheric fissure. The area labeled e is occasionally seen in fMRI finger tapping tasks, where it has been assigned to the premotor area. Thus Fig. 24.2 suggests that the entire motor system may exhibit significant functional connectivity from which the task selects a subset.

XIONG et al. (1998a, b) extended the work of BISWAL et al. (1995c). They analyzed resting state fluctuations and identified six areas of the motor system that exhibit significant inter-regional connectivity: primary motor cortex, primary somatosensory cortex, premotor cortex, secondary somatosensory cortex, anterior cingulate cortex, and posterior cingulate. These authors commented on the fact that analysis of resting state physiological fluctuations reveals many more activations than the usual task-induced activation analysis. They make the hypothesis that task-induced activation maps underestimate the size and number of areas involved in a task and that those areas are more fully revealed by fluctuation analysis of activity during rest. This hypothesis raises several issues: (a) the need to develop objective measures of coincidence of maps produced by different methods. HYDE and BISWAL (1997a) introduced the spatial coincidence coefficient (SCC) as one such measure. (b) The need to develop objective methods for setting the threshold. (c) The careful use of graded tasks of progressively increasing difficulty. The authors have noticed the presence of some of the regions mentioned by these authors in task activation maps produced at lower than normal threshold. The provocative hypothesis

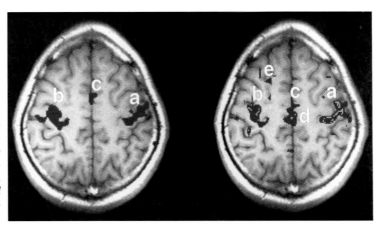

Fig. 24.2. fMRI task activation response to bilateral left and right finger movement, superimposed on a GRASS anatomic image (*left*). Fluctuation response using the methods of BISWAL et al. (1995c) (*right*). See Sect. 24.2 for assignment of labeled regions. *Red* is positive correlation, and *yellow* is negative

of XIONG et al. (1998a, b) should stimulate a considerable amount of future research.

The question then became, does coherence of physiological fluctuations between well separated focal regions occur only within the motor system, or do similar coherences exist in other functionally related brain systems? BISWAL et al. (1995a, 1996a) addressed this question by studying the visual cortex and the auditory cortex (BISWAL et al. 1996c). The auditory cortex was defined by periodic text reading. Analysis of resting state physiological fluctuations was carried out in a manner that was modeled after the previous motor cortex studies, and results were essentially similar. The visual cortex was defined by a black and white checkered annulus flickering at 8 Hz surrounding a fixation dot, alternating with steady gaze at the dot. This task defines area V1. Resting state data were obtained while the subject maintained steady gaze at the fixation dot. Analysis of resting state fluctuations not only showed a high degree of spatial coincidence with area V1, but also showed correlations with visual area MT, which does not respond to this particular task. In retrospect, this finding closely parallels the work of XIONG et al. (1998a, b) on the motor system and is supportive of their hypothesis: task-induced maps underestimate the size and number of areas involved in a task.

Low-frequency fluctuations that are the subject of this chapter have periods of the order of 10 s. Even with fairly long periods of acquisition of resting state data, such low frequencies are sampled sparsely. A further question of interest is whether fluctuations in different brain systems are asynchronous, and even if they are, whether the sampling is sufficiently dense to distinguish two or more brain systems in the same data set. This question was addressed quite early in an abstract by BISWAL et al. (1995a), and in a full paper by LOWE et al. (1998) that followed an early abstract (LOWE et al. 1996). BISWAL et al.. (1995a) placed an axial slice in the motor cortex and another one in the visual cortex within the same sequence. Motor and visual cortices were identified by separate tasks and coincidence with resting state maps demonstrated. Intersystem correlations across slices were not observed. LOWE et al. (1998) obtained whole-brain data (i.e., 15 slices) using a TR value of 2 s. Their data were somewhat compromised by two technical issues: aliasing of the heart rate and interslice phase differences because the various slices in the gradient-recalled EPI sequence were acquired at slightly different times. Nevertheless, they acquired satisfactory data both within and across slices. Complicated patterns of correlations were re-

ported. This important paper opens the opportunity to study patterns of functional connectivities across the entire brain. It defines a significant area for future development of image-processing tools designed to characterize these patterns.

24.3
Biophysical Characterization

In this section, experiments are described which address the hypothesis that the linkage between periodic task-induced neuronal activity and the observed periodic changes in MRI signal intensity is also the linkage that is responsible for asynchronous low-frequency physiological fluctuations observed in the absence of synchronized brain activity. That is, it is hypothesized that it should in principle make no difference whether a neuronal event occurs spontaneously or in response to an external demand. In either case there is a concomitant change in local blood flow, blood oxygenation, and blood volume. Five specific biophysical indicators or probes are discussed.

1. Low-frequency physiological fluctuations occur on the same time scale as the hemodynamic response to a task. Analysis of physiological fluctuations begins by applying to the resting state pixel time courses a low-pass 3 dB per octave digital filter that has the 3 dB point set at 0.08 Hz. This is a Wiener filter in the sense that the Fourier transform of a representative task activation pixel time course was obtained and the time constant of the filter adjusted so that it would pass this time course with minimal distortion. If the hypothesis is valid, low-frequency fluctuations in the local hemodynamics of the microcirculation that occur in response to spontaneous neuronal activity must also pass this filter.

2. Maps of low-frequency physiological fluctuations obtained from data collected during rest have a high degree of coincidence with maps produced in response to task activation, and in both cases only pixels lying in gray matter are active. Custom and experience has led to a consensus that a correlation coefficient threshold of 0.5 is a suitable choice for production of a task activation map. It is also necessary to set the resting state threshold. An objective strategy was introduced by HYDE and BISWAL (1997a) for this purpose, which is reviewed in Sect. 24.6.2 of this chapter. The spatial coincidence coefficient that was introduced in this method provides

an objective measure of the similarity of the two maps. This coefficient is calculated as a function of resting state correlation coefficient threshold. A well-defined maximum is observed across all subjects and studies that occurs at a threshold of about 0.35. When this procedure is carried out, some well-defined areas nevertheless appear in the resting state functional connectivity maps that are not present in the task activation maps. This result is consistent with the hypothesis of XIONG et al. (1998a, b) that task-induced maps underestimate the size and number of areas involved in a task. Good spatial coincidence including interhemispheric coincidence, gray matter specificity, consistency across subjects, and overall consistency with the expectations of systems neuroscience are powerful arguments that low-frequency resting state physiological fluctuations and response-to-task have a common neuronal basis and share a common biophysical linkage with the observed MRI signals.

Table 24.2. Motor cortex percent enhancement at 3 Tesla

TE (ms)	Full k-space			Half k-space		
	Task	Resting	Ratio	Task	Resting	Ratio
27	5.3±1.4	1.4±0.8	3.9±2.1	5.9±1.4	1.5±0.9	3.4±2.3
40	7.3±1.8	2.5±1.0	2.9±1.9	7.3±1.9	2.9±1.1	2.5±2.0
60	9.0±2.1	3.1±1.2	2.2±1.7	11.4±3.1	3.4±1.3	3.3±2.2

3. Using gradient-recalled echo-planar imaging, which is T2* sensitized for BOLD contrast, task activation response and low-frequency physiological fluctuations exhibit a similar dependence on the echo time, TE. The amount of data on this point is small and as yet unpublished. Nevertheless, this is a key technical test of the hypothesis of this section. Available data are given in Table 24.2. Half k-space and full k-space acquisition (see Jesmanowicz et al. 1998) are also compared in the table. These data were obtained from a single subject at 96×96 matrix, 5 mm slice thickness at 3 T. It is apparent that both resting state and task activation percent enhancements are proportional to TE for both half and full k-space acquisition and that the ratio of task activation response to physiological noise is approximately unchanged across the entire table. The standard deviations in the table were calculated across all active pixel time courses.

4. Hypercapnia reversibly suppresses low-frequency fluctuations in the human motor cortex during rest. Task activation response in humans to hypercapnia behaves similarly. In addition, the effects are similar to those observed in rats. This was the subject of an extended paper in the *Journal of Cerebral Blood Flow and Metabolism*, by BISWAL et al. (1997a; see also BISWAL et al. 1996b). Fourier analysis is essential in these experiments in order to control for changes in the heart rate and for the marked increase in the amplitude of the band at the respiration frequency. Representative images are shown in Fig. 24.3. The figure caption gives experimental details. Data were consistent across six subjects. This study not only establishes the similarity of the response to hypercapnia for both physiological fluctuations and task-activated fMRI signals, but also provides a linkage to the extensive body of literature on spontaneous oscillations in rats.

5. Flow fluctuations can be used to produce resting state functional connectivity maps in a manner that parallels the production of BOLD-sensitized task activation maps. This was the subject of an article by BISWAL et al. (1997d) in *NMR in Biomedicine* (see also BISWAL et al. 1997c). An embedded pulse sequence was used for simultaneous acquisition of BOLD-weighted and flow-weighted resting state data. As in task activation studies, the flow signals were of the order of one third of the BOLD signals, which further demonstrates the similarity of the biophysical basis of modulation of capillary hemodynamics by task-induced neuronal activity and spontaneous neuronal activity. The flow-weighted signals were sufficiently small that detailed comparison of maps produced by BOLD- and flow-weighted fluctuation data was difficult. Nevertheless, it could be concluded that they were essentially similar.

The authors are satisfied that the similarity of the biophysical linkage that connects neuronal activity with observed MRI signals comparing task-activated response with spontaneous neuronal activity has been established.

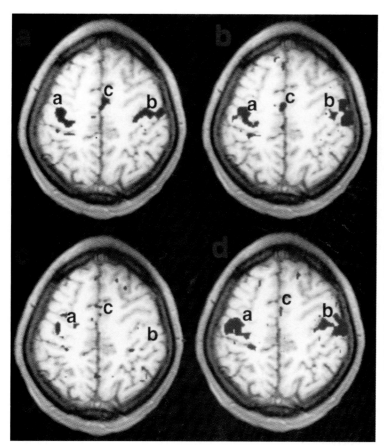

Fig. 24.3. a fMRI task activation response to bilateral left and right finger movement superimposed on a GRASS anatomic image. b Functional connectivity map obtained by choosing a reference waveform from the left motor cortex. c Functional connectivity map obtained during hypercapnia using the time course in the same pixel location as the reference waveform. d Functional connectivity map obtained after resumption of breathing room air. Regions a, b, and c in each of the images represent left primary motor cortex, right primary motor cortex, and supplementary motor areas (SMA), respectively. A substantial overlap between the task activation map and the functional connectivity map during each of the room-air scans was obtained. However, maps generated during hypercapnia had less overlap. Overlaps between the task activation and the first rest scan while breathing room air for the left motor cortex, right motor cortex, and SMA were 74%, 67%, and 53%, respectively. These dropped to 48%, 26%, and 31%, respectively, during hypercapnia. (From BISWAL et al. 1997a)

24.4
Clinical Reports

LOWE et al. (1997b) studied a subject with almost complete agenesis of the corpus callosum using an fMRI noise correlation protocol. They compared interhemisphere functional connectivity of the auditory cortex of a normal control with the connectivity in this patient, with impressive results. Callosal agenesis substantially eliminated interhemisphere auditory cortex connectivity. The result supports the hypothesis that the observed correlations are indicative of neuronal connectivity.

The authors and their colleagues have carried out a study on a diverse group of five patients with Tourette syndrome (TS). The results of their investigations are reported in a paper in *American Journal of Neuroradiology* (BISWAL et al. 1998), which describes motor task activation studies, and in two abstracts (BISWAL et al. 1997e, f) that report on functional connectivity using analysis of physiological fluctuations. Comparisons were made with age- and gender-matched controls. A bilateral finger tapping paradigm was used for task activation.

In normal subjects, typical signal intensities vary by about 5% and 1.5% during bilateral finger tapping and resting state, respectively. Both values were substantially higher in TS subjects: 7% and 2.5%, respectively. If normal and TS subjects are compared at constant threshold, the area of activation in response to task increased by 75% in the sensorimotor cortex and 60% in the supplementary motor area in TS subjects. Resting state maps were substantially coincident with task activation maps in both TS subjects and controls. Similarly, during the presentation of common English words, the spatial extent of activation in the auditory and associated cortex increased by about 25% in TS subjects. These results are generally consistent with the PET study of STERN et al. (1996).

This TS patient population has been extended to ten subjects in work-in-progress. The difference between patients and controls for both task and physiological fluctuation analyses is robust and readily apparent (see, for example, Fig. 24.4). The close parallelism between the results of task and fluctuation analyses supports the hypothesis that both have the same biophysical linkage between neuronal activity and observable MRI signal.

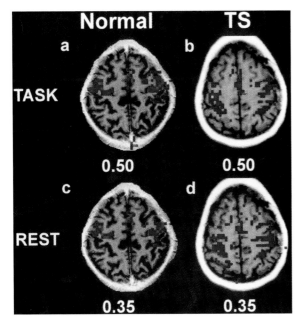

Fig. 24.4. Comparison of motor cortex images from an age-matched normal and a Tourette syndrome (TS) subject using task activation and resting state fMRI. A series of 90 sequential axial slices passing through the motor cortex was acquired for each of the four images using identical parameters: TR=2 sec, TE=40 ms, slice thickness=8 mm, FOV=24 cm, flip angle=90°. Thresholds for task activation and resting state connectivity maps for the TS and the normal subject were 0.5 and 0.35, respectively. In all ten subject pairs studied thus far, activation is greater in TS subjects

24.5
Effect of Low-Frequency Fluctuations on Task Activation Signals

It is apparent that the concept of "resting state" is not well defined. In the context of fMRI, all it really means is the absence of periodic or time encoded stimulation. Three preliminary reports have appeared in which functional connectivity studies were carried out in the presence of sustained stimulation.

BISWAL and HYDE (1998a) studied physiological fluctuations in the motor cortex during a sustained 6-min period of bilateral finger tapping. It was observed in each of the four subjects that were studied that the magnitude of the low-frequency physiological fluctuations was enhanced during continuous finger tapping. In addition, maps produced by analysis of these low-frequency fluctuations had an improved coincidence with task activation maps. These authors remark that the data were consistent with the hypothesis that attention to a prolonged task spontaneously fluctuates.

SKUDLARSKI and GORE (1998) compared fluctuations during three sustained passive stimuli: a pleasant odor, an unpleasant odor, and no odor. They report that the presentation of odor changed the strength of correlation between some regions in the human cortex, although the effect was weak.

LOWE et al. (1997a) presented the subject with a random sequence of either an auditory tone or a circular symbol and asked the subject to press a button when the auditory tone was heard. Subsequently, the identical sequence was presented but the instructions were to press the button when the visual symbol appeared. The repetition rate was 750 ms. The hypothesis of the experiment was the following: since all external stimuli were identical between the two scans, and the stimulus presentation was fast compared to the sampling rate, any change in correlation between the cortical areas controlling motor, vision, and auditory function across the two scans should be due to a change in neuronal connectivity from attention effects. Only three subjects were studied, and the effects were small. Nevertheless, it was concluded that the data were significant and consistent with the hypothesis.

These three studies involved a sustained active task or a sustained change in environment or a sustained task that was repeated twice with different instructions. Numerous other variants and extensions of these ideas are immediately apparent. However, in each case one is comparing differences between small effects. There is a significant challenge to improve experimental methodologies for these kinds of experiments.

It is apparent from these and other studies that low-frequency physiological fluctuations are superimposed on the data when conventional task activation experiments are performed. The nature of the task may affect the magnitude of these superimposed fluctuations, either up or down, but probably by a factor that does not exceed 30%. On the basis of this observation, a mathematical model of fMRI task activation contrast-to-noise ratio, CNR, has been developed in the research group of the authors in which the noise arises not only from thermal sources, but also from physiological fluctuations and other sources.

fMRI BOLD contrast was predicted by BANDETTINI (1994) and by MENON et al. (1993) to vary with respect to TE as:

$$S \propto \exp(-TE / T2^*) - \exp(-TE / T2'^*) \quad (24.1)$$

where T2*, T2'* are values of T2* in the presence and absence (Eq. 24.1) of task activation. This equation is plotted in Fig. 24.5. An optimum occurs at TE=T2*. A central finding of the work discussed in this article is that the task-induced response is superimposed on internally generated neuronally induced BOLD signals that vary asynchronously with the task and appear as noise. The CNR model is written as:

$$CNR = A_k \frac{\exp(-TE/T2^*) - \exp(TE/T2^{'*})}{\left\langle \left\{ N_B[\exp(-TE/T2^*) - \exp(-TE/T2^{'*})] + N_O + N_T + N_{SC} \right\}^2 \right\rangle^{1/2}}$$

(24.2)

where N_B, N_O, N_T, N_{SC} stand, respectively, for physiological noise of BOLD origin, other physiological noise, thermal noise, and scanner noise arising from system instabilities, and the brackets $\langle \rangle$ denote time course averaging.

It is important to emphasize that Eq. 24.2 implies that fMRI filtering has been done such that the fMRI signal and the noise are in a narrow bandwidth centered around 0.1 Hz. If physiological noise is much larger than thermal or system noise, Eq. 24.2 predicts that the exponential terms in the numerator and denominator will cancel, since they arise from the same neuronal-hemodynamic linkage, and CNR will be independent of TE.

This model must still be considered a hypothesis that requires detailed confirmation. Nevertheless, the authors are convinced of its general validity. There are a number of counterintuitive consequences of our study of physiological fluctuations that can profoundly affect the way in which task activation fMRI experiments are performed. Some of these ways are:

1. The CNR will tend to be independent of TE.
2. If the signal is increased by use of a surface coil, the CNR will be independent of TE over a wider range.

3. The signal-to-noise ratio (SNR) will tend to be independent of voxel size, including both in-plane matrix and slice thickness.
4. If the signal is increased by use of a surface coil, the CNR will be independent of TE over a wider range of voxel size.
5. If two decoupled RF coils receive signals from the same voxel, physiological noise will be correlated and thermal noise will be uncorrelated.
6. When using a surface coil, the CNR will be constant over a larger region even though the intensity varies substantially over that region.
7. Good coils do not give better CNR; they do permit increase of the resolution until physiological noise and thermal noise become comparable.
8. Half k-space acquisition is preferable to full k-space acquisition when physiological noise dominates.
9. EDELSTEIN et al. (1986) showed that if one compares an image acquired at lower resolution with one acquired at higher resolution that is subsequently averaged to lower resolution, the former is always better. This proof is valid only when thermal noise dominates, and should be reexamined for the CNR model. When physiological noise dominates, it is likely to be better to acquire data at the highest possible resolution, and average in order to achieve lower resolution, although spatial correlations of physiological noise are a potential complication.

24.6
Acquisition and Processing of Resting State Data

Four aspects of MR physics that are relevant to the experimental acquisition and processing of resting state data sets are considered in this section.

24.6.1
Motion Detection and Image Registration

The subject of this section is particularly important in the study of physiological fluctuations not only because the contrast is low, but also because the frequencies that characterize human motions when in the scanner tend to be in the same range as the physiological fluctuations that are of interest. An immediate requirement is that all image registration strategies be at the sub-pixel level. In general, inten-

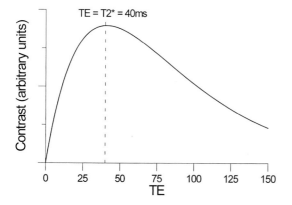

Fig. 24.5. Plot of Eq. 24.1

sity-based registration methods seem inappropriate at the level of accuracy that is being sought because physiological fluctuations are fluctuations in intensity that introduce noise into the registration algorithm.

BISWAL and HYDE (1997b) described a contour-based registration technique that was designed to differentiate between task-induced and motion-induced signal variations in fMRI. The method involved the following steps:

1. Generation of contour images by convolution with a Laplacian-of-Gaussian operator. The Laplacian operator produces the edges or features and the Gaussian operator smoothes the noise.
2. Identification and use of closed-loop contours that have an intensity above a set threshold; the intensities of all other contours are set to zero. The consequence of this step is that image registration is based only on major well-defined features.
3. Cross-correlation in two dimensions of the pair of images to be registered. The calculation is in the Fourier domain following the method of CONNAUGHTON et al. (1992). This method lends itself conveniently to sub-pixel registration utilizing the shift theorem of the Fourier transform.

Procedures used for image registration by the authors continue to evolve. The strategy currently in use was described by BISWAL and HYDE (1998b). Each image is registered to the first image of the series using the contour-based method, as a first step. This step is used to detect gross motion. Any image in the time course that requires more than two pixels of shift is discarded, since image registration of grossly misaligned images seems impossible – perhaps because of out-of-plane motional components. The next step is to identify and discard those pixel time courses that fluctuate in intensity. A sub-pixel intensity-based algorithm is then applied for fine registration. These last two steps are applied iteratively and continue until both the pattern of activation and the registration parameters converge.

24.6.2
Formation of Functional Connectivity Maps

Analytical tools are needed to facilitate recognition of patterns of correlations in EPI time courses from resting brain. If there are, for example, 1000 pixels, 1000 correlation coefficient images can be formed by cross-correlation of each pixel time course with all other pixel time courses. The search for patterns

is formidable. An initial strategy is to search for coincidence of an image obtained using periodic task activation with an image formed by analysis of a time course of resting state images. Spatial coincidence of these two images depends on the thresholds used for each. An objective procedure was introduced by HYDE and BISWAL (1997a-c). The method was illustrated using resting state auditory cortex data to set the resting correlation coefficient (RCC) threshold for a given activation correlation coefficient (ACC) threshold for optimum spatial coincidence.

The notation introduced in Sect. 24.2 was used where n_L and n_R are the number of activated pixel time courses in the left, L, and right, R, sides above the ACC threshold, n_O is the number of pixels in brain tissue below this threshold, and $n=n_L+n_R+n_O$. A matched *resting state* time course of images is obtained, and the pairwise correlation coefficient (PCC) matrix is formed. This matrix is of dimensionality n×n with entry of the ij element given by the correlation coefficient of the ith resting state pixel time course with the jth. The spatial coincidence coefficient (SCC) is defined in Eq. 24.3.

$$SCC = 1/3\left[\frac{n_{LL}}{n_L^2+n_{LO}}+\frac{n_{RR}}{n_R^2+n_{RO}}+\frac{2n_{LR}}{2n_Ln_R+n_{LO}+n_{RO}}\right]$$
(24.3)

Here n_{LL} is the number of off-diagonal entries in the $n_L×n_L$ PCC submatrix above the RCC threshold, and similarly for n_{RR}, n_{LO}, and n_{RO}. SCC lies between zero and one. The value of SCC was calculated as a function of the RCC threshold for a given ACC threshold by HYDE and BISWAL (1997a); well-defined maxima were observed, permitting determination of an optimum RCC value. Measures of ipsilateral and contralateral coincidence are given by Eqs. 24.4–24.6, and of spuriously correlated pixel time courses by Eq. 24.7. Images can be formed from any row of the $(n_L+n_R)×n$ submatrix of the PCC matrix or by averaging the correlation coefficients in each column.

$$SCC_{LL}=n_{LL}/(n_L^2+n_{LO})$$
(24.4)

$$SCC_{RR}=n_{RR}/(n_R^2+n_{RO})$$
(24.5)

$$SCC_{LR}=SCC_{RL}=2n_{LR}/(2n_Ln_R+n_{LO}+n_{RO})$$
(24.6)

$$SCC_{RLO}=(n_{LO}/n_On_L)+(n_{RO}/n_On_R)$$
(24.7)

The analysis of Eqs. 24.3–24.7 assumes a "hard" threshold, with a single color assigned to all pixels that have a CCC (see Sect. 24.2) above this value.

BISWAL et al. (1995c) found a few pixels adjacent to the task-defined regions that exhibited resting state pairwise correlation coefficients above threshold. An alternative approach was developed by HYDE and BISWAL (1997a) to include these clustered pixels in the analysis. Regions of interest centered on the task-defined regions, but oversize by one or two pixels, were defined and the pairwise correlation coefficient matrix formed. This alternate formulation is equivalent to assuming that resting state correlation coefficients that are above threshold with indices i and j corresponding to pixels that are adjacent to the region defined by task activation are valid rather than extraneous. Equations analogous to Eqs. 24.3–24.7 can be written by inspection for this alternate formulation.

In a study of the auditory cortices using a 64×64 matrix, representative values $n_R=15$, $n_L=15$, $n_O=1000$ were obtained for an ACC threshold of 0.5. The RCC threshold using the optimization method described here ranged from 0.28 to 0.34 over five subjects (average 0.31) and increased by 10% when the alternate formulation was used. Average values of spatial coincidence over all subjects were $SCC_{LL}=0.6\pm0.05$, $SCC_{RR}=0.58\pm0.04$, $SCC_{LR}=0.49\pm0.04$ and $SCC_{RLO}=0.02\pm0.01$. SCC values with subscripts LL, RR and LR increased by 10% using the alternate formulation and SCC_{RLO} was reduced by 50%. The average correlation coefficient of all pixel pairs in the auditory cortex, averaged across all subjects, was 0.37 ± 0.08 during rest, while during task activation the average across subjects and pixels of the correlation coefficient with an ideal reference waveform was 0.58 ± 0.11.

24.6.3
Whole Brain and High Spatial Acquisition

In order to avoid aliasing of the heart rate into the low-frequency range, $(TR)^{-1}$ should be shorter than one half of the heart rate, which approximately corresponds to TR<400 ms. In practice, a TR value of 250 ms has often been used. A low-pass digital filter is then applied to remove the cardiac frequency from the pixel time course. A representative cutoff frequency that has been used is 0.08 Hz.

It is apparent that one direction for future research is the acquisition of whole brain resting state data, following the work of LOWE et al. (1998). Another direction is acquisition of a smaller number of slices, but at higher spatial resolution. Partial k-space acquisition, as described by JESMANOWICZ et al. (1998), seems to be an essential sequence in such studies within the constraint that TR<400 ms. Data presented in their paper show that 15-slice 64×64 matrix data sets can be acquired within 400 ms or alternatively that two to three slices at 192×192 matrix size can be acquired. This is an important direction for future research.

All studies performed by the authors have used local gradient coil technology, as introduced by WONG et al. (1992a, b, 1993), with switching rise times of 96 µs, gradient strength of 2 G/cm, and dB/dt<20 T/s for all three gradients. It is technically possible in our apparatus to drop the rise time to 50 µs and to hold the x and y dB/dt values to <60 T/s, which is consistent with the 1988 FDA guidelines. This would give additional benefit in acquiring either whole volume or high resolution resting state data. Local gradient coil technology has substantial advantages over whole body gradient coil technology within the condition that aliasing of the cardiac rate should be avoided. Acquisition of resting state data with cardiac gating is an alternative approach that has not yet been investigated. Several distinct aspects of cardiac contributions to the resting state pixel time course intensities are listed in the Introduction (Sect. 24.1) of this article. These include both T1 in-flow effects that would not be eliminated by gating, and motional effects that would not be eliminated by filtering. Thus both techniques, high speed acquisition with filtering and cardiac gating, may be of value.

24.6.4
The Static Field Strength

The authors have substantial experience in the study of physiological fluctuations at both 1.5 and 3 T field strengths and have observed a clear qualitative benefit of the higher field strength. The theoretical model for this observation is that the NMR signal tends to increase linearly with field strength, the BOLD susceptibility fluctuations that are the origin of the low-frequency physiological fluctuations discussed in this article also increase linearly with field strength, and the noise is thermal in origin and independent of field strength. Thus one would expect a factor of 4 improvement in detection of low-frequency physiological fluctuations upon going from 1.5 T to 3 T. Rigorous experimental testing of this model has not yet been carried out. It is possible that physiological fluctuations in a given region of brain tissue can be divided into two or more components and that if one is interested in one of the components, the other components become noise.

The contrast-to-noise model described in Sect. 24.5 (Eq. 24.2) predicts that for task activation experiments there is no benefit in going to higher field strength unless the conditions are such that physiological noise is comparable to or less than thermal noise. This situation can occur if the TE value is sufficiently short or the voxel is sufficiently small. Primarily the use of high field strength modulates the word "sufficiently" in the previous sentence. Higher field strength permits TE to be shorter or the spatial resolution to be higher. In addition, the TR value can be shorter, in order to avoid aliasing of the cardiac rate, without loss of contrast.

A particular problem of high field strength fMRI is intravoxel dephasing because of air-tissue-bone susceptibility effects. The difficulty is largely in the slice selection direction. Under conditions of dominant physiological noise, the slice thickness can be reduced without loss of CNR. There can even be a net benefit by the use of thinner slices that arises from reduction of partial volume and leads to higher percent enhancements.

The partial k-space sequence introduced by JESMANOWICZ et al. (1998) is central to the discussion of field strength effects, since it permits the use of short TE values and single-slice single-shot resolution at 3 T up to 192×192 over 16×16 cm². In summary, high field strength in fMRI is definitely advantageous, but the presence of physiological fluctuations means that the benefit lies in improved resolution rather than higher CNR.

24.7
Conclusions

The major conclusion of this review is that it has been established that work directed at improved understanding and use of low-frequency physiological fluctuations has become a significant field of research in its own right.

It is customary to begin every task activation fMRI scanning session by acquisition of a high resolution whole brain anatomic data set, usually requiring about 15 min. It is suggested that a routine part of every scanning session might well be, in addition, to obtain a whole-brain, resting state, low-frequency physiological-fluctuation data set, which would require about five more minutes. These two reference data sets would characterize the anatomic and neurological state of the brain and both would serve to enhance interpretation of subsequent task activation experiments.

Low-frequency physiological fluctuations constitute the limiting noise source in most task activation experiments. The magnitude of these fluctuations can be somewhat affected by attention, but not by much more than about 30%. This has profound implications about how one thinks about fMRI CNR and the associated magnetic resonance physics. The most significant conclusion is that the CNR is independent of spatial resolution of task activation experiments over a wide range. Much higher resolution can be used than was previously thought possible. Partial k-space acquisition, following the work of JESMANOWICZ et al. (1998), or alternatively, the use of interleaved EPI, are strategies for achieving higher resolution. Whole-brain spatial resolution in task activation experiments at the cortical column level is within reach.

The three one-page abstracts that were concerned with attentional modulation of low-frequency physiological fluctuations, as reviewed in Sect. 24.4, are of interest from a systems neuroscience perspective. It would seem that interesting new paradigms can be designed that combine techniques used in these three abstracts with task activation experiments.

New clinically relevant strategies for investigating the brain of patients who are either unable to respond to tasks or who respond poorly are likely to develop based on measurement of low-frequency fluctuations.

The local gradient coil/local brain coil technology that has been developed at the Medical College of Wisconsin is advantageous for the studies that have been reviewed in this article.

Acknowledgement. This work was supported by grant MH51358 from the National Institutes of Health

References

Bandettini PA (1994) Magnetic resonance imaging of human brain activation using endogenous susceptibility contrast. PhD thesis, Medical College of Wisconsin
Biswal BB, Hudetz AG (1996) Synchronous oscillations in cerebrocortical capillary red blood cell velocity after nitric oxide synthase inhibition. Microvasc Res 52:1–12
Biswal B, Hyde JS (1997a) Physiological fluctuations in FMRI: effects of inspired oxygen. Proc 5th ISMRM, Vancouver, p 728

Biswal B, Hyde JS (1997b) Contour-based registration technique to differentiate between task-activated and head motion-induced signal variations in fMRI. Magn Reson Med 38:470–476

Biswal BB, Hyde JS (1998a) Functional connectivity during continuous task activation. Proc 6th ISMRM, Sydney, p 1410

Biswal BB, Hyde JS (1998b) A novel image registration technique for fMRI. Proc 6th ISMRM, Sydney, p 2132

Biswal B, Bandettini PA, Jesmanowicz A, Hyde JS (1993) Time-frequency analysis of functional EPI time-course series. Proc 12th SMRM, New York, p 722

Biswal B, DeYoe EA, Yetkin FZ, Haughton VM, Rao S, Hyde JS (1995a) Temporal correlation of fMRI signals may reveal brain connectivity. Soc Neurosci Abstr 21:905

Biswal B, Yetkin FZ, Haughton VM, Hyde JS (1995b) Functional connectivity of the resting human brain using echo-planar MRI. Proc 3rd ISMRM, Nice, p 400

Biswal B, Yetkin FZ, Haughton VM, Hyde JS (1995c) Functional connectivity in the motor cortex of resting human brain using echo-planar MRI. Magn Reson Med 34:537–541

Biswal BB, DeYoe EA, Anderson BJ, Beauchamp MS, Hyde JS (1996a) Functional connectivity in the human visual cortex using FMRI. Proc 4th ISMRM, New York, p 291

Biswal B, Hudetz AG, Yetkin FZ, Haughton VM, Hyde JS (1996b) Hypercapnia reversibly diminishes low-frequency fluctuations in the human motor cortex using EPI. Proc 4th ISMRM, New York, p 1760

Biswal B, Yetkin FZ, Hyde J, Haughton VM (1996c) Functional connectivity of the auditory cortex studied with FMRI. Neuroimage 3:S305

Biswal B, Hudetz AG, Yetkin FZ, Haughton VM, Hyde JS (1997a) Hypercapnia reversibly suppresses low-frequency fluctuations in the human motor cortex during rest using echo-planar MRI. J Cereb Blood Flow Metab 17:301–308

Biswal BB, Shen H, Hudetz AG (1997b) Spatio-temporal analysis of multiple site LDF spontaneous oscillations. Proc 25th ISOTT, Milwaukee, p 106

Biswal B, Van Kylen J, Hyde JS (1997c) Simultaneous assessment of flow and BOLD signal in resting state functional connectivity maps. Proc 5th ISMRM, Vancouver, p 1643

Biswal BB, Van Kylen J, Hyde JS (1997d) Simultaneous assessment of flow and BOLD signals in resting state functional connectivity maps. NMR Biomed 10:165–170

Biswal B, Yetkin FZ, Ulmer JL, Haughton VM, Hyde JS (1997e) Detection of abnormal functional connectivity in Tourette syndrome using FMRI. Proc 5th ISMRM, Vancouver, p 733

Biswal BB, Yetkin FZ, Ulmer JL, Haughton VM, Hyde JS (1997f) Detection of abnormal task-induced signal changes in Tourette syndrome using FMRI. Neuroimage 5:308

Biswal B, Jesmanowicz A, Hyde JS (1997g) High temporal resolution FMRI. Proc 5th ISMRM, Vancouver, p 1629

Biswal B, Ulmer JL, Krippendorf RL, Harsch HH, Daniels DL, Hyde JS, Haughton VM (1998) Abnormal cerebral activation associated with a motor task in Tourette syndrome. Am J Neuroradiol 19:1509–1512

Connaughton PV, Jesmanowicz A, Froncisz W, Hyde JS (1992) Two applications of cross-correlation in MRI: image registration of CT, PET, and/or MR images of the brain. Proc 11th SMRM, Berlin, p 4219

Cooper R, Crow HJ, Walter WG, Winter WL (1966) Regional control of cerebral vascular reactivity and oxygen supply in man. Brain Res 3:174–191

Dora E, Kovach AGB (1980) Metabolic and vascular volume oscillations in the cat cerebral cortex. Acta Physiol Acad Sci Hung 57:261–275

Edelstein WA, Glover GH, Hardy CJ, Redington RW (1986) The intrinsic signal-to-noise ratio in NMR imaging. Magn Reson Med 3:604–618

Friston KJ, Frith CD, Liddle PF, Frackowiak RSJ (1993) Functional connectivity: the principle-component analysis of large (PET) data sets. J Cereb Blood Flow Metab 13:5–14

Golanov EV, Yamamoto S, Resi DJ (1994) Spontaneous waves of cerebral blood flow associated with patterns of electrocortical activity. Am J Physiol 266:R204–R214

Halsey JH Jr, McFarland S (1974) Oxygen cycles and metabolic autoregulation. Stroke 5:219–225

Hudetz AG, Roman RJ, Harder DR (1992) Spontaneous flow oscillations in the cerebral cortex during acute changes in mean arterial pressure. J Cereb Blood Flow Metab 12:491–499

Hudetz AG, Smith JJ, Lee JG, Bosnjak ZJ, Kampine JP (1995) Modification of cerebral laser-Doppler flow oscillations by halothane, PCO_2, and nitric oxide synthase. Am J Physiol 269(1 Pt 2):H114–H120

Hyde JS, Biswal B, Yetkin FZ, Haughton VM (1995) Functional connectivity determined from analysis of physiological fluctuations in a series of echo-planar images. Human Brain Mapping [Suppl] 1:287

Hyde JS, Biswal B (1997a) Analysis of physiological fluctuations in a time course of echo-planar images. Proc 5th ISMRM, Vancouver, p 352

Hyde JS, Biswal B (1997b) Basal signal fluctuations in fMRI. Proc 25th ISOTT, Milwaukee, p 101

Hyde JS, Biswal BB (1997c) Analysis of low frequency physiological fluctuation in fMRI. Neuroimage 5:478

Jesmanowicz A, Bandettini PA, Hyde JS (1998) Single-shot half k-space high resolution gradient recalled EPI for fMRI at 3 Tesla. Magn Reson Med 40:754-762

Jezzard P, LeBihan D, Cuenod C, Pannier L, Prinster A, Turner R (1993) An investigation of the contribution of physiological noise in human functional MRI studies at 1.5 Tesla and 4 Tesla. Proc 12th SMRM, New York, p 1392

Lowe MJ, Mock BJ, Sorenson JA (1996) Resting state fMRI signal correlations in multi-slice EPI. Neuroimage 3(2):S257

Lowe MJ, Davidson RJ, Orendi J (1997a) Intra-hemispheric functional connectivity of fMRI physiological noise correlations: dependence on attention. Proc 5th ISMRM, Vancouver, p 1688

Lowe MJ, Rutecki P, Turski P, Woodard A, Sorenson J (1997b) Auditory cortex fMRI noise correlations in callosal agenesis. Neuroimage 5(2):S194

Lowe MJ, Mock BJ, Sorenson JA (1998) Functional connectivity in single and multislice echoplanar imaging using resting state fluctuations. Neuroimage 7:119–132

Menon RS, Ogawa S, Tank DW, Utmurbil K (1993) 4 Tesla gradient recalled echo characteristics of photic stimulation-induced signal changes in the human primary visual cortex. Magn Reson Med 30:380–386

Moskalenko YE (1980) Biophysical aspects of cerebral circulation. Pergamon, Oxford

Ogawa S, Tank DW, Menon R, Ellermann JM, Kim SG, Merkle H, Ugurbil K (1992) Functional brain mapping using MRI: intrinsic signal changes accompanying sensory stimulations. Proc 11th SMRM, Berlin, p 303

Skudlarski P, Gore JC (1998) Changes in the correlations in the fMRI physiological fluctuations may reveal functional connectivity within the brain. Neuroimage 7:S37

Stern E, Silbersweig DA, Chee K-Y, Frith CD, Frackowiak RSJ, Dolan RJ (1996) A functional neuroanatomy of involuntary action in Tourette's syndrome. Neuroimage 3:S600

Vern BA, Schuette WH, Leheta B, Juel VC, Radulovacki M (1988) Low-frequency oscillations of cortical oxidative metabolism in waking and sleep. J Cereb Blood Flow Metab 8:215–226

Vern BA, Leheta BJ, Juel VC, LaGuardia J, Graupe P, Schuette WH (1997) Slow oscillations of cytochrome oxidase redox state and blood volume in unanesthetized cat and rabbit cortex: interhemispheric synchrony. Proc 25th ISOTT, Milwaukee, p 103

Weisskoff RM, Baker J, Belliveau J, Davis TL, Kwong KK, Cohen MS, Rosen BR (1993) Power spectrum analysis of functionally-weighted MR data: what's in the noise? Proc 12th SMRM, New York, p 7

Wong EC, Bandettini PA, Hyde JS (1992a) Echo-planar imaging of the human brain using a three axis local gradient coil. Proc 11th SMRM, Berlin, p 105

Wong EC, Boskamp E, Hyde JS (1992b) A volume optimized quadrature elliptical endcap birdcage brain coil. Proc 11th SMRM, Berlin, p 4015

Wong EC, Tan G, Hyde JS (1993) A quadrature transmit-receive endcapped birdcage coil for imaging of the human head at 125 MHz. Proc 12th SMRM, New York, p 1344

Xiong J, Parson LM, Pu Y, Gao J-H, Fox PT (1998a) Improved interregional connectivity mapping by use of covariance analysis within rest condition. Proc 6th ISMRM, Sydney, p 1480

Xiong J, Parsons LM, Pu Y, Gao J-H, Fox PT (1998b) Covarying activity during rest reveals improved connectivity maps. Neuroimage 7:S771

25 Field Strength Dependence of Functional MRI Signals

J.S. Gati, R.S. Menon, B.K. Rutt

CONTENTS

25.1 Introduction

The strength of the main magnetic field (B_0) is an important factor in determining the magnitude of blood oxygenation level-dependent (BOLD)-based (Ogawa et al. 1990a) functional MRI signal changes. The BOLD technique involves complex changes in regional cerebral blood volume, blood flow and deoxyhemoglobin levels, associated with neuronal activation, that result in altered signal intensity in T_2^* or T_2 weighted MR images within anatomically distinct regions during motor, sensory or cognitive function (Ogawa et al. 1990b; Kwong et al. 1992). This is due to the fact that the bulk magnetic susceptibility difference between blood containing paramagnetic deoxyhemoglobin and surrounding diamagnetic tissue increases with main magnetic field strength, creating larger MR signal changes between baseline and activated states. The BOLD signal responses in large venous vessels and cortical gray matter (cGM) capillaries have been theorized to be field-dependent to different degrees. Ogawa et al. (1993) have shown, using numerical modeling tech-

niques, that the contribution to the apparent transverse relaxation rate (R_2^*) due to the BOLD effect is proportional to B_0 for large vessels (venules and veins; d>10 μm) and to B_0^2 for small vessels (capillaries; d<10 μm). Attempts to experimentally quantify these BOLD field dependencies have been made using low-resolution echo planar imaging (EPI) or fast low angle shot (FLASH) (Turner et al. 1993; McKenzie et al. 1994; Bandettini et al. 1994). However, separation of voxels containing large venous vessels from those containing primarily venules and smaller vessels was not attempted in these studies, because of the low in-plane resolution. Large vessels contribute to a significant blood volume fraction and thus to the majority of the signal change within each voxel (Lai et al. 1993; Menon et al. 1993; Segebarth et al. 1994). Therefore, the large vessel BOLD field dependence will dominate in studies which do not exclude voxels containing larger vessels. The small vessel BOLD response, however, is important to characterize since it is this effect which will presumably indicate local neuronal activity.

The optimal field strength for performing BOLD-based fMRI experiments has been a matter of some debate (Cohen and Bookheimer 1994; Kwong 1995; Menon et al. 1995). More importantly, field strength dependence is central to mechanistic considerations of the BOLD effect. This chapter will examine the BOLD field dependence in two categories: (1) those that contain venous vessels of diameter equal to or greater than the voxel, and (2) those that contain a mixture of capillaries, venules and small veins with diameters less than the voxel itself. These field dependencies are presented from high resolution experiments (Gati et al. 1997) on human volunteers over widely varying field strengths (0.5T–4.0 T). A robust photic stimulation paradigm was used to induce brain activation within the area of the primary visual cortex (V1). The study was conducted in two parts. In the first part, single-echo gradient echo images were acquired with a FLASH pulse sequence using an echo time approximately equal to the T_2^* of gray matter at each field strength. Relative func-

J.S. Gati, MSc; R.S. Menon, PhD; B.K. Rutt, PhD; The Laboratory for Functional Magnetic Resonance, John P. Roberts Research Institute, PO Box 5015, 100 Perth Drive, London, Ontario, Canada N6A 5K8

tional signal changes (ΔS/S) were measured within regions of activated visible veins ("vessels") and cortical gray matter ("tissue"), and used to estimate the field dependence of ΔR_2^*, the change between activated and baseline states. In the second part, multi-echo gradient echo images were acquired using the same visual stimulation paradigm. Values for the apparent transverse relaxation rate (R_2^*) were measured in the vessel and tissue regions and compared as a function of field strength. We measured both ΔR_2^* and R_2^* vs B_0, since the ratio of ΔR_2^* to R_2^* is a fundamental quantity in determining the ultimate sensitivity, functional contrast-to-noise ratio and optimal field strength for BOLD experiments.

25.2
Imaging Considerations

25.2.1
In-Flow Suppression

Neuronal activation alters the vascular physiology leading to increased flow, both in the resistance pial arteries which feed the activated capillary beds (IADECOLA 1993) and in the venules which drain these beds. The MRI signal is inherently sensitive to in-flowing fully magnetized spins, so the hemodynamic changes, especially in larger arterial and venous vessels, can create signal fluctuations coincident with neuronal activation due to this in-flow effect. The in-flow effect is usually considered to be an undesirable contribution to the fMRI signal response, since it can produce large signal changes in regions remote from the actual site of neuronal activity. The in-flow effect can be eliminated by utilizing low flip

angles, centrically ordered k-space trajectories and inter-image delays (MENON et al. 1993; FRAHM et al. 1994). The intercept at TE=0, according to the line of best fit, in the signal decay vs TE curves in Fig. 25.1 indicate that there are no activation-induced changes in signal due to the in-flow effect since the activated signal at TE=0[S_0(activated)]=the baseline signal at TE=0[S_0(baseline)] at the field strengths shown. The effectiveness of this flow-suppression technique is due to the fact that tissue longitudinal magnetization is allowed to recover nearly completely prior to each collection of the center of k-space. With no magnetization saturation, there can be no in-flow enhancement.

25.2.2
Optimal Echo Time

It has been shown experimentally (GATI et al. 1997) that if the MRI signal decays mono-exponentially with TE in an experiment, and in-flow effects are negligible, the maximum signal difference between the activated and baseline states will occur when the echo time is equal to the apparent baseline transverse relaxation (TE=T_{2b}^*). These data confirm earlier predictions (MENON et al. 1993) that tissue BOLD signal changes are maximized by operating at the optimal TE at each field strength.

25.3
Fractional BOLD Signal Change

This section is intended to illustrate the field strength dependence of the BOLD signal response during cortical activation specifically within voxels containing large vessels and those which contain small vessels. With sufficiently high resolution it is possible to separately delineate and evaluate the signal response within regions of cortical gray matter and venous vasculature. The functional maps shown in Fig. 25.2 from a robust visual stimulus paradigm are found to be anatomically consistent with previous PET (Fox et al. 1987) and fMRI (BELLIVEAU et al. 1991; MENON et al. 1992) experiments during full-field visual stimulation of the human striate cortex. The average percentage signal change observed at the optimal echo time in vessel regions is large (13.3±2.3%, 18.4±4.0% and 15.1±1.2%) compared to that in tissue (1.4±0.7%, 1.9±0.7% and 3.3±0.2%) at 0.5 T, 1.5 T and 4 T, respectively.

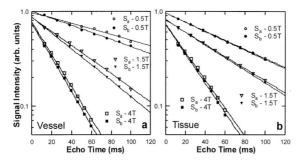

Fig. 25.1a, b. Signal decay within regions of vessel (**a**) and tissue (**b**) at each field during activated (*Sa*) and baseline (*Sb*) states. The lines indicate the best linear fit to each curve assuming a mono-exponential decay with T2*. The extrapolated line in each case intercepts so that Sa=Sb in both the vessel and tissue plots, indicating negligible in-flow effects

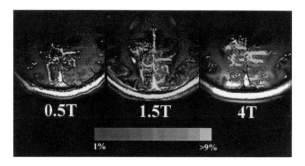

Fig. 25.2. Axial-oblique images through the primary visual cortex showing function during a simple visual paradigm (described in text). Color activation maps represent percent signal change and overlayed onto high resolution snapshot FLASH T1-weighted anatomical images, for reference, which were acquired during the same experimental session. Function was assessed using a Student's paired *t* test (p<0.01)

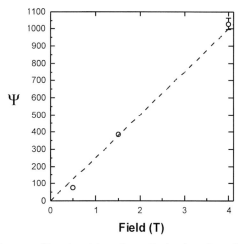

Fig. 25.3. The signal-to-noise ratio is plotted vs the field strength in the BOLD functional images. Signal was measured as the mean signal intensity of a region of interest (ROI) within the region of analysis in the primary visual cortex. Noise was measured as the average signal in a ROI outside the head in air

25.4
Intrinsic BOLD Parameters

25.4.1
Signal-to-Noise Ratio (Ψ)

The signal-to-noise ratio can be measured in fully relaxed, proton density-weighted gradient echo images (TR>5T_1, α=90°). This image signal intensity can then be extrapolated to TE=0(S_0) using experimental measures of T_2^* to estimate the fully relaxed BOLD signal-to-noise ratio (Ψ). One of the main advantages of imaging at higher fields is the increase in the intrinsic signal-to-noise ratio that is predicted and observed to be linear with field (Edelstein et al. 1986; Hoult et al. 1976) for human NMR imaging experiments. This linear relationship is typically true, assuming the RF coil geometry, quality factor (Q), imaging parameters and sample geometry are held constant. The measured Ψ obtained from fully relaxed images is found to increase linearly with field (Fig. 25.3) and indicates that a linear field dependence for Ψ is a good assumption with regard to predictions of the upper bound on BOLD contrast-to-noise ratio.

25.4.2
R$_2$* Contrast ($\Delta R_2^*/R_2^*$)

The signal difference between the activated and baseline states in a fully relaxed BOLD experiment can be given by:

$$\Delta S = S_0 \cdot \left\{ \exp\left(-TE \cdot R_{2b}^*\right) \cdot \left[\exp\left(-TE \cdot \Delta R_2^*\right) - 1 \right] \right\} \quad (25.1)$$

where S_0 is the fully relaxed signal at TE=0 and R_{2b}^* is the apparent transverse relaxation rate in the baseline state. This expression is true assuming the differential in-flow effects are suppressed and the signal in each state decays mono-exponentially with TE. From BOLD images the fractional signal change ($\Delta S/S$) can be measured, and therefore the apparent transverse relaxation rate (ΔR_2^*) can be given by:

$$\Delta R_2^* \approx -\frac{\Delta S / S}{TE} \quad (25.2)$$

This is an excellent approximation, from Eq. (25.1), if TE$\cdot\Delta R_2^* <<$1, which is always true in BOLD experiments, and if in-flow suppression is effective.

In considering the field dependence of the R_2^* contrast term ($\Delta R_2^*/R_2^*$), it is useful to consider separately the field dependence of ΔR_2^* and R_2^*. We have shown that the vessel baseline relaxation rate, R_{2vb}^*, follows a hyper-linear field strength dependence up to 4 T according to the following fit to experimental data shown in Fig. 25.4a:

$$R_{2vb}^* = 1.27 B_0^2 + 5.46 B_0 + 7.25 \quad (25.3)$$

In a quadratic fit, the linear term dominates at 0.5 T and 1.5 T, while the linear and quadratic terms contribute equally to the total R_{2vb}^* at 4 T. The tissue baseline relaxation rate, R_{2tb}^*, also shows a hyper-linear field dependence (Fig. 25.4a) according to:

$$R_{2tb}^* = 1.09 B_0^2 + 0.81 B_0 + 10.72 \qquad (25.4)$$

In the quadratic fit to this data, the linear and quadratic terms contribute approximately equally between 0.5 T and 1.5 T, while the quadratic term dominates at 4 T. The significance of these responses and the interpretation of the quadratic vs linear components of the fitted field strength relationships are not clear. There are other underlying biophysical mechanisms, besides the BOLD effect, determining these R_{2vb}^* and R_{2tb}^* field strength relationships. Extrapolating the tissue R_{2tb}^* quadratic fit to zero field, we find $R_{2tb}^*(B_0=0)=10.72\,s^{-1}$, a value which is 11% greater than the measured intrinsic T_2 relaxation rate for gray matter, $R_2=9.64\,s^{-1}$ (OGAWA et al. 1993).

Now, in considering the ΔR_2^* response with field we notice that the tissue signal demonstrates a consistently smaller magnitude than that in vessel, by a factor of five to ten over the 0.5–4 T field strength range (Fig. 25.4b). This is consistent with the observation that BOLD signal changes can be dominated by large vessel effects, unless care is taken to exclude these large vessel effects (HAACKE et al. 1994). Quadratic fits to the experimental data yield the following:

$$-\Delta R_{2v}^* = -0.33 B_0^2 + 2.61 B_0 \qquad (25.5)$$

$$-\Delta R_{2t}^* = 0.016 B_0^2 + 0.206 B_0$$

It can be seen that the linear term of the tissue ΔR_2^* response dominates at 0.5 T and 1.5 T, accounting for 90% or more of the total ΔR_2^*. On the other hand, at 4 T the quadratic term contributes a significant fraction, approximately 30% to the total ΔR_2^*. This finding is consistent with Ogawa's model for BOLD-specific relaxation rate, which predicts a linear response with field for vessels larger than 10 μm, and a quadratic response for capillaries. Given the inevitable mixture of venules/veins (up to ~0.5 mm) and capillaries in these tissue voxels, we expect a mixture of linear and quadratic contributions in the measured tissue response (OGAWA et al. 1993). With higher resolution voxels, it may be possible to further increase the relative proportion of non-capillary vasculature in the vessel voxels and capillaries in the tissue voxels, in which case we would expect cleaner separation of the linear from quadratic terms of the BOLD field dependence.

The vessel ΔR_2^* magnitude increases with field strength somewhat less than linearly over the 0.5–4 T range. An experimental finding of $\Delta R_2^*=-3.1\pm0.3\,s^{-1}$ in vessel voxels at 1.5 T agrees well with values predicted theoretically (YABLONSKIY and HAACKE 1994, Eq. (22), $\Delta R_2^*=-3.4\,s^{-1}$; BOXERMAN et al. 1995, $\Delta R_2^*=-3.5\,s^{-1}$) for randomly oriented cylindrical vessels of diameter greater than 10 μm. Previous experimental findings (TURNER et al. 1993; BANDETTINI et al. 1994; MCKENZIE et al. 1994) can also be compared to these field strength results. Turner's measurements at 1.5 T and 4 T show a hyper-linear ΔR_2^* field strength dependence, while those of BANDETTINI and MACKENZIE show approximately linear field strength dependence. The measured values of ΔR_2^* in all of these experiments fall between our measures of ΔR_2^* in vessel and tissue regions except for Turner's 4 T result, which is slightly greater than our vessel value. These previous experimental studies all employed lower image resolution than ours and therefore did not allow for the same delineation of vessel from tissue voxels. Because of this, there is likely a larger mixing of the large and small vessel ΔR_2^* responses in each of the measured voxels compared to our study. Thus, high resolution experiments are better able to delineate the upper and lower bounds for BOLD-based ΔR_2^* due to functional stimulation of the human brain.

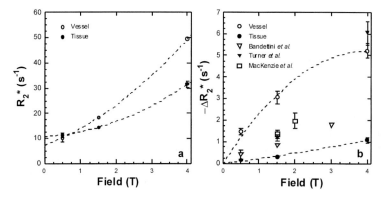

Fig. 25.4a, b. Apparent relaxation rates for vessel and tissue (a) at three field strengths measured during the resting state of the multi-echo BOLD experiments. The change in R_2^* (b) is measured the fractional signal change in the single-echo BOLD experiments normalized by the echo time that they were acquired at. *Error bars* represent the standard error for the measurements at each field. The data presented have been age matched

Our data indicate that tissue R_2^* contrast ($\Delta R_2^*/R_2^*$) increases monotonically with field strength, at least up to 4 T. By contrast, vessel R_2^* contrast increases between 0.5 T and 1.5 T but falls below the 1.5 T value at 4 T. It is clear that R_2^* contrast depends in a complex way on tissue type. Given the desirability of vessel BOLD response for accurate localization of brain function, the "relevant" (i.e., tissue) R_2^* contrast behavior in the relevant clinical range (1.5–4 T) can be described as weakly increasing with field strength.

25.4.3
Contrast-to-Noise Ratio (ΔS/N)

The sensitivity and accuracy of BOLD-based fMRI experiments are ultimately determined by the functional contrast-to-noise ratio (ΔS/N) between activated and baseline states, and this quantity has been hypothesized theoretically and also shown experimentally to depend on field strength. The measured Ψ, R_{2b}^* and ΔR_2^* can be used to estimate the maximal functional contrast-to-noise ratio (ΔS/N) field strength dependence for fully relaxed BOLD imaging. The "noise" term (N) in this ratio includes contributions from random noise, instrument instabilities and physiological fluctuations. The upper bound of ΔS/N can be obtained from experimental data if we assume the noise term is dominated by random (thermal) noise and TE»TE$_{opt}$. Under these conditions, $S_0/N\approx\Psi\exp(1)$, and the maximum available BOLD ΔS/N can be estimated from Eq. (25.1) as:

$$\left.\frac{\Delta S}{N}\right|_{max} = \Psi \cdot \frac{\Delta R_2^*}{R_{2b}^*} \qquad (25.6)$$

From the experimental measures of Ψ, ΔR_2^* and R_2^* we predict the field dependence for the maximum available BOLD ΔS/N in vessel to be less than the linear field dependence, while the tissue response is clearly greater than linear (Fig. 25.5). The strongly increasing field strength dependence of this maximal BOLD contrast-to-noise ratio, particularly for tissue, obviously depends to a large extent on the Ψ field strength response (since in both vessel and tissue cases, the R_2^* contrast term is not strongly increasing with B_0). In our experiments we have made an estimate for the maximal ΔS/N based upon the assumption that thermal noise will ultimately dominate the noise term and that magnetization is fully relaxed. In fact we know that "physiological" noise dominates in all present-day BOLD fMRI experiments (WEISKOFF

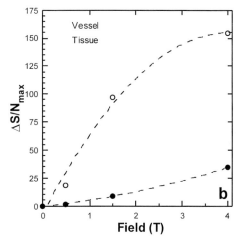

Fig. 25.5. The maximal DS/N is plotted vs field based upon the calculation from Eq. 25.6 based upon the experimental measures of R_2^*, ΔR_2^* and Ψ_{BOLD} (for further details, see text)

et al. 1993; JEZZARD et al. 1993; BISWAL et al. 1995). The degree to which this physiological noise dominates will depend upon the imaging system stability, volunteer stability (motion) and the specific image acquisition techniques. With further understanding of the sources of physiological noise, and further development of imaging systems, motion correction schemes and fast acquisition techniques, it is conceivable that the physiological noise contributions will be reduced to the range of thermal noise, or at least to the stage that the ratio of signal to total noise scales linearly with B_0. In this limit, then, the experimental data reported in this chapter would predict a strong BOLD contrast-to-noise advantage of operating at the highest available magnetic field strength, particularly for fMRI studies which require the highest spatial and/or temporal resolution.

References

Bandettini PA, Wong EC, Jesmanowicz A, Prost R, Cox RW, Hinks RS, Hyde JS (1994) MRI of human brain activation at 0.5 T, 1.5 T and 3.0 T: Comparisons of ΔR_2^* and functional contrast to noise ratio. In: Proc SMR 2nd Annu Meeting, San Francisco, p. 434

Belliveau JW, Kennedy DN, McKinstry RC et al (1991) Functional mapping of the human visual cortex by magnetic resonance imaging. Science 254:716–719

Biswal B, Yetkin FZ, Haughton VM, Hyde JS (1995) Functional connectivity of the resting human brain using echo-planar MRI. In: Proc SMR 3rd Annu Meeting, Nice, p. 400

Boxerman JL, Hamberg LM, Rosen BR, Weiskoff RM (1995) MR contrast due to intravascular magnetic susceptibility perturbations. Magn Res Med 34:555–566

Cohen MS, Bookheimer SY (1994) Localization of brain function using magnetic resonance imaging. Trends Neurosci 17:268–277

Edelstein WA, Glover GH, Hardy CJ, Redington RW (1986) The intrinsic signal-to-noise ratio in NMR imaging. Magn Res Med 3:604–618

Fox PT, Miezen FM, Allman JM, Van Essen DC, Raichle ME (1987) Retinotopic organization of human visual cortex mapped with positron-emission tomography. J Neurosci 7:913–922

Frahm J, Merboldt K-D, Hanicke W, Kleinschmidt A, Boecker H (1994) Brain or vein - oxygenation or flow? On signal physiology in functional MRI of human brain activation. NMR Biomed 7:45–53

Gati JS, Menon RS, Ugurbil K, Rutt BK (1997) Experimental determination of the BOLD field strength dependence in vessels and tissue. Magn Res Med 38:296–302

Haacke EM, Hopkins A, Lai S et al (1994) 2D and 3D high resolution gradient echo functional imaging of the brain: venous contributions to signal in motor cortex studies. NMR Biomed 7:54–62

Hoult DI, Richards RE (1976) The signal-to-noise ratio of the nuclear magnetic resonance experiment. J Magn Res 24:71–85

Hoult DI, Chen C-N, Sank VJ (1966) The field dependence of NMR imaging. II. Arguments concerning an optimal field strength. Magn Res Med 3:730–746

Iadecola C (1993) Regulation of the cerebral microcirculation during neural activity: is nitric oxide the missing link? Trends Neurosci 16:206–214

Jezzard P, LeBihan D, Cuenod C, Pannier L, Prinster A, Turner R (1993) An investigation of the contribution of physiological noise in human functional MRI studies at 1.5 Tesla and 4 Tesla. In: Proc SMRM 12th Annu Meeting, New York, p. 1392

Kwong KK (1995) Functional magnetic resonance imaging with echo planar imaging. Magn Res Q 11:1–20

Kwong KK, Belliveau JW, Chesler DA et al (1992) Dynamic magnetic resonance imaging of human brain activity during primary sensory stimulation. Proc Natl Acad Sci USA 89:5675–5679

Lai S, Hopkins A, Haacke E et al (1993) Identification of vascular structures as a major source of signal contrast in high resolution 2D and 3D functional activation imaging of the motor cortex at 1.5 T: preliminary results. Magn Reson Med 30:387–392

McKenzie CA, Drost DJ, Carr TJ (1994) The effect of magnetic field strength on signal change ΔS/S in functional MRI with BOLD contrast. In: Proc SMR 2nd Annu Meeting, San Francisco, p. 433

Menon RS, Ogawa S, Kim S-G, Ellermann JM, Merkle H, Tank DW, Ugurbil K (1992) Functional brain mapping using magnetic resonance imaging: signal changes accompanying visual stimulation. Invest Radiol 27:S47–S53

Menon RS, Ogawa S, Tank DW, Ugurbil K (1993) 4 Tesla gradient recalled echo characteristics of photic stimulation induced signal changes in the primary visual cortex. Magn Res Med 30:380–386

Menon RS, Ogawa S, Hu X, Strupp JP, Anderson P, Ugurbil K (1995) BOLD based functional MRI at 4 Tesla includes capillary bed contribution: echo-planar imaging correlates with previous optical imaging using intrinsic signals. Magn Res Med 33:453–459

Ogawa S, Lee T-M, Kay AR, Tank DW (1990a) Brain magnetic resonance imaging with contrast dependent on blood oxygenation. Proc Natl Acad Sci USA 87:9868–9872

Ogawa S, Lee T-M, Nayak AS, Glynn P (1990b) Oxygenation-sensitive contrast in magnetic resonance image of rodent brain at high magnetic fields. Magn Res Med 14:68–78

Ogawa S, Menon RS, Tank DW, Kim S-G, Merkle H, Ellerman JM, Ugurbil K (1993) Functional brain mapping by blood oxygenation level-dependent contrast magnetic resonance imaging. A comparison of signal characteristics with a biophysical model. Biophys J 64:803–812

Segebarth C, Belle V, Delon C et al (1994) Functional MRI of the human brain: predominance of signals from extracerebral veins. Neuroreport 5:813–816

Turner R, Jezzard P, Wen PH, Kwong KK, LeBihan, Zeffiro T, Balaban RS (1993) Functional mapping of the human visual cortex at 4 and 1.5 tesla using deoxygenation contrast EPI. Magn Reson Med 29:277–279

Weisskoff RM, Baker J, Belliveau J, Davis TL, Kwong KK, Cohen MS, Rosen BR (1993) Power spectrum analysis of functionally-weighted MR data: what's in the noise. In: Proc SMRM 12th Annu Meeting, New York, p. 7

Yablonsky DA, Haacke EM (1994) Theory of NMR signal behaviour in magnetically inhomogeneous tissues: the static dephasing regime. Magn Res Med 32:749–763

Data Processing
and Practical Issues

26 Image Registration

J. Ashburner and K.J. Friston

CONTENTS

26.1 Introduction

Image registration is important in many aspects of functional image analysis. In imaging neuroscience, particularly for functional magnetic resonance imaging (fMRI), the signal changes due to any hemodynamic response can be small compared to signal changes that can result from subject motion, so prior to performing any statistical tests, it is important that the images are aligned as closely as possible. Subject head movement in the scanner cannot be completely eliminated, so motion correction needs to be performed as a preprocessing step on the image data. The first step in the correction is image registration, which involves determining the parameter values for a rigid body transformation that optimize some criteria for matching each image with a reference image (see Sect. 26.3). Following this registration, the images are transformed by resampling according to the determined parameters.

J. Ashburner; K.J. Friston, MD; The Wellcome Department of Cognitive Neurology, Institute of Neurology, 12 Queen Square, London WC1N 3BG, England

Sometimes it is desirable to warp images from a number of individuals into roughly the same standard space to allow signal averaging across subjects. Because different people may have different strategies for performing tasks in the scanner, spatial normalization of the images is useful for determining what happens generically over individuals. A further advantage of using spatially normalized images is that activation sites can be reported according to their Euclidian coordinates within a standard space (Fox 1995). The most commonly adopted coordinate system within the brain imaging community is that described by Talairach and Tournoux (1988). The spatial normalization usually begins by matching the brains to a template image using an affine transformation (see Sect. 5.3), followed by introducing nonlinear deformations described by a number of smooth basis functions (Friston et al. 1995) (see Sect. 26.5.4). Matching is only possible on a coarse scale, since there is not necessarily a one-to-one mapping of the cortical structures between different brains. Because of this, the images are smoothed prior to the statistical analysis in a multi-subject study, so that corresponding sites of activation from the different brains are superimposed.

For studies of a single subject, the sites of activation can be accurately localized by superimposing them on a high resolution structural image of the subject (typically a T_1-weighted MRI). This requires the registration of the functional images with the structural image. As in the case of movement correction, this is normally performed by optimizing a set of parameters describing a rigid body transformation, but the matching criterion needs to be more complex since the images are often acquired using different modalities or MR contrasts (see Sect. 26.4). A further use for this registration is that a more precise spatial normalization can be achieved by computing it using a more detailed structural image. With the functional and structural images in register, the computed warps can be applied to the functional images.

The sections in this chapter are arranged as follows: "Basic Principles" gives a brief introduction to some of the concepts that are used throughout the rest of the chapter. In order to register images, it is necessary to describe the required spatial transformations by a set of parameters. Spatially transforming an image, involves resampling it according to the parameters describing the transformation. The subsection on "Resampling Images" describes a number of different interpolation methods that can be used for this.

This chapter will concentrate upon automatic methods of estimating the parameters describing the transformations. A method of "Optimization" is necessary for automatically determining the best parameters for matching images together. The optimization framework that is used throughout the rest of the chapter is introduced in this subsection.

"Within Modality Image Coregistration" is probably the simplest form of image registration. It involves finding the best six-parameter rigid body transformation to minimize the difference between two images of the same subject.

"Between Modality Image Coregistration" again involves rigid body transformations, but in this case – since the images to be matched appear completely different – different matching strategies need to be used.

"Spatial Normalization" describes the steps involved in registering images of different subjects into roughly the same coordinate system. The spatial normalization begins by matching the brains to a template image by using an affine transformation. Unlike the previous two sections – where the images to be matched together are from the same subject – zooms and shears are needed to register heads of different shapes and sizes. Following the affine registration, gross differences in head shapes, which cannot be accounted for by affine normalization alone, are corrected by a nonlinear spatial normalization step. These nonlinear warps are modeled by linear combinations of smooth basis functions.

26.2
Basic Principles

For every image registration, the spatial transformation should be described by a set of parameters. For rigid body registration, the parameters are typically three orthogonal translations and three rotations. The parameters for the spatial normalization ap-

proach described in this chapter are twelve parameters describing an affine transformation and a number of coefficients for nonlinear basis functions describing nonlinear transformations. There are two steps involved in registering images together. There is the registration itself, whereby the parameters describing a transformation are determined. Then there is the transformation, in which one of the images is transformed according to the set of parameters. This section will touch first on how the images are transformed via the process of resampling, and then the general principal of how the parameters describing the transformations are determined automatically.

26.2.1
Resampling Images

Once there is a mapping between the original and transformed coordinates of an image, it is necessary to resample the image in order to apply the spatial transform.

Spatially transforming images is usually implemented as a "pulling" operation (in which pixel values are pulled from the original image into their new location) rather than a "pushing" one (in which the pixels in the original image are pushed into their new location). This involves determining for each voxel in the transformed image, the corresponding intensity in the original image. Usually, this requires sampling between the centers of voxels, so some form of interpolation is needed.

The simplest approach is to take the value of the closest neighboring voxel. This is referred to as nearest neighbor or zero-order hold resampling. This has the advantage that the original voxel intensities are preserved, but the resulting image can be degraded quite considerably.

Another approach is to use trilinear interpolation (first-order hold) to resample the data. This is slightly slower than nearest neighbor, but the resulting images have a less "blocky" appearance. However, trilinear interpolation has the effect of losing some high frequency information from the image.

Figure 26.1 will be used to illustrate bilinear interpolation in two dimensions. Assume that there is a regular grid of pixels at coordinates x_a, y_a to x_p, y_p, having intensities v_a to v_p, and that the point to resample is at t. The value at points r and s are first determined (using linear interpolation) as follows:

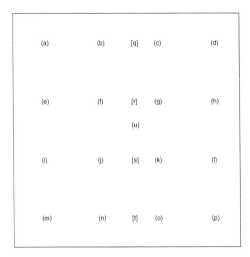

Fig. 26.1. Illustration of image interpolation in two dimensions. Points *a* through to *p* represent the original regular grid of pixels. Point *u* is the point whose value is to be determined. Points *q* to *t* are used as intermediates in the computation

$$v_r = \frac{(x_g - x_r)v_f + (x_r - x_f)v_g}{x_g - x_f} \qquad (26.1)$$

$$v_s = \frac{(x_k - x_s)v_j + (x_s - x_j)v_k}{x_k - x_j} \qquad (26.2)$$

Then v_u is determined by interpolating between v_r and v_s:

$$v_u = \frac{(y_u - y_s)v_r + (y_r - y_u)v_s}{y_r - y_s} \qquad (26.3)$$

The extension of the approach to three dimensions is trivial. Rather than using only the eight nearest neighbors (in 3D) to estimate the value at a point, more neighbors can be used in order to fit a smooth function through the points, and then read off the value of the function at the desired location. Polynomial interpolation is one such approach (zero-order and first-order hold interpolation are simply low order polynomial interpolations). We now illustrate how v_q can be determined from pixels *a–d*. The coefficients (q) of a polynomial that runs through these points can be obtained by computing:

$$q = \begin{pmatrix} 1 & 0 & 0 & 0 \\ 1 & (x_b - x_a) & (x_b - x_a)^2 & (x_b - x_a)^3 \\ 1 & (x_c - x_a) & (x_c - x_a)^2 & (x_c - x_a)^3 \\ 1 & (x_d - x_a) & (x_d - x_a)^2 & (x_d - x_a)^3 \end{pmatrix}^{-1} \begin{pmatrix} v_a \\ v_b \\ v_c \\ v_d \end{pmatrix}$$
$$(26.4)$$

Then v_q can be determined from these coefficients by:

$$v_q = (1 \ (x_q - x_a) \ (x_q - x_a)^2 \ (x_q - x_a)^3)q \qquad (26.5)$$

To determine v_u, a similar polynomial would be fitted through points *q*, *r*, *s* and *t*. Polynomial interpolation is normally performed using Lagrange polynomials. See PRESS et al. (1992) or JAIN (1989) for more information on this or on interpolation in general.

The optimum method of applying rigid body transformations to images with minimal interpolation artifact is to do it in Fourier space (EDDY et al. 1996). In real space, the interpolation method that gives results closest to a Fourier interpolation is sinc interpolation. To perform a pure sinc interpolation, every voxel in the image should be used to sample a single point. This is not feasible due to speed considerations, so an approximation using a limited number of nearest neighbors is used. Because the sinc function extends to infinity, it is truncated by modulating with a Hanning window (Fig. 26.2). The implementation of sinc interpolation is similar to that for polynomial interpolation, in that it is performed sequentially in the three dimensions of the volume. For one dimension the windowed sinc function using the *I* nearest neighbors would be:

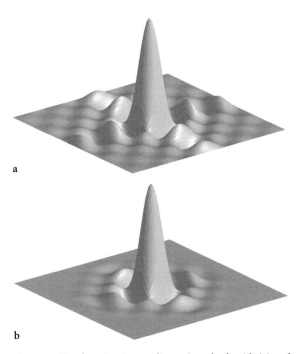

Fig. 26.2. Sinc function in two dimensions, both with (**a**) and without (**b**) a Hanning window

$$\sum_{i=1}^{I} v_i \frac{\dfrac{\sin(\pi d_i)}{\pi d_i}\dfrac{1}{2}(1+\cos{(2\pi d_i \,/\, I)})}{\sum_{j=1}^{I}\dfrac{\sin(\pi d_j)}{\pi d_j}\dfrac{1}{2}(1+\cos{(2\pi d_j \,/\, I)})} \qquad (26.6)$$

where d_i is the distance from the center of the ith voxel to the point to be sampled, and v_i is the value of the ith voxel. Sinc interpolation is slow when many neighboring voxels are used. A slightly better alternative is to use Fourier interpolation for effecting a rigid body transformation. In one dimension, a translation is simply a convolution with a translated delta function. For translations that are not whole numbers of pixels, the delta function is replaced by a sinc function centered at the translation distance. The use of fast Fourier transforms means that the convolution can be performed most rapidly as a multiplication in Fourier space. It is clear how translations can be performed in this way, but rotations are less obvious. One way that rotations can be done involves replacing each rotation by three sheers. For a simple two-dimensional case, a matrix encoding a rotation of q radians about the origin (see Sect. 26.3) can be constructed by multiplying together three matrices that effect shears:

$$\begin{pmatrix} \cos(\theta) & \sin(\theta) & 0 \\ -\sin(\theta) & \cos(\theta) & 0 \\ 0 & 0 & 1 \end{pmatrix} \equiv \begin{pmatrix} 1 & \tan(\theta/2) & 0 \\ 0 & 1 & 0 \\ 0 & 0 & 1 \end{pmatrix}\begin{pmatrix} 1 & 0 & 0 \\ \sin(\theta) & 1 & 0 \\ 0 & 0 & 1 \end{pmatrix}\begin{pmatrix} 1 & \tan(\theta/2) & 0 \\ 0 & 1* & 0 \\ 0 & 0 & 1 \end{pmatrix}$$
$$(26.7)$$

A shear simply involves translating different rows or columns of an image by different amounts, so each shear can be performed by a series of one dimensional convolutions in Fourier space. For more information on this approach, see EDDY et al. (1996).

26.2.2
Optimization

The objective of optimization is to determine the values for a set of parameters for which some function of the parameters is minimized (or maximized). One of the simplest cases is determining the optimum parameters for a model in order to minimize the sum of squared differences between the model and a set of real world data (χ^2). Usually there are many parameters in the model, and it is not possible to exhaustively search through the whole parameter space. The usual approach is to make an initial pa-

rameter estimate and begin iteratively searching from there. At each iteration, the model is evaluated using the current estimates, and χ^2 computed. A judgment is then made about how the parameters should be modified, before continuing on to the next iteration. The optimization is terminated when some convergence criterion is achieved (usually when χ^2 stops decreasing).

The image registration approach described here is essentially an optimization. One image (the object image) is spatially transformed so that it matches another (the template image), by minimizing χ^2. The parameters that are optimized are those that describe the spatial transformation (although there are often other nuisance parameters required by the model, such as intensity scaling parameters). The algorithm of choice (FRISTON et al. 1995) is one that is similar to Gauss-Newton optimization (see PRESS et al. 1992, Sect. 15.5, for a fuller explanation of the approach), and it is illustrated here:

Suppose that $e_i(\mathbf{p})$ is the function describing the difference between the object and template images at voxel i, when the vector of model parameters have values $\mathbf{p}$. For each voxel (i), a first approximation of Taylor's Theorem can be used to estimate the value that this difference will take if the parameters $\mathbf{p}$ are increased by $\mathbf{t}$:

$$e_i(\mathbf{p}+\mathbf{t}) \cong e_i(\mathbf{p}) + t_1\frac{\partial e_i(\mathbf{p})}{\partial p_1} + t_2\frac{\partial e_i(\mathbf{p})}{\partial p_2}\cdots \qquad (26.8)$$

This allows the construction of a set of simultaneous equations (of the form $\mathbf{Ax}\cong\mathbf{e}$) for estimating the values that t should assume to in order to minimize $\sum_i(\mathbf{p}+\mathbf{t})^2$:

$$\begin{pmatrix} \dfrac{\partial e_1(\mathbf{p})}{\partial p_1} & \dfrac{\partial e_1(\mathbf{p})}{\partial p_2} & \cdots \\ \dfrac{\partial e_2(\mathbf{p})}{\partial p_1} & \dfrac{\partial e_2(\mathbf{p})}{\partial p_2} & \cdots \\ \vdots & \vdots & \ddots \end{pmatrix}\begin{pmatrix} t_1 \\ t_2 \\ \vdots \end{pmatrix} \cong \begin{pmatrix} e_1(\mathbf{p}) \\ e_2(\mathbf{p}) \\ \vdots \end{pmatrix} \qquad (26.9)$$

From this we can derive an iterative scheme for improving the parameter estimates. For iteration n, the parameters $\mathbf{p}$ are updated as:

$$\mathbf{p}^{(n+1)}=\mathbf{p}^{(n)}-(\mathbf{A}^T\mathbf{A})^{-1}\mathbf{A}^T\mathbf{e} \qquad (26.10)$$

$$\text{where } \mathbf{A} = \begin{pmatrix} \dfrac{\partial e_1(\mathbf{p})}{\partial p_1} & \dfrac{\partial e_1(\mathbf{p})}{\partial p_2} & \cdots \\[2ex] \dfrac{\partial e_2(\mathbf{p})}{\partial p_1} & \dfrac{\partial e_2(\mathbf{p})}{\partial p_2} & \cdots \\[2ex] \vdots & \vdots & \ddots \end{pmatrix} \text{ and } \mathbf{e} = \begin{pmatrix} e_1(\mathbf{p}) \\ e_2(\mathbf{p}) \\ \vdots \end{pmatrix}$$

(26.11)

This process is repeated until χ^2 can no longer be decreased – or for a fixed number of iterations. There is no guarantee that the best global solution will be reached, since the algorithm can get caught in a local minimum (Fig. 26.3). To reduce this problem, the starting estimates for $\mathbf{p}$ should be set as close as possible to the optimum solution. The number of potential local minima can also be decreased by working with smooth images. This also has the effect of making the first order Taylor approximation more accurate for larger displacements. Once the registration is close to the final solution, the registration can continue with less smooth images.

In practice, $\mathbf{A}^T\mathbf{A}$ and $\mathbf{A}^T\mathbf{e}$ from Eq. 26.10 are computed "on the fly" for each iteration. By computing these matrices using only a few rows of $\mathbf{A}$ and $\mathbf{e}$ at a time, much less computer memory is required than is necessary for storing the whole of matrix $\mathbf{A}$. Also, the partial derivatives $\partial e_i(\mathbf{p})/\partial p_j$ can be rapidly computed from the gradients of the images using the chain rule. These calculations will be illustrated more fully in the next few sections.

26.3
Within Modality Image Coregistration

The most common application of within modality coregistration is in motion correction of series of images. It is inevitable that a subject will move slightly during a series of scans, so prior to performing any statistical tests, it is important that the images are as closely aligned as possible. Subject head movement in the scanner cannot be completely eliminated, so motion correction needs to be performed as a preprocessing step on the data.

Accurate motion correction is especially important for fMRI studies with paradigms in which the subject may move in the scanner in a way that is correlated with the different experimental conditions (HAJNAL et al. 1994). Even tiny systematic differences can result in a significant signal accumulating over numerous scans. Without suitable corrections, artifacts arising from subject movement correlated with the paradigm may appear as activations.

A second reason why motion correction is important is that it increases sensitivity. Statistical tests used to localize activations are usually based on the signal change relative to the residual variance – which is computed from the sum of squared differences between the data and the linear model to which it is fitted. Movement artifacts add to this residual variance, and so reduce the sensitivity of the test to true activations.

Most current algorithms for movement correction consider the head as a rigid object. In three dimensions, six parameters are needed to define a rigid body transformation (three translations and three rotations). These transformations are a subset of the more general affine transformations. For each point (x_1, x_2, x_3) in an image, an affine mapping can be defined into the coordinates of another space (y_1, y_2, y_3). This is expressed as:

$$y_1 = m_{11}x_1 + m_{12}x_2 + m_{13}x_3 + m_{14}$$

$$y_2 = m_{21}x_1 + m_{22}x_2 + m_{23}x_3 + m_{24}$$

$$y_3 = m_{31}x_1 + m_{32}x_2 + m_{33}x_3 + m_{34}$$

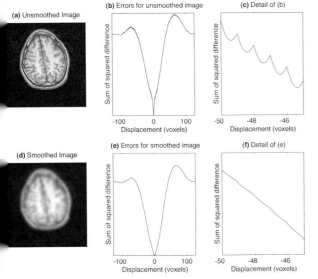

Fig. 26.3a–f. The sum of squared differences between an image and itself translated by different amounts in one direction, using bilinear interpolation. The original image is shown in (a). Sum of squared difference is plotted against translation in (b), and a detail of this is shown in (c), where a periodic effect arising from the interpolation can clearly be seen. This effect is reduced when the procedure is repeated with a smoothed image, as illustrated in (d), (e) and (f). This figure shows that an optimization of this parameter would only converge to the optimal solution if the starting estimates are within certain bounds

This mapping is often expressed as a simple matrix multiplication ($\mathbf{y}=\mathbf{Mx}$):

$$\begin{pmatrix} y_1 \\ y_2 \\ y_3 \\ 1 \end{pmatrix} = \begin{pmatrix} m_{11} & m_{12} & m_{13} & m_{14} \\ m_{21} & m_{22} & m_{23} & m_{24} \\ m_{31} & m_{32} & m_{33} & m_{34} \\ 0 & 0 & 0 & 1 \end{pmatrix} \begin{pmatrix} x_1 \\ x_2 \\ x_3 \\ 1 \end{pmatrix} \qquad (26.12)$$

The elegance of formulating these transformations in terms of matrices is that several transformations can be combined simply by multiplying the matrices together to form a single matrix. This means that repeated resampling of the data can be avoided when re-orienting an image.

In three dimensions a rigid body transformation is described by six parameters. These parameters are, typically, three translations and three rotations about orthogonal axes. A matrix that implements the translation is:

$$\begin{pmatrix} 1 & 0 & 0 & p_1 \\ 0 & 1 & 0 & p_2 \\ 0 & 0 & 1 & p_3 \\ 0 & 0 & 0 & 1 \end{pmatrix} \qquad (26.13)$$

Matrixes that carry out rotations (p_4, p_5 and p_6 – in radians) about the X, Y and Z axes respectively are:

$$\begin{pmatrix} 1 & 0 & 0 & 0 \\ 0 & cos(p_4) & sin(p_4) & 0 \\ 0 & -sin(p_4) & cos(p_4) & 0 \\ 0 & 0 & 0 & 1 \end{pmatrix} \begin{pmatrix} cos(p_5) & 0 & sin(p_5) & 0 \\ 0 & 1 & 0 & 0 \\ -sin(p_5) & 0 & cos(p_5) & 0 \\ 0 & 0 & 0 & 1 \end{pmatrix} and \begin{pmatrix} cos(p_6) & sin(p_6) & 0 & 0 \\ -sin(p_6) & cos(p_6) & 0 & 0 \\ 0 & 0 & 1 & 0 \\ 0 & 0 & 0 & 1 \end{pmatrix}$$

$$(26.14)$$

The combined transformation is achieved by multiplying these matrices together in the appropriate order. The order in which the operations are performed is important. For example, a rotation about the X axis of $\pi/2$ radians followed by an equivalent rotation about the Y axis would produce a very different result if the order of the operations was reversed.

Voxel sizes of images need to be considered in order to register them using a rigid body transformation. Often, the images (say, $\mathbf{f}$ and $\mathbf{g}$) will have voxels that are anisotropic. The dimensions of the voxels are also likely to differ between images of different modalities. For simplicity, a Euclidian space is used, where measures of distances are expressed in millimeters. Rather than interpolating the images such that the voxels are cubic and have the same dimensions in all images, one can simply define affine

transformation matrices that map from voxel coordinates into this Euclidian space. For example, if image $\mathbf{f}$ is of size 128×128×43 and has voxels that are 2.1×2.1×2.45 mm, we can define the following matrix:

$$\mathbf{M_f} = \begin{pmatrix} 2.1 & 0 & 0 & -134.4 \\ 0 & 2.1 & 0 & -134.4 \\ 0 & 0 & 2.45 & -52.675 \\ 0 & 0 & 0 & 1 \end{pmatrix} \qquad (26.15)$$

This transformation matrix maps voxel coordinates to a Euclidian space whose axes are parallel to those of the image and whose distances are measured in millimeters, with the origin at the center of the image. A similar matrix can be defined for $\mathbf{g}$ ($\mathbf{M_g}$). Because modern image formats such as SPI (standard product interconnect) generally contain information about image orientations in their headers, it is possible to extract this information to automatically compute values for $\mathbf{M_f}$ or $\mathbf{M_g}$. This makes it possible to easily register images together that were originally acquired in completely different orientations.

The objective of any coregistration is to determine the rigid body transformation that maps the coordinates of image $\mathbf{f}$ to that of $\mathbf{g}$. To accomplish this, a rigid body transformation matrix $\mathbf{M_r}$ is determined, such that $\mathbf{M_g}^{-1}\mathbf{M_r}\mathbf{M_f}$ will register the images. Once $\mathbf{M_r}$ has been determined, $\mathbf{M_f}$ can be set to $\mathbf{M_r}\,\mathbf{M_f}$.

From there onwards the mapping between the images can be achieved by $\mathbf{M_g}^{-1}\mathbf{M_f}$. Similarly, if another image ($\mathbf{h}$) is also coregistered to image $\mathbf{g}$ in the same manner, then not only is there a mapping between $\mathbf{g}$ and $\mathbf{h}$ ($\mathbf{M_g}^{-1}\mathbf{M_h}$, but there is also one between $\mathbf{f}$ and $\mathbf{h}$ which is simply $\mathbf{M_f}^{-1}\mathbf{M_h}$ (derived from $\mathbf{M_f}^{-1}\mathbf{M_g}\mathbf{M_g}^{-1}\mathbf{M_h}$.

The objective of realignment is to determine rigid body transformations that best map the series of functional images to the same space. This can be achieved by minimizing the sum of squared differences between each of the images and a reference image, for which the reference image could be one of the images in the series. For slightly better results, this procedure could be repeated, but instead of matching to one of the images from the series, the images would be registered to the mean all the realigned images. Because of the nonstationary variance in the images, a variance image could be computed at the same time as the mean, in order to provide better weighting for the registration. Voxels with a lot of variance should be given lower weighting, whereas those with less variance should be weighted more highly.

To fit an image **f** to the reference image **g**, a six-parameter rigid body transformation (parameters p_1–p_6) would be used. The images may be scaled slightly differently, so an additional intensity scaling parameter (p_7) is included in the model. The parameters (**p**) are optimized by minimizing the sum of squared differences between the images according to the algorithm described in Sect. 26.2.2 (Eq. 26.10). The function that is minimized is:

$$\sum_i (f(\mathbf{Mx}_i) - p_7 g(\mathbf{x}_i))^2 \qquad (26.16)$$

where $\mathbf{M} \equiv \mathbf{M}_g^{-1} \mathbf{M}_r \mathbf{M}_f$, and $\mathbf{M}_r$ is constructed from parameters **p**. Vector **e** is generated for each iteration as:

$$e_i = f(\mathbf{Mx}_i) - p_7 g(\mathbf{x}_i) \qquad (26.17)$$

Matrix A is constructed by differentiating Eq. 26.17 with respect to parameters p_1–p_6. However, this involves recomputing the gradients of image **f** at different sampled points at each iteration. Because the affine transformation matrices are invertible, a more efficient method can be achieved by computing the derivatives of **f** only once, and transforming image **g** by the inverse of **M** at each iteration. Because low order interpolation methods are faster than high order interpolation, another modification to facilitate faster realignment is to use a low order method (such as trilinear interpolation) for the early iterations and to obtain the final estimates using a higher order sinc or polynomial interpolation.

26.3.1
Residual Artifacts

Even after realignment, there may still be some motion related artifacts remaining in the data. There are a number of sources of these motion related artifacts:

1. Interpolation error from the resampling algorithm used to transform the images is one of the main sources of motion related artifacts. When the image series is resampled, it is important to use a very accurate interpolation method such as sinc or Fourier interpolation.
2. When MR images are reconstructed, the final images are usually the modulus of the initially complex data, resulting in any voxels that should be negative being rendered positive. This has implications when the images are resampled, because it

leads to errors at the edge of the brain that cannot be corrected however good the interpolation method is. Possible ways to circumvent this problem are to work with complex data, or possibly to apply a low pass filter to the complex data before taking the modulus.
3. The sensitivity (slice selection) profile of each slice also plays a role in introducing artifacts (NOLL et al. 1997).
4. fMRI images are spatially distorted, and the amount of distortion depends partly upon the position of the subject's head within the magnetic field. Relatively large subject movements result in the brain images changing shape, and these shape changes cannot be corrected by a rigid body transformation.
5. Each fMRI volume of a series is currently acquired a plane at a time over a period of a few seconds. Subject movement between acquiring the first and last plane of any volume leads to another reason why the images may not strictly obey the rules of rigid body motion.
6. After a slice is magnetized, the excited tissue takes time to recover to its original state, and the amount of recovery that has taken place will influence the intensity of the tissue in the image. Out of plane movement will result in a slightly different part of the brain being excited during each repeat. This means that the spin excitation will vary in a way that is related to head motion, and so leads to more movement related artifacts.
7. Ghost artifacts in the images do not obey the same rigid body rules as the head, so a rigid rotation to align the head will not mean that the ghosts are aligned.
8. The accuracy of the estimated registration parameters is normally in the region of tens of microns. This is dependent upon many factors, including the effects just mentioned. Even the signal changes elicited by the experiment can have a slight effect (a few microns) on the estimated parameters.

These problems cannot be corrected by rigid body registration, and so may be sources of possible stimulus correlated motion artifacts. Systematic movement artifacts resulting in a signal change of only 1%–2% can lead to highly significant false positives over an experiment with many scans. This is especially important for experiments in which some conditions may cause slight head movements (such as motor tasks, or speech), because these movements are likely to be highly correlated with the experimental design. In cases like this, it is extremely difficult to separate true activations from stimulus correlated motion artifacts. Providing that there are enough images in the series and the movements are small, some of these artifacts can be removed by using an ANCOVA model to remove any signal that is correlated with functions of the movement parameters (FRISTON et al. 1996). However, when the estimates of the movement parameters are related to the experimental design, it is likely that much of the true fMRI signal will also be lost. At the time of writing, these are still unresolved problems.

26.4
Between Modality Image Coregistration

The coregistration of brain images of the same subject acquired in different modalities has proved itself to be useful in many areas, both in research and clinically. Intermodality registration of images is less straightforward than that of registering images of the same modality. Two images from the same subject acquired using the same scanning sequences generally look similar, so it suffices to find the rigid-body transformation parameters that minimize the sum of squared differences between them. However, for coregistration between modalities there is nothing quite so obvious to minimize. Older methods of registration involved the manual identification of homologous landmarks in the images. These landmarks are aligned together, thus bringing the images into registration. This is time-consuming, requires a degree of experience, and can be rather subjective. More recently, the idea of matching images by maximizing the mutual information in their histograms is becoming more widespread (COLLIGNON et al. 1995). For this approach, the histogram (H, see Fig. 26.4) is considered as an M by N matrix, and the registration involves maximizing the following objective function:

$$\sum_{j=1}^{J} \sum_{i=1}^{I} h_{i,j} \log \left(\frac{h_{i,j}}{(\sum_{k=1}^{J} h_{i,k})(\sum_{l=1}^{I} h_{l,j})} \right) \quad (26.18)$$

Maximizing mutual information is a very general approach, which has been successfully applied to registering a wide variety of images. The within modality registration model described in this chapter also maximizes mutual information, but more assumptions are made about the images and the type of noise they contain.

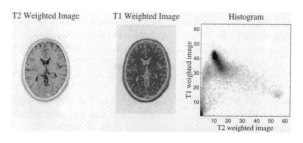

Fig.26.4. The two dimensional histogram of registered T2- and T1-weighted images. When the images are less well registered, the clusters in the histogram become less "tight"

The next section describes the first step of an alternative approach (ASHBURNER and FRISTON 1997) for between modality registration. The whole procedure normally involves two additional steps which refine the parameters, but it is possible to obtain a reasonable match using the first step alone.

26.4.1
One Method of Between Modality Registration

This method requires images other than the images to be registered (**f** and **g**).

These are template images of the same modalities as **f** and **g** (**t**$_f$ and **t**$_g$), which should conform to the same anatomical space.

For simplicity, we work in a Euclidian space, where measures of distances are expressed in millimeters. To facilitate this, we need to define matrices M_f, M_g and M_t that map from the voxel coordinates of images **f**, **g** and the templates, into their own Euclidian space. The objective is to determine the affine transformation that maps the coordinate system of **f** to that of **g**. To accomplish this, we need to find a rigid body transformation matrix M_r, such that $M_g^{-1} M_r M_f$ will coregister the images.

It is possible to obtain a reasonable match of images of most normal brains to a template image of the same modality using just a twelve- (or even nine) parameter affine transformation. One can register image **g** to template t_g, and similarly register **f** to t_f using this approach. We will call these transformation matrices M_{gt} and M_{ft} respectively. Thus a mapping from **f** to **g** now becomes $M_g^{-1} M_{gt} M_{ft}^{-1} M_f$. However, this affine transformation between f and g has not been constrained to be rigid body. We modify this simple approach in order to incorporate this constraint, by decomposing matrix M_{gt} into matrices that perform a rigid body transformation (M_{gr}), and one that performs the scaling and shearing (M_{ta}), i.e.

$M_{gt}=M_{gr}M_{ta}$, and similarly $M_{ft}=M_{fr}M_{ta}$. Notice that M_{ta} is the same for both f and g. Now the mapping becomes $M_g^{-1}M_{gr}(M_{ta}M_{ta}^{-1})M_{fr}^{-1}M_f$, and is a rigid body transformation. The construction of matrices M_{gr}, M_{fr} and M_{ta} is shown in Fig. 26.5.

We can now optimize the parameter set $q=(q_1 q_2 \ldots)$ in order to determine the transformations that minimize the sum of squared differences between the images and templates. The basic optimization method has been described in previous sections and involves generating matrix $A^T A$ and vector $A^T e$ for each iteration, solving the equations and incrementing the parameter estimates. Matrices A and e are described in Fig. 26.6.

The parameters describing the non-rigid transformations (q_{13}–q_{18}) could in theory be derived from either f or g. In practice, we obtain a better solution by estimating these parameters using both images and by biasing the result so that the image that fits the template better has a greater influence over the parameter estimates. This is achieved by weighting the rows of A and e that correspond to the different images. The weights are derived from the sum of squared differences between the template and object images, obtained from the previous solution of q. These are:

$$\frac{I}{\sum_{i=1}^{I}(f(M_1x_i)-q_{19}t_f(x_i))^2} \quad \text{and} \quad \frac{I}{\sum_{i=1}^{I}(g(M_2x_i)-q_{20}t_g(x_i))^2}$$

(26.19)

where $M_1=(M_t^{-1}M_{ft}M_f)^{-1}$, and $M_2=(M_t^{-1}M_{gt}M_g)^{-1}$. Even more robust parameter estimates can be

$$M_{gr} = \begin{pmatrix} 1 & 0 & 0 & q_1 \\ 0 & 1 & 0 & q_2 \\ 0 & 0 & 1 & q_3 \\ 0 & 0 & 0 & 1 \end{pmatrix} \times \begin{pmatrix} 1 & 0 & 0 & 0 \\ 0 & cos(q_4) & sin(q_4) & 0 \\ 0 & -sin(q_4) & cos(q_4) & 0 \\ 0 & 0 & 0 & 1 \end{pmatrix} \times \begin{pmatrix} cos(q_5) & 0 & sin(q_5) & 0 \\ 0 & 0 & 0 & 0 \\ -sin(q_5) & 0 & cos(q_5) & 0 \\ 0 & 0 & 0 & 1 \end{pmatrix} \times \begin{pmatrix} cos(q_6) & sin(q_6) & 0 & 0 \\ -sin(q_6) & cos(q_6) & 0 & 0 \\ 0 & 0 & 1 & 0 \\ 0 & 0 & 0 & 1 \end{pmatrix}$$

$$M_{fr} = \begin{pmatrix} 1 & 0 & 0 & q_7 \\ 0 & 1 & 0 & q_8 \\ 0 & 0 & 1 & q_9 \\ 0 & 0 & 0 & 1 \end{pmatrix} \times \begin{pmatrix} 1 & 0 & 0 & 0 \\ 0 & cos(q_{10}) & sin(q_{10}) & 0 \\ 0 & -sin(q_{10}) & cos(q_{10}) & 0 \\ 0 & 0 & 0 & 1 \end{pmatrix} \times \begin{pmatrix} cos(q_{11}) & 0 & sin(q_{11}) & 0 \\ 0 & 0 & 0 & 0 \\ -sin(q_{11}) & 0 & cos(q_{11}) & 0 \\ 0 & 0 & 0 & 1 \end{pmatrix} \times \begin{pmatrix} cos(q_{12}) & sin(q_{12}) & 0 & 0 \\ -sin(q_{12}) & cos(q_{12}) & 0 & 0 \\ 0 & 0 & 1 & 0 \\ 0 & 0 & 0 & 1 \end{pmatrix}$$

$$M_{ta} = \begin{pmatrix} q_{13} & 0 & 0 & 0 \\ 0 & q_{14} & 0 & 0 \\ 0 & 0 & q_{15} & 0 \\ 0 & 0 & 0 & 1 \end{pmatrix} \times \begin{pmatrix} 1 & q_{16} & q_{17} & 0 \\ 0 & 1 & q_{18} & 0 \\ 0 & 0 & 1 & 0 \\ 0 & 0 & 0 & 1 \end{pmatrix}$$

Fig. 26.5. The construction of affine transformation matrices M_{gr}, M_{fr} and M_{ta} from the parameters q

$$A = \begin{pmatrix} -\frac{df(M_1x_1)}{dq_1} & \cdots & -\frac{df(M_1x_1)}{dq_6} & 0 & \cdots & 0 & -\frac{df(M_1x_1)}{dq_{13}} & \cdots & -\frac{df(M_1x_1)}{dq_{18}} & t_f(x_1) & 0 \\ -\frac{df(M_1x_2)}{dq_1} & & -\frac{df(M_1x_2)}{dq_6} & 0 & \cdots & 0 & -\frac{df(M_1x_2)}{dq_{13}} & \cdots & -\frac{df(M_1x_2)}{dq_{18}} & t_f(x_2) & 0 \\ \vdots & \ddots & \vdots & \vdots & & \vdots & \vdots & \ddots & \vdots & \vdots & \vdots \\ 0 & \cdots & 0 & -\frac{dg(M_2x_1)}{dq_7} & \cdots & -\frac{dg(M_2x_1)}{dq_{12}} & -\frac{dg(M_2x_1)}{dq_{13}} & \cdots & -\frac{dg(M_2x_1)}{dq_{18}} & 0 & t_g(x_1) \\ 0 & \cdots & 0 & -\frac{dg(M_2x_2)}{dq_7} & \cdots & -\frac{dg(M_2x_2)}{dq_{12}} & -\frac{dg(M_2x_2)}{dq_{13}} & \cdots & -\frac{dg(M_2x_2)}{dq_{18}} & 0 & t_g(x_2) \\ \vdots & \ddots & \vdots & \vdots & & \vdots & \vdots & \ddots & \vdots & \vdots & \vdots \end{pmatrix}$$

$$e = \begin{pmatrix} f(M_1x_1) - q_{19}t_f(x_1) \\ f(M_1x_2) - q_{19}t_f(x_2) \\ \vdots \\ g(M_2x_1) - q_{20}t_g(x_1) \\ g(M_2x_2) - q_{20}t_g(x_2) \\ \vdots \end{pmatrix}$$

Fig. 26.6. Matrices A and e used for estimating the constrained affine mappings described in Sect. 26.4.1. We utilize the notation that $f(x)$ is the intensity of image f at position x, and similarly for $g(x)$, $t_f(x)$ and $t_g(x)$. For the purpose of this optimization, we define two matrices, $M_1=(M_t^{-1}M_{ft}M_f)^{-1}$, and $M_2=(M_t^{-1}M_{gt}M_g)^{-1}$

achieved by incorporating some of the ideas that will be discussed in Sect. 26.5.3.

Once the optimization has converged to the final solution, we can obtain the rigid body transformation that approximately maps between **f** and **g**, and we also have affine transformation matrices that map between the object images and the templates.

26.5
Spatial Normalization

This section concerns the problem of spatial normalization, namely, how to map a single subject's brain image into a standard space. The solution of this problem, assuming that the standard space adopted has a known relationship to other standard spaces, allows for a wide range of voxel-based analyses and facilitates the comparison of different subjects and databases. The nature of this comparison is determined by the modality of the images and the question asked of the data. The problem of spatial normalization is not a trivial one; indeed at some anatomical scales it is not clear that a solution even exists.

In the domain of imaging neuroscience, the operation of spatial normalization facilitates inter-subject averaging of data. This means that it is often necessary to average signals over a number of subjects in order to obtain a meaningful result. A further advantage of using spatially normalized images is that activations can be reported according to their Euclidian coordinates within a standard space (Fox 1995). New results can be readily incorporated into ongoing brain atlas and database projects such as that being developed by the International Consortium for Human Brain Mapping (ICBM) (Mazziotta et al. 1995). The most commonly adopted coordinate system within the brain imaging community is that described by the atlas of Talairach and Tournoux (1988).

This section has four main components. We start with the theoretical background to spatial normalization and make a distinction between label- and non-label-based approaches. Most routine spatial normalization is automatic and therefore eschews the identification of labeled landmarks in the brain that are required in label-based approaches. We will therefore concentrate on non-label-based approaches. There are a variety of approaches to these types of spatial normalization. These include the use of spatial basis functions, viscous fluid models, elastic models and multi-resolution approaches. In this

section we concentrate on techniques that use spatial basis functions because this is the approach adopted by the most widely used algorithms. There are a number of themes that are common to all the approaches and, where possible, these will be emphasized (e.g., the minimization of some bending or elastic energy to ensure smooth deformations).

The second subsection introduces the Bayesian framework used to find maximum a posteriori (MAP) estimates of the deformation fields. MAP schemes can be used to embody prior knowledge about the shape or size of brains during the normalization or to incorporate some constraint (e.g., a minimization of bending energy).

The remainder of the section describes some specific details about how the spatial deformations are modeled and estimated. The first stage of the spatial normalization is an affine registration by matching to a template image. In this instance we use some simple observations about the normal variation in the size of people's heads in order to incorporate this information into a MAP scheme. This is followed by describing the method of nonlinear normalization (to remove shape differences) using exactly the same formalism as used to determine the linear or affine components.

26.5.1
Background

The process of spatial normalization involves matching the object image to some form of standardized template image. Unlike in the work of Christensen et al. (1994, 1996) or the segmentation work by Collins et al. (1994a, 1995), spatial normalization requires that the images themselves are transformed to the space of the template, rather than a transformation being determined that transforms the template to the individual images.

Spatial transformations can be broadly divided into label-based and non-label-based. Label-based techniques identify homologous features (labels) in the image and template and find the transformations that best superpose them. The labels can be points, lines or surfaces. Homologous features are often identified manually, but this process is time consuming and subjective. Another disadvantage of using points as landmarks is that there are very few readily identifiable discrete points in the brain. A similar problem is faced during identification of homologous lines. However, surfaces are more readily identified, and in many instances they can be extracted automatically (or at least semi-automatically). Once they are identified, the spatial transformation is effected by bringing the homologies together. If the labels are points, then the required transformations at each of those points is known. Between the points, the deforming behavior is not known, so it is forced to be as "smooth" as possible. There are a number of methods for modeling this smoothness. The simplest models include fitting splines through the points in order to minimize bending energy (BOOKSTEIN 1989). More complex forms of interpolation are often used when the labels are surfaces. For example THOMPSON et al. (1996) map surfaces together using a fluid model.

Non-label-based approaches identify a spatial transformation that minimizes some index of the difference between an object and a template image, in which both are treated as unlabeled continuous processes. The matching criterion is usually based upon minimizing the sum of squared differences or maximizing the correlation coefficient between the images. For this criterion to be successful, it requires the template to appear like a warped version of the image. In other words, there must be correspondence in the gray levels of the different tissue types between the image and template.

There are a number of approaches to non-label-based spatial normalization. A potentially enormous number of parameters are required to describe the nonlinear transformations that warp two images together (i.e., the problem is very high dimensional). The forms of spatial normalization tend to differ in how they cope with the large number of parameters.

Some have abandoned conventional optimization approaches and use viscous fluid models (CHRISTENSEN et al. 1994, 1996) to describe the warps. In these models, finite element methods are used to solve the partial differential equations that model one image as it "flows" to the same shape as the other. The major advantage of these methods is that they are able to account for large nonlinear displacements and also ensure that the topology of the warped image is preserved, but they do have the disadvantage that they are computationally expensive. Not every unit in the imaging neuroscience field has the capacity to routinely perform spatial normalizations using these methods.

Others adopt a multi-resolution approach whereby only a few of the parameters are determined at any one time (COLLINS et al. 1994a). Usually, the entire volume is used to determine parameters that describe global low frequency deformations. The volume is then subdivided, and slightly higher frequency deformations are found for each subvolume. This continues until the desired deformation precision is achieved.

Another approach is to reduce the number of parameters that model the deformations. Some groups use only a nine- or twelve-parameter affine transformation to spatially normalize their images, accounting for differences in position, orientation and overall brain size. Low spatial frequency global variability in head shape can be accommodated by describing deformations by a linear combination of low frequency basis functions. The small number of parameters will not allow every feature to be matched exactly, but it will permit the global head shape to be modeled. The method described in this section is one such approach. The rational for adopting a low dimensional approach is that there is not necessarily a one-to-one mapping between any pair of brains. Different subjects have different patterns of gyral convolutions and even if gyral anatomy can be matched exactly, this is no guarantee that areas of functional specialization will be matched in a homologous way. For the purpose of averaging signals from functional images of different subjects, very high resolution spatial normalization may be unnecessary or unrealistic.

The deformations required to transform images to the same space are not clearly defined. Unlike rigid body transformations, in which the constraints are explicit, those for nonlinear warping are more arbitrary. Without any constraints it is of course possible to transform any image such that it matches another exactly. The issue is therefore less about the nature of the transformation and more about defining constraints or priors under which a transformation is effected. The validity of a transformation can usually be reduced to the validity of these priors. Priors are normally incorporated using some form of Bayesian scheme, using estimators such as the MAP estimate or the minimum variance estimate (MVE). The MAP estimate is the single solution that has the highest a posteriori probability of being correct.

26.5.2
A Maximum A Posteriori Solution

Bayes rule is generally expressed in the continuous form:

$$p(a_\mathrm{p}|b) = \frac{p(b|a_\mathrm{p})p(a_\mathrm{p})}{\int_\mathrm{q} p(b|a_\mathrm{q})\mathrm{p}(a_\mathrm{q})d\mathbf{q}} \qquad (26.20)$$

where $p(a_p)$ is the prior probability of a_p being true, $p(b|a_p)$ is the conditional probability that b is observed given that a_p is true and $p(a_p|b)$ is the posterior probability of a_p being true, given that measurement b has been made. The MAP estimate for parameters $\mathbf{p}$ is the mode of $p(a_p|b)$. For our purposes, $p(a_p)$ represents a known prior probability distribution from which the parameters are drawn, $p(b|a_p)$ is the likelihood of obtaining the data b given the parameters (the maximum likelihood estimate), and $p(a_p|b)$ is the function to be maximized. The optimization can be simplified by assuming that all probability distributions are multidimensional and normal (multi-normal) and can therefore be described by a mean vector and a covariance matrix.

When close to the minimum, the optimization becomes almost a linear problem. This allows us to assume that the errors of the fitted parameters ($\mathbf{p}$) can be locally approximated by a multi-normal distribution with covariance matrix $\mathbf{C}$.

We assume that the true parameters are drawn from a known underlying multi-normal distribution of mean $\mathbf{p}_0$ and covariance matrix $\mathbf{C}_0$. By using the a priori probability density function (p.d.f) of the parameters, we can obtain a better estimate of the true parameters by taking a weighted average of $\mathbf{p}$ and $\mathbf{p}_0$:

$$\mathbf{p}_b=(\mathbf{C}_0^{-1}+\mathbf{C}^{-1})^{-1}(\mathbf{C}_0^{-1}\mathbf{p}_0+\mathbf{C}^{-1}\mathbf{p}) \qquad (26.21)$$

An estimation of $\mathbf{C}$ is required in order to employ this approach. This is the estimated covariance matrix of the standard errors of the fitted parameters and is derived from the data itself. If the observations are independent, and each has unit standard deviation, then $\mathbf{C}$ is given by $(\mathbf{A}^T\mathbf{A})^{-1}$. In practice, the standard deviations of the observations are unknown, so we assume they are equal for all observations, and estimate this value from the sum of squared differences:

$$\sigma^2 = \sum_{i=1}^{I} e_i(\mathbf{p})^2 / v \qquad (26.22)$$

where v refers to the degrees of freedom. This gives a covariance matrix:

$$\mathbf{C}=(\mathbf{A}^T\mathbf{A})^{-1}\sigma^2 \qquad (26.23)$$

By combining Eqs. 26.10, 26.16 and 26.23, we obtain the following scheme:

$$\mathbf{p}_b^{(n+1)}=\mathbf{C}_0^{-1}+\mathbf{A}^T\mathbf{A}/\sigma^2)^{-1}(\mathbf{C}_0^{-1}\mathbf{p}_0+\mathbf{A}^T\mathbf{A}\mathbf{p}_b^{(n)}/\sigma^2-\mathbf{A}^T\mathbf{e}/\sigma^2) \qquad (26.24)$$

Another way of thinking about this optimization scheme, is that two criteria are simultaneously being minimized. The first is the sum of squared differences between the images, and the second is a squared distance between the parameters and their known expectation $\mathbf{p}_b^T\mathbf{C}_0^{-1}\mathbf{p}_b$.

26.5.3
Affine Spatial Normalization

Almost all between subject coregistration or spatial normalization methods for brain images begin by determining the optimal nine- or twelve-parameter affine transformation that registers the images together. This step is normally performed automatically by minimizing (or maximizing) some mutual function of the images.

The objective of affine registration is to fit the image to a template image, using a twelve-parameter affine transformation. The images may be scaled quite differently, so an additional intensity scaling parameter is included in the model.

Without constraints and with poor data, the simple parameter optimization approach can produce some extremely unlikely transformations. For example, when there are only a few transverse slices in the image (spanning the X and Y dimensions), it is not possible for the algorithms to determine an accurate zoom in the Z direction. Any estimate of this value is likely to have very large errors. When the MAP approach is not used, it may be better to assign a fixed value for this difficult to determine parameter and simply fit for the remaining ones. By incorporating prior information into the optimization procedure, a smooth transition between fixed and fitted parameters can be achieved (ASHBURNER et al. 1997). When the error for a particular fitted parameter is known to be large, then that parameter will be based more upon the prior information.

In order to adopt a MAP approach, the prior distribution of the parameters should be known. A suitable a priori distribution of the parameters relating to brain shape and size ($\mathbf{p}_0$ and $\mathbf{C}_0$ from Eq. 26.24) can easily be determined from affine transformations estimated from a large number of images using the basic least squares optimization algorithm.

26.5.4
Nonlinear Spatial Normalization

Following affine registration, more subtle differences in global brain shape can be corrected by nonlinear spatial normalization. One approach involves describing the spatial transformations by a linear combination of smooth basis functions. The choice of basis functions depends partly upon how translations at the boundaries should behave. If points at the boundary over which the transform is computed are not required to move in any direction, then the basis functions should consist of the lowest frequencies of the three-dimensional discrete sine transform (DST). If there are to be no constraints at the boundaries, then a three-dimensional discrete cosine transform (DCT) is more appropriate. Both of these transforms use the same set of basis functions to represent warps in each of the directions. Alternatively, a mixture of DCT and DST basis functions can be used to constrain translations at the surfaces of the volume to be parallel to the surface only (sliding boundary conditions). By using a different combination of DCT and DST basis functions, the corners of the volume can be fixed and the remaining points on the surface can be free to move in all directions (bending boundary conditions) (CHRISTENSEN 1994). A schematic example of a deformation based upon these principles is shown in Fig. 26.7. The optimization involves determining the set of coefficients that minimizes the sum of squared differences between the warped object image and the template image. Further implementational details can be found in ASHBURNER and FRISTON (1998).

Without using the MAP formulation, it is possible to introduce unnecessary deformations that only reduce the residual sum of squares by a tiny amount (Fig. 26.8). This could potentially make the algorithm very unstable. The first requirement for the MAP approach is to define some form of prior distribution for the parameters in order to regularize the optimization. For a simple linear approach, the priors consist of an a priori estimate of the mean of the parameters (assumed to be zero) and also a covariance matrix describing the distribution of the parameters about this mean. There are many possible forms for modeling these priors, each of which refers to some type of "energy" term. Possible forms for these energy terms include the membrane energy (or Laplacians) of the deformation field (AMIT et al. 1991; GEE et al. 1997), the bending energy (BOOKSTEIN 1997a, b) and the linear-elastic energy (MILLER et al. 1993). None of these schemes enforce a strict one to one mapping between the object and template images, but this makes little

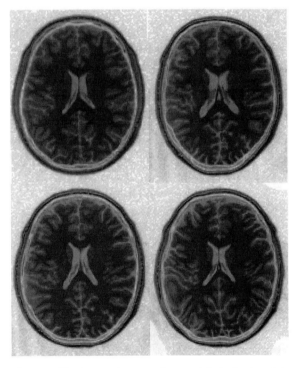

Fig. 26.8. The image shown at the *top, left,* is the template image. At the *top, right,* is an image that has been registered with it using a 12-parameter affine registration. The image at the *bottom, left,* is the same image registered using the 12-parameter affine registration, followed by a regularized global nonlinear registration. It should be clear that the shape of the image approaches that of the template much better after nonlinear registration. At the *bottom, right,* is the image after the same affine transformation and nonlinear registration, but this time without using any regularization. The mean squared difference between the image and template after the affine registration was 472.1. After the regularized nonlinear registration this was reduced to 302.7. Without regularization, a mean squared difference of 287.3 is achieved, but this is at the expense of introducing a lot of unnecessary warping

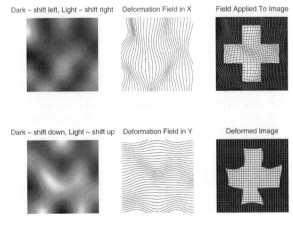

Fig. 26.7. For the two-dimensional case, the deformation field consists of two scalar fields. One for horizontal deformations, and the other for vertical deformations. The images on the *left* show the deformation fields as a linear combination of the basis images. The *center* column shows the deformations in a more intuitive sense. The deformation field is applied by overlaying it on the object image, and re-sampling (*right*)

difference for the small deformations that we are interested in here.

26.6
Summary

Prior to any statistical analysis of fMRI data, it is important that all the images from each subject are aligned together. This step is performed by determining a rigid body transformation for each of the images that registers them to the first in the series. This step is a within modality procedure and results in an optimization of the parameters by minimizing the residual sum of squares.

Often, it is desirable to register a structural image to the functional image series. Again, this is a rigid body registration, but because the structural image is acquired in a different modality to the functional images, the registration cannot simply be performed by minimizing the residual sum of squares. These between modality registrations can be performed by first partitioning the images into gray and white matter and then simultaneously registering the partitions together.

Images from several subjects can be analyzed together by first normalizing them all to the same space. In order to facilitate reporting of significant activations by their location within a standard coordinate system, this space is usually that described by TALAIRACH and TOURNOUX (1988). Brains vary in shape and size so more parameters are needed to describe the spatial transformations. The spatial normalization usually begins by determining the optimum twelve-parameter affine transformation to register the brain with a template image. The template image is of the same modality as the image to be registered, so the optimization is simply done by minimizing the residual sum of squares. This twelve-parameter transformation corrects for the variation in position and size of the image, before more subtle differences are corrected by a nonlinear registration. In order to reduce the number of parameters to be fitted, only smoothly varying deformations are determined by the nonlinear registration. These deformations are modeled by a linear combination of smooth basis functions. Once the transformation parameters have been determined from one image, they can be applied to any other image that is in register with it.

References

Amit Y, Grenander U, Piccioni M (1991) Structural image restoration through derormable templates. J Am Stat Assoc 86:376–387

Ashburner J, Friston KJ (1997) Multimodal image coregistration and partitioning – a unified framework. NeuroImage 6:209–217

Ashburner J, Friston KJ (1998) Nonlinear spatial normalization using basis functions. (submitted)

Ashburner J, Neelin P, Collins DL, Evans AC, Friston KJ (1997) Incorporating prior knowledge into image registration. NeuroImage 6:344–352

Bookstein FL (1989) Principal warps: thin-plate splines and the decomposition of deformations. IEEE Trans Pattern Anal Machine Intelligence 11:567–585

Bookstein FL (1997a) Landmark methods for forms without landmarks: Morphometrics of group differences in outline shape. Med Image Anal 1: 225–243

Bookstein FL (1997b) Quadratic variation of deformations. Information Processing in Medical Imaging, Proceedings 15th International Conference. June 9–13, 1997, Putney, Vermont, USA p. 1–14

Christensen GE (1994) Deformable shape models for anatomy. Doctoral thesis. Sever Institute of Technology, Washington University

Christensen GE, Rabbitt RD, Miller MI (1994) 3D brain mapping using a deformable neuroanatomy. Phys Med Biol 39: 609–618

Christensen GE, Rabbitt RD, Miller MI (1996) Deformable templates using large deformation kinematics. IEEE Transactions on Image Processing 5: 1435–1447

Collignon A, Maes F, Delaere D, Vandermeulen D, Suetens P, Marchal G (1995) Automated multi-modality image registration based on information theory. Information Processing in Medical Imaging, pp 263–274

Collins DL, Peters TM, Evans AC (1994a) An automated 3D non-linear image deformation procedure for determination of gross morphometric variability in human brain. Proc Conference on Visualisation in Biomedical Computing, pp 180–190

Collins DL, Neelin P, Peters TM, Evans AC (1994b) Automatic 3D intersubject registration of MR volumetric data in standardized Taliarach space. J Comput Assist Tomogr 18: 192–205

Collins DL, Evans AC, Holmes C, Peters TM (1995) Automatic 3D segmentation of neuro-anatomical structures from MRI. Information Processing in Medical Imaging, pp 139–152

Eddy WF, Fitzgerald M, Noll DC (1996) Improved image registration by using Fourier interpolation. Magn Res Med 36:923–931

Fox PT (1995) Spatial normalization origins: Objectives, applications, and alternatives. Human Brain Mapping 3 161–164

Friston KJ, Ashburner J, Frith CD, Poline J-B, Heather JD, Frackowiak R SJ (1995) Spatial registration and normalization of images. Human Brain Mapping 2:165–189

Friston KJ, Williams S, Howard R, Frackowiak RSJ, Turner R (1996) Movement-related effects in fMRI time-series. Magn Res Med 35:346–355

Gee JC, Haynor DR, Le Briquer L, Bajcsy RK (1997) Advances in elastic matching theory and its implementation. In: P.

Cinquin, R. Kikinis, S. Lavalée (eds) CVRMed-MRCAS'97. Springer, Berlin, Heidelberg, New York

Hajnal JV, Mayers R, Oatridge A, Schwieso JE, Young JR, Bydder GM (1994) Artifacts due to stimulus correlated motion in functional imaging of the brain. Magn Res Med 31:289–291

Jain AK (1989) Fundamentals of digital image processing. Prentice-Hall, Englewood Cliffs, New Jersey

Mazziotta JC, Toga AW, Evans A, Fox P, Lancaster J (1995) A probablistic atlas of the human brain: Theory and rationale for its development. NeuroImage 2 89–101

Miller MI, Christensen GE, Amit Y, Grenander U (1993) Mathematical textbook of deformable neuroanatomies. Proc Natl Acad Sci USA 90: 11944–11948

Noll DC, Boada FE, Eddy WF (1997) A spectral approach to analyzing slice selection in planar imaging: Optimization for through-plane interpolation. Magn Res Med 38:151–160

Press WH, Teukolsky SA, Vetterling WT, Flannery BP (1992) Numerical recipes in C (second edition). Cambridge, Cambridge, England

Talairach J, Tournoux (1988. Coplanar stereotaxic atlas of the human brain. Thieme Medical, New York

Thompson PM, Toga AW (1996) Visualization and mapping of anatomic abnormalities using a probabilistic brain atlas based on random fluid transformations. Proceedings of the International Conference on Visualization in Biomedical Computing, pp 383–392

27 Statistical Procedures for Functional MRI

N. Lange

CONTENTS

27.1 Introduction

The foci of this chapter are statistical procedures for fMRI of the human brain, or neuro-fMRI. Neuro-fMRI data consist of collections of space-time series arranged in a matrix $\mathbf{Y} = [y_{tv}]$ of dimension $T{\times}V$, where T is the number of time points and V is the number of brain locations (voxels). Element y_{tv} of matrix $\mathbf{Y}$ is the value of the signal at time t and voxel v. For the present discussion, rows index time and columns index space, so that when $T{<}V$, as is generally the case, matrix $\mathbf{Y}$ is "long and flat" rather than "tall and narrow." Neither orientation of the data matrix, $\mathbf{Y}$ nor $\mathbf{Y}^{\mathrm{T}}$, is optimal in all situations; choices vary in statistical and fMRI literature, the present choice being perhaps the more common of the two. In the discussion of the singular value decomposition in Sect. 27.3.4.2, orientation $\mathbf{Y}^{\mathrm{T}}$ is conventional. Each column of $\mathbf{Y}$ is a $T{\times}1$ time series:

$$\mathbf{y}_v = (y_{1v},...,y_{Tv})^{\mathrm{T}}$$

N. Lange, ScD; Dept. of Psychiatry, Faculty of Medicine, Harvard University, and Chief Biostatistician, Brain Imaging Center, McLean Hospital, 115 Mill Street, Belmont, MA 02178, USA

at brain location $v = 1,...V$; each row of $\mathbf{Y}$ is a $1{\times}V$ spatial pattern $\mathbf{y}_t = (y_{t1}...,y_{tV})$ at time $t = 1,...T$. One dimensional (1-D) vector ordering of three dimensional (3-D) brain locations along the columns of $\mathbf{Y}$ is simply a convenient way of storing such data. Coordinates of original spatial locations, i.e., slice number and voxels within slices, may be reconstructed easily given the voxel dimensions of the original images and the order in which the data were read from the RF coil. Context and running subscripts distinguish rows from columns. Study design determines a known reference function:

$$\mathbf{x} = (x_1,...,x_T)^{\mathrm{T}}$$

applying, potentially, at every spatial location (hence no subscript on $\mathbf{x}$). Note that reference function $\mathbf{x}$ is by no means restricted to the simple *on* and *off* states of simple block designs for fMRI stimuli, but instead can take on a wide range of values that vary in time.

The statistical procedures for fMRI research discussed in this chapter help decide what is and is not relevant in $\mathbf{Y}$ and $\mathbf{x}$. Neuro-fMRI statistics generally take advantage of some form of data averaging and aggregation when possible and advisable to reduce extraneous sources of variance and thus increase signal-to-noise ratio. Classes of procedures discussed encompass a large part of current practice and are described with enough detail for the reader to learn key ideas and to know where to look for further study.

27.2 Preliminaries

Descriptions of statistical procedures for neuro-fMRI in this chapter presume reader familiarity with vectors and matrices and operations upon these elements (linear algebra), some introductory calculus, and basic statistical thinking. Likelihood-based methods are discussed only indirectly through least-squares solutions under Gaussian ("normality") assumptions. LARSEN and MARX (1986) is a good text for least-squares, likelihood and other general statistical approaches; FISHER and VAN BELLE (1993) is an encyclopedic, modern treatment; MILLER (1996) is also useful; MOSTELLER and TUKEY (1977) takes a data-driven approach to modern statistical practice. Specialized statistical bibliographic resources on linear models, time series, multivariate analysis and other topics are cited in the following sections dealing with these procedures.

A consistent notation that conforms to standard conventions in journals and texts is employed throughout the chapter. In general, scalars are denoted by lower-case italics (e.g., b), vectors by bold face (**b**) and matrices by upper-case and bold face (**B**). Except for known constants, such as π, Greek characters denote unknown scalar parameters to be estimated (β), bold face Greek characters denote vector parameters ($\boldsymbol{\beta}$) and upper case bold Greek characters denote matrix parameters (**B**), which may appear to be Roman and not Greek for some characters, as in the present example. Subscripts on any of these characters in general denote a running index over time or space (e.g., $\boldsymbol{\beta}_v$, $v = 1,...,V$ voxels).

27.2.1
Experimental Design

Classical statistics is populated by numerous texts on experimental design, a very important aspect of any neuro-fMRI study; Box et al. (1978) is a useful general reference. A formal survey and comparison of neuro-fMRI study designs does not yet appear to exist, neither do specific guidelines for designing a neuro-fMRI study. Experimental design for neuro-fMRI is not an aim of the present chapter. The currently predominant neuro-fMRI study design is of the block trial type, in which reference function **x** consists of temporal blocks of stimuli and baseline conditions. Block designs do not consist necessarily of simple alternating on/off patterns, for they also include more elaborate stimulus presentation schemes, as described in Chap. 29 of this volume. Alternatives to the block trial design, limited as it is in temporal resolution by the hemodynamic response function, are currently being explored through the advent of single-trial or event-related designs BUCKNER et al. 1996; DALE and BUCKNER 1997; FRISTON et al. 1998a,b; for further discussion, see Sect. 27.3.1.6). While post-hoc deconvolution and other statistical procedures applied in these newer designs are less understood than

the more standard variety, neither design is excluded in the present discussion (see the Chap. 36 in the present volume for a detailed treatment of single-trial designs).

27.2.2
Reliability and Reproducibility

Since to date there is little published work on reliability and reproducibility assessment for neuro-fMRI, it is perhaps tacitly assumed by most researchers that neuro-fMR images are both sufficiently reliable and reproducible. Yet these images are measurements and, as such, lend themselves to statistical inquiry and analysis. There is a plethora of possible sources of noise (extraneous variability) and artifact (bias) from the subject, from the instrumentation, and from the method of statistical analysis itself. The same subject repeating his/her performance under identical experimental conditions may yield quite different measurements, or, conversely, different subjects performing under identical experimental conditions may yield quite similar measurements. Tradeoffs in terms of net information gain between imaging a single person multiple times and imaging multiple persons a single time are not yet well understood. There is a large body of statistical work on intra- and inter-subject reliability and reproducibility in other fields, deriving mainly from quality control and experimental design contexts in industry, educational testing, and controlled clinical trials. These methods will not be reviewed here. Some examples of applications of quality control methodology in neuro-fMRI can be found in Chap. 28 of this volume. CONSTABLE et al. (1995), LANGE et al. (1995), XIONG et al. (1996) and LANGE et al. (1998) employ receiver-operating characteristic curves in their comparisons of a wide variety of activation detection methods for neuro-fMRI; GENOVESE et al. (1997) propose applications of test-retest reliability procedures. These works and the references therein provide a full, current background to readers interested in this important aspect of neuro-fMRI statistics.

27.2.3
Preprocessing

From the perspective of an MR physicist, clinician, engineer or computer scientist, the majority of procedures described in this chapter may comprise what to him/her is neuro-fMRI "post-processing." At present, aspects of neuro-fMRI research are not clearly separated; lines drawn for convenience differ by researcher background and viewpoint in this highly multi-disciplinary field. The term "preprocessing" in this chapter refers to operations performed on neuro-fMRI data after signals in k-space have been reconstructed in image space by Fourier methods, prior to their statistical analysis. Preprocessing issues and methods could occupy a small chapter in their own right. Some salient points and procedures will be discussed only briefly here.

Perhaps the most prevalent preprocessing procedure for neuro-fMRI data, if not the most important and feasible issue, involves realignment of image volumes to correct for rigid body motions of the subject's head while in the magnet. A similar yet actually quite different problem of this type involves the "warping" or "deformation" of an individual subject's anatomical MRI brain volume to a template, reference brain volume (e.g., TALAIRACH and TOURNOUX 1988). Stimulus correlated motion (HAJNAL et al. 1994; BULLMORE et al. 1998)) is also a major potential problem in neuro-fMRI data analysis, in studies of schizophrenic subjects for instance. Surface matching methods (e.g., PELIZZARI et al. 1989) and landmark-based methods developed for MR, CT, SPECT and PET applications have given way in neuro-fMRI to global, automatic methods requiring little operator assistance and few subjective judgments and interactions. The automated image registration (AIR) of WOODS et al. (1992, 1993) is one such method. AIR's statistical objective is to minimize the sampling coefficient of variation of ratios of voxel values between successive fMR images, or between the first image and each successive image. For each pair of fMR image volumes, AIR computes ratios

$$r_{tv} = y_{tv} / y_{t'v} \qquad (27.1)$$

for two different time points $t \neq t'$ over all voxels $v = 1,\dots,V$. The coefficient of variation is itself a ratio of standard deviation to mean, namely:

$$\theta_t = \bar{r}_t^{-1} \left[\sum_{v=1}^{V} \left(r_{tv} - \bar{r}_t \right)^2 / (V-1) \right]^{1/2}$$

where $\bar{r}_t = \sum_{v=1}^{V} r_{tv} / V$. Since it should not matter which voxel value at either time point is numerator or denominator in the ratio of Eq. 27.1, AIR seeks to minimize the average coefficient of variation $(\theta_t + \theta_{t'})/2$ where, for $\theta_{t'}$, $r_{t'v} = y_{t'v}/y_{tv}$. This seems a reasonable criterion by which to minimize the dif-

ferences in two images due to rigid body motion, yet perhaps a logarithmic variance-stabilizing transformation could improve the overall performance of the method. In further and more recent work (Woods et al. 1998a,b), different cost functions, different minimization methods, and various sampling, smoothing, and editing strategies were compared, with brain phantoms for PET and structural MRI, not neuro-fMRI. As expected, linear or nonlinear automated inter-subject registration of PET and MRI data from 22 healthy subjects produced more accurate alignment of homologous landmarks than manual nine-parameter Talairach registration. Nonlinear models provided better registration than linear models but were of course slower, indicating the expected tradeoff of speed against accuracy.

An alternative yet related method (LANGE 1994) parametrizes an estimate $\hat{y}_{t'v}$ of y_{tv} in terms of $y_{t'v}$ by a set of unknown constants that quantify changes in voxel values due to rigid body motion. The method operates on the spatial coordinates themselves in addition to the voxel values at the spatial coordinates. This approach has been developed by FRISTON et al. (1995a) for the registration of PET and fMR images and by ASHBURNER et al. (1997) to determine the affine transformation[1] that best maps a brain volume to a template image in a standard space, as mentioned previously. These are simpler instances of general deformable template methods, developed by GRENANDER (1970), AMIT et al. (1991), and MILLER et al. (1993, 1997), and are described here in two spatial dimensions only. By writing voxel subscript v as a 2-D vector $\mathbf{v} = (v_1, v_2)^T$ so that $\mathbf{y}_t[\mathbf{v}] = \mathbf{y}_{tv}$ and $\mathbf{y}_t[\mathbf{v}'] = \mathbf{y}_{t'v'}$, this slight change of notation emphasizes the dependence of voxel values in the two images on their spatial coordinates. Consider the simple equation:

$$\hat{\mathbf{y}}_t[\mathbf{v}] = \mathbf{y}_{t'}[\mathbf{A}\mathbf{v}' + \mathbf{b}] \cdot c + d \qquad (27.2)$$

which expresses an estimate of the image at time t in terms of the image at time t' and unknown constants $\mathbf{A}, \mathbf{b}, c, d$. In Eq. 27.2, rotation matrix

$$\mathbf{A} = \begin{bmatrix} \cos\alpha & -\sin\alpha \\ \sin\alpha & \cos\alpha \end{bmatrix}$$

---

[1] A transformation $\mathbf{T}$ of vectors $\mathbf{x}$ in the euclidean plane to other vectors $\mathbf{y}$ in the plane is affine if there is an invertible 2×2 matrix $\mathbf{A}$ and a vector $\mathbf{b}$ in the plane such that for every vector $\mathbf{x}$ in the plane, $\mathbf{y} = \mathbf{T}\mathbf{x} = \mathbf{A}\mathbf{x} + \mathbf{b}$

captures in-plane rotations and involves a single angle α, parameter $\mathbf{b} = (b_1, b_2)^T$ accounts for in-plane translations, and parameters c and d account for differences in voxel values due to changes in scale and level respectively. Note that the parametric representation of the rigid body motion is nonlinear: a main component of Eq. 27.2, the $\mathbf{Av}' + \mathbf{b}$ part, is a transformation of the pixel coordinates themselves and not of the pixel values at the coordinates.

In addition to spatial registration of images, another body of statistical preprocessing procedures involves estimation and correction of physiological fluctuation in fMR images. By monitoring respiration and heart beat simultaneously during fMR image acquisition, and then synchronizing these two data sets retrospectively, such physiological effects can be estimated and removed (see, for instance, Hu et al. 1995; Le and Hu 1996). Through fitting truncated Fourier series (see Sect. 27.3.1.3), the statistical procedures in the cited literature are performed in k-space and assume quasi-periodic physiological signal structure in order to be effective. Observed fMR signal improvements in neuro-fMRI summary maps from a visual stimulation study are modest (see, for example, Fig. 10 of Hu et al. 1995). Greater artifacts in fMR summaries due to physiological fluctuations may occur in subcortical and cerebellar structures.

27.3
A Plurality of Analyses

Some readers may be of the skeptical initial opinion that "If you can't see it in the data, then statistics can't help you, and if you can see it in the data, then you don't need statistics!" Yet, in this familiar conundrum, what exactly is meant by "seeing" an effect in a collection of functional neuroimages? By classical definition, a statistic is any function of the data, and this definition implies that to "see" an effect one always employs some statistic, such as a mean, variance, maximum, minimum, correlation coefficient and coefficient of variation, or more subjective measures such as degree of belief and prior probability. A statistical procedure is defined here as any effectively computable rule or algorithm that combines data and assumptions as input to yield a result, an output that we can "see." This broad definition includes closed-form computations (e.g., linear and Gaussian random field models; Sect. 27.3.1.5), simulations (e.g., Monte Carlo and deterministic mathematical models), genetic algorithms, and iterative

or recursive reuse of previous outputs as current inputs to form cascading series of results. Given the infinite number of statistical procedures that combine data and assumptions to yield statistics, essential features of useful and effective statistical models for functional brain imaging include parsimony – an application of Occam's razor to arrive at simplicity without becoming simplistic – and elegance. One cannot avoid making assumptions when interpreting experimental data. Statistical models help to make implicit assumptions explicit so that they can be discarded, enlarged and refined.

Other readers who already see the utility of statistical procedures for neuro-fMRI perhaps feel that there may exist a single "best" statistical procedure for the analysis of a particular neuro-fMRI study. While it is indeed true that in a particular context some statistical procedures are better than others, it is nearly always the case that many different procedures apply equally well. This is particularly true in the present stage of development of neuro-fMRI methods and analyses of their results. During the beginnings of the presently highly developed and regulated field of controlled clinical trials, no predominant mode of analysis was adopted across the field. Yet, from the advent of the Cox proportional hazards model (Cox 1972) onward, one sees a progressively more uniform and effective statistical treatment of clinical trials data. One can perhaps anticipate development of such a unifying statistical approach in our field, but it appears too far off to speculate at present regarding what future form statistical procedures for neuro-fMRI will take.

Thus, in the meantime and perhaps well into the future, one may best adopt an attitude toward statistical procedures for neuro-fMRI that is pragmatic, pluralistic and empirical: pragmatic in that one judges the effectiveness of a statistical procedure for neuro-fMRI according to its consequences in application, pluralistic in that multiple perspectives are supported and encouraged by denying that any single statistical procedure or computer program can fully "explain" neuro-fMRI data, and empirical in that all supposed "facts" about the neuro-fMRI signal are regarded as hypotheses to be tested in a changing and rapidly evolving research environment.

Design and construction of statistical procedures for neuro-fMRI and comparative evaluation of their performance usually involves some form of prediction. One way to assess predictive performance is to estimate the "generalization ability" of the method, that is, how well a statistical procedure performs on an entirely new set of neuro-fMRI data examples (called a test set) after having been constructed and tuned using previous, similar examples (called a training set). Some form of bias/variance tradeoff is required in order to avoid too much variance, or overfitting, on the one hand, and too much bias, or underfitting, on the other. Such a bias/variance tradeoff is a type of statistical model selection. For a fixed number of neuro-fMRI examples, bias/variance tradeoffs within families of statistical procedures relate to their complexities: if a statistical procedure is too simple it is biased and makes systematic prediction errors, whereas if it is too complex it will make unreliable, highly variable predictions. An additional and somewhat complementary way of assessing predictive performance is to fix procedural complexity and to graph generalization error as a function of training set size. This produces a "learning curve," a generally decreasing function. Constructing learning curves for two statistical procedures of different complexity enables a comparison: when learning curves cross, one procedure outperforms the other for small vs large numbers of examples. Neuro-fMRI researchers, in general, seem to favor simple yet not simplistic approaches that have good predictive performance as measured in these two ways.

27.3.1
Parametric Methods

Parametric methods dominate the current world of neuro-fMRI statistical procedures. In general, the parametric methods described in this section all attempt to determine the value of an index, i.e., a parameter, that identifies a particular member among a large parametric family of plausible probability distributions that could have generated the neuro-fMRI data, i.e., a model. The identifying index for a particular neuro-fMRI study is often not a single number but is instead a small collection of numbers: a parameter is often a vector or a matrix and not simply a scalar. In this section, the reader will see many practical examples of parameters and the neuro-fMRI data distributions they identify.

27.3.1.1
General Linear Model

The most frequently occurring parametric statistical procedures in current neuro-fMRI literature employ linear methods. While for some researchers

"linearity breeds contempt," the general linear model is used so often because it works so well in a wide range of applied areas. Its application often results in closed-form, i.e., noniterative, adequate solutions to complex problems (see, for instance, BOYNTON et al. 1996; COHEN 1997). It is noted that the term "linear," as used in statistics and as used here, almost invariably applies not to images, on the left-hand side of the regression equation, but to parameters, on the right-hand side: a linear model is linear in its parameters. In statistical modeling, "linear" generally implies "additive" and "Gaussian," the latter term referring to the familiar bell-shaped curve or error function:

$$\mathrm{erf}(x, \mu, \sigma) = 1 / \left(\sqrt{2\pi}\sigma\right) \cdot \exp\left[-(x - \mu / \sigma)^2 / 2\right]$$

with mean (location) μ and variance (scale) σ^2, two parameters that uniquely identify members of this parametric family of probability distributions.

Perhaps the simplest linear procedure employed in neuro-fMRI is the linear model underlying Student's two-sample t statistic and simple correlation analyses. The two-sample problem in neuro-fMRI involves a binary reference function $\mathbf{x}$, which takes on only two values according to whether the controlled stimulus is *off* or *on*. For simplicity, binary reference function $\mathbf{x}$ is "centered" so that its components sum to zero. One can also assume for simplicity that each neuro-fMRI time series $\mathbf{y}_v$ has been centered so that its components also sum to zero. Such centering in no way diminishes the generality of the approach to be described. Computation of Student's two-sample t statistic as a summary of the neuro-fMRI signal at each voxel may be defined by the collection of simple linear regression models:

$$y_{tv} = x_t \beta_v + \varepsilon_v \tag{27.3}$$

for time points $t = 1, ..., T$, at brain locations $v = 1, ..., V$. The models at Eq. 27.3 are regressions through the origin that involve an unknown scalar slope parameter β_v and no intercept parameter. In vector form, these models are:

$$\mathbf{y}_v = \mathbf{x}\beta_v + \boldsymbol{\epsilon}_v \tag{27.4}$$

where β_v remains an unknown parameter to be estimated at each voxel and where $\boldsymbol{\epsilon}_v$ is a vector of T independent and identically distributed, mean-zero Gaussian errors with assumed common variance σ_v^2 at each voxel yet with potentially different variances across voxels. The least-squares regression estimate of β_v is the simple linear combination of xs and ys given by:

$$\hat{\beta}_v = \sum_{t=1}^{T} x_t y_{tv} / \sum_{t=1}^{T} x_t^2$$
$$= \mathbf{x}^T \mathbf{y}_v / \mathbf{x}^T \mathbf{x}. \tag{27.5}$$

The predicted value of the neuro-fMRI time series is:

$$\hat{\mathbf{y}}_v = (\hat{y}_{v1}, \dots, \hat{y}_{vT})^T$$

where

$$\hat{y}_{tv} = x_t \hat{\beta}_v.$$

Residual differences between observed and predicted values provide a corresponding estimate of error variance σ_v^2 given by:

$$\hat{\sigma}_v^2 = \sum_{t=1}^{T} (y_{tv} - \hat{y}_{tv})^2 / (T-1). \tag{27.6}$$

Estimated error variances are the average squared vertical distance from the predicted values to the observed data.[2] An estimate of the uncertainty in the mean parameter estimate employs estimated error variance, namely:

$$\hat{\text{var}}(\hat{\beta}_v) = \hat{\sigma}_v^2 / \sum_{t=1}^{T} x_t^2. \tag{27.7}$$

Expressing $\hat{\beta}_v$ in units of its standard deviation yields Student's familiar pooled two-sample t statistic:

$$t_v = \hat{\beta}_v / \hat{\text{se}}(\hat{\beta}_v)$$

where:

$$\hat{\text{se}}(\hat{\beta}_v) = \sqrt{\hat{\text{var}}(\hat{\beta}_v)} \tag{27.8}$$

The probability distribution for t_v is a Student's t distribution on $T-1$ degrees of freedom (subtract 1 from the number of time points for estimating β_v) and not a Gaussian distribution because, essentially, σ_v^2 has been estimated and plugged in. Thus, simple linear regression of each observed neuro-fMRI time

series on a binary regressor $\mathbf{x}$, with different variances at each voxel but equal residual variances at off and on states, is equivalent to Student's pooled two-sample t test.

A little further algebra shows that Student's t is equivalent to Pearson's product-moment estimate in simple correlation analysis by the relationship:

$$\hat{\varrho}_v = k_{1v} \hat{\beta}_v = k_{2v} t_v$$

where: $k_{1v} = \left[\left(\sum_{t=1}^{T} x_t^2 \right) / \left(\sum_{t=1}^{T} y_{tv}^2 \right) \right]^{1/2}$ is the ratio of reference function and time series standard deviations and $k_{2v} = \hat{\sigma}_v / \left(\sum_{t=1}^{T} y_{tv}^2 \right)^{1/2}$ is the ratio of residual and time series standard deviations. One can also show that:

$$t_v = \hat{\varrho}_v \left[(T-2) / (1 - \hat{\varrho}_v^2) \right]^{1/2}$$

(MONTGOMERY and PECK 1982, pp 47–48; LANGE 1996; COHEN 1997).

The estimated standard error $\hat{\text{se}}(\hat{\beta}_v)$, from Eq. 27.8, is the unit of measurement for $\hat{\beta}_v$. As such, $\hat{\text{se}}(\hat{\beta}_v)$ can be used to construct a confidence interval for the true value $\hat{\beta}_v$ of neuro-fMRI signal magnitude. For instance, the interval:

$$\left[\hat{\beta}_v - t_{T-1}^{(\alpha/2)} \cdot \hat{\text{se}}(\hat{\beta}_v), \quad \hat{\beta}_v + \tau_{T-1}^{(\alpha/2)} \cdot \hat{\text{se}}(\hat{\beta}_v) \right] \tag{27.9}$$

covers $\hat{\beta}_v$ with probability $1-\alpha$, where $t_{T-1}^{(\alpha/2)}$ is the $100 + (\alpha/2)$th percentile of Student's t distribution on $T-1$ degrees of freedom. When $\alpha = 0.05$, the interval given by Eq. 27.9 has 90% coverage probability. Emphases in the neuro-fMRI literature to date have been more on hypothesis tests and p-values than on confidence intervals, which are their inversion (see, for instance, FISHER and VAN BELLE 1993, pp. 138–43). It is highly likely that confidence intervals will play a more central role in future neuro-fMRI statistics as researchers becomes less concerned with the transformation of complex brain signals into binary summaries (e.g., by thresholding a summary statistical image of $\hat{\beta}_v$s for instance), resultant p-values and the like. Future neuro-fMRI may be more concerned with measuring and modeling properties of the neuro-fMRI signals themselves, asking not only "is there activity at this brain location in response to stimuli?" but also, "*how much* activity is there?"

The preceding development has shown two things: that three apparently different statistical pro-

---

[2] The available degrees of freedom, being equal initially to the number of time points before any model is fit, is decreased by 1 for estimation of the mean $\hat{\beta}_v$ in order to make the resulting estimate "unbiased," so that, on average, through repetitions of the experiment, the estimand equals the true value of the parameter, in this case σ_v^2.

cedures for binary block study designs (simple regression through the origin on a binary covariate, Student's t and Pearson's ϱ) are in fact equivalent, and that all three may be inadequate. The simple linear regression model makes assumptions that may not be valid for neuro-fMRI time series, namely: (1) that the serial observations are independent of one another, (2) that their common error distribution is Gaussian, (3) that there are equal variabilities about averages in off and on states, and (4) that these averages are adequate descriptive constants for summary of local neuro-fMRI signal behavior. The importance and correction of potential mismatches of model to data are addressed in following sections of this chapter.

By thinking of each neuro-fMRI time series as a finite sequence of discrete elements, model (4) employs three closely associated linear vector spaces: an image or outcome space (represented symbolically by $\mathbf{y}_v$), a design space ($\mathbf{x}$) and a parameter space (β_v). By thinking of neuro-fMRI time series as continuous curves in time and space, methods for functional data analysis in (infinite dimensional) Hilbert space apply (see Sect. 27.2.2). Some intuition for the geometry of finite-dimensional vector spaces and of least squares projection in particular is depicted in Fig. 27.1. The regression involves a single parameter β for a single voxel v (suppressed for notational simplicity). A neuro-fMRI time series $\mathbf{y}$ may be imagined as a single point Y in T-dimensional euclidean space. Any particular value of parameter β^* defines a vector of fitted values $\mathbf{x}\beta^*$, which is another point Y^* in that same space. As β ranges over all of its possible values, $\mathbf{x}\beta$ traces out a linear subspace, a locus of possible predictions, which in this one-dimensional case consists of all points on a line through origin O in direction $\mathbf{x}$. No value of β reproduces the data exactly; a model is only a model. Parameter β can also be thought of as a direction, in that it gives the direction from vantage point Y in which the data are projected onto line $\mathbf{x}$. The point on $\mathbf{x}$ nearest $\mathbf{y}$ is found by dropping a perpendicular $Y\hat{Y}$ onto $\mathbf{x}\beta$, an orthogonal projection. The coordinates of point $\hat{Y}$ are the vector $\mathbf{x}\hat{\beta}$ where $\hat{\beta}$ is the least-squares solution given by Eq. 27.5. The vector $Y\hat{Y} = \mathbf{y}-\mathbf{x}\hat{\beta}$ is the residual vector in the residual or error space populated by differences between observed and expected images.

The orthogonality of vectors $O\hat{Y}$ and $Y\hat{Y}$ is expressed algebraically as $\mathbf{x}^T(\mathbf{y}-\mathbf{x}\hat{\beta}) = 0$, which indeed implies that $\hat{\beta} = \mathbf{x}^T\mathbf{y}/\mathbf{x}^T\mathbf{x}$ (see Eq. 27.5). Further insight into least-squares geometry can be gained through inspection of triangle $Y\hat{Y}Y^*$. The

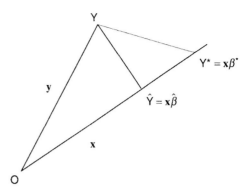

Fig. 27.1. Least squares geometry for a single parameter. (Adapted from McCULLAGH and NELDER 1989, p. 72)

Pythagorean theorem in T dimensions applied to triangle $Y\hat{Y}Y^*$ shows that:

$$(\mathbf{y} - \mathbf{x}\beta^*)^T(\mathbf{y} - \mathbf{x}\beta^*) = (\mathbf{y} - \mathbf{x}\hat{\beta})^T(\mathbf{y} - \mathbf{x}\hat{\beta}) + (\hat{\beta} - \beta^*)\mathbf{x}^T\mathbf{x}(\hat{\beta} - \beta^*)$$

$$(27.10)$$

As a function of $\hat{\beta}^*$, the left-hand side of Eq. 27.10 is a parabola whose minimum is achieved at $\hat{\beta}^* = \hat{\beta}$. The second derivative of the parabola at its minimum is $\mathbf{x}^T\mathbf{x}$. When scaled by units of error variance σ^2, the quantity $\mathbf{x}^T\mathbf{x}/\sigma^2$ is known as the Fisher information[3] for parameter β, being the reciprocal of the variance of $\hat{\beta}$ given at Eq. 27.7. All of the preceding geometric observations generalize to linear vector spaces of $P>1$ dimensions. In a way, simple or "ordinary" least squares regression, as depicted in Fig. 27.1, is to statistics what the on/off block design is to neuro-fMRI.

The general linear model takes the following scalar form:

$$y_{tv} = x_{1t}\beta_{v1} + x_{2t}\beta_{v2} + \dots + x_{Pt}\beta_{vP} + \varepsilon_{tv} \qquad (27.11)$$

for $t = 1,\dots,T$, $v = 1, \dots ,V$, and $1 \leq P \leq T$ measured covariates. In Eq. 27.11, the xs are values of factors assumed to have some effect on y_{tv}, such as the stimuli themselves, which can be thought of as the first few factors (the order of the xs is irrelevant), detrending factors such as sine and cosine waveforms (HOLMES et al. 1997), and background covariates such as cardiopulmonary and other

---

[3] The geneticist and statistician R. A. Fisher, the inventor of analysis of variance (ANOVA) and for whom the F test is named, developed many of the theoretical and applied statistical procedures employed in neuro-fMRI and many other modern scientific areas.

physiological measures that change with time. Those covariate values that do not change with time can simply be repeated as constants across time. This is the case for a constant mean term for overall level, which is often encoded as $x_{1t} = 1$ for all t. As a rule of thumb, the number of degrees of freedom available for hypothesis tests and construction of confidence intervals in each voxel-specific regression is equal to the number of data points (T) minus the number of estimated parameters (P) minus the number of constraints. Dimension P of the parameter space varies by how the design matrix is constructed and by conventions on how its associated parameter values are constrained so that a unique solution to the linear system exists. Detailed descriptions of the general linear model and its uses can be found, for instance, in DRAPER and SMITH (1966); MONTGOMERY and PECK (1982); SEBER (1977); FRISTON et al. (1995); FRISTON (1996); MAYHEW et al. (1998), and will not be repeated here. Current neuro-fMRI researchers advocate the use of linear systems models, while checking assumption validity, as more powerful alternatives to simplistic t statistics, probability levels and correlation coefficients.

As in Fig. 27.1 for a single parameter, the general linear model captures important image and signal structure through discovering informative projections of originally high-dimensional image data onto linear subspaces of lower dimension. For each voxel, if parameter dimension P equals outcome dimension T, then nothing has been gained by the model besides an ineffectual one-to-one swap of data points for estimated parameters. However, an economical representation of image signal structure has been found for small P and large T if the least-squares distance between observed and expected images defined at Eq. 27.6 is sufficiently small. Such residual error distance can be made artificially small by increasing P arbitrarily through addition of extra design terms that bear no actual relation to images. Vector space geometry guarantees that overly complex predictions will always be closer to actual values than predictions based on fewer covariates. Considerable skill is required to find an optimal parameter dimension P and its associated covariates in design space that does not miss important structure (minimal bias) yet is not too complicated (minimal variance). This is an example of the bias/variance tradeoff described in the beginning of this section. Such thinking motivates one interpretation of a p-value for choosing between design space dimensions P–1 and P by asking the question: Are the chances small enough (e.g., $p<0.05$) that the model has

"spent" available resources wisely, in terms of increasing or decreasing design space dimension, by including or excluding this additional covariate and thus improving predictions?

The general linear model, as its name suggests, covers a very broad range of possibilities, including analysis of variance (ANOVA) methods as special cases. For instance, in one-way, two-way, ..., k-way ANOVAs, all covariates x_{tP} are indicator variables that encode levels of factors and their interactions. Analysis of covariance (ANCOVA) is also a special case of the general linear model. For instance, when a single continuous covariate is included among factor-level indicators and their interactions, the effects of these factors are estimated as if a simpler linear model that includes only the continuous covariate is fit first, and then the full ANOVA model is fit next to residuals $y_{tv}-\hat{y}_{tv}$ from the first regression without the continuous covariate, for all time points and voxels.

An equivalent vector form for the model of Eq. 27.11 is:

$$\mathbf{y}_v = \mathbf{x}_1\beta_{v1} + \mathbf{x}_2\beta_{v2} + ... + \mathbf{x}_P\beta_{vP} + \boldsymbol{\epsilon}_v$$

where $\mathbf{x}_p=(x_{p1},...x_{pT})^T$ for all p and $\boldsymbol{\epsilon}_v=(\varepsilon_{1v},...,\varepsilon_{Tv})^T$ for all v. More compactly:

$$\mathbf{y}_v = \mathbf{X}\boldsymbol{\beta}_v + \boldsymbol{\epsilon}_v \qquad (27.12)$$

where $\mathbf{X}=(\mathbf{x}_1,...,\mathbf{x}_P)$ is the $T{\times}P$ matrix formed by concatenating covariate vectors across columns and $\boldsymbol{\beta}\hat{v}=(\beta_{v1},...,\beta_{vP})^T$ is the P-vector formed by concatenating parameters. A fully compact matrix form of the general linear model is:

$$\mathbf{Y} = \mathbf{XB+E} \qquad (27.13)$$

where $\mathbf{Y}$ is the original fMR image matrix, $\mathbf{B}=(\boldsymbol{\beta}_1,...,\boldsymbol{\beta}_V)$ is the $P{\times}V$ matrix formed by concatenating parameter vectors across columns, and likewise for $\mathbf{E}=(\boldsymbol{\epsilon}_1,...,\boldsymbol{\epsilon}_V)$. Assumptions identical to those for the model of Eq. 27.3 apply in equivalent Eq. 27.13: it is assumed that mean function $\mathbf{XB}$ is adequate and thus that errors $\mathbf{E}$ have expectation zero, that these errors are Gaussian and independent, with equal variance across time at the same voxel yet potentially different variances across different voxels.

The linear vector space projections introduced earlier can also be expressed compactly when using Eq. 27.13. Namely, the estimated element of the parameter space is given succinctly by the expression:

$$\hat{\mathbf{B}} = \left(\mathbf{X}^T\mathbf{X}\right)^{-1}\mathbf{X}^T\mathbf{Y} \qquad (27.14)$$

provided that $(\mathbf{X}^T\mathbf{X})^{-1}$ exists. Note that Eq. 27.14 is equivalent to Eq. 27.5) when $\mathbf{X}=\mathbf{x}=(x_1,...,x_T)^T$. Using linear operator theory, one can show that the variance-covariance matrix for $\hat{\boldsymbol{\beta}}$ is:

$$\mathrm{var}\!\left(\hat{\mathbf{B}}\right)=\left(\mathbf{X}^T\mathbf{X}\right)^{-1}\mathbf{x}\;\mathrm{diag}\!\left(\boldsymbol{\sigma}^2\right) \tag{27.15}$$

where $\mathbf{x}$ denotes Kronecker's product and $\mathrm{diag}(\boldsymbol{\sigma}^2)$ is a $V\mathbf{x}V$ diagonal matrix with $\boldsymbol{\sigma}^2=(\sigma_1^2,...,\sigma_V^2)$ along its diagonal.[4] It is thus seen that if errors $\mathbf{E}$ are serially independent, so that $\mathrm{diag}(\boldsymbol{\sigma}^2)$ is an adequate error structure, then $(\mathbf{X}^T\mathbf{X})^{-1}$ has diagonal elements that are proportional to the variances of parameter estimates $\hat{\mathbf{B}}$, and off-diagonal elements that are proportional to the covariances between parameter estimates. Predicted neuro-fMRI images are:

$$\hat{\mathbf{Y}}=\mathbf{X}\hat{\mathbf{B}}=\mathbf{X}\left(\mathbf{X}^T\mathbf{X}\right)^{-1}\mathbf{X}^T\mathbf{Y}=\mathbf{H}\mathbf{Y}$$

and the estimated residuals are:

$$\hat{\mathbf{E}}=\mathbf{Y}-\hat{\mathbf{Y}}=(\mathbf{I}-\mathbf{H})\mathbf{Y}$$

Matrix $\mathbf{H}$ is a projection operator possessing some very useful properties (see, for instance, MONTGOMERY and PECK 1982). For an excellent yet accessible further development of general linear model theory along these lines, see Seber (1977).

Patterned Variance-Covariance Matrices. While the assumptions for the general linear model permit a very flexible range of mean functions $\mathbf{XB}$, they induce some restrictions on allowable patterns for variance-covariance matrices associated with image matrix $\mathbf{Y}$. Patterned variance-covariance matrices play an important role in the development of all of the statistical models for neuro-fMRI space-time series in the following sections of this chapter. A variance-covariance matrix $\boldsymbol{\Sigma}$ for the model of Eq. 27.13 is of dimension $TV+TV$ and consists of a diagonally symmetric and positive semi-definite arrangement of non-negative elements.[5] Variance terms populate the diagonal of $\boldsymbol{\Sigma}$ and covariances populate its off-diagonal elements. The most restrictive pattern for $\boldsymbol{\Sigma}$ sets all of its diagonal elements σ_v^2 to σ^2 for all v, and sets all off-diagonal elements to zero. This unrealistic and overly restrictive pattern, governed by a

single parameter σ^2, records an assumption of error distribution equality (no v subscript) and independence (off-diagonal elements zero) across both time and space. The least restrictive pattern for $\boldsymbol{\Sigma}$ is a completely arbitrary yet symmetric and positive semi-definite matrix involving $TV(TV+1)/2$ parameters. A statistical model for neuro-fMRI space-time series employs a variance-covariance matrix whose complexity, in terms of parameter dimension, places it somewhere in between these two extremes. Just as Occam's razor helps find a compromise between bias and variance for complexity of the mean function $\mathbf{XB}$, so too does this principle of parsimony aid the neuro-fMRI model builder in choosing one patterned $\boldsymbol{\Sigma}$ over another.

A less restrictive pattern allows error variances to differ across voxels and arranges σ_v^2 parameters along the diagonal of $\boldsymbol{\Sigma}$ in groups of length T starting with the first voxel, second voxel, and so forth. Such verbal descriptions quickly become unwieldy. The direct sum operator provides a convenient notation for describing $\boldsymbol{\Sigma}$.[6] The previous variance-covariance matrix is written as $\boldsymbol{\Sigma}=\boldsymbol{\Sigma}_1\oplus...\oplus\boldsymbol{\Sigma}_V$, where each $\boldsymbol{\Sigma}_v$ is a diagonal matrix with σ_v^2 repeated along its diagonal, or $\boldsymbol{\Sigma}_v=\mathrm{diag}/\sigma_v^2,...,\sigma_v^2)$ and requires exactly V free parameters. However, consider a simple binary block design in which the mean function $\mathbf{XB}$ appears to change under the stimulus condition and, in addition, that underlying signals exhibit greater residual variability about their means during stimulation. A common σ_v^2 and the previous $\boldsymbol{\Sigma}_v$ across all time points for activating voxels would be inadequate. One would perhaps do better by modeling two variances to reflect this behavior, σ_{0v}^2 corresponding to baseline time points and σ_{1v}^2 corresponding to stimulation time points, with a constraint that $\sigma_{1v}^2>\sigma_{0v}^2$.

Non-zero off-diagonal $\boldsymbol{\Sigma}$ elements within blocks capture temporal autocorrelation across time points. Non-zero elements between blocks capture spatial autocorrelation across voxels. One may enlarge the range of choices for possible $\boldsymbol{\Sigma}$s by modeling patterns of temporal autocorrelation explicitly (see Sect. 27.3.1.2 on time series methods). One may enlarge possibilities further through similar explicit pattern modeling for spatial autocorrelations (see Sect. 27.3.1.5 on random field models). Judicious selection of patterned $\boldsymbol{\Sigma}$ matrices is a major aspect of

---

[4] The Kronecker product of $a\times b$ matrix $\mathbf{A}_1$ and $c\times d$ matrix $\mathbf{A}_2$ is the $ac\times bd$ matrix $\mathbf{A}_3=\mathbf{A}_1\mathbf{x}\mathbf{A}_2$ in which each element of $\mathbf{A}_1$ is replaced by a matrix which is the element's scalar product with $\mathbf{A}_2$
[5] Matrix $\boldsymbol{\Sigma}$ is positive semi-definite if $\mathbf{u}^T\mathbf{S}\mathbf{u}\geq 0$ for all non-zero vectors $\mathbf{u}$.

[6] The direct sum of two $T\times T$ matrices $\mathbf{A}_1$ and $\mathbf{A}_2$ is defined as the $2T\times 2T$ block-diagonal matrix $\mathbf{A}_3=\mathbf{A}_1\oplus\mathbf{A}_2$ obtained by lining up $\mathbf{A}_1$ and then $\mathbf{A}_2$ as blocks along a common diagonal and filling off-diagonal blocks with zeroes.

statistical procedures for neuro-fMRI analysis and in some cases can be as important as modeling the mean function. As noted in the Introduction, the total amount of data variance is split by a statistical model into components deriving from specified mean and variance-covariance functions, that is, between signal and noise. Similar to the way that the σ_v^2 terms at the beginning of this section were seen to affect the magnitudes of Student t statistics and correlation coefficients, the choice of patterned variance-covariance matrix is important because its elements affect estimates of neuro-fMRI mean function summaries derived from the general linear model.

Smoothing. Various modifications of the general linear model, beyond the generality supported by Eq. 27.13, appear in current neuro-fMRI literature. An important class of modifications involves application of a smoothing operator on both sides of regression Eq. 27.13 (e.g., MAYHEW et al. 1998):

$$KY = K(XB+E)$$

where matrix K is a known convolution matrix (see Sect. 27.3.1.6), to form another linear model:

$$\mathbf{Y}_K = \mathbf{X}_K \mathbf{B}_K + \mathbf{E}_K \tag{27.16}$$

Comparison of the models of Eqs. 27.13 and 27.16 reveals that smoothing by K induces autocorrelation in the variance-covariance matrix S_K for the noise term E_K. Off-diagonal elements associated with temporal and/or spatial error covariances that were previously zero are now no longer zero. In essence, the presence of such autocorrelations reduces the number of effective degrees of freedom available for hypothesis tests (see Sect. 27.3.1.2 on time series models and Sect. 27.3.1.6 on modeling brain physiology for more on this point). In addition, the smoothed least-squares estimate:

$$\hat{\mathbf{B}}_K = \left(\mathbf{X}_K^T \mathbf{X}_K\right)^{-1} \mathbf{X}_K^T \mathbf{Y}_K$$

is biased. If the actual model is not Eq. 27.16 but is Eq. 27.13 instead, then, on average, $\hat{\mathbf{B}}_K \neq \mathbf{B}$. Whether to smooth or not to smooth is another instance of the bias/variance tradeoff: Adding a little bias (by smoothing) may achieve a favorable decrease variance and may therefore yield mean function estimates that are more interpretable. In a pair of articles, ZARAHN et al. (1997) and AGUIRRE et al. (1997) compare and contrast unsmoothed and smoothed analyses of neuro-fMRI data using the

general linear model and thresholds of random fields (see Sect. 27.3.1.5). Parameter estimation and hypothesis testing for the model of Eq. 27.16 is discussed in detail by WORSLEY and FRISTON (1995), correcting and expanding on earlier related work (FRISTON et al. 1995d).

27.3.1.2
Univariate Time Series Models

A natural domain of statistical procedures for neuro-fMRI is the large body of sophisticated methods developed for the analysis of univariate time series. A spatial ensemble of neuro-fMRI time series can be analyzed in two stages: first by time and then by space. That is, one can first treat each neuro-fMRI time series $y_v, v = 1,...V$, independently, even though they are spatially dependent, and then accommodate spatial autocorrelations among the collection of univariate series by analysis and modeling of residuals. The present section deals solely with statistical procedures for such first-stage analyses (see Sect. 27.3.1.5 and Sect. 27.3.1.6 for the second stage spatial component). The applied statistical literature on the analysis of time series is enormous; BOX and JENKINS (1976) is a classic; DIGGLE (1990) is an accessible biostatistical introduction to many central ideas which will be addressed only briefly here.

A general aim of time series methods in the analysis of neuro-fMRI data is to discover time trends in the presence of serial dependence – temporal autocorrelation – under an assumption of stationarity, or, equivalently, time invariance. The mean function of a general linear model as defined in the preceding section is equivalent to a trend in a time series. Temporal autocorrelation implies that voxel values in the same location and nearby in time tend to be alike, so that y_{tv} and $y_{t'v}$ are similar when their temporal lag $u = |t-t'|$ is small. Of course, series values at the same brain location and nearby each other in time may be similar due to the mean function of the process. Accommodation of temporal autocorrelation in a statistical model refers not to its systematic mean function component but instead to its random error component after the mean function has been removed.

Formally, the autocovariance function $\varrho(u,t,\lambda)$ of the time series may depend on lag u, on time t, and on some parameter λ to be estimated. Errors in the general linear model were assumed to be independent and identically distributed; the autocovariance function was zero. Independent Gaussian noise is "white"; temporally autocorrelated noise is "colored": "correlation" is "coloration." Assuming (second-order) stationarity means that the auto-covariance function of the time series depends only on lag u and not on time t: once temporal trend has been removed, the time series looks the same at whatever point one chooses to observe it. It is perhaps fair to say that observed time series are rarely, if ever, truly perfectly stationary in this sense and that assumptions of time invariance are made on primarily pragmatic grounds.

An example of coloration, stationarity and non-stationarity is found in a simple random walk at brain location v given by:

$$y_{tv} = y_{t(v-1)} + z_{tv} \qquad (27.17)$$

for $t = 1,\dots,T$, where noise z_{tv} has mean zero and variance σ_v^2 for all t; that is, z_{tv} is white noise. Successive values in the series are clearly correlated in this example of a non-stationary, autoregressive integrated moving average (ARIMA) process (Box and Jenkins 1976). Realizations of this random walk will appear to possess time trends when in fact no trends are present. Taking first-order differences of its successive terms transforms the series into a stationary time series. Such differencing can be expressed compactly through use of backshift operator B:

$$(1 - B)y_{tv} = z_{tv} \qquad (27.18)$$

where $By_{tv} = y_{t(v-1)}$ is equivalent to Eq. 27.17 without the error term. More generally, higher-order polynomial differencing on both sides of Eq. 27.18 can be expressed succinctly as:

$$\phi(B)y_{tv} = \theta(B)z_{tv} \qquad (27.19)$$

where $\phi(B)$ and $\theta(B)$ are polynomials of order p and q, respectively. For instance, if $\theta(B) = 6+5B+B^2$, then $\theta(B)z_{tv} = 6z_{tv}+5z_{t(v-1)}+z_{t(v-2)}$. Putting Eqs. 27.18 and 27.19 together, one defines an ARIMA(p,d,q) process as:

$$\phi(B)(1 - B)^d y_{tv} = \theta(B)z_{tv}$$

where d is the number of times the series need to be differenced to yield a stationary series (e.g., first-order differences, second-order differences of differences, etc.). Thus, the simple random walk (Eq. 27.18) is an ARIMA(0,1,0) process with $\phi(B) = \theta(B) = 1$.

One way to determine differencing order d is to plot the partial autocorrelation function (PACF) of the series against lag. The PACF at lag u is defined as Pearson product-moment correlation between shifted residual time series after removal of the non-stationary mean function and lower-order lags by least-squares regression as defined in the previous section. For instance, the random walk $(1-\varrho)y_{tv} = z_{tv}$ yields a significant PACF coefficient equal to ϱ at lag 1 only and not at any higher lags. Bullmore et al. (1996a) use the PACF method in their analysis of neuro-fMRI time series collected during periodic visual and auditory stimulation. In order to correct for AR(1) errors once identified, these authors used a adjustment technique (Cochrane and Orcutt 1949) that applies the general linear model to shifted versions of the image and design matrices of the model of Eq. 27.13 given by:

$$\mathbf{Y}_B = (1 - \varrho B)\mathbf{Y}$$

and

$$\mathbf{X}_B = (1 - \varrho B)\mathbf{X}$$

where ϱ is the first-order autoregressive coefficient estimated from the PACF analysis, and where B is understood to apply element-wise to each series (see the original work, or, for instance, Montgomery and Peck 1982, pp 347–360). Even though the preceding transformation of image and design space depends on the unknown parameter ϱ, regressions of form $\varepsilon_{tv} = \varrho\varepsilon_{tv-1}+z_{tv}$ are regressions through the origin, as those in Eq. 27.3, so that ordinary least-squares methods apply. A test that residuals from these regressions are indeed white (Durbin and Watson 1950, 1951; Box and Pierce 1970) should be applied and the method iterated if necessary. The iteration may not always be successful, in part because the estimate of ϱ is lower on average than the true value (biased). If a few iterations do not produce white noise, then perhaps the frequency domain methods discussed in Sect. 27.3.1.6 of this chapter should be employed. Tagaris et al. (1997) provide an example of an ARIMA model analysis of neuro-fMRI time series which includes detailed decision tree guidelines to procedural stages of Box-Jenkins intervention analysis. Box-Jenkins intervention analysis seeks to determine whether reference function $\mathbf{x}$, the intervention, has a significant effect on the time series, with the pre-intervention series being the baseline series void of stimuli. These authors find that effects which appear statistically significant by simple Student's t tests vanish under these more sophisticated and realistic time series methods.

There is a duality between trend and serial dependence which is sometimes overlooked and which is often resolved through assuming, either explicitly or implicitly, that the mean function is "smooth" while the error function is "rough." Such splits between smooth and rough time series components are similar to compromises made by the general linear model, yet now under autocorrelated error structures. Resolution of this duality clearly depends on the scale at which the series are observed. Temporal smoothing as a preprocessing step in neuro-fMRI data analysis carries with it such an assumption.

Temporal autocorrelation, whether induced by smoothing or inherent in the unprocessed series themselves, inflates the variance of the mean function estimator relative to the variance of the least-squares estimator from the general linear model. This fact implies, in several following realistic examples, that a simple Student t statistic computed under an independence assumption will be larger than it should be and that the neuro-fMRI researcher will deem "significant" some observed effects which are actually no different from noise. Consider a simple example of the effects of autocorrelated errors in time series y_v having mean function equal to the series average. That is, let $y_{tv}=b_v+\varepsilon_{tv}$, so that $x_t=1$ for all t. From Eq. 27.5 $\hat{\beta}_v=\bar{y}_v=\sum_{t=1}^{T}y_{tv}/T$. If var$(y_{tv})=s_v^2$ and if errors are independent, then, from Eq. 27.7, var $\hat{\beta}_v=\sigma_v^2/T$. Now suppose that errors are exponentially autocorrelated according to an autocorrelation function given by:

$$\varrho(u,\lambda) = \exp(-\lambda u) \tag{27.20}$$

which says that autocorrelation between values ε_{tv} and $\varepsilon_{t'v}$ decreases monotonically proportional to a fixed value λ as lag u increases. This correlation does not affect the value of the mean function estimator, yet its variance now becomes $k \cdot \text{var}(\hat{\beta}_v)$, where:

$$k = 1 + \sum_{u=1}^{T-1}(T-u)\exp(-\lambda u),$$

which is a factor clearly greater than one. In fact, when $T = 100$ and $\lambda = 1.0$, the variance of $\bar{y}_v$ is about twice as large as that under independence, and when $\lambda=0.5, 0.2, 0.1$, variances are inflated by factors of 4, 10 and 18, respectively. On the standard error scale, such variance inflation due to temporal autocorrelations yields Student t statistics that are roughly 2, 3 and 4 times larger than they should be, respectively, producing falsely "significant" results that can be seriously misleading.

For the more complex and realistic general linear model $\mathbf{Y}=\mathbf{XB}+\mathbf{E}$ with autocorrelated errors and equally spaced time points, almost invariably the case in neuro-fMRI, the mean function estimator remains equal to Eq. 27.14, yet its variance is incorrect because variance-covariance matrix $\mathbf{\Sigma}$ is no longer diagonal. Introduction of the autocorrelation function $\varrho(u,\lambda)$ at Eq. 27.20 enables a variety of low-dimensional parametrizations of the variance-covariance matrix for image matrix $\mathbf{Y}$ that expand patterns possibilities beyond those described previously in the general linear model section. Specifically, instead of spending $(T-1)^2/2$ additional parameters to move from a diagonal $\mathbf{\Sigma}_v$ that requires independent errors to an arbitrary $\mathbf{\Sigma}_v$ that allows all manner of possible autocorrelations among neuro-fMRI time series elements, one can spend only one additional parameter to define the patterned variance-covariance matrix for $y_v, v=1,...,V$, as:

$$\Sigma(\lambda_v) = [\sigma_{tt'}(\lambda_v)] \tag{27.21}$$

where

$$\sigma_{tt'}(\lambda_v) = \begin{cases} \varrho(u,\lambda_v) \cdot \sigma_v^2 \text{ when } t \neq t' \\ \sigma_v^2 \text{ otherwise.} \end{cases}$$

Such a model as in Eq. 27.21 for non-zero, off-diagonal elements can express many useful patterns of temporal autocorrelation, where lag u is now seen to indicate distance from the matrix diagonal. For instance, letting $\varrho(u,\lambda_v) = \lambda_v$ for all lags gives rise to a "compound symmetric" or "exchangeable" pattern in which all errors are equally correlated regardless of their temporal separation. The AR(1) process of the simple random walk possesses autocorrelation function $\varrho(u,\lambda_v) = \lambda_v^u$ in which correlations die off geometrically as temporal separation increases. Two additional parametric forms are the previous exponential autocorrelation function $\varrho(u,\lambda) = \exp(-\lambda u)$, which dies off rapidly nearby $u = 0$, and its Gaussian cousin $\varrho(u,\lambda_v) = \exp(-\lambda_v u^2)$ which decreases less sharply at the origin. This is one of the methods employed by Lange and Zeger (1997) described in the next section. The empirical distribution of simulated Student's t statistics for a linear time trend under the exponential autocorrelation model is much more "heavy tailed," i.e., more spread out, than the theoretical yet incorrect t distribution under independence (Diggle 1990, pp. 92–93). Such evidence suggests that the same pattern of variance inflation under autocorrelated errors as that known exactly in the simpler, constant mean case.

27.3.1.3
Analyses in the Frequency Domain

A special case of the general linear model with autocorrelated errors involves statistical procedures whose design space is spanned by covariates that are sines and cosines, the simple trigonometric functions employed in the discrete Fourier transform (DFT) of the neuro-fMRI signal. Trigonometric bases are useful when reference function $\mathbf{x}$ is periodic and/or when there are quasi-periodic background effects to be removed from the analysis. The following is a simple development of the DFT of a univariate time series as a statistical "harmonic regression" model.

Recall that the general linear model at a single voxel v is of the following form:

$$y_{tv} = c_{0t}w_{v0} + c_{1t}w_{v1} + \ldots + c_{(P-1)t}w_{v(P-1)} + \varepsilon_{tv} \quad (27.22)$$

for $t=0,\ldots,T-1$. The xs of Eq. 27.11 are replaced by cs, bs by ws, and the index starts at 0 instead of 1 for reasons that become clear in what follows and further in Sect. 27.3.1.6. At present, reference function $\mathbf{x}$ is not included as one of the covariates. When $P=T$, the model is "saturated," swapping data points $y_{tv}, t = 0,\ldots,T-1$ for estimated parameters w_{vp}, $p = 0,\ldots,T-1$, and the error term vanishes. If one is willing to assume that covariates c_{pt} exhibit regular, periodic behavior over time that can be expressed by simple trigonometric functions, one can define complex-valued covariates:

$$c_{pt} = \cos(\omega_p t) + i \sin(\omega_p t) \quad (27.23)$$

for $t = 0,\ldots,T-1$ where $i = \sqrt{-1}$ and where $\omega_p = 2\pi p/T$ are integer-valued Fourier frequencies at which the sines and cosines are orthogonal to one another (hence the "i") . If the signal oscillates with period T, then all other components besides those in Eq. 27.23 vanish, and $p = 1$ corresponds to the fundamental signal frequency and $p = 2,3\ldots$ corresponds to its higher-order harmonics. Aliasing due to discrete sampling of the neuro-fMRI signal limits consideration of frequencies within the range $0 \leq \omega_p \leq \pi$.[7] The complex number representation enables a compact expression of this trigonometric basis as:

$$c_{pt} = \exp(i \omega_p t)$$

(Note that when one multiplies two complex numbers together one simply multiplies amplitudes and adds angles, exactly what one does when multiplying two exponentials.) In addition, re-express parameters ω_{vp} as $\phi_v(\omega_p)$ to emphasize the dependence of these coefficients on Fourier frequencies ω_p. Hence, with this notation, the present, saturated case of the general linear model with periodic covariates becomes:

$$y_{tv} = \sum_{p=0}^{T-1} \phi_v(\omega_p) \exp(i \omega_p t) \quad (27.24)$$

in which $\phi_v(w_p)$ are Fourier coefficients at Fourier frequencies w_p. These coefficients are an exact one-to-one swap for data points (e.g., Bloomfield 1976; Bracewell 1986):

$$\phi_v(\omega_p) = \sum_{t=0}^{T-1} y_{tv} \exp(-i \omega_p t) \quad (27.25)$$

The DFT is fully invertible: one can pass easily from the original temporal domain of Eq. 27.24 to the frequency domain of Eq. 27.25 and back again with ease and little computational burden.

In the frequency domain, series magnitudes at each frequency are given by the empirical power spectrum, empirical spectral density, or periodogram (all equivalent terms) of the signal whose ordinates are given by:

$$I_v(\omega_p) = \phi_v^2(\omega_p) / \sum_{p=0}^{T-1} \phi_v^2(\omega_p)$$

Plots of $I_v(\omega_p)$ against frequency, one plot for each voxel v arranged in a spatial grid corresponding to a brain region of interest, yield spectral-spatial displays which are paired with corresponding temporal-spatial displays of the time courses themselves, as, for instance, in the early neuro-fMRI work of Bandettini et al. (1993). Frequency domain plots can in many cases yield representations that are more compact than their time domain counterparts. The DFT of a narrow function is a broad function, and vice versa. Periodograms exhibit sharp peaks at those Fourier frequencies that carry dominant periodic signal components and are very useful in suggesting forms for statistical models of neuro-fMRI space-time processes (see Sect. 27.3.1.6).

In addition to providing compact representations of neuro-fMRI signals, the DFT can also simplify certain integrations, convolutions in particular, that are useful in statistics. For instance, consider two

---

[7] Instead of expressing covariates c_{pt} as complex numbers initially, as in Eq. 27.23, some authors instead write Eq. 27.22 as a sum over pairs of terms $a_{vp}\cos(\omega_p t)+b_{vp}\sin(w_p t)$ that range over only one-half of the time points. The approaches are identical since $w_{vp}=a_{vp}-ib_{vp}$.

samples $\mathbf{x}=(x_1,...,x_T)$ and $\mathbf{y}=(y_1,...,y_T)$ with sample means $\bar{x}_T$ and $\bar{y}_T$ and DFTs denoted by:

$$d_x\left[\omega_p\right]=\left[d_x(\omega_1),...,d_x(\omega_p)\right]$$

and

$$d_y\left[\omega_p\right]=\left[d_y(\omega_1),...,d_y(\omega_p)\right]$$

respectively. Consider the convolution summation given by:

$$C_{xy}(u)=\sum_{0\leq t, t-u\leq T-1}\left(x_t-\bar{x}_T\right)\left(y_{t-u}-\bar{y}_T\right) \qquad (27.26)$$

at lags $u=0,\pm1,\pm2,...$ in the time domain. As discussed by BRILLINGER (1975), the DFT of $C_{xy}(u)$ becomes the multiplication:

$$d_c(\omega,u)=d_X(\omega)d_Y^*(\omega)\exp(i\omega h')$$

where the asterisk denotes complex conjugation. This result shows, for instance, that in lieu of shifting the two series and calculating correlations at all lags to compute the partial autocorrelation function (PACF) of Sect. 27.3.1.2, one can instead use the inverse DFT:

$$C_{xy}(u)=\sum_{p=0}^{S-1}d_X\left(\omega_p\right)d_Y^*\left(\omega_p\right)\exp\left(i\omega u'\right)/S \qquad (27.27)$$

for $u'=0,\pm1,\pm2,...(S-T)$ and some integer $S>T$ to obtain the PACF in a much more expedient manner. Equation 27.27 can also be very useful for estimating sample moments, such as Pearson product-moment correlation, and ordinary least-squares regression of Sect. 27.3.1.1.

There is an additional advantage of working with neuro-fMRI time series in the frequency domain concerning temporal autocorrelation. Autocorrelated errors in the time domain become approximately independent errors in the frequency domain with different variances at the Fourier frequencies. This means that one can diagonalize an arbitrary variance-covariance matrix for a statistical model by re-expressing the model in the frequency domain and thus, potentially, model $(T-1)^2/2$ fewer parameters while incurring only slightly more computational cost (see Sect. 27.3.1.6 for some examples).

27.3.1.4
Longitudinal Data Analysis

Longitudinal data consist of series of scalar- or vector-valued measurements recorded repeatedly over time for each of a moderate to large number of subjects. Biostatistical applications usually involve large numbers of short time series, e.g., blood pressure measurements over several successive days from 100 or more subjects in a multi-center controlled clinical trial. Longitudinal studies are in contrast to cross-sectional studies, in which data are available at only a single point in time, such as in FDG PET studies. Classical ^{15}O[water] PET studies are examples of highly multivariate longitudinal studies involving short time series and more than a handful of subjects. Neuro-FMRI space-time series are a somewhat atypical instance of longitudinal data since the typical number of subjects studied currently is very small, the time series are lengthy and the dimension of vector-valued measurements is very large, being equal to the number of imaged brain voxels. When neuro-fMRI time series are treated not as individual time points but instead as spatially correlated samples of related curves, methods of functional data analysis apply (see Sect. 27.2.2).

Longitudinal data analysis (LDA) for neuro-fMRI is relatively underdeveloped at present yet can be expected to grow as neuro-fMRI methods move into clinical contexts. This is not to say that statistical tools for LDA are not employed in neuro-fMRI. On the contrary, existing neuro-fMRI literature contains rudimentary applications of these techniques, consisting of simple two-stage derived variable procedures which date at least from WISHART (1938). In a two-stage, derived variable procedure, data reduction at stage I is followed by data aggregation at stage II. In stage I, the researcher fits his/her statistical model of choice, applied voxel-by-voxel or perhaps to neuro-fMRI time series aggregated regionally into functional-neuroanatomic sets, to yield a small number of summary statistics for each series. Examples of summary statistics include regression slope estimates in an instance of general linear model (Eq. 27.13) that correspond to the controlled reference function(s) and a few interesting discrete factors and continuous covariates, and/or statistical summaries from a time series model accommodating autocorrelated errors. The stage I model is applied separately for each subject. Although these low-dimensional summaries in current neuro-fMRI often consist only of mean-function effects estimates, there is no reason why an individual subject's variance and covariance summaries could not also be carried along into the next stage. Stage II then combines individual subject summary statistics across subjects by use of a new model to arrive at a statistical conclusion that is applicable not only to an individual subject but also to the population of subjects to which he/she belongs.

Recent work by Courtney et al. (1997) provides an example of such a two-stage, derived variable LDA. These researchers first fit an ANCOVA model to each of eight subjects' neuro-fMRI time series in a regional analysis that included contrasts between non-selective visual stimulation vs no stimulation and memory vs control tasks (face-selective vs memory-delay regressors). Each of three mean-function parameter estimates from this multiple regression model were normalized by their sum and the resulting derived variables fed into a three-way ANOVA for a between-subjects aggregation and summary that included region, hemisphere and regressor as discrete factors along with their interactions. If this entire process were to be repeated across a number of separate fMR imaging occasions, as in a crossover drug trial or long-term learning or plasticity study, then an appropriate stage II model could perhaps be a classical repeated measures ANOVA. Statistical procedures for neuro-fMRI in this context could thus be termed "hyper-longitudinal" since they would involve repeated imaging occasions, each with a lengthy within-subject longitudinal component, for moderate to large numbers of subjects. The important point here is that a stage I "micro-level" model is fit at the individual level and these results are aggregated across individuals by a stage II "macro-level" model. Consistency of patterns in functional brain activity so aggregated, if any, enables the stage II model to "borrow strength" across people and thus to enrich statistical conclusions. Similar borrowing strength methods are developed for combinations of many small studies by meta-analysis (see Sect. 27.4, which discusses this topic briefly). Methods of LDA enable study of changes over time, in particular the brain changes induced by controlled temporal stimuli, for both the individual and the population(s) of study subjects.

A common way to formalize the preceding notion of borrowing strength across people in two-stage procedures for neuro-fMRI studies is to employ a particular class of LDA methods known as random effects models (Laird and Ware 1982; Lange and Laird 1989; Lange and Ryan 1989; Diggle et al. 1994). Consider a region of interest neuro-fMRI study involving T time points, repeated measures y_i for subjects $i = 1,...,N$, and some reference function x whose values increase over time, so that a simple Student's t test is inapplicable. Common voxel subscript v is suppressed for simplicity, being replaced by a subscript i for individuals. Although not strictly

necessary, the number of time points and their spacings are assumed to be shared by all subjects, again for simplicity, in a "balanced and complete" design with common $T \times 2$ individual design matrix $X = [1x]$, where 1 is the T-vector of ones corresponding to an individual intercept parameter, and where x corresponds to an individual slope parameter. Generalizations of the following development exist when $X_i \neq X$ for all subjects (see, for instance, Laird et al. 1987). Interest thus centers on individual intercept and slope estimates from the simple linear regression model:

$$y_i = X\beta_i + \epsilon_i$$

for $i = 1,...,N$, where $\beta_i = (\beta_{0i}, \beta_{1i})^T$ are individual intercepts and slopes, respectively, and where errors ϵ_i are assumed to be independently and identically distributed as Gaussian random variable with mean zero and common variance σ^2. Summary statistics from each stage I regression are the vectors $\hat{\beta}_i = (\hat{\beta}_{0i}, \hat{\beta}_{1i})^T$ and estimated error variances $\hat{\sigma}_i^2, i =,...,N$, as in Eq. 27.6.

Random effects for individuals enter in the stage II aggregation step when one assumes that study subjects have been drawn from a larger population of individuals who share unobserved factors. Represent these unobserved factors by latent variables δ_i that are common to all repeated measurements from each individual yet which vary across subjects, inducing correlation among repeated responses. Latent variables δ_i for the present example are interpreted as random individual offsets, i.e., individual intercepts and slopes, to common population trajectories. Formally, one assumes that:

$$\beta_i = \beta + \delta_i$$

where the δ_i are drawn from a common bivariate Gaussian distribution with mean 0 and variance-covariance matrix Δ. This assumption induces the following linear model:

$$y_i = \beta + X\beta_i + \epsilon_i \qquad (27.28)$$

with patterned variance-covariance matrix:

$$\text{var}(y_i) = X\Delta X^T + \sigma^2 I \qquad (27.29)$$

possessing common between-subjects variance component Δ and common within-subject variance component σ^2. Note that the presence of design term X in Eq. 27.29, not present in previous variance-covariance patterns, suggests that the neuro-fMRI researcher's choice of experimental design can emphasize the importance of either intercept or slope terms by minimizing respective variances of their estimates, a point developed in detail for this model by Lange and Laird (1989).

Note also that one is able to generalize the common mean function parameter β in Eq. 27.28 by absorbing this constant as a common intercept effect in a between-subjects design matrix that enables estimation of additional covariate effects such as age, sex, handedness, etc. That is, define between-subjects design matrix $Z_i = [A_i X]$ to contain covariate values A_i and the common X and replace β in Eq. 27.28 by $Z_i \alpha$ to write:

$$y_i = Z_i \alpha + X \beta_i + \epsilon_i \qquad (27.30)$$

for $i=,...N$. In the present case, the model of Eq. 27.30 is termed a "growth curve" model with fixed effects a when the design space spanned by the between-subjects matrix Z_i contains the design space spanned by the within-subject matrix X. Such growth curve models support the following natural interpretation: the study population "tracks" across time according to parameter a, which contains group effects for age, sex, handedness, etc., as in the general linear model, and individual trajectories across time are given by random offsets β_i to the population trajectories.

One final point concerns incorporation of serial autocorrelation in LDA, a feature not accommodated by the model of Eq. 27.30. A richer patterned variance-covariance matrix such as:

$$\text{var}(y_i) = X \Delta X^T + \Sigma(\lambda) + \sigma^2 I$$

in which $\Sigma(\lambda)$ arises from autocorrelation function $\varrho(u,\lambda)$ discussed at Eq. 27.20 and Eq. 27.21. Such extended models, applicable to lengthy neuro-fMRI time series aggregated across subjects, are described, for instance, by Azzalini (1987) and Diggle et al. (1994), as well as the state-space approach developed by Jones (1993). It seems reasonable to predict that, as neuro-fMRI research increases its average numbers of subjects per study and moves more fully into the clinical realm, growth curve models and other forms of random effects models such as those described here will occupy a more central role in statistical procedures for neuro-fMRI.

27.3.1.5
Thresholds of Random Fields

In preceding sections, neuro-fMRI time series at different brain locations have been treated separately. In this section, spatial autocorrelations among summary statistics at different voxels, such as Student's two-sample t statistic, are accommodated by thinking of these numbers as constituting a random field defined over space. The innovative work of Friston et al. (1991), Worsley et al. (1992, 1993) and Poline and Mazoyer (1993) in PET, building on the earlier theoretical work of Adler (1981), Adler and Hasofer (1976) and Hasofer (1978), has led over recent years to extensions and refinements of these procedures to neuro-fMRI (see, for instance, Friston et al. 1994b; Worsley 1994; Forman et al. 1995; Worsley and Friston 1995; Poline et al. 1997b; Cao et al. 1997). Summaries for the Gaussian case are provided by Friston (1996), Lange (1996) and Rabe-Hesketh et al. (1997) and will not be repeated here. Brain activity as measured by neuro-fMRI can be rendered graphically as rising swells in a choppy (noisy) sea whose undulations possess intrinsic smoothness (and roughness) modeled as a Gaussian random field. A small Gaussian random field is a 3×3 voxel patch whose intensities are governed by random variables that follow a nine-dimensional multivariate Gaussian distribution that is correlated spatially by a 9×9 variance-covariance matrix. As alternatives to overly conservative Bonferroni corrections for multiplicity, mathematically and statistically sophisticated methodologies now exist to ensure that p-values attached to spatial regions of suspected activity evoked by controlled stimuli are approximately correct through adjustments for spatial autocorrelations under a wide variety of situations.

27.3.1.6
Modeling Brain Physiology

Neuro-fMRI researchers very often direct their attention to substantive considerations involving underlying brain physiology and hemodynamics (e.g., Friston et al. 1994a, 1995c; Hu et al. 1995; Kim et al. 1997; Lange and Zeger 1997; Le and Hu 1996; Mitra et al. 1997; Richter et al. 1997). Aspects of brain physiology affecting neuro-fMRI signals involve local hemodynamic delays and cardiopulmonary processes and are not yet fully understood (Villringer and Dirnagel 1995; see chapters 1,

22, and 23 in the present volume for more detailed treatment of this aspect of neuro-fMRI research). Effects of cardiopulmonary processes were mentioned in Sect. 27.2.3, on preprocessing. Regarding local hemodynamic delays, many view the neuro-fMRI signal as a convolution of an unobservable hemodynamic response function (HRF) and reference function **x**, a very reasonable assumption. Equation 27.26 gave one example of a convolution when dealing with correlations of time-shifted series. When local neuronal activity is initiated by the controlled stimulus, the brain region requires an increased supply of fresh oxygenated blood to continue its work. Oxygenated blood is delayed by the transit time through the cerebral vasculature to a degree that depends on how far it has traveled from the site of flow regulation (LEE et al. 1995). The process that controls this supply is governed by hemodynamic responses that are not directly observable in humans. This fresh supply may actually cover a region in the brain wider than the activation site, by a process likened to "watering the entire garden for the sake of a single flower bed" (R. Turner). The HRF limits the temporal resolution of neuro-fMRI time series, defined as the time between two separable tasks. KIM et al. (1997) found that without averaging repeated trials of the same task, a sequence of four single-finger movements with an execution time of approximately 2 s can be resolved when the delay time between consecutive sequences is at least 3 s. With averaging and by allowing for variable delay time in a similar series of experiments, this resolution could be reduced to 2 s.

Further improvements in effective temporal resolution can be gained by increasing B_0 field strength and/or using event-related, single trial neuro-fMRI experimental designs, as mentioned in Sect. 27.2.1. These considerations of effective temporal resolution show that, even though neuro-fMRI time series may be nominally very lengthy, involving hundreds of time points, these series may be effectively very short. As pointed out by THOMSON (1982), a short series is one in which the resolution required is of the same order as the reciprocal of series length. If the true spectrum is complex, the number of time points in short series may still be large. Thomson cautions further that added complexities arise when the spectra themselves are mixed, as they are in neuro-fMRI. In an important paper, MITRA et al. (1997) find that changes in the neuro-fMRI signal evoked by a simple visual stimulus in a single-trial neuro-fMRI experiment at 4.0 Tesla possess complex spatio-temporal structure. After motion suppression (Sect. 27.2.3),

these authors employ singular value decomposition (Sect. 27.3.4.2), Slepian multi-taper methods, (being discrete prolate spheroid sequences; see SLEPIAN and POLLACK 1961; THOMSON 1982, 1995; PERCIVAL and WALDEN 1993), and narrow-band frequency projections to concentrate empirical power of the neuro-fMRI spectra within a narrow frequency band of 0–0.2 cycles/s (Hz). These authors find two frequency domain transfer functions, which are akin to HRFs in the time domain, operating coherently at two different frequencies in two distinct spatial regions in visual cortex, and, in addition to cardiopulmonary fluctuations, find vasomotor oscillations in neuro-fMRI signals at about 0.1 Hz having complex spatio-temporal structure.

Convolution of reference function **x** with a voxel-specific HRF $\lambda_v = (\lambda_{v1}, ..., \lambda_{vT})$ results in a smoothed version of the reference function denoted by $\mathbf{x} \otimes \lambda_v$, with $\otimes$ denoting convolution. Each HRF λ_v may have a temporal delay that varies with spatial location and hence the smoothed reference function also may vary spatially. FRISTON et al. (1994a) employed a spatially invariant global λ modeled as a Poisson density; BULLMORE et al. (1996a) also estimated global hemodynamic delay by a phase-shifted sine wave in a trigonometric regression model. Yet from the preceding comments, both the delay and the dispersion of the HRF depend on location, and neuro-fMRI time series models need to take account of this fact. Toward this end, the HRF may be modeled parametrically as a two-parameter gamma density (LANGE and ZEGER 1997):

$$\lambda_v\left(\alpha_v, \gamma_v\right) = \gamma_v\left(\gamma_v t\right)^{\alpha_v - 1} \exp\left(-\gamma_v\right) / \Gamma\left(\alpha_v\right) \qquad (27.31)$$

where $\Gamma(\alpha_v)$ is Euler's gamma function. Voxel-specific shape and scale parameters, α_v and γ_v, respectively, identify each member of this flexible parametric family at each spatial location. The expectation of each gamma density is α_v / γ_v, a quantity having direct interpretation as a voxel-specific neuro-fMRI signal delay.

One way to model hemodynamic effects on the neuro-fMRI signal in the time domain is through the following convolution model (LANGE and ZEGER 1997):

$$\mathbf{y}_v = \left(\mathbf{x} \otimes \lambda_v\right)\beta_v + \boldsymbol{\epsilon}_v \qquad (27.32)$$

where λ_v is from Eq. 27.31 and thus the design term is the result of the convolution summation of reference function **x** with HRF λ_v. Parameter β_v quantifies the magnitude of the delayed signal. Error terms $\boldsymbol{\epsilon}_v$

are temporally and spatially autocorrelated with other errors nearby in time and space. The model of Eq. 27.32 is fit in the frequency domain by use of a DFT(see Sect. 27.3.1.2). Representation in the frequency domain enables autocovariance functions at each Fourier frequency included in the block-diagonal variance-covariance matrix of the residuals to be modeled separately. Random field models for patterns in spatial autocovariance functions can be discerned through inspection of residual images, one image for each Fourier frequency, as discussed in Sect. 27.3.1.2, yet spatially instead of temporally (LANGE and ZEGER 1997). The parametric gamma density convolution model has been compared with a finite impulse response convolution model that accounts for HRFs nonparametrically (NIELSEN et al. 1997).

Blocked vs Rapid Mixed Trials. Furthering the work of BUCKNER et al. (1996), DALE and BUCKNER (1997) assumed validity of the linear systems assumption common to convolution models, such as that given by Eq. 27.32. As employed previously, this assumption states that the neuro-fMRI signal is well-approximated by the convolution of an experimentally controlled condition $e(t)$ and an unobservable hemodynamic response function $h(t)$, written simply as $s(t)=e(t)\otimes h(t)$. The temporal resolution of the commonly used blocked designs for $e(t)$, for instance repeated cycles of a series of off condition images followed by a series of on condition images, are limited by $h(t)$. Therefore, one customarily spaces the repeated images far apart by choosing a long, fixed time to repetition (TR). Yet such a long inter-stimulus interval limits the possible number of images collected, approaching the smaller number of neuroimages recorded in PET studies in some cases. A way around this limitation is to try to deconvolve a series of rapidly mixed trials collected with variable inter-stimulus intervals. DALE and BUCKNER (1997) demonstrated initial success with such an approach, in which an apparently bimodal $h(t)$ in two trials spaced 5 s apart was separated into two functions of nearly identical shape. Some evidence of stationarity was thus provided, yet the second $h(t)$ possessed a slight undershoot not present in the first. For further work on event-related, single-trial neuro-fMRI, see BIRN et al. (1998); FRISTON et al. (1998a,b).

Models for effects of brain physiology and hemodynamics can contain further substantive components. The disproportionate change in cerebral blood flow (CBF) and cerebral oxygen metabolic rate

(CMRO$_2$) observed in PET studies, on the order of 30%–50% changes for CBF compared with only 5% changes for CMRO$_2$, has been interpreted as an uncoupling of flow and oxidative metabolism (Fox and RAICHLE 1986). This is to say that the increase/decrease in blood flow exceeds the increase/decrease in oxygen consumption due to increases/decreases in neuronal activity. This feature may be the brain's way of maintaining oxygen availability and not uncoupling in the strict historical sense as it was once meant. The phenomenon could arise from a nonlinear coupling or recoupling with a different gain, yet there have been too few studies and too few data points in existing studies to use parametric curve-fitting to detect subtle nonlinearities. BUXTON and FRANK (1997) argue that because MR signal changes measured in neuro-fMRI by long time-to-echo (TE) of 30–50 ms to accentuate T_2^* sensitivity depends of relative changes on CBF and CMRO$_2$, stating that "*any* [italics added] quantitative interpretation of neuro-fMRI data requires, first, a theory of the physiological relationship between CBF and CMRO$_2$ changes during neural stimulation." Because the implications of their statement affect the potential relevance of much statistical preprocessing of neuro-fMRI data (Sect. 27.2.3), it is important to study in more detail the physiological model put forth by these authors to account for coupling/uncoupling phenomena.

In a series of related papers, BUXTON and Frank (1993, 1997) and BUXTON et al. (1997) suggest that the large imbalance of CBF and CMRO$_2$ changes reflects a tight coupling due to limited availability of fresh oxygen. These authors support their claim by citing evidence from the literature suggesting that: (1) CBF increases reflect increased flow velocity rather than capillary recruitment, so that all brain capillaries are assumed to be perfused, and (2) there is a small rate of return of unmetabolized O$_2$ from brain tissue to the capillary bed, so that oxygen metabolism in the brain is assumed to be highly efficient. The decrease in total capillary O$_2$ concentration $C_T(t)$ is assumed to be proportional to plasma O$_2$ concentration $C_p(t)$ as governed by the differential equation:

$$dC_T(t)/dt = -kC_p(t) \qquad (27.33)$$

Equation 27.33 implies simple exponential decay when $C_p(t)/C_T(t)$ is constant and when all capillaries have the same transit time. The overall oxygen extraction fraction E is the extraction fraction for transit time t averaged against $h(t,\theta)$, the distribution of transit times:

$$E(\theta) = \int_0^\infty E_t(t) h(t,\theta) dt, \qquad (27.34)$$

where $E_t(t) = [C_T(0) - C_T(t)]/C_T 0$. In Eq. 27.34, BUXTON and FRANK (1997) assumed $h(t,\theta)$ to be a gamma density, as in Eq. 27.31 yet without formal accommodation of spatial variability, so that $\theta = (\alpha, \gamma)$ indexed pairs of shape and scale parameters. In order to investigate the sensitivity of the extraction fraction to choice of h, these authors fixed α and varied γ so that $h(t,\theta)$ took on various approximate functional shapes (exponential, Weibull, Gaussian). They found that only the exponential form ($\alpha = 1$), which they felt to be unlikely physiologically, appeared to deviate from the simple model of the relationship between oxygen extraction fraction and CBF implied by Eq. 27.33 when the extraction fraction is high and percent flow decreases. Solving Eq. 27.33 for k in terms of local cerebral blood flow f yielded:

$$E(f) = 1 - (1 - E_0)^{f_0/f} \qquad (27.35)$$

for which E_0 and f_0 are boundary values for extraction fraction and flow, respectively, at time $t = 0$. BUXTON and FRANK (1997) noted that an assumption of exponential transit times is equivalent to assuming a one-compartment model of blood exchanges between capillaries and tissue.

That the exponential assumption is unlikely appears to be at some odds with its adoption by BUXTON et al. (1997) in their development of a "balloon" model to accommodate the initial stimulus "dip," "overshoot" and post-stimulus "undershoot" observed. The dip in particular is controversial; some researchers claim it can be seen only at high field (≥ 3.0 Tesla); others deny its existence. Taking the exponential assumption at face value, BUXTON et al. (1997) assumed that blood oxygen level-dependent (BOLD) signal changes arise from predominantly venous blood changes with both extra- and intravascular components (BOXERMAN et al. 1995; OGAWA et al. 1993) as a function of two time-dependent quantities, $q(t)$ and $v(t)$, the total local tissue deoxyhemoglobin and the venous blood volume, respectively. They model the venous compartment as an expandable balloon fed downstream by the output of the capillary bed whose volume changes when compartment input and output are mismatched. Compartment pressure increases until a new steady-state equilibrium is reached. Balloon expansion depends on the pressure/volume curve of the compartment. Assuming a well-mixed compartment, i.e., common exponential transit time, gave rise to the following pair of differential equations:

$$\begin{cases} \dfrac{dq}{dt} = \left[f_{\rm in}(t) \dfrac{E[f_{\rm in}(t)]}{E_0} - f_{\rm out}(v) \dfrac{q(t)}{v(t)} \right] / t_0 \\ \dfrac{dv}{dt} = [f_{\rm in}(t) - f_{\rm out}(v)] / t_0. \end{cases} \qquad (27.36)$$

Assumed tight coupling between flow and oxygen extraction enables $E[f_{\rm in}(t)]$ to be well approximated by Eq. 27.35. Equation 27.36 shows the extreme sensitivity of the assumed system on initial conditions E_0, the extraction fraction, t_0, the mean transit time through the venous compartment, and with respect to different pressure/volume curves as represented by $f_{\rm out}$. Indeed, through small perturbations in these components BUXTON et al. (1997) demonstrated that a wide variety of time-activity curve shapes observed in neuro-fMRI can be obtained from their model.

27.3.2
Functional Data Analysis

A newly emerging area in statistics is the field of functional data analysis (FDA) (RAMSAY and SILVERMAN 1997). The spirit of this line of statistical research is to think of observed neuro-fMRI time series $y_v = (y_{1v},...,y_{Tv})^T$, $v = 1,...,V$, as single entities rather than as merely a sequence of individual observations. The term "functional" in this context refers to the intrinsic structure of the data rather than their explicit form, although for neuro-fMRI the term is quite apt. In practice, the observed data are discretely sampled versions of true underlying continuous functions. If these discrete values are assumed falsely to be errorless, then conversion of raw data points to true functional form involves interpolation; otherwise, one employs smoothing techniques to remove observational errors that cause the data to be rougher than the true functions (see, for instance, GREEN and SILVERMAN 1994; HASTIE and TIBSHIRANI 1990; RAMSAY and SILVERMAN 1997). That is, one posits a model:

$$y_{tv} = f(\tau, v) + \varepsilon_{tv}$$

where $f(\tau, v)$ is a latent function defined on the tensor product domain $\Pi = (\tau, v)$, where τ represents time (moment at which activity at the brain location is sampled) and v represents space (location in the brain). The sampling rate or temporal resolution of the observed data, whose limits arise from constraints on the duration for which the magnetic gradient coils of the imaging device can run their duty cycles continuously, is a key determinant of what is possible in FDA above what is already available through existing statistical procedures. Another determinant of what FDA can do lies in the local curvature of the functions themselves, defined as the second temporal derivative of $f(\tau,u)$. Where curvature is high, it is essential to have enough data points to estimate the function effectively, where "enough" depends on errors ε_{tv}. For instance, for study of the previous balloon model and shape of the HRF in Sect. 27.3.1.6, data should be acquired at the most rapid rate the gradient coils will allow. FDA may comprise a particularly useful collections of statistical procedures for neuro-fMRI space-time series with high temporal resolution.

Many standard statistical quantities and procedures developed for finite dimensional vector spaces, "finite" because the number of data points is finite, have their direct counterparts in infinite dimensional (Hilbert or Banach) spaces for FDA, "infinite" because the number of points at which the functions take on values is infinite. Procedures for matrix and vector multiplication are seen as special cases of more general inner products defined on these spaces. For instance, the cross-product terms at Eq. 27.5 used in the linear regressions of Sect. 27.3.1.1 may be written as:

$$\langle \mathbf{x}, \mathbf{y}_v \rangle = \sum_{t=1}^{T} x_t y_{tv} = \mathbf{x}^{\mathrm{T}} \mathbf{y}_v$$

as an example of a so-called euclidean inner product. But there is no reason why one is limited to inner products of this type alone. In fact, the weighted least-squares regression at Eq. 27.16 arising from the smoothing operation involves another inner product:

$$\langle \mathbf{x}, \mathbf{y}_v \rangle = \sum_{t=1}^{T} k_{tv} x_t y_{tv}$$

where k_{tv} is a non-negative weight arising from the pre-multiplication of both sides of the regression equation by smoothing matrix $\mathbf{K}$. When corresponding elements of the neuro-fMRI data analysis are considered as functional entities $x(\tau)$ and $y_v(\tau)$, where τ takes on an infinity of values over $[0,\mathrm{T}]$, then the preceding inner products take on the integral forms:

$$\langle \mathbf{x}, \mathbf{y}_v \rangle = \int_0^{\mathrm{T}} x(\tau) y_v(\tau) d\tau$$

and

$$\langle \mathbf{x}, \mathbf{y}_v \rangle = \int_0^{\mathrm{T}} w_v(\tau) x(\tau) y_v(\tau) d\tau$$

respectively. In FDA, predictions from the usual linear model (Eq. 27.12) become:

$$\hat{y}_v(t) = \mu(t) + \int_{\mathrm{T}_X} x_v(p) \beta(p,t) dp$$

where $\hat{y}_u(t)$, $x_v(t)$, and $\beta(p,t)$ are now considered as functions instead of as multivariate vectors. For much more on correspondences between FDA and classical statistics, see RAMSAY and SILVERMAN (1997); RAMSAY (1982); RAMSAY and DALZELL (1991) and RICE and SILVERMAN (1991).

As discussed by LANGE (1998a), the recent article by BRUMBACK and RICE(1998) provides functional data analytic methods that appear very useful for neuro-FMRI data aggregation across subjects, shifting some attention away from too close a focus by some researchers on microstructure of within-subject signals. Consider, for instance, the rich data structure that emerges when the neuro-fMRI study imposes a multi-factor ANOVA design on collections of curves grouped according to distinct brain regions (e.g., temporal and frontal lobes) both within and between individuals. The reader may refer to BRILLINGER (1973) and DIGGLE and AL WASEL (1997) for approaches to frequency domain analyses of such replicated time series. Moreover, "hyper-longitudinal" study designs, as mentioned briefly in Sect. 27.3.1.4, arise when clinical subjects are observed on multiple imaging occasions under different treatment states (e.g., drug vs no drug). For instance, suppose that neuro-fMRI signals are recorded from two brain regions $R = i$, $i \in \{1,2\}$, in subject $S = j$, $j \in \{1,\dots,N\}$ in drug state $D = k$, $k \in \{1,2\}$. These data consist of functions $f_{ijk}(t,v)$, where coordinates t and u denote discretely sampled subsets of the positive real line and 3-D euclidean space, respectively. Approximately two dozen (or more) positions in each brain region may be sampled at 100 or more time points each for every combination of region, subject, and drug state to yield two dozen curves sampled at 100 time points; alternately, this data structure may be viewed as 100 surfaces sampled at two dozen brain locations. Subject j_0 contributes four such functions $f_{ij0k}(t,v)$, one function from each of the four brain region and drug state combinations (i,k). These functions are thus the observational units of a three-way ANOVA where region (R) is a two-level factor that is crossed with the N-level subject factor (S) which is then crossed with the two-level drug state factor (D); one observational unit is contained in each cell of the three-way table representing $R \times S \times D$. In one analysis, measurements at different brain positions (P) within a given region, subject and drug state could be treated as repeated realizations of the same temporal process, so that each observational unit can be viewed as a sample of two dozen similar curves measured through time. When viewed in this manner, the entire data set consists of an even larger sample of curves stratified on the crossed factors $R \times S \times D \times P$, where v in the tensor product space is replaced by the discrete index domain $P = \{1, ..., 24\}$. The new methodology developed by BRUMBACK and RICE (1998) for handling such stratified samples of curves appears ideally suited for these kinds of analyses. The basic idea would be to model a curve $f_{ijkl}(t,v)$ sampled at $R = i$, $S = j$, and $P = l$ as an additive decomposition of smooth functions on τ, as:

$$f_{ijkl}(t) = f_i(t) + f_j(t) + f_k(t) + f_l(t) + \varepsilon_{ijkl}(t),$$

where the curve is presumed to be observed with noise $\varepsilon_{ijkl}(t)$. To compare data across the two drug states, for instance, is thus to compare estimates of $f_{ij1l}(t)$ and $f_{ij2l}(t)$.

In a further analysis, observational units could be thought of as smooth functions defined on the entire domain Π. Statistical methodology in this context is known as smoothing spline ANOVA (SS ANOVA), generalized recently by WANG (1998). SS ANOVA accommodates functions measured on tensor products of arbitrary domains, including mixtures of discrete and continuous domains. Using Wang's generalization, the models of BRUMBACK and RICE (1998) can be viewed as SS ANOVA models over tensor product domains (R,S,D,P,τ) or even (R,S,D,τ,v) where now both position and time may be viewed as continuous domains albeit sampled discretely. SS ANOVA seeks to estimate smooth functions of the continuous domains that are indexed by the other domains. As demonstrated in their current work, this methodology is directly applicable in exploratory functional ANOVA. Rather than estimating the contribution to data variance between each of the two drug states through use of functionals chosen a priori, as in classical growth curve analyses (e.g., REINSEL 1982, 1984, 1985; LANGE and LAIRD 1989), exploratory functional ANOVA could be employed to allow the data to suggest new functionals that account for drug state differences. Such functional ANOVA could also be used in tests for overall functional differences with inferences based on bootstrap distributions (see Sect. 27.2.3). As discussed by LANGE and ZEGER (1997) and MITRA et al. (1997), spatio-temporal autocorrelations in neuro-fMRI are particularly complex. There is some concern that the

forms of inter-curve correlations supported by the methods of BRUMBACK and RICE may be inadequate, in particular when employing the recommended eigenimage preprocessing steps to lighten computational burden. One can anticipate particular interest in richer covariance structures that depend on more than one or two variance components, especially since this structure strongly affects the variances of estimated fixed effects, and hence practical conclusions drawn from the analyses (see Sect. 27.3.1.4).

27.3.3
Nonparametric Methods

As noted in the introduction to Sect. 27.3.1 on parametric methods, a parameter is an index by which one identifies a data-generating distribution from among members of parametric family of possible distributions. Student's t statistic was an example of how one uses a parametric approach in a simple on/off block design assuming a Gaussian model to assess whether changes in the neuro-fMRI signal are due to stimulus-related changes. By computing the mean difference in signal between on and off states and standardizing the mean differences by a pooled estimate of standard deviation, the resultant Student t statistic is used to choose between two t distributions: one with zero mean ($\hat{\beta}_v = 0$) and one with positive mean ($\hat{\beta}_v \geq 0$). (Recall that plugging in an estimate of the variance converts a Gaussian distribution to a t distribution with appropriate degrees of freedom.) Relating the standardized mean difference to a Student t distribution made this choice easy (although not necessarily good), in the sense that the range of possible choices was narrowed dramatically by the equivariant Gaussian distribution assumption dependent on only two parameters, the mean and the variance.

Nonparametric methods make no assumptions about the possible parametric families of distributions generating the neuro-fMRI data and are thus less dependent on a specific statistical model. It is for this reason that nonparametric methods are sometimes termed "distribution free." While such freedom seems attractive, there is another side to the offer: if parametric assumptions are roughly correct, then a parametric, model-based approach (not necessarily Gaussian) is superior to one that does not employ these assumptions (ALTHAM 1984); nonparametric freedom has not gained anything in such a case. The difficulty is that one rarely, if ever, fully knows the properties of the true data-generating mechanism, and some statistical compromise between knowns and unknowns is often a pragmatic course of action.

Nonparametric statistical procedures have found some place in current neuro-fMRI literature, perhaps the most prevalent being the Kolmogorov-Smirnov (KS) procedure (see, for instance, PRESS et al. 1992). The KS procedure has limited utility outside of simple on/off block designs, being a nonparametric alternative to Student's t statistic in such cases. KS yields a statistic that is the maximum deviation between empirical cumulative distributions for neuro-fMRI time series in on and off states, making no assumptions about the shapes of these two distributions. In order to produce the KS statistic at voxel location v, first rank from smallest to largest the values in $\mathbf{y}_v$ for which x_t is off to obtain the empirical cumulative distribution $G_v^{off}(t)$. The empirical cumulative distribution $G_v^{off}(t)$ is a partial sum that accumulates the probability mass of the ordered values up to and including time point t, with probability mass for each value being equal to the reciprocal of the number of time points in the off state, i.e., values at all time points are deemed equally likely. Next, obtain the empirical cumulative distribution $G_v^{on}(t)$ for the neuro-fMRI signal in the on state, and compute the maximum difference:

$$D_v = \max_t \left[G_v^{on}(t) - G_v^{off}(t) \right]$$

Repeat this procedure for all voxel locations $v=1,\ldots,V$ of interest and display the result as a KS-field summary image, just as one would display a Student t field derived from application of the Student procedure discussed in Sect. 27.3.1.1.

The KS procedure for neuro-fMRI has recently come under severe criticism AGUIRRE et al. (1998). These authors point to empirical evidence in their laboratory that suggests that BOLD neuro-fMRI distributions are only slightly non-Gaussian, making nonparametric alternatives less attractive, and also present further evidence that temporal autocorrelations, such as those discussed in Sect. 27.3.1.2, yield false-positive rates (saying there is significant activation when in fact there is none) that are excessively and unacceptably high.

27.3.3.1
Permutation, Jackknife and Bootstrap Techniques

Whether the KS procedure is valid for neuro-fMRI data analysis or not, there are additional nonpara-

metric methods that may have something to offer. Three methods discussed here, which actually cover quite a lot of modern computational nonparametric statistics, are permutation, jackknife and bootstrap procedures.

Permutation. One can continue with the Student t statistic example to develop neuro-fMRI nonparametrics further through introduction of permutation techniques. Interestingly, a permutation argument was first introduced by Fisher as a theoretical basis to support Student's method (EFRON and TIBSHIRANI 1993). Permutation tests, also called randomization tests, are described by many authors since Fisher; EDGINGTON (1987) is a comprehensive overview. Statistical inference via permutation tests for PET has been proposed by HOLMES (1994), HOLMES et al. (1996) and STROTHER et al. (1997) and for neuro-fMRI by BULLMORE et al. (1996a).

Consider once again the on/off block design. Instead of ranking the on and off parts of $\mathbf{y}_v$ separately, rank the entire set of values in $\mathbf{y}_v$ from lowest to highest. Carry along the corresponding reference function $\mathbf{x}$ in the ranking, so that the on and off indicators in $\mathbf{x}$ change vector position according to the ranks of their associated values in $\mathbf{y}_v$. If there is an increase in neuro-fMRI signal due to stimulation, most of the higher-ranked values of $\mathbf{y}_v$ will be associated with an on value in $\mathbf{x}$. For an neuro-fMRI time series of length T in which T_0 elements correspond to the off state and T_1 elements correspond to the on state, with $T=T_0+T_1$, the number of distinct orderings of the elements in $\mathbf{x}$ is:

$$\binom{T}{T_1} = \binom{T}{T_0} = \frac{T!}{(T_0)!(T_1)!} \tag{27.37}$$

where ! is the factorial function, $n! = 1+2\ldots(n-1)\cdot n$[8]. If there is no actual difference between the neuro-fMRI signal in on and off states, then each of these permutations is equally likely with probability equal to the reciprocal of Eq. 27.37. This fact, true under the null hypothesis of no activation, may be used as a basis for attaching a nonparametric, empirical p-value to the average difference:

$$\bar{d} = \bar{y}_1 - \bar{y}_0$$

between the neuro-fMRI signal observed in the two states (subscript v is suppressed). Observed differ-

---

[8] Euler's gamma function (see Sect. 27.3.1.6) applies for real-valued n, a special case of which is $n!$ for integer n.

ence $\bar{d}$ occurred when one of the possible permutations of $\mathbf{x}$ was in effect, namely the actual $\mathbf{x}$ in force when the study was conducted. Generating the permutation distribution of $\bar{d}$, from which the empirical p-value is calculated, is simple and computationally straightforward. First, if the number of time points T is at all large, the total number of possible permutations in Eq. 27.37 is enormous. In such cases, one needs to determine how many permutations are actually required in order to obtain a reasonable estimate of the distribution. For the present suppose that some large number B of permutations are required; how to choose B will be resolved shortly. Next, shuffle the elements of $\mathbf{x}$ to obtain a permuted copy $\mathbf{x}_1^*$, and repeat this shuffling independently for $b = 2,...,B$ times to obtain the set $\{\mathbf{x}_b^*, b = 1,...,B\}$. This form of sampling is called "sampling without replacement" because each value in $\mathbf{x}$ appears only once in the shuffle; by way of contrast, "sampling with replacement" is the method underlying the following "bootstrap" procedure in the next subsection. Associated with each resampled copy $\mathbf{x}_b^*$ of $\mathbf{x}$ is a permutation replication $\bar{d}_b^*$ of d, for $b = 1,...,B$. Each permutation replication $\bar{d}_b^*$ is the value of the mean difference computed under a fictitious, simulated relabeling of time points as on or off states according to $\mathbf{x}_b^*$. The desired empirical p-value is simply the number of $\bar{d}_b^*$ that are greater than or equal to the $\bar{d}$ actually observed, divided by the total number of permutation replications, B. Under the null hypothesis of no activation, the labeling of time points as on or off is irrelevant. A large value for $\bar{d}$ is therefore unlikely and the empirical p-value is a measure of the probability of such an unlikely event, as is any p-value regardless of whether it was derived by a parametric or nonparametric procedure.

How many permutation replications are required? To answer this question, one needs to consider the variability in the permutation distribution that is due to the simulation itself, as opposed to inherent variability in the observed data. By way of example, if $T = 100$ and half of the time is spent in the on state ($T_1 = T_0 = 50$), there are more than 10^{29} possible permutations and repeated samples of much smaller size, $B = 1000$ for instance, will vary from sample to sample, an effect that is not present if one were able to work with the entire permutation distribution. As shown by EFRON and TIBSHIRANI (1993), the coefficient of variation of the empirical p-value, being a binomial random variable, is $[(1-p)/(pB)]^{1/2}$, where p is the true p-value. If one requires that simulation variation be limited to less than 10%, as quantified by the coefficient of variation, then the number of

samples from the permutation distribution needs to be at least $B = 1901$ for $p \leq 0.05$; when $p \leq 0.025$, the minimum increases to $B = 3894$. These authors also note the accuracy of the permutation procedure: empirical p-values so derived have a false-positive rate that is equal to the nominal rate, unlike the findings reported by AGUIRRE et al. (1998) for applications in neuro-fMRI of the KS procedure.

Jackknife. Jackknife procedures (QUENOUILLE 1949; TUKEY 1958) are also known as "leave-one-out" or cross-validation techniques and provide additional computer-intense, nonparametric approaches useful in neuro-fMRI statistics that are free of distributional assumptions. Consider again a neuro-fMRI time series $\mathbf{y}_v$, although the jackknife method is very general and could apply to the entire data matrix $\mathbf{Y}$. Subscript v will continue to be suppressed for notational simplicity. Another way to assess variability of *any* neuro-fMRI statistic $\hat{\theta}$, i.e., any function of the data, is to delete each time point in turn from $\mathbf{y}_v$ and recompute the statistic on the remaining $T-1$ data points. Denote the resultant "jackknife" replication of $\hat{\theta}$ by $\hat{\theta}_{(t)}$, $t = 1,...,T$. A jackknife estimate of standard error for $\hat{\theta}$ is:

$$\tilde{\sigma} = \left\{ \frac{T-1}{T} \sum_{t=1}^{T} \left[\hat{\theta}_{(t)} - \hat{\theta}_{(\cdot)} \right]^2 \right\}^{1/2} \tag{27.38}$$

where $\hat{\theta}_{(\cdot)} = \sum_{t=1}^{T} \hat{\theta}_{(t)} / T$. When the statistic θ is the mean difference $\bar{d}$ for a simple blocked on/off neuro-fMRI study design, then a little algebra shows that the formula of Eq. 27.38 equals the unbiased estimate of the standard error of the mean.

The jackknife begins to show its utility when more complicated statistics, such as the sample variance itself, ratios of means, spectra, coherences and transfer functions (THOMSON and CHAVE 1991), are required to quantify local brain activity by neuro-fMRI, as demonstrated recently by MITRA et al. (1997). However, while it may seem attractive to build confidence intervals for $\hat{\theta}$ using Eq. 27.38 instead of the classical Student interval, a preferable "bootstrap" method of resampling generally yields superior results.

Bootstrap. A revolutionary approach to statistical data analysis that goes far beyond limitations imposed by Gaussian and other parametric assumptions is developed through a recent series of articles and books (EFRON 1979a,b, 1982; EFRON and TIBSHIRANI 1991, 1993). These authors' method, termed the "bootstrap," is closely related to the permutation and jackknife methods discussed previously. For the bootstrap, neuro-fMRI data are sampled *with* replacement instead of without replacement as in permutation methods or by leave-one-out sampling as in the jackknife. Just as there are permutation replications and jackknife replications, there are bootstrap replications of a statistic $\hat{\theta}$, denoted by $\hat{\theta}_b$, $b=1,...,B$, for some large number of replications, B. Each bootstrap replication $\hat{\theta}_b$ is the result of applying the same statistical procedure that yielded the original statistic $\hat{\theta}$ to a resampled neuro-fMRI data vector $\mathbf{y}_v$ that is not a shuffled version of $\mathbf{y}_v$, as in the permutation method, but consists instead of T draws from $\mathbf{y}_v$ that are completely independent and random (sampled with replacement). There is some small probability that all of the values in $\mathbf{y}_b^*$ will be identical if the same value happens to be drawn T times, or that $\mathbf{y}_b^*$ will equal $\mathbf{y}_v$.

The bootstrap shows its superior performance over classical parametric, permutation and jackknife methods for neuro-fMRI data analysis when the statistic in question is not a simple linear, "smooth" statistic such as a mean. As an example, consider a bootstrap alternative to the classical Gaussian confidence intervals discussed at the beginning of Sect. 27.3.1.1 at Eq. 27.9. As discussed by EFRON and TIBSHIRANI (1993), the so-called BC_a (bias-corrected and accelerated) interval possesses excellent statistical properties under *both* nonparametric and parametric situations. Letting $\hat{\theta}^*\alpha$ denote the 100+ath percentile of the empirical distribution of bootstrap replications $\{\hat{\theta}_b, b=1,...,B\}$, the BC_a interval is defined as:

$$\left[\hat{\theta}^*(\alpha_1),\ \hat{\theta}^*(\alpha_2)\right]$$

where

$$\alpha_1 = \Phi\left[\hat{z}_0 + \frac{\hat{z}_0 + z^{(\alpha)}}{1 - \hat{a}\left(\hat{z}_0 + z^{(\alpha)}\right)}\right]$$

$$\alpha_2 = \Phi\left[\hat{z}_0 + \frac{\hat{z}_0 + z^{(1-\alpha)}}{1 - \hat{a}\left(\hat{z}_0 + z^{(1-\alpha)}\right)}\right] \qquad (27.39)$$

In Eq. 27.39, $\Phi[\cdot]$ is the standard normal cumulative distribution function and $z^{(\alpha)}$ is the 100+αth percentile of a standard normal distribution, e.g., $z^{(0.95)}=1.645$ and F[1.645]=0.95. The BC_a interval depends on two constants, "bias-correction" $\hat{z}_0$ and "acceleration" $\hat{a}$, which are estimated from the data to correct for deficiencies of confidence intervals based on simple percentiles of the bootstrap distribution (see EFRON and TIBSHIRANI 1993 for details).

27.3.4
Multivariate Methods

In one sense, all of neuro-fMRI statistics is multivariate. There are many time points and many spatial locations which are high-dimensional, multivariate data ensembles. Differences between multivariate and univariate statistical approaches reside generally in the manner in which the left-hand side of the statistical equation, not the right-hand side, is treated. The regression models of Sect. 27.3.1.1 are generally univariate models, even though their right-hand sides may be quite complex, because their left-hand sides are composed of single variables that are treated separately and independently since the associated variance-covariance matrix for the ensemble is assumed by these models to be diagonal. The neuro-fMRI time series models in Sect. 27.3.1.2 are also largely univariate because each series is also treated independently, although autocorrelations within each series imply a variance-covariance matrix for the data ensemble which is block-diagonal. The frequency domain and random field models of Sect. 27.3.1.3 and Sect. 27.3.1.5, respectively, are multivariate in nature. The longitudinal models of Sect. 27.3.1.4 make a step toward multivariate statistical procedures by modeling inter-series correlations, that is, modeling patterns of variance and covariance in off-diagonal blocks. Functional data analysis for neuro-fMRI, as outlined in Sect. 27.2.2, is a beginning of a method that treats collections of curves as single entities in function space instead of as discrete points, standing apart from both univariate and multivariate approaches.

The following section describes several additional multivariate statistical procedures for neuro-fMRI, discriminant analysis and singular value decomposition, taking a course in between univariate and functional procedures. Discrimination and singular value decomposition are central to many multivariate methods, such as principal component analysis and canonical correlation. These and other methods are very ably described in much more detail and with many examples in the classical texts by MARDIA et al. (1979) and GNANADESIKAN (1997). This section assumes some familiarity with eigenvalues and eigenvectors from linear algebra (see DUDA and HART (1973), STRANG (1980) and the next section on the singular value decomposition of a matrix).

27.3.4.1
Discriminants

An important class of dimension reduction methods are known as discriminants: Fisher's linear discriminant (FISHER 1936, 1938), quadratic discriminant, generalized linear discriminant, etc. These multivariate techniques all aim to find optimal projections of original high-dimensional neuro-fMRI data onto subspaces of lower dimension (see Fig. 27.1 and Sect. 27.3.1.1 for least-squares regression of y on x as a projection). For simplicity, one can reduce the rather large dimension V, equal to the number of voxels, to only one dimension by projecting the data onto a line. That is, data matrix $\mathbf{Y}$ may be viewed as a set of T samples $\mathbf{y}_t = (y_{t1},...y_{tV})^{\mathrm{T}}$ for $t = 1,...,T$, each of dimension V. Fisher's linear discriminant (FLD) can be written as a projection of each $\mathbf{y}_t$ onto a line in direction β, and is given by the scalar:

$$\xi_t = \boldsymbol{\beta}^{\mathrm{T}}\mathbf{y}_t \qquad (27.40)$$

which is a linear combination of voxel values at time t. Geometrically, only the direction of β is important, not its magnitude; setting $\|\beta\|=1$ loses no generality and makes Eq. 27.40 a true projection. Consider again a simple situation when reference function $\mathbf{x}$ has only two distinct elements indicating baseline and stimulus states. Just as each V-vector $\mathbf{y}_t$ belongs to one of two groups according to x_t, so does its corresponding scalar ξ_t belong in one of these same two groups lying on the line with direction $\boldsymbol{\beta}$. If the predicted group indicator z_t matches the actual group indicator x_t with very low error rate for every t, then the entire sample of fMR images $\mathbf{Y}$ is said to be linearly separable. Thus, in such cases, the aim of FLD is to find a projection direction $\boldsymbol{\beta}$ that causes the groups of ξ_ts to be well-separated when viewed from that direction. The optimal viewing direction is the value of $\boldsymbol{\beta}$ that maximizes the objective function given by:

$$F_\beta = \frac{\boldsymbol{\beta}^{\mathrm{T}}\mathbf{S}_{\mathrm{B}}\boldsymbol{\beta}}{\boldsymbol{\beta}^{\mathrm{T}}\mathbf{S}_{\mathrm{W}}\boldsymbol{\beta}} \qquad (27.41)$$

where $\mathbf{S}_{\mathrm{B}}$ and $\mathbf{S}_{\mathrm{W}}$ are between-group and within-group mean sums of squares matrices.
The ratio of Eq. 27.41 is known as the generalized Rayleigh quotient in mathematical physics or as Fisher's F ratio in statistics. The optimal $\boldsymbol{\beta}$ satisfies the generalized eigenvalue problem:

$$\mathbf{S}_{\mathrm{B}}\boldsymbol{\beta} = \lambda\mathbf{S}_{\mathrm{W}}\boldsymbol{\beta}$$

which, if $\mathbf{S}_{\mathrm{W}}$ is nonsingular, is converted to the ordinary eigenvalue problem:

$$\mathbf{S}_{\mathrm{W}}^{-1}\mathbf{S}_{\mathrm{B}}\boldsymbol{\beta} = \lambda\boldsymbol{\beta}$$

In the simple two-group case, it is unnecessary to find the eigenvalues of $\mathbf{S}_{\mathrm{W}}^{-1}\mathbf{S}_{\mathrm{B}}$ because $\mathbf{S}_{\mathrm{B}}\boldsymbol{\beta}$ is always along the direction of the vector difference of group centroids $\bar{\mathbf{y}}_1 - \bar{\mathbf{y}}_0$, where $\bar{\mathbf{y}}_g = \sum_{\{t:x_t=g\}}\mathbf{y}_t / \sum_{\{t:x_t=g\}}1$, $g = 0,1$. Also, as has been noted, the scale of $\boldsymbol{\beta}$ is unimportant. Hence, the optimal $\boldsymbol{\beta}$ is proportional to:

$$\hat{\boldsymbol{\beta}} = \mathbf{S}_{\mathrm{W}}^{-1}(\bar{\mathbf{y}}_1 - \bar{\mathbf{y}}_0)$$

Equation 27.40 is reminiscent of the linear regression models of Sect. 4.1.2, yet with the roles of $\mathbf{x}$ and $\mathbf{y}$ reversed and without the error term. That is, it appears as though one may write:

$$x_t = \beta_0 + \boldsymbol{\beta}^{\mathrm{T}}\mathbf{y}_t + \varepsilon_t$$

assume independent Gaussian errors and fit this model to obtain $\hat{x}_t = \hat{\beta}_0 + \hat{\boldsymbol{\beta}}^{\mathrm{T}}\mathbf{y}_t + \varepsilon_t$, $t = 1,...,T$. This intuition is valid: FLD is indeed equivalent to the simple least-squares regression of $\mathbf{x}$ on $\mathbf{Y}$ when the variance-covariance matrices of the two groups of voxel values are equal (see Fisher's original work, or, for instance, MCLACHLAN 1992, p. 63). Another way of looking at this same situation in the multivariate Gaussian case with two equal group variance-covariance matrices is to notice that Fisher's linear discriminant defines an optimal decision surface, or hyperplane, whose equation is:

$$\hat{x}_t = \hat{\beta}_0 + \hat{\boldsymbol{\beta}}^{\mathrm{T}}\mathbf{y}_t + \varepsilon_t, \quad t = 1,...,T$$

where scalar β_0 is the location or threshold for the decision surface and $\mathbf{b}$ is its orientation (direction). This hyperplane separates fMR images assigned to the baseline and stimulus groups according to whether $d(\mathbf{y},\beta)>0$ or $d(\mathbf{y},\beta)<0$. When the equal variance-covariance matrices for the two groups are diagonal, isocontours of equal probability are circles and the hyperplane is orthogonal to the vector difference of group centroids. When the variance-covariance matrices are equal yet arbitrary, isoprobability contours are ellipses and the hyperplane is not necessarily orthogonal to the group centroid difference but is oriented in the same direction as the major axes of the ellipses.

Fisher's linear discriminant provides a basis for generalizations of the classification problem in at least two directions: increased complexity of the decision surface and increased complexity of the reference function. First, a quadratic decision surface arises when the variance-covariance matrices for the two groups are completely arbitrary. Isoprobability contours remain ellipses, yet the decision boundary is no longer a hyperplane. It is instead a "hyperquadratic" surface, being a member of the more set general of conic sections (pairs of hyperplanes, "hyperspheres," "hyperellipsoids," "hyperparabolas," etc.). Second, when study design dictates more complex stimuli than a simple baseline vs single stimulus comparison, there are more than two groups of fMR images to be classified. One useful way to proceed in such cases is to define G different discriminant functions:

$$d_g(\mathbf{y}, \boldsymbol{\beta}) = \beta_{g0} + \boldsymbol{\beta}_g^T \mathbf{y}, \qquad g = 1, \dots, G,$$

where $G > 2$ is the number of distinct stimulus states, including baseline. The linear classifier so defined operates in a similar manner to the two-group case: assign fMR image $\mathbf{y}$ to group g if $d_g(\mathbf{y},\beta) > d_{g'}(\mathbf{y},\beta)$ for all g'. This procedure partitions image space into a set of mutually exclusive and exhaustive regions with piecewise linear hyperplane boundaries, and thus the problem may remain linearly separable if misclassification error probabilities are very low.

27.3.4.2
Singular Value Decomposition

One of the most frequently employed statistical procedures for neuro-fMRI data re-expression and dimension reduction is the singular value decomposition (SVD). This procedure has a long history, first published by BELTRAMI (1873) and developed independently since then by a variety of mathematicians, numerical analysts and computer scientists. The utility of the SVD for a wide range of applied problems was not appreciated fully until it was shown in the 1960s that it could be computed effectively and efficiently and used as the basis of stable numerical algorithms. Important theoretical developments and applications of the SVD can be found in numerous articles and textbooks, such as ECKART and YOUNG (1936); GOLUB and LOAN (1996); GOOD (1969); STRANG (1980) and TREFETHEN and BAU (1997). Use of the SVD for ascribing physical interpretations to complexes of variables such as those of present interest is pre-dated in the statistical literature by the related principal component transformation of such complexes (see HOTELLING 1933, 1936; PEARSON 1901). For more recent discussion of statistical applications of the SVD, see for instance MARDIA et al.

(1979) and GNANADESIKAN (1997). For applications of the SVD in neuro-fMRI and optical imaging, see FRISTON et al. (1995b); FRISTON (1996); BULLMORE et al. (1996b); MAYHEW et al. (1998); MITRA and PESARAN (1997); MITRA et al. (1997); POLINE et al. (1997a); RABE-HESKETH et al. (1997); WORSLEY et al. (1997). The role of the SVD in neuro-fMRI data analysis is so important that this statistical procedure should be well understood by every researcher who employs it.

The idea behind the SVD in two dimensions is simple enough, as the following abstraction attempts to demonstrate. Consider a 2×2 matrix $\mathbf{M}$ which maps points in the 2-D euclidean plane to other points in this plane[9]. Consider two sets of points in the plane, a circle of unit radius and an ellipse, as depicted in Fig. 27.2. Matrix $\mathbf{M}$ maps points on the circle to points on the ellipse. Two points on the circle are depicted by vectors $\mathbf{b}_1$ and $\mathbf{b}_2$ of unit length and at right angles to each other (orthogonal). The two corresponding points on the ellipse are depicted by vectors $\mathbf{a}_1$ and $\mathbf{a}_2$, also of unit length and orthogonal, multiplied by two non-negative scalars σ_1 and σ_2 to become the major and minor semi-axes of the ellipse. Matrix $\mathbf{M}$ takes each vector, stretches or shrinks it and changes its direction as seen by the equations:

$$\begin{cases} \mathbf{M}\mathbf{b}_1 = \sigma_1 \mathbf{a}_1 \\ \mathbf{M}\mathbf{b}_2 = \sigma_2 \mathbf{a}_2 \end{cases} \qquad (27.42)$$

A more compact way of writing Eq. 27.42 is:

$$\mathbf{M}\mathbf{B} = \mathbf{A}\Sigma$$

where

$$\mathbf{A} = \begin{bmatrix} \mathbf{a}_1 & \mathbf{a}_2 \end{bmatrix}, \; \Sigma = \begin{bmatrix} \sigma_1 & 0 \\ 0 & \sigma_2 \end{bmatrix}, \; \mathbf{B} = \begin{bmatrix} \mathbf{b}_1 & \mathbf{b}_2 \end{bmatrix}.$$

Scalars and σ_1 and σ_2 are the non-negative singular values of $\mathbf{M}$ and are numbered, by convention, in descending order according to their magnitudes. Because vectors $\mathbf{a}_1$ and $\mathbf{a}_2$ are of unit length and at right angles to each other, matrix $\mathbf{A}$ is orthonormal, meaning that $\mathbf{A}^T\mathbf{A} = \mathbf{I}_2$, where $\mathbf{I}_2$ is the 2×2 identity matrix with 1s on its diagonal and 0s elsewhere; the identity matrix, in any dimension, "leaves everything where

---

[9] The SVD applies more generally to complex-valued matrices, in which, for instance, transposition is replaced by Hermitian conjugation and orthonormal matrices replaced by unitary matrices, yet in this discussion all matrices and vectors are real-valued.

it is." Similarly, **B** is also orthonormal, so that $\mathbf{B}^T\mathbf{B} = \mathbf{I}_2$. It is also the case that $\mathbf{BB}^T=\mathbf{I}_2$. Using this latter fact, one may multiply each side of Eq. 27.42 by $\mathbf{B}^T$ to obtain the explicit decomposition:

$$\mathbf{M} = \mathbf{A}\Sigma\mathbf{B}^T \qquad (27.43)$$

Equation 27.43 is the SVD of **M**, which, for any matrix **M**, always exists and is unique. Matrix **A** consists of left singular vectors, Σ consists of singular values sorted in descending order along its diagonal, and **B** consists of right singular vectors[10]. Another way of expressing Eq. 43 shows why this decomposition is called "singular." Matrix **M** can be written as a sum of 2×2 matrices that each have only a single effective dimension (they are matrices of rank one), being the outer product of left and right singular vectors:

$$\mathbf{M} = \sigma_1\mathbf{a}_1\mathbf{b}_1^T + \sigma_2\mathbf{a}_2\mathbf{b}_2^T \qquad (27.44)$$

These ideas can be generalized to apply to any $R\times C$ matrix, where R and C are not necessarily equal and possibly much greater than 2; at present **M** is a stand-in for the neuro-fMRI data matrix $\mathbf{Y}^T$ treated subsequently. Any $R\times C$ matrix **M** can be thought of as providing basis vectors for two spaces, a row space and a column space. The row space of **M** (also called the domain of **M**) is the space spanned by its rows, being the collection of all vectors r that can be expressed as a linear combination of rows $\mathbf{m}^T_i$, $i=1,...,R$, of M. This collection thus consists of all vectors **r** such that:

$$\mathbf{r} = \mathbf{M}^T\mathbf{c} = \sum_{i=1}^{R} c_i\mathbf{m}_i^T \qquad (27.45)$$

for some vector **c**. Similarly, the column space of **M** (also called the range of **M**) is the space spanned by its columns, being the collection of all vectors that can be expressed as a linear combination of the columns of **M**, that is, all vectors **c** such that:

$$\mathbf{c} = \mathbf{Mr} = \sum_{j=1}^{C} r_j\mathbf{m}_j \qquad (27.46)$$

for some vector **r**. The row space of **M** is denoted span($\mathbf{M}^T$) and the column space of **M** is denoted

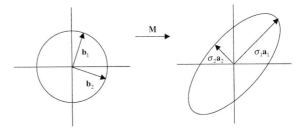

Fig. 27.2. Singular value decomposition (SVD) of a 2×2 matrix M. (Adapted from TREFETHEN and BAU 1997)

span(M). The common dimension of these two spaces is equal to the number of linearly independent row or columns and is called the rank of **M**. Since the number of linearly independent row or columns of **M** can be no greater than the lesser of its two dimensions, the dimension of span(M) is no greater than the lesser of R and C. There is also a third space, called the null space of M and denoted null(M), that consists of all vectors that **M** maps to zero, that is, all vectors **r** that satisfy **Mr**=0, where **0** is the vector of length R consisting entirely of 0s.

Notice that Eqs. 27.45 and 27.46 are *not* written as

$$r_j = \sum_{i=1}^{R} m_{ij}c_i, \ i=1,...,R \text{ and}$$

$$c_i = \sum_{j=1}^{C} m_{ij}r_j,$$

$j=1,...,C$ an equivalent and more customary way to write a matrix-vector product. (One standard way to picture this operation is to fix a row of the matrix, multiply elements in the vector by corresponding elements of that row, add them up to obtain one element of the result, and then proceed through rows.) A conventional way of thinking about the operation c=Mr in Eq. 27.46 is that **M** acts on **r** to produce **c**. However, for understanding the SVD, a preferable way of thinking about the matrix-vector product c=Mr in Eq. 27.46 is that **r** *acts on* **M** *to produce* **c**. A different way to picture a matrix-vector product is to place **r**, not to the right of **M**, but instead on top of **M**, fix an element of **r**, multiply the corresponding column of **M** by that element to obtain one columnar component of the result, and then proceed through columns by adding up these components. Similarly, **c** acts on $\mathbf{M}^T$ to produce **r**. This way of interpreting **M** is particularly helpful when **M** is an neuro-fMRI data matrix.

By use of the SVD one can also show how any matrix is a diagonal matrix depending on how one looks at it, that is, by how the bases for its row and column spaces are chosen. This fact is important for

---

[10] The adjectives "left" and "right" when applied to singular vectors refer to the conventional placements of **A** and **B** in Eq. 27.43 and not to their placements in Fig. 27.2, in which the mapping of **B** to **A** by matrix **M** is also, unfortunately, drawn according to convention from left to right.

the interpretation of neuro-fMRI data, as discussed subsequently. Specifically, suppose one has SVD $M = A\Sigma B^T$ where A is $R \times C$, Σ is $C \times C$ and B $C \times C$.[11] In addition, suppose that:

$$c' = A^T c \quad \text{and} \quad r' = B^T r$$

for some vectors r and c. The matrix-vector product $c = Mr$ can be re-expressed in terms of r' and c' by use of the SVD to diagonalize M. Use the orthonormal property of A to write the matrix-vector product as (Trefethen and Bau 1997, p. 32):

$$c = Mr \iff A^T c = A^T Mr = A^T A\Sigma B^T r = \Sigma B^T r \iff c' = \Sigma r' \tag{27.47}$$

Eq 27.47 says that whenever $c = Mr$ one knows that $c' = \Sigma r'$, the only difference being the change of bases from M to A and B. That is, matrix M reduces to the diagonal matrix Σ when the basis for the column space of M is chosen to be the columns of A and when the basis for the row space of M is chosen to be the columns of B.

Expressing M as a diagonal matrix, in light of Eq. 27.44 and the preceding discussion, separates its components into singular, independent terms each having dimension one. Such decomposition increases interpretability of its potentially highly complex structure. By employing the SVD, one may write partial sums $\hat{M}_p$, where:

$$\hat{M}_p = \sigma_1 a_1 b_1^T + \sigma_2 a_2 b_2^T + \cdots + \sigma_p a_p b_p^T, \quad \text{for } p = 1, \ldots, C. \tag{27.48}$$

Each $\hat{M}_p$ is still $R \times C$, yet the "^"over M_p indicates that choice of partial sum p, or for that matter any subset of the C columns, is a statistical estimation problem. One may generalize the ellipse of Fig. 27.2 by considering a hyperellipsoid in C dimensions, for $C>2$. When $p=1$, the best approximation to the hyperellipsoid Y^T is its longest axis; when $p=2$, the best approximation to the hyperellipsoid is the ellipse formed by its longest and second-longest axes; and so forth.

The SVD demonstrates its power for increasing interpretability of complex structure when matrix M is replaced by the $V \times T$ neuro-fMRI data matrix Y^T. Convention dictates that the matrix to which the SVD is applied be oriented as "tall and narrow" rather than "long and flat." As mentioned in the Introduction, neither orientation, Y or Y^T, is optimal in all situations, and this is one situation in which Y^T is generally preferred. Prior to taking the SVD, a first step is often performed to remove temporal and spatial drifts from Y^T that are not of primary interest. This is done through subtraction of row and column means from Y^T to obtain its row- and column-centered version, Y_0^T, with elements in each row summing to 0 and elements in each column also summing to 0. Although the centering step is not strictly necessary, it has often been found in neuro-fMRI that the doubly-centered matrix Y_0^T contains the spatio-temporal interactions of primary interest. As depicted in Fig. 27.3, Y_0^T can be decomposed uniquely by the SVD into the following product of an orthonormal matrix, a diagonal matrix and another orthonormal matrix:

$$Y_0^T = A_0 \Sigma_0 B_0^T \tag{27.49}$$

In Eq. 27.49, columns of the $V \times T$ matrix $A_0 = (a_1, \ldots, a_T)$ are the left singular vectors of Y_0^T, or, equivalently, its "singular images" of length $V \times 1$. (Recall that the 2-D or 3-D structure of each image is easily reconstructed from these 1-D data columns structures.) Since A_0 is orthonormal $A_0^T A_0 = I_T$: each singular image has unit length and carries an independent, principal spatial component of brain activation that is fundamentally different from components carried by other singular images. Corresponding to each singular image a_t is a singular value σ_t positioned on the diagonal of the $T \times T$ diagonal matrix $\Sigma_0 = \text{diag}(\sigma_1, \ldots, \sigma_T)$. As was seen in Fig. 27.2, since the singular values are multipliers of unit vectors, these scalars are interpreted as the amount of deviation or spread of their associated singular vectors. Columns of the $T \times T$ matrix $B_0 = (b_1, \ldots, b_T)$ are the right singular vectors of Y_0^T, or, equivalently, its "singular time trends" of length $T \times 1$. As with A_0, B_0 is also orthonormal, so that $B_0^T B_0 = I_T$, yet note that while $B_0^T B_0 = I_T$, $A_0 A_0^T \neq I_V$. Each singular time trend also has unit length and carries an independent, principal temporal component of brain activation that is fundamentally different from components carried by other singular time trends.

The singular values $(\sigma_1, \ldots, \sigma_T)$ are the eigenvalues of the $T \times T$ cross-product matrix $Y_0 Y_0^T$ and are also the eigenvalues of the much larger $V \times V$ cross-product matrix $Y_0^T Y_0$. Singular images $(a_1, \ldots, a_T)$ and singular time trends $(b_1, \ldots, b_T)$ are the eigenvectors of $Y_0 Y_0^T$ and $Y_0^T Y_0$, respectively. These facts allow one to

---

[11] Technically, the SVD expressed here is a *reduced* singular value decomposition, since A and Σ are $R+C$ and $C+C$, respectively, and not $R+R$ and $R+C$. This makes little difference in practice since the $R-C$ "missing" rows and columns in A and Σ are "silent."

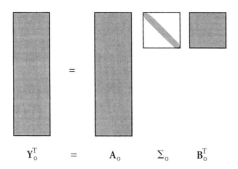

$$\mathbf{Y}_0^{\mathrm{T}} \quad = \quad \mathbf{A}_0 \quad \Sigma_0 \quad \mathbf{B}_0^{\mathrm{T}}$$

Fig. 27.3. Singular value decomposition (SVD) of the doubly-centered $V \times T$ matrix

work with the smaller and more easily computed matrix $\mathbf{Y}_0 \mathbf{Y}_0^{\mathrm{T}}$ and not $\mathbf{Y}_0^{\mathrm{T}} \mathbf{Y}_0$.

Some singular vectors may contain only noise and not any "interesting" neuro-fMRI signal structure, where "interesting" is necessarily vague in this abstraction yet clearly has a very specific definition depending on the goals and aims of the neuro-fMRI experiment. To remove such noise from further consideration, the next statistical procedure in application of the SVD to neuro-fMRI data is generally a dimension reduction step. This step smoothes $\mathbf{Y}_0^{\mathrm{T}}$ by using its factored representation to choose a subset of size $P < T$ from among the columns of $\mathbf{B}_0$, much in the way that the partial sums of Eq. 27.48 approximated the hyperellipsoid by ellipsoids of lower dimension. The number P is the estimated numerical rank of column space of neuro-fMRI data matrix $\mathbf{Y}_0^{\mathrm{T}}$; that is, the dimension of span($\mathbf{Y}_0^{\mathrm{T}}$) is P. Denote the subset of column indices of size P by index vector $\tau_P \subset \{1,...,T\}$. Objective methods exist for choice of τ_P (see, for instance, DENBY and MALLOWS 1991; HANSEN et al. 1997; MITRA and PESARAN 1997). Subset selection is not simply a matter of choosing the singular vectors associated with the P largest singular values. For physical interpretation of results, it may well be that the relations associated with the *smallest* singular values are those of greatest interest (GNANADESIKAN 1997 p. 11).

Denote the smoothed and centered $V \times P$ image matrix by

$$\hat{\mathbf{Y}}^{\mathrm{T}} = \hat{\mathbf{A}} \hat{\mathbf{\Sigma}} \hat{\mathbf{B}}^{\mathrm{T}} \tag{27.50}$$

dropping the subscript "0" for simplicity and where the $V \times P$ matrix $\hat{\mathbf{A}}$ is defined as:

$$\hat{\mathbf{A}} = \left(\mathbf{a}_{\tau_1}, ..., \mathbf{a}_{\tau_P} \right)$$

the $P \times P$ matrix $\hat{\mathbf{\Sigma}}$ is defined as:

$$\hat{\mathbf{\Sigma}} = \mathrm{diag} \left(\sigma_{\tau_1}, ..., \sigma_{\tau_P} \right)$$

and the $T \times P$ matrix $\hat{\mathbf{B}}$ is defined as:

$$\hat{\mathbf{B}} = \left(\mathbf{b}_{\tau_1}, ..., \mathbf{b}_{\tau_P} \right)$$

This new smoothed setup is depicted in Fig. 27.4. Vector elements of $\hat{\mathbf{A}}, \hat{\mathbf{\Sigma}}$, and $\hat{\mathbf{B}}$ are indexed subsequently without the awkward $\tau_1,...,\tau_P$ subscripts but rather simply as $1,...,P$, it being understood that the subset included in these matrices may be any subset of $\{1,...,T\}$ of size P. As with each $\hat{\mathbf{M}}_p$ at Eq. 27.48, $\hat{\mathbf{Y}}^{\mathrm{T}}$ is still $V \times T$ yet the "∧" indicates that the estimated version of the neuro-fMRI data matrix on the left-hand side of Eq. 27.50 has been doubly centered and that a subset τ_P has been selected from the complete set of left and right singular vectors available from the SVD. All matrices in Eq. 27.50 are of full rank. This means that all "uninteresting" and "silent" columns of $\mathbf{A}$ and $\mathbf{M}$ corresponding to diagonal elements of Σ_c that are effectively zero have been eliminated from further consideration. In the decomposition of Eq. 27.50, $\hat{\mathbf{A}}$ and $\hat{\mathbf{B}}$ remain orthonormal so that $\hat{\mathbf{A}}^{\mathrm{T}} \hat{\mathbf{A}} = \hat{\mathbf{B}}^{\mathrm{T}} \hat{\mathbf{B}} = \mathbf{I}_P$. However, now both $\hat{\mathbf{A}} \hat{\mathbf{A}}^{\mathrm{T}} \neq \mathbf{I}_V$ and $\hat{\mathbf{B}} \hat{\mathbf{B}}^{\mathrm{T}} \neq \mathbf{I}_T$; prior to smoothing by choosing column subset τ_P, recall that $\mathbf{B}_0 \mathbf{B}_0^{\mathrm{T}} = \mathbf{I}_T$. The P-dimensional "temporal space" spanned by the columns of $\hat{\mathbf{B}}$ is denoted span($\hat{\mathbf{B}}$), and the P-dimensional "image space" spanned by the columns of $\hat{\mathbf{A}}$ is denoted span($\hat{\mathbf{A}}$).

One can move easily between span($\hat{\mathbf{B}}$) and span($\hat{\mathbf{A}}$) by the projection, scaling and orthogonal transformation operations afforded by Eq. 27.50. These operations are smoothed versions of the diagonalization argument for the SVD given previously at Eq. 27.47. For instance, any vector $\mathbf{r}$ of length T may be projected onto span($\hat{\mathbf{B}}$) of dimension $P < T$, the result being written as:

$$\hat{\mathbf{r}} = \hat{\mu}_1 \mathbf{b}_1 + \cdots + \hat{\mu}_P \mathbf{b}_P.$$

The vector $\mathbf{r}$ is simply the "shadow" of $\mathbf{r}$ in span($\hat{\mathbf{B}}$) produced from the ordinary least-squares regression of $\mathbf{r}$ on $\hat{\mathbf{B}}$ with fitted regression coefficients $\hat{\mu}_1,...,\hat{\mu}_P$ (Fig. 27.1). In other words, similar to the matrix representation of linear regression estimates given in Sect. 27.3.1.1:

$$\hat{\mu} = \left(\hat{\mu}_1, ..., \hat{\mu}_P \right) = \left(\hat{\mathbf{B}}^{\mathrm{T}} \hat{\mathbf{B}} \right)^{-1} \hat{\mathbf{B}}^{\mathrm{T}} \mathbf{r} = \hat{\mathbf{B}}^{\mathrm{T}} \mathbf{r} \tag{27.51}$$

and:

$$\hat{\mathbf{r}} = \hat{\mathbf{B}} \left(\hat{\mathbf{B}}^{\mathrm{T}} \hat{\mathbf{B}} \right)^{-1} \hat{\mathbf{B}}^{\mathrm{T}} \mathbf{r} = \hat{\mathbf{B}} \hat{\mathbf{B}}^{\mathrm{T}} \mathbf{r} = \mathbf{P} \mathbf{r} \tag{27.52}$$

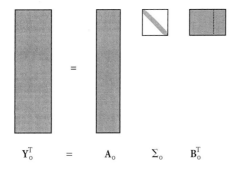

$$\mathbf{Y}_o^T \quad = \quad \mathbf{A}_o \quad \Sigma_o \quad \mathbf{B}_o^T$$

Fig. 27.4. Smoothing the singular value decomposition (SVD) of $\mathbf{Y}_o^T$

where $\mathbf{P} = \hat{\mathbf{B}}\,\hat{\mathbf{B}}^T$ is a $T \times T$ projection operator of rank $P < T$. Residuals from the regression in Eq. 27.51 lie in null($\hat{\mathbf{B}}$), being forced by the projection to be orthogonal to span($\hat{\mathbf{B}}$). The estimated $\hat{\mathbf{r}}$ can then be re-expressed in span($\hat{\mathbf{A}}$) by scaling and orthogonal transformation, to write:

$$\hat{\mathbf{c}} = \mathbf{a}_1 \sigma_1 \hat{\mu}_1 + \cdots + \mathbf{a}_P \sigma_P \hat{\mu}_P \qquad (27.53)$$

or, more compactly by Eq. 27.50:

$$\hat{\mathbf{c}} = \hat{\mathbf{A}}\hat{\Sigma}\hat{\mathbf{r}}$$

While each combined spatio-temporal component ($\hat{\mathbf{r}}, \hat{\mathbf{c}}$) consists of a collection of $T+V$ numbers, $\hat{\mathbf{c}}$ is often the element of primary interest in current neuro-fMRI work, for this element can be displayed as an image.

When the vector $\mathbf{r}$ in Eq. 27.51 is chosen to be the reference function $\mathbf{x}$, or some function of $\mathbf{x}$, the associated image $\hat{\mathbf{c}}$ in Eq. 27.53 is of greatest interest, for this image contains spatial regions of brain activity closely associated with the controlled stimuli encoded in $\mathbf{x}$.

27.3.4.3
Adaptive Techniques

The nonparametric methods of Sect. 27.2.3, Fisher's linear discriminant of Sect. 27.3.4.1 and the singular value decomposition of Sect. 27.3.4.2 are introductory examples of a much broader and richer class of adaptive statistical procedures that do not adhere closely to a priori modeling assumptions but instead adapt to local neuro-fMRI data features in time and space. These procedures also fall under the heading of statistical pattern recognition; see, for instance, McLachlan (1992) and Lange (1999). Some re-

searchers use the term "statistical pattern recognition" to describe lines of investigation that probe structure and pattern in very large data sets without recourse to classical assumptions that they feel may be too inflexible for practical use. Artificial neural networks embody many key pattern recognition ideas and principles (see for instance Ripley 1996; Bishop 1995). Independent component analysis (Bell and Sejnowski 1995) is one such instance, recently applied to neuro-fMRI (McKeown et al. 1998).

"Recognition" often means "classification," as in Sect. 27.3.4.1, and is an exercise in learning from examples. Under supervised learning, the statistical procedure is "trained" with a labeled collection of examples. In neuro-fMRI, the examples are the time series of images and the labels are encoded in reference function $\mathbf{x}$. Training usually involves some form of cross-validation (see Sect. 27.3.3.1). Unsupervised learning, which occurs less frequently in practice, refers to a statistical pattern recognition exercise that does not involve pre-assigned labels in either training or test phases of algorithm development. The emphasis in unsupervised learning for neuro-fMRI is on discovery of new groupings and common characteristics amongst previously unclassified ensembles of examples, that is, to see if the procedure can "guess" $\mathbf{x}$ given only the neuro-fMRI time series. A loss function is defined through consideration of losses incurred by making different sorts of classification errors, such as false positives and false negatives. A classification rule is then chosen which minimizes total risk, that is, total expected loss, when assigning class labels. Criteria for label assignment can be parametric or nonparametric. Nonparametric "nearest neighbor" pattern recognition assigns labels to new examples by measuring distances to their nearest neighbors under some particular metric. Metrics for determining nearness may either be fixed or adaptive, euclidean or non-euclidean. Class labels are determined by assigning a new example to that class that minimizes the combined distance from the example to a fixed number of previous examples of that same class over all possible class assignments. Adaptive systems built according to well established criteria from statistical decision and information theory are known to outperform simplistic models and ad hoc methods in other application areas, and thus appear to offer some promise for future neuro-fMRI research.

27.4
Meta-Analysis

Given that many current neuro-fMRI study designs employ very few subjects, the formal combination of results from many small studies by statistical procedures – meta-analysis – is often ill advised. Variability between studies is often likely to be so high that data aggregation at this level may not gain much additional power to detect important differences, and, if done properly, could actually *decrease* the statistical significance of results. One can identify several pre-conditions that enable a valid meta-analysis (FISHER and VAN BELLE 1993): (1) All of the studies conducted in the area of interest need to be available; that is, there is no publication bias (BEGG and BERLIN 1988), so that the likelihood of publication is independent of the significance of the result, a condition that is unfortunately not often met in much current neuro-fMRI literature. (2) The studies must be of sufficient quality, perhaps determined through review by knowledgeable experts. (3) Results should be moderately homogeneous so that their combination can yield an informative result.

However, there may be contexts in which meta-analysis for neuro-fMRI is, or will become, both feasible and advisable. As one looks to the future of statistical procedures for neuro-fMRI, in clinical settings for instance, neuro-fMRI study protocols will of necessity become more rigorous and will involve larger samples. In such cases, FISHER (1954) proposed one simple method for combining *p*-values from separate yet moderately homogeneous studies. Fisher's meta-analysis employs the following basic idea. Suppose that *k* comparable yet independent studies have each yielded *p*-value p_j, $j=1,...,k$, through application of some not necessarily identical statistical procedures. Since $-2\ln p_j$ is distributed as a χ^2 random variable on 2 degrees of freedom regardless of the procedure from which each *p*-value was derived, the sum $P_k = -2\sum_{j=1}^{k} \ln p_j$ is distributed as a χ^2 random variable on $2k$ degrees of freedom. Neuro-fMRI studies need to be independent in order for $2k$ degrees of freedom to be available for the combined test. This simple idea can be used to perform a quick and easy test of combined significance. For instance, suppose that $k=5$ independent neuro-fMRI studies of visual attention have shown evidence of marginal activation in the fusiform gyrus dorsal to the calcarine fissure after lower visual field stimulation, with associated *p*-values of 0.077, 0.093, 0.13, 0.082, and 0.065 from a *t* test, KS-test, repeated measures ANOVA, Fisher's linear discriminant and nonparametric resampling test. Since the value of the combined test statistic $P_k=24.43$ exceeds a 0.01-level critical value of $\chi^2_{0.01}(10)=23.21$, one rejects the null hypothesis of no activation to conclude that neurons in this portion of the fusiform gyrus are sensitive to activity in the lower visual hemifield. The available degrees of freedom drops, as does the significance of the combined result, if the previous results were not gleaned from independent sources or if fewer results were available. This example shows the power of Fisher's simple method to combine "insignificant" (*p*>0.05) results, the importance of reporting results from all comparable studies regardless of their statistical significance, and the strength of independent information.

27.5
Bayesian Paradigm

A statistical formalism for combining subject-matter knowledge with current data to yield new results is given by the following equation: (a posteriori distribution)=(data likelihood)·(a priori distribution) or, in symbols:

$$p(\theta|\text{data}) = \frac{p(\text{data}|\theta)}{\int p(\text{data}|\theta) \cdot p(\theta)} \cdot p(\theta). \qquad (27.54)$$

In the right-hand side of Eq.27.54 is the product of a data-model term and a prior knowledge term. The data-model term is a statistical likelihood expressed as $p(\text{data}|\theta)$, being a conditional probability density function of the data given θ, a symbol representing a scalar or vector-valued parameter that identifies the member of a specified model family which best approximates the observed data; nonparametric and functional data analytic models are included by allowing θ to be of infinite dimension. The prior knowledge term is an unconditional a priori probability distribution $p(\theta)$ that quantifies the degree of belief in the values of θ prior to seeing results of the current data-model. The integral in the denominator of Eq. 27.54 is required so that its left-hand side is also a probability density function. The Bayesian paradigm updates prior information about a parameter of interest by current data to yield new a posteriori information about that parameter. For instance, before one conducts an neuro-fMRI study of primary motor cortex the magnitude and location of the neuro-fMRI signal may be assumed to be distributed evenly across a preselected imaging region.

New data provided by the study update this "flat" prior distribution for the parameter of interest as its distribution takes on shape to become high and peaked in some locations and low and broad in others, indicating increased chances of activity in some regions compared to others.

As knowledge of the neuro-fMRI signal increases through application of statistical procedures to greater numbers of studies of human brain function in highly focused areas involving larger numbers of subjects, it is perhaps a reliable prediction that prior distributions which quantify prior degrees of belief about the properties of the neuro-fMRI signal will become much sharper and consistent across varieties of subject-matter experts than they are at present, thus making Bayesian methods a viable choice for future work in statistical procedures for neuro-fMRI.

References

Adler R (1981) The geometry of random fields. Wiley, New York

Adler R, Hasofer A (1976) Level crossings of random fields. Ann Prob 4:1–12

Aguirre GK, Zarahn E, D'Esposito M (1997) Empirical analyses of BOLD fMRI statistics: II. Spatially smoothed data collected under null-hypothesis and experimental conditions. NeuroImage 5:199–212

Aguirre GK, Zarahn E, D'Esposito M (1998) A critique of the use of the Kolmogorov-Smirnov (KS) statistic for the analysis of BOLD fMRI data. Magn Res Med 39:500–505

Altham PME (1984) Improving the precision of estimation by fitting a model. J Roy Stat Soc, Series B 46:118–119

Amit Y, Grenander U, Piccioni M (1991) Structural image restoration through deformable templates. J Amer Stat Assoc 86:376–387

Ashburner J, Neelin P, Collins DL, Evans A, Friston K (1997) Incorporating prior knowledge into image registration. NeuroImage 6:344–352

Azzalini A (1987) Growth curves analysis for patterned covariance matrices. In: Puri M, Vilaplana J, Wertz W (eds) New perspectives in theoretical and applied statistics. Wiley, New York, pp 61–74

Bandettini PA, Jesmanowicz A, Wong EC, Hyde JS (1993) Processing strategies for time-course data sets in functional MRI of the human brain. Magn Res Med 30:161–173

Begg C, Berlin J (1988) Publication bias: a problem in interpreting medical data. J Royal Stat Soc, Series A 151:419–463

Bell A, Sejnowski T (1995) An information-maximization approach to blind separation and blind deconvolution. Neural Computation 7:1129–1159

Beltrami E (1873) Sulle funzioni bilineari. Gionale di Mathematiche 11:98–106

Birn RM, Bandettini PA, Cox RW, Shaker R, Event-Related fMRI of Tasks Involving Brief Motion. Human Brain Mapping, Volume 7, issue 2, p. 106–114 (1999)

Bishop CM (1995) Neural networks for pattern recognition. Oxford University, Oxford

Bloomfield P (1976) Fourier analysis of time series. Wiley, New York

Box G, Hunter W, Hunter J (1978) Statistics for experimenters. Wiley, New York

Box G, Pierce D (1970) Distribution of residual autocorrelations in autoregressive integrated moving average time series models. J Amer Stat Assoc 65:1509–1526

Box GEP, Jenkins GM (1976) Time series analysis: forecasting and control. Holden-Day, San Francisco, CA

Boxerman JL, Hamberg LM, Rosen BR, Weisskoff RM (1995) MR contrast due to intravascular magnetic susceptibility perturbations. Magn Reson Med 34:555–566

Boynton G, Engel S, Glover G, Heeger D (1996) Linear systems analysis of functional magnetic resonance imaging in human V1. J Neurosci 16:4207–4221

Bracewell R (1986) The Fourier transform and its applications. Second revised edition. McGraw Hill, New York

Brillinger D (1973) The analysis of time series collected in an experimental design Multivariate Analysis, vol III. Academic, New York, pp 241–256

Brillinger D (1975) Time series data analysis and theory. Wiley, New York

Brumback BA, Rice JA (1998) Smoothing spline models for the analysis of nested and crossed samples of curves (with discussion). J Amer Stat Assoc 93:961–976

Buckner R, Bandettini P, O'Craven K, Savoy R, Petersen S, Raichle M, Rosen B (1996) Detection of cortical activation during averaged single trials of a cognitive task using functional magnetic resonance imaging. Proc Natl Acad Sci USA 93:14878–14883

Bullmore E, Brammer M, Williams SCR, Rabe-Hesketh S, Janot N, David A, Mellers J, Howard R, Sham P (1996a) Statistical methods of estimation and inference for functional MR images. Magn Reson Med 35:261–277

Bullmore ET, Brammer MJ, Rabe-Hesketh S, Curtis VA, Morris RG, Williams SCR, Sharma T, McGuire PK (1999) Methods for the diagnosis and treatment of stimulus correlated motion in generic brain activation studies using fMRI. Human Brain Mapping 7:38–48

Bullmore ET, Rabe-Hasketh S, Morris RG, Williams SCR, Gregory L, Gray JA, Brammer MJ (1996b) Functional magnetic resonance image analysis of a large-scale neurocognitive network. NeuroImage 4:16–33

Buxton RB, Frank LR (1993) A physiological model for the interpretation of functional MRI brain activation studies. 12th Annual Meeting of the SMRM, New York, p. 4

Buxton RB, Frank LR (1997) A model for the coupling between cerebral blood flow and oxygen metabolism during neural stimulation. J Cereb Blood Flow Metab 17:64–72

Buxton RB, Wong EC, Frank LR (1997) A biomechanical interpretation of the BOLD signal time course: the balloon model

Cao J, Worsley KJ, Liu C, Collins L, Evans AC (1997) New statistical results for the detection of brain structural and functional changes using random field theory. NeuroImage 5:S512

Cochrane D, Orcutt G (1949) Application of least squares regression to relationships containing autocorrelated error terms. J Amer Stat Assoc 44:32–61

Cohen MS (1997) Parametric analysis of fMRI data using linear systems methods. NeuroImage 6:93–103

Constable RT, Skudlarski P, Gore JC (1995) An ROC approach for evaluating functional brain MR imaging and postprocessing protocols. Magn Reson Med 34:57–64

Courtney SM, Ungerleider LG, Keil K, Haxby JV (1997) Transient and sustained activity in a distributed neural system for human working memory. Nature 386:608–611

Cox D (1972) Regression models and life tables. J Roy Stat Soc, Ser B 34:187–220

Dale AM, Buckner RL (1997) Selective averaging of rapidly presented individual trials using fMRI. Human Brain Mapping 5:329–340

Denby L, Mallows C (1991) Singular values of large matrices subject to Gaussian perturbations. Computing Science and Statistics: Proceedings of the 23rd Symposium on the Interface, pp 54–57

Diggle PJ (1990) Time series: a biostatistical introduction. Oxford University, Oxford

Diggle PJ, Liang K-Y, Zeger SL (1994) Analysis of longitudinal data. Oxford University, Oxford

Draper N, Smith H (1966) Applied regression analysis. Wiley, New York

Duda RO, Hart PE (1973) Pattern classification and scene analysis. Wiley, New York

Durbin J, Watson G (1950) Testing for serial correlation in least squares regression I. Biometrika 37:409–438

Durbin J, Watson G (1951) Testing for serial correlation in least squares regression II. Biometrika 38:159–178

Eckart C, Young G (1936) The approximation of one matrix by another of lower rank. Psychometrika 1:211–218

Edgington E (1987) Randomization tests, 2nd edn. Decker, New York

Efron B (1979a) Bootstrap methods: another look at the jackknife. Annals of Statistics 7:1–26

Efron B (1979b) Computers and the theory of statistics: thinking the unthinkable. SIAM Review 21:460–480

Efron B (1982) The jackknife, the bootstrap and other resampling plans. Society for Industrial and Applied Mathematics, Philadelphia, PA

Efron B, Tibshirani R (1991) Statistical data analysis in the computer age. Science 253:390–395

Efron B, Tibshirani RJ (1993) An introduction to the bootstrap. Chapman and Hall, New York

Fisher L, van Belle G (1993) Biostatistics. Wiley, New York

Fisher RA (1936) The use of multiple measurements in taxonomic problems. Ann Eugen 7:179–188

Fisher RA (1938) The statistical utilization of multiple measurements. Ann Eugen 8:376–386

Fisher RA (1954) Statistical methods for research workers, 12th edn. Oliver and Boyd, Edinburgh

Forman SD, Cohen JD, Fitzgerald M, Eddy WF, Mintun MA, Noll DC (1995) Improved assessment of significant change in functional magentic resonance imaging (fMRI): use of a cluster size threshold. Magn Reson Med33:636–647

Fox P, Raichle M (1986) Focal physiological uncoupling of cerebral blood flow and oxidative metabolism during somatosensory stimulation in human subjects. Proc Natl Acad Sci USA 83:1140–1144

Friston K, Ashburner J, Frith C, Poline J-B, Heather J, Frackowiak R (1995a) Spatial registration and normalization of images. Human Brain Mapping 2:165–189

Friston KJ (1996) Statistical parametric mapping and other analyses of functional imaging data. In: Toga AW, Mazziotta JC (eds) Brain mapping: the methods. Academic, New York, pp 363–386

Friston KJ, Fletcher P, Josephs O, Holmes A, Rugg MD, Turner R (1998a) Event-related fMRI: characterizing differential responses. NeuroImage 7:30–40

Friston KJ, Frith CD, Frackowiak RSJ, Turner R (1995b) Characterizing dynamic brain responses with fMRI: a multivariate approach. NeuoImage 2:166–172

Friston KJ, Frith CD, Frackowiak RSJ, Turner R (1995c) Characterizing evoked hemodynamics with fMRI. NeuroImage 2:157–165

Friston KJ, Frith CD, Liddle PF, Frackowiak RSJ (1991) Comparing functional (PET) images: the assessment of significant change. J Cereb Blood Flow Metab 11:690–699

Friston KJ, Holmes AP, Poline J-B, Glasbey B, Williams C, Frackowiak RSJ, Turner R (1995d) Analysis of fMRI time-series revisited. NeuroImage 2:45–53

Friston KJ, Jezzard P, Turner R (1994a) Analysis of functional MRI time series. Human Brain Mapping 1:153–171

Friston KJ, Josephs O, Rees G, Turner R (1998b) Nonlinear event-related responses in fMRI. Mag Resn Med 39:41–52

Friston KJ, Worsley KJ, Frackowiak RSJ, Mazziotta JC, Evans AC (1994b) Assessing the significance of focal activations using their spatial extent. Human Brain Mapping 1:210–220

Genovese CR, Noll DC, Eddy WF (1997) Estimating test-retest reliability in functional MR imaging I: statistical methodology. Magn Reson Med 38:497–507

Gnanadesikan R (1997) Methods for statistical analysis of multivariate observations, 2nd edn. John Wiley and Sons, New York

Golub GH, Loan CFV (1996) Matrix computations, 3rd edn. Johns Hopkins University Press, Baltimore, MD

Good IJ (1969) Some applications of the singular decomposition of a matrix. Technometrics 11:823–831

Green PJ, Silverman BW (1994) Nonparametric regression and generalized linear models. Chapman and Hall, New York

Grenander U (1970) A unified approach to pattern analysis. Advances in Computers 10:175–216

Hajnal J, Myers R, Oatridge A, Schwieso J, Young I, Bydder G (1994) Artifacts due to stimulus correlated motion in functional imaging of the brain. Magn Res Med 31:283–291

Hansen LK, Nielsen FA, Toft P, Strother SC, Lange N, Morch N, Svarer C, Paulson OB (1997) How many principal components? NeuroImage 5:S474

Hasofer A (1978) Upcrossings of random fields. Adv Appl Prob (Supp) 10:14–21

Hastie T, Tibshirani R (1990) Generalized Additive Models. Chapman and Hall, London

Holmes A, Josephs O, Buchel C, Friston KJ (1997) Statistical modeling of low-frequency confounds in fMRI. NeuroImage 5:S480

Holmes AP (1994) Statistical issues in functional brain mapping. PhD Thesis, Department of Statistics. University of Glasgow

Holmes AP, Blair RC, Watson JDG, Ford I (1996) Nonparametric analysis of statistic images from functional mapping experiments. J Cereb Blood Flow Metab 16:7–22

Hotelling H (1933) Analysis of a complex of statistical variables in principal components. J Educ Psych 24:417–441, 498–520

Hotelling H (1936) Relations between two sets of variates. Biometrika 28:321–377

Hu X, Le TH, Parrish T, Erhard P (1995) Retrospective estimation and correction of physiological fluctuation in functional MRI. Magn Reson Med 34:201–212

Jones R (1993) Longitudinal data with serial correlation: a state-space approach. Chapman and Hall, London

Kim S-G, Richter W, Ugurbil K (1997) Limitations of temporal resolution in functional MRI. Mag Res Med 37:631–636

Laird N, Lange N, Stram D (1987) Maximum likelihood computations with repeated measures: application of the EM algorithm. J Amer Stat Assoc 82:97–105

Laird N, Ware J (1982) Random-effects models for longitudinal data. Biometrics 38:963–974

Lange N (1994) Some computational and statistical tools for paired comparisons of digital images. Stat Meth Med Res 3:23–40

Lange N (1996) Statistical approaches to human brain mapping by functional magnetic resonance imaging. Statistics in Medicine 15:389–428

Lange N (1998a) Discussion of Brumback and Rice: smoothing spline models for the analysis of nested and crossed samples of curves. J Amer Stat Assoc 93:986–988

Lange N (1999) Pattern recognition. In: Armitage P (ed) Encyclopedia of Biostatistics. John Wiley & Sons, New York

Lange N, Bandettini PA, Baker JR, Rosen BR (1995) A comparison of activation detection methods in functional MRI Soc Magn Resonance, Nice, France, pp 828

Lange N, Hansen LK, Anderson JR, Nielsen FA, Savoy R, Kim S-G, Strother SC (1998) An empirical study of statistical model complexity in neuro-fMRI. Fourth International Conference on the Functional Mapping of the Human Brain, Montreal, Canada

Lange N, Laird NM (1989) The effect of covariance structure on variance estimation in balanced growth curve models with random parameters. J Amer Stat Assoc 84:241–247

Lange N, Ryan L (1989) Assessing normality in random effects models. Annals of Statistics 17:624–642

Lange N, Zeger SL (1997) Non-linear Fourier time series analysis for human brain mapping by functional magnetic resonance imaging (with discussion). J Roy Stat Soc, Ser C 46:1–29

Larsen R, Marx M (1986) An introduction to mathematical statistics and its applications, 2nd edn. Prentice-Hall, New York

Le TH, Hu X (1996) Retrospective estimation and correction of physiological artifacts in fMRI by direct extraction of physiological activity from MR data. Magn Reson Med35:290–298

Lee AT, Glover GH, Meyer CH (1995) Discrimination of large venous vessels in time-course spiral blood-oxygen-level-dependent magnetic-resonance functional neuroimaging. Magn Reson Med 33:745–754

Mardia KV, Kent JT, Bibby JM (1979) Multivariate analysis. Academic, London

Mayhew J, Hu D, Zheng Y, Askew S, Hou Y, Berwick J, Coffey PJ (1998) An evaluation of linear model analysis techniques for processing images of microcirculation activity. Neuroimage 7:49–71

McCullagh P, Nelder J (1989) Generalized Linear Models, Second edn. Chapman and Hall, London

McKeown MJ, Makeig S, Brown GG, Jung T-P, Kinderman SS, Bell AJ, Sejnowski TJ (1998) Analysis of fMRI data by blind separation into independent spatial components. Human Brain Mapping 6:160–188

McLachlan GJ (1992) Discriminant analysis and statistical pattern recognition. Wiley, New York

Miller M, Banerjee A, Christensen G, Joshi S, Khaneja N, Grenander U, Matejic L (1997) Statistical methods in computational anatomy. Stat Meth Med Res 6:267–299

Miller M, Christensen G, Amit Y, Grenander U (1993) Mathematical textbook of deformable neuroanatomies. Proc Natl Acad Sci USA 90:11944–11948

Miller RG, Jr. (1996) Beyond ANOVA: basics of applied statistics, 2nd edn. John Wiley and Sons, New York

Mitra P, Pesaran B (1997) Analysis of dynamic brain imaging data. Bell Laboratories, Lucent Technologies, Murray Hill

Mitra PP, Ogawa S, Hu X, Ugurbil K (1997) The nature of spatiotemporal changes in cerebral hemodynamics as manifested in functional magnetic resonance imaging. Magn Reson Med 37:511–518

Montgomery D, Peck E (1982) Introduction to linear regression analysis. Wiley, New York

Mosteller F, Tukey J (1977) Data analysis and regression: a second course in statistics. Addison-Wesley, New York

Nielsen FA, Hansen LK, Toft P, Goutte C, Lange N, Strother SC, Rottenberg D, Morch N, Svarer C, Paulson OB, Savoy R, Rosen B, Rostrup E, Born P (1997) Comparison of two convolution models for fMRI time series. NeuroIm 5:S47

Ogawa S, Menon R, Tank D, Kim S, Merkle H, Ellerman J, Ugurbil K (1993) Functional brain mapping by blood oxygenation level-dependent contrast magnetic resonance imaging. A comparison of signal characteristics with a biophysical model. Biophys J 64:808–13

Pearson K (1901) On lines and planes of closest fit to systems of points in space. Phil Mag [6] 2:559–572

Pelizzari C, Chen G, Spelbring D, Weichselbaum R, Chen C-T (1989) Accurate three-dimensional registration of CT, PET and/or MR images of the brain. J Comp Assist Tomography 13:20–26

Percival D, Walden A (1993) Spectral analysis for physical applications: multitaper and conventional univariate techniques. Cambridge University, New York

Poline JB, Worsley KJ, Evans A, Friston KJ (1997a) Issues in the use of two multivariate analyses for fMRI data. NeuroImage 5:S472

Poline J-B, Mazoyer BM (1993) Analysis of individual positron emission tomography activation maps by detection of high signal-to-noise pixel clusters. J Cereb Blood Flow Metab 13:425–437

Poline J-B, Worsley KJ, Evans AC, Friston KJ (1997b) Combining spatial extent and peak intensity to test for activations in functional imaging. NeuroImage 5:83–96

Press WH, Teukolsky SA, Vettering WT, Flannery BP (1992) Numerical recipes in C: the art of scientific computation, 2n edn. Cambridge University, Cambridge

Quenouille M (1949) Approximate tests of correlation in time series. J Roy Stat Soc, Ser B 11:18–84

Rabe-Hesketh S, Bullmore ET, Brammer MJ (1997) The analysis of functional magnetic resonance images. Stat Meth Med Res 6:215–237

Ramsay J, Silverman B (1997) Functional data analysis. Springer, Berlin, Heidelberg, New York

Ramsay JO (1982) When the data are functions. Psychometrika 47:379–396

Ramsay JO, Dalzell CJ (1991) Some tools for functional data analysis. J Roy Stat Soc, Ser B 53:539–561

Reinsel G (1982) Multivariate repeated-measurement or growth curve models with multivariate random effects covariance structure. J Amer Stat Assoc 77:190–195

Reinsel G (1984) Estimation and prediction in a multivariate random effects generalized linear model. J Amer Stat Assoc 79:406–414

Reinsel G (1985) Mean squared error properties of empirical Bayes estimators in a multivariate random effects general linear model. J Amer Stat Assoc 80:642–650

Rice JA, Silverman BW (1991) Estimating the mean and covariance structure nonparametrically when the data are curves. J Roy Stat Soc, Ser B 53:233–243

Richter W, Andersen PM, Georgopoulos AP, Kim S-G (1997) Sequential activity in human motor areas during a delayed cued finger movement task studied by time-resolved fMRI. NeuroReport 8:1257–1261

Ripley BD (1996) Pattern recognition and neural networks. Cambridge University, Cambridge

Seber CAF (1977) Linear regression analysis. Wiley, New York

Slepian A, Pollack H (1961) Prolate spheroidal wave functions, Fourier analysis and uncertainty–I. Bell Syst Tech 40:43–64

Strang G (1980) Linear algebra and its applications. Academic, New York

Strother SC, Lange N, Anderson JR, Schaper KA, Rehm K, Hansen LK, Rottenberg DA (1997) Activation pattern reproducibility: measuring the effects of group size and data analysis models. Human Brain Mapping 5:312–316

Tagaris GA, Richter W, Kim S-G, Georgopoulos AP (1997) Box-Jenkins intervention analysis of functional magnetic resonance imaging data. Neurosci Res 27:289–294

Talairach J, Tournoux P (1988) Co-planar stereotaxic atlas of the human brain. Thieme, New York

Thomson D (1995) The seasons, global temperature and precession. Science 268:59–68

Thomson DJ (1982) Spectrum estimation and harmonic analysis. Proceedings of the IEEE 70:1055–1096

Thomson DJ, Chave AD (1991) Jackknifed error estimates for spectra, coherences and transfer functions. In: Haykin S (ed) Advances in spectrum analysis and array processing, vol. 1. Prentice Hall, New York, pp 58–113

Trefethen LN, Bau D (1997) Numerical linear algebra. SIAM, Philadelphia, PA

Tukey J (1958) Bias and confidence in not quite large samples. Annals of Mathematical Statistics 29:614

Villringer A, Dirnagel U (1995) Coupling of brain activity and cerebral blood flow: basis of functional neuroimaging. Cereb Brain Metab Rev 7:240–276

Wang Y (1998) Mixed-effects smoothing spline ANOVA. J Royal Stat Soc, Series B 60 60:159–174

Wishart J (1938) Growth rate determinations in nutrition studies with the bacon pig, and their analyses. Biometrika 30:16–28

Woods R, Cherry S, Mazziotta J (1992) Rapid automated algorithm for aligning and reslicing PET images. J Comp Assist Tomogr 16:620–633

Woods R, Grafton S, Holmes C, Cherry S, Mazziotta J (1998a) Automated image registration: I. General methods and intrasubject, intramodality validation. J Comp Assist Tomogr 22

Woods R, Grafton S, Watson J, Sicotte N, Mazziotta J (1998b) Automated image registration: II. Intersubject validation of linear and nonlinear models. J Comp Assist Tomogr 22:153–165

Woods R, Mazziotta J, Cherry S (1993) MRI-PET registration with automated algorithm. J Comp Assist Tomogr 17:536–546

Worsley K (1994) Local maxima and the expected Euler characteristic of excursion sets of χ^2, F, and t fields. Adv Appl Prob 26:13–42

Worsley K, Evans A, Marrett S, Neelin P (1993) Detecting and estimating the regions of activation in CBF activation studies in human brain. In: Uemura K, Lassen N, Jones T, Kanno I (eds) Qualification of brain function: tracer kinetics and image analysis in brain PET. Excerpta Medica, London, pp 535–548

Worsley KJ, Evans AC, Marrett S, Neelin P (1992) Determining the number of statistically significant areas of activation in subtracted studies from PET. J Cereb Blood Flow Metab 12:900–918

Worsley KJ, Friston KJ (1995) Analysis of fMRI time series revisited-again. NeuroImage 2:173–181

Worsley KJ, Poline J-B, Friston KJ, Evans AC (1997) Characterizing the response of fMRI data using multivariate linear models. NeuroImage 6(4):305–319

Xiong J, Gao J-H, Lancaster JL, Fox PT (1996) Assessment and optimization of functional MRI analyses. Human Brain Mapping 4:153–167

Zarahn E, Aguirre GK, D'Esposito M (1997) Empirical analyses of BOLD fMRI statistics: I. Spatially unsmoothed data collected under null-hypothesis conditions. NeuroImage 5:179–197

28 Quality Assurance in Clinical and Research Echo Planar Functional MRI

K.R. Thulborn

CONTENTS

28.1
Introduction

As the signal changes detected by blood oxygenation level-dependent (BOLD) contrast fMRI are small (OGAWA et al. 1990, 1992; KWONG et al. 1992), usually requiring statistical methods to process many images acquired over periods of many minutes, many sources of signal variation contribute to the resultant activation patterns. The sources of these variations should be understood for the instrumentation being used and for the paradigm under investigation if the interpretation of the resultant data is to be meaningful. Two steps are involved in this process. The first is an intensive cataloging of the many sources of noise relevant to the entire site, including mechanical stability of building, quality of electrical power, as well as the scanner electronics. Although some noise sources are likely to be common to all sites, there are sources that may be expected to vary. Examples of site-specific noise may be the instrument itself or the structural integrity, electrical power stability or radiofrequency noise isolation of the site. Having identified and characterized these noise sources, the second step is to implement less time consuming measures of daily

quality assurance that reflect overall system performance and stability relevant to the fMRI method. This quality assurance is a necessary (although not sufficient) element underpinning the interpretation of the results of the fMRI technique. This chapter will describe the steps taken to ensure optimal site performance at the time of construction, instrument design to maximize performance, characterization of noise sources and methods of daily quality assurance that have been used in the MR Research Center at the University of Pittsburgh Medical Center. Elements of this process have been discussed in part elsewhere (THULBORN et al. 1996a–e, 1998a). This experience, accumulated over 5 years, is presented to serve as a model on which other fMRI sites may build and hopefully continue to improve. As my site has nearly identical 1.5 Tesla and 3.0 Tesla scanners, the influence of magnetic field strength is highlighted where important differences have been identified. The data presented are relevant to resonant gradient, echo planar imaging (COHEN and WEISSKOFF 1991) although the principles should generalize across other ultrafast imaging strategies. An important parameter in the construction and operation of such a facility of this magnitude that will not be discussed further is the cost of strategies designed to enhance performance. Such costs are local variables that cannot be generalized over time or site.

28.2
Site Design and Performance

The suitability of a site is determined by many factors although the choice is often based on conveniently available space. Careful examination of the site is required to ensure that the appropriate measures are taken to prepare the site for optimal performance.

The required floor space is mandated by the manufacturer for a particular magnet and field strength. As high field magnets are usually designed

K.R. THULBORN, MD, PhD; MR Research Center, 8th Floor, B wing, Presbyterian University Hospital, 200 Lothrop Street, Pittsburgh, PA 12153, USA

as horizontal superconducting solenoid coils, the magnetic field is always present. The magnetic field lines are highly homogeneous and concentrated within the coil. They form closed loops that extend great distances outside the coil. Because these fringe magnetic fields have adverse effects on cardiac pacemakers, mechanical wrist watches, computer screens and magnetic media, the fringe magnetic field must be contained within a protected space to avoid potential mishaps. Coupling of the fringe field to moving masses can also disrupt the homogeneity of the main field within the magnet and thereby degrade performance. A safe magnetic field is usually considered to be 5 Gauss. As the magnetic field increases for a fixed diameter magnet, the fringe field expands. Although the fringe field of an unshielded 1.5 Tesla magnet extends for several meters, it can be contained by either active shielding or by a passive iron yoke. The active shielding system uses an opposing magnetic field to counterbalance the fringe field. The passive yoke is a large mass of iron placed closely around the magnet to confine the fringe field within the yoke. The walls of the room can also be lined with iron to further contain the fringe field. These choices are site-specific. Both the 1.5 and 3.0 Tesla scanners have passive yokes and similar site footprints for the fringe fields. This was possible by reducing the superconducting solenoid coil of the 3.0 Tesla magnet to 80 cm, as compared to 100 cm for the 1.5 Tesla magnet. Although this reduction could be considered to compromise the homogeneity of the magnetic field, the use of both superconducting and passive shimming allowed similar homogeneity performance (0.5 ppm over 22 cm diameter spherical volume) to be achieved for both scanners. The greater weight (35 tonnes) of the passive yoke over the active shielding imposes requirements for the structural support. This is not a great engineering challenge as demonstrated by placing both passively shielded 1.5 and 3.0 Tesla scanners on the 8th floor of the hospital. The success of such shielding is also reflected in that the positron emission tomography (PET) cameras on the 9th floor immediately above the 3.0 Tesla magnet continue to function without influence despite the requirement of a magnetic environment of less than 1 Gauss. The containment of the fringe field by the passive yoke yields a 50 (30) Gauss line at the end of the patient table on the 3.0 (1.5) Tesla scanner allowing the use of a LCD projector with accessory equipment such as fans at the end of the patient table. This is a great practical convenience for the stimulus presentation system to be described below.

The mechanical stability of the site is not only important to support the weight of the magnet but vibrations from the building can be a concern. The manufacturers provide guidelines for vibration limits and have test procedures that can aid in identifying sources of potentially troublesome vibrations. The sources of vibration may be from machinery such as elevators, the ventilation system, building motion and geological movements. These sources may vary with time of day, day of week and season unless appropriate site preparation and structural support are provided.

The electrical power that is required to run the site should be as stable as possible. This stability influences the precision of the imaging gradients as well as the radiofrequency (RF) power that is essential for long-term stability of series of images. Power lines from the electrical substation should not be shared with other heavy equipment. Power conditioning is mandatory. Uninterruptible power supplies in some settings may be necessary. During installation, the input lines should be monitored over at least 24 h periods to ensure that daily power instabilities are not a source of MR signal variation. The need for power conditioning can then be determined.

The thermal and humidity stability of the equipment room must be ensured over all seasons irrespective of the load, especially if the system is shared with other spaces. Temperature gradients are detrimental to scanner performance and can be avoided by distributing the heat exchangers around the room. Isolation of the room from the mechanical effects of the fans of these systems is also mandatory. Although the manufacturers have recommended temperature and humidity ranges, greater stability was achieved by reducing the temperature several degrees below that recommended. To ensure adequate circulation of air over the electronics, the electronic equipment rack covers should always be in place when experiments are being performed.

Although most magnet rooms of clinical sites have adequate isolation from environmental RF noise for clinical imaging (ca. 70 dB), the RF isolation of the magnet room is easily improved (over 100 dB). There are several types of RF shielding but the fully soldered solid copper room has proven performance at my site. This shield, tested before perforation (except for the door which must be fully occluded at testing), should be well over 120 dB isolation at all frequencies of interest. Perforations for window, penetration panel, ventilation, sprinkler system, wave guides and electrical wiring should not reduce isolation below 100 dB. Window dimensions should be chosen to avoid optimal transmission of observation frequencies and further screened with wire mesh. The door seal that I have found optimal for maintaining RF isolation performance for over 4 years without replacement is a custom designed, pneumatically inflatable, continuous seal surrounding the door. This means that no step is present at the door, which eases movement of the patient table in and out of the room. Care must be taken to avoid the accumulation of floor polish over the metal door frame which can prevent adequate electrical contact. This door is closed with a simple switch thereby avoiding the mechanical wearing experienced with more traditional doors at many clinical sites. The finishing of the room must not compromise the RF isolation and should be independent of the copper surface. Electrical power, required in the scan room for lighting and other equipment, must be filtered for RF noise. Lighting should follow the manufacturers' guidelines and usually requires a direct current supply. The copper shield should have a single ground at the penetration panel to avoid ground loops. This can be difficult to ensure without careful supervision of the construction.

Because of the considerable acoustical noise produced by high speed gradients, the magnet room requires acoustical dampening. This need increases as the field strength increases, especially for echo planar imaging. Double glazing of the windows and sound proofing of the door must be considered along with the walls, ceiling and floor. These details not only are required to meet Occupational Safety and Health Act (OSHA) standards for the staff but also for the use of auditory stimuli in paradigms for fMRI.

28.3
Scanner Design and Performance

Several features of a fMRI scanner distinguish it from a clinical scanner. Clinical scanners rarely need more than 256 images for an entire patient study taking 45–60 min. A single series of consecutive images rarely exceeds 128 individual images as in three-dimensional acquisitions. In marked contrast, a fMRI study with a single paradigm lasts less than 10 min but produces more than 2500 images. These capabilities require stability of signal intensity over time (typically, <1% peak-to-peak signal variation over 30 min using echo planar gradient echo imaging at 3.0 Tesla). Representative stability plots for both the 3.0 and 1.5 Tesla scanners are shown in Fig. 28.1. The quality assurance criterion is less than 1.0% peak-to-peak variation over 30 min on the 3.0 Tesla scanner using a standard phantom and spin-echo echo planar imaging (EPI; 450 axial images, TR=4 s, TE=20 ms/45 ms and slice thicknesses=5 mm/10 mm at 3.0 and 1.5 Tesla, respectively, field of view=40×20 cm, matrix size=128×64).

Large and efficient data handling capabilities in terms of acquisition, reconstruction, transfer and storage are essential. With 0.5 GB of random access memory (RAM) and close to 9 GB of on-line hard disk storage, a schedule with high throughput can be maintained without compromising data acquisition. Subject setup time can be minimized using the efficient subject positioning and landmarking capabilities that are familiar to clinical scanners. Ultrafast imaging techniques, such as EPI, are essential for fMRI to minimize motion artifacts within single images. As subject motion must be limited to much less than a voxel dimension, head immobilization must be achieved with complete subject comfort (THULBORN et al. 1998a). Discomfort not only results in head motion but distracts from cognitive performance on test paradigms. Different forms of real-time registration (THULBORN et al. 1998a; LEE et al. 1996, 1998) have been reported and promise to be

Fig. 28.1a, b. Normalized signal intensity, measured with a standardized protocol, for the **a** 3.0 Tesla and **b** 1.5 Tesla scanners. Peak-to-peak signal variations of less than 1% and 1.5% are demonstrated for the 3.0 Tesla and 1.5 Tesla scanners, respectively. The 3.0 Tesla scanner continues to show stability at ~0.6% over 2 years. Note that the range of the ordinate scales are different to show the minute-to-minute variation

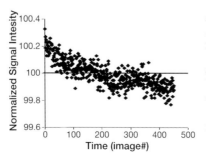
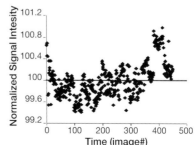

important innovations when used routinely. An alternative approach of image re-registration during post-processing (Woods et al. 1993; Cox 1996; Eddy et al. 1996; Friston et al. 1996; Strupp 1996; Maas et al. 1997) may improve the data but should not overshadow all attempts to reduce unnecessary motion during the acquisition.

Automated shimming for each subject is important (Reese et al. 1995). Although the magnetic field can be highly homogeneous in the absence of a sample, the human body introduces marked distortions. Correction of these distortions by adjustment of at least first-, and if available, second-order shims improves the signal-to-noise ratio (SNR) with minimal loss of time. Initial adjustment of the magnet homogeneity should be done on a spherical phantom if the scanner is to be used primarily for head imaging. The use of a cylindrical phantom introduces a z^2 gradient on human heads that should be avoided.

The imaging x, y and z gradients can be of several types. Resonant gradients (Advanced NMR, Inc. Wilmington, MA) offer fixed gradient switching rates in a sinusoidal wave form at high SNR. Nonresonant gradients allow greater control over the gradient wave form and offer an apparent simplification of sampling under a constant gradient. The gradient switching rates used by the manufacturers reflect Food and Drug Administration (FDA) guidelines. Gradient strength and rise times are considerations but improved performance is achieved usually by decreasing the dimensions over which the gradients must function. For whole body scanners, a separate gradient set can be inserted into the main magnet to improve performance.

Although fMRI may be the primary reason for an investigator to be performing a MRI examination, other features of the scanner may be useful for interpretation of the fMRI data. MR angiography (MRA), using either time-of-flight or phase contrast techniques, may be worthy of consideration for evaluation of vascular structures. In patient studies, it is often useful to use clinical sequences for delineation of anatomic changes. Although not discussed further in this chapter, these aspects of neuroimaging also require quality assurance. Given the clinical use of these sequences, the quality assurance program of the manufacturer is usually efficient and, in my experience, adequate.

28.4
Paradigm Presentation and Subject Monitoring Control System

During imaging acquisition, the fMRI experiment engages the subject in a paradigm that involves two or more tasks differing only by the functional aspect under investigation. The paradigm involves the presentation of a sensory input, usually visual or auditory, but results from novel somatosensory, olfactory and gustatory stimuli are being reported. The performance and degree of difficulty of the task for the subject have been shown to influence the activation patterns (Just et al. 1996). As well as synchronizing stimulus presentation and imaging acquisition, the behavioral responses should be monitored throughout the task. These are experimental design issues that are well established in neuropsychology. The implementation of these requirements for fMRI concerns compatibility of presentation and monitoring equipment with the MR scanner. No losses in SNR of the images need be tolerated from this accessory equipment. Similarly, the presentation and recording equipment also cannot be compromised by the magnetic field. Such equipment has been designed and used on a routine basis (Thulborn et al. 1996b). The quality assurance can be as simple as an overall SNR measurement on a standard phantom in a standard RF coil while all the accessory equipment is operational. A useful measure of SNR has been reported (Weisskoff 1996). My experience has been that for a standard protocol (General Electric Medical Systems spherical phantom and head coil, echo planar, gradient-echo sequence, TR=4 ms, TE=45 ms, single slice, thickness=10 mm for 1.5 Tesla and 5 mm for 3.0 Tesla, field of view=40×20 cm, matrix=128×64), established through discussions with the manufacturer at the time of initial acceptance testing, if the SNR falls below the guideline of 280 (at 3.0 Tesla) service should be initiated. In practice, numbers are routinely above 300 and averaged 340 and 309 over the course of 2 years, as shown in Fig. 28.2 for the 3.0 Tesla and 1.5 Tesla scanners, respectively. The 1.5 Tesla scanner is matched to similar values as the 3.0 Tesla scanner by increasing the slice thickness. The specific numbers and protocol are not as important as ensuring reproducibility of SNR over time.

In addition to the behavioral measures, the cardiac and respiratory cycles have been shown to affect fMRI data and can be used in the analysis. Monitoring of these physiological changes can be used for retrospective corrections or for gating the scanner

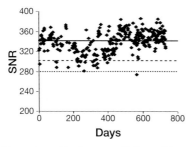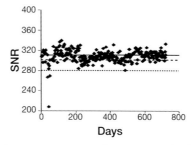

Fig. 28.2a, b. Signal-to-noise ratio for a 3.0 Tesla and b 1.5 Tesla scanners measured over 2 years in the standard quality assurance protocol. The mean signal-to-noise ratio (SNR) values of 340 and 309 for the 3.0 and 1.5 Tesla scanners use 5 and 10 mm slice thicknesses, respectively. This is above the manufacturer's specification of 280. These SNR values are site-specific, but the general approach for quality assurance is important. The time of the low SNR, below the guideline value on the 1.5 Tesla scanner, required a preamplifier replacement service

prospectively. Such gating requires a known longitudinal relaxation rate to correct for the changing longitudinal magnetization with variable excitation rate. The importance of cardiac gating at 1.5 Tesla has been reported (GUIMARAES et al. 1996). Respiratory effects seem to be more important at higher field strengths (HU et al. 1995; THULBORN et al. 1998b). Figure 28.3 demonstrates activation in the primary (V1/V2) and association (V5/MT) visual cortex for a paradigm comparing central fixation on vertically moving black and white strips to the same stationary strips. The activation pattern (Fig. 28.3a) without regard to cardiac and respiratory cycles shows activation and deactivation distributed across nine images (each 3 mm in thickness separated by 1 mm) or 36 mm. The respiratory and cardiac responses were recorded during the image acquisition to allow grouping of images corresponding to specific phases of the respiratory and cardiac cycles. The activation maps (limited to the central three slices of Fig. 28.3b) from the uncensored data at both normal and high t values (t values of 4.5 and 6.0 for Fig. 28.3b, 28.3c, respectively) can be compared to those obtained from the physiologically censored data (images confined to end expiration and diastole phases in Fig. 28.3d, 28.3e, respectively). The more focal activation for the physiologically confined data at the same statistical significance ($t>4.5$) is not due to loss of statistical significance from the reduced number of images (20% and 25% of the images available in the uncensored data for respiratory and cardiac phases, respectively). This is evident from the widely distributed activation pattern even when using the very high threshold ($t>6.0$) for the uncensored data (Fig. 28.3c). These data suggest that removing these sources of physiological variance reduces the total number of images required to obtain activation maps of the same quality. Although the total ac-

quisition times may not be markedly shortened with prospective gating due to the long respiratory time, the much smaller size of the data sets does reduce the not insignificant requirements for computational power and data storage. Clearly prospective censor-

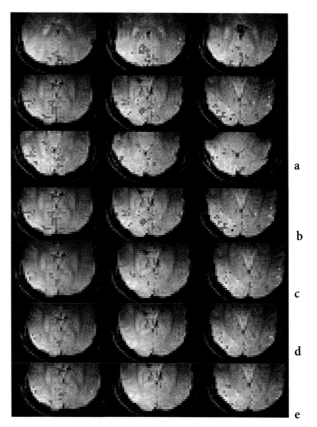

Fig. 28.3a–e. Activation maps for the motion detection paradigm without regard to physiological cycles a over nine slices ($t>4.5$, $t<-4.5$) and then for the three middle slices: b without physiological censorship $t>4.5$, $t<-4.5$), c without physiological censorship ($t>6$, $t<-5$), d with end expiration respiratory censorship ($t>4.5$, $t<-4.5$), and e with diastole cardiac censorship ($t>4.5$, $t<-4.5$)

ship with physiological gating has a role in fMRI strategies.

The quality assurance of these issues involve the automation and precision of time recording, flexibility of the paradigm software and an operating system that allows the entire experiment to be performed by one technologist. As precision and accuracy of timing are high in standard computers, tests can be as simple as checking the timing of paradigms over extended periods of time.

28.5
Subject Preparation

The fact that the performance by the subject of the task to be studied in a fMRI experiment strongly influences the activation patterns obtained is obviously central to this technique. Performance has many influences and is not necessarily constant during an experiment. Sources of variation in performance of a subject include novelty effects from the fMRI environment, anxiety arising from the test itself, training effects and attention to the task over the duration of the examination. Such considerations and experience with subjects across the pediatric to geriatric age range have indicated that a scanner simulator (Fig. 28.4) to acclimate subjects to the scanner environment combined with task training are essential preparation (ROSENBERG et al. 1997).

The most common reason for low quality activation maps to be obtained from a well designed fMRI experiment performed on high quality equipment is head motion (COHEN 1996). Training and preparation in the simulator decreases the problem as does reducing the duration of the paradigm. Many strategies for reducing head motion have been reported including thermoplastic masks and bite bars. Such methods are not suitable for some patient populations where safety may be compromised. Various packing materials have been used to improve head immobilization as have positioning devices (THULBORN et al. 1998a). A universally superior solution is not apparent at this time. My experience is that a cooperative and informed subject comfortably positioned with a positioning feedback system is essential. This is particularly true for high resolution fMRI (THULBORN et al. 1997a). Measurement of head motion is useful to quantify the extent of movement and several methods are available, often linked to correction algorithms (EDDY et al. 1996). Head mo-

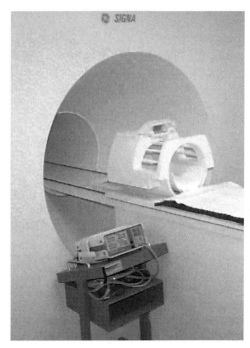

Fig. 28.4. The scanner simulator is a safe and economical means of acclimating subjects to the scanner environment, thereby reducing the novelty effects of the confined space and the imaging sounds. Vital signs (blood pressure, heart rate, arterial oxygen saturation) can be monitored (equipment in foreground) to follow anxiety levels. Paradigms can also be demonstrated in the simulator

tion with peak-to-peak variation of less than 0.3 voxel dimensions produces satisfactory activation maps. Although correction schemes can be used, reacquisition of the data, if possible, is my approach.

28.6
Acquisition of Images

The enormous variety of questions that can be asked with fMRI has an equivalent number of ways in which an experiment can be designed. The choice of RF coil is usually between a volume coil with a uniform large field of view and a surface coil with a non-uniform localized field of view but high SNR. The choice of coil is determined by the question being asked. The phase array of surface coils recently reported produces high SNR over a non-uniform wide field of view (THULBORN et al. 1998a). The issues of quality assurance must be addressed with each type of coil. An important issue is the sensitivity of BOLD contrast across a non-uniform field of view. The sensitivity profile is reflected in the B1 field distribution of the coil, which can be measured rapidly with EPI (THULBORN et al. 1998b).

The imaging sequence most often used for fMRI is some variant of a gradient-echo pulse sequence due to its sensitivity to BOLD contrast (BANDETTINI et al. 1992). The influence of large veins on the activation patterns must always be considered in this setting. At higher field strengths (THULBORN et al. 1996a, b), the SNR is sufficient to allow use of the more selective spin-echo sequence (BOXERMAN et al. 1995). The imaging parameters are determined by matching the echo time, TE, to transverse relaxation time, T2*, to optimize sensitivity to the T2* processes. This implies that T2* is known in each location of interest. A better approach is to measure T2* over the entire field of view, readily done with EPI. The repetition time, TR, is usually determined by a compromise between the duty cycle of the scanner gradients and the number of slices desired. Whole brain coverage requires more than 20 slices at a slice thickness of 3 mm and duty cycle limitations of the gradients can impose TR values of 4 s or longer. The spatial resolution used by most investigators has voxel dimensions of 3×3×3–8 mm^3 reflecting a bias to maintain the SNR at 1.5 Tesla. At 3.0 Tesla, it has been shown that percent signal change for BOLD contrast actually increases as the voxel dimensions are made smaller despite the expected decrease in SNR. This is presumably due to the voxel size matching the functional unit of the cortex (THULBORN et al. 1997a).

28.7
Statistical Methods

As summarized elsewhere (GOLD et al. 1998), no universally accepted statistical method has ascended from the multitude of analysis techniques used for fMRI data (BANDETTINI et al. 1993; FRISTON et al. 1995; BACKFRIEDER et al. 1996; EDDY et al. 1996; BAUMGARTNER et al. 1997; GENOVESE et al. 1997). This is so unlike PET data analysis, in which statistical parametric mapping (SPM) (FRISTON et al. 1995) has become the PET research community standard, that it is worthy of further comment. The data from fMRI varies dramatically amongst laboratories, from scanner instrumentation, magnetic field strength and image acquisition schemes to paradigm design and stimulus presentation equipment. The richness of the data in terms of spatial, temporal and behavioral information obtained on single indi-

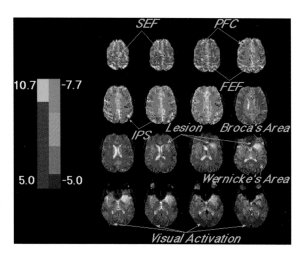

Fig. 28.5. Activation map for the language comprehension paradigm using a t-threshold of 5 and –5 superimposed over a single set of images from the same functional image set. The network of activation includes the eye movement network (supplementary eye fields, *SEF*; frontal eye fields, *FEF*; prefrontal cortex, *PFC*; intraparietal sulcus, *IPS*; visual cortex, *V1/V2*) and the language network (Wernicke's area; Broca's area and homologous areas in the right hemisphere)

viduals is likely to continue to encourage innovative customizing of statistical techniques. The Student *t* test represents the simplest approach to analysis of fMRI data although a Gaussian distribution of noise and the independence of each voxel across the field of view must be assumed. These assumptions have been demonstrated to be reasonable experimentally for EPI (Eddy, personal communication). If the data are of sufficient quality, this test produces informative activation maps, as shown in Fig. 28.5. This example was derived from mapping Broca's area in a patient with a left frontal tumor as a part of presurgical planning. The language reading comprehension paradigm required the patient to silently read word lists and to read sentences and answer questions about each sentence projected onto the viewing screen inside the magnet. This paradigm activates Broca's area in the left frontal lobe, which appears to be displaced anteriorly and laterally from the tumor mass. There is also activation in the homologous region in the right frontal lobe, indicating bilateral language function in this patient. Other areas of activation include Wernicke's area in the left superior temporal gyrus (JUST et al. 1996) and the eye movement pathway of supplementary eye fields (SEF), frontal eye fields (FEF) and intraparietal sulcus (IPS) (LUNA et al. 1998).

One important assumption that is made when applying BOLD fMRI to patient populations is that the hemodynamic response is unchanged from normal subjects used to establish the paradigm. Perfusion and diffusion MRI studies can be used to investigate such assumptions (THULBORN et al. 1997c).

28.8
Display of Multidimensional Data

Given the variety in analysis of fMRI data, the desire to communicate the results back to the research community imposes certain requirements. The location, volume, distribution and generalizability of individual activation patterns must be defined. Location of the nodes of an activation pattern may be reported in several ways. The coordinate system of the Talairach atlas is commonly employed (TALAIRACH and TOURNOUX 1988). This system requires the anatomy of the individual brain to be transformed into the coordinate system of the atlas. Although satisfactory for low resolution image data, the data available from high resolution fMRI are not optimally displayed in this way. Parcellation schemes are also used in which the individual topography of the brain is used to define regions to which activation can be attributed (RADEMACHER et al. 1992). This is a labor intensive and skillful process that reflects the richness of the data. Variations between functional and morphometric anatomy may also decrease the accuracy of such parcellation schemes. However once the method is defined and the limitations appreciated, either method facilitates communication between researchers.

The point to be emphasized from a quality assurance perspective is that fMRI data are often acquired at a low resolution (voxel dimensions of approx. $3\times3\times4$–8 mm^3) and superimposed over high resolution images acquired using a different acquisition scheme, sometimes even with entirely different gradients. Although such enhanced activation maps are aesthetically pleasing, the distortions that occur between image types must be calibrated to ensure fidelity in reporting results. This is particularly revealing for patients with distorted anatomy when data are transformed into Talairach coordinates. An alternative approach has been to acquire high resolution structural data using the same sequence as the functional data so that any distortions are the same in both images sets. The optimal result is obtained when the functional images are of sufficient resolution to provide the structural information. Such activation maps in the visual cortex have been reported elsewhere (THULBORN et al. 1997a).

Either parcellation or Talairach coordinate systems can be used to pool results from individual subjects into group data to investigate generality of results across populations. Such comparisons should report the matching of performance parameters (e.g., response time, accuracy) between the individuals of the group before conclusions are drawn. Although the generality of an activation pattern can be examined using grouped data, a major distinction from other imaging modalities must be made. It is not necessary to group data to obtain a result, i.e., an activation map. Thus, the spatial resolution is that of the imaging scheme and not that of the anatomic variability amongst individual subjects. Group activation maps are most appropriately reported superimposed over group structural maps (LUNA et al. 1998).

The display of activation maps is another means to communicate such patterns but must confront the difficulty of displaying multidimensional data in limited space. Three-dimensional rendered images of the highly convoluted brain surface may fail to provide detailed information even with various strategies of partial transparency and multiple rotated views. Flattened two-dimensional maps based on an atlas (VAN ESSEN and DRURY 1997) or, better, taken from the individual subject (DALE and SERENO 1993) provide an informative display once experience has been gained with the interpretation of this format.

28.9
Conclusions

Quality assurance for fMRI commences with preparation of the site and installation of the scanner. Overall system performance as described in terms of SNR and signal stability should be measured routinely and is an essential part of being able to interpret functional data. Choices of RF coils, acquisition parameters and the quality assurance associated with each are dependent on the question at hand. Subject preparation and training is essential to ensure complete cooperation and an interpretable result. BOLD contrast is enhanced at high field and is the single most effective means of providing technically successful fMRI studies routinely.

Acknowledgments. The author gratefully acknowledges the technical support from General Electric Medical Systems, Advanced NMR Systems, Inc. and

Magnex Scientific and financial support from Public Health Services grant PO1 NS35949-01A1 and General Electric Medical Systems. The enthusiastic help of Densie Davis and Tanya Gindin with preparation of figures in this manuscript is thankfully acknowledged.

References

Backfrieder W, Baumgartner R, Samal M, Moser E, Bergmann H (1996) Quantification of intensity variations in functional MR images using rotated principal components. Phys Med Biol 41:1425–1438

Bandettini PA, Wong EC, Hinks RS, Tikofsky RS, Hyde JS (1992) Time course EPI of human brain function during task activation. Magn Reson Med 25:390–397

Bandettini PA, Jesmanowicz A, Wong EC, Hyde JS (1993) Processing strategies for time-course data sets in functional MRI of the human brain. Magn Reson Med 30:161–173

Baumgartner R, Scarth G, Teichtmeister C, Somorjai R, Moser E (1997) Fuzzy clustering of gradient-echo functional MRI in the human visual cortex. Part 1: reproducibility. J Magn Reson Imaging 7:1094–1101

Boxerman JL, Bandettini PA, Kwong KK, Baker JR, Davis TL, Rosen BR, Weisskoff RM (1995) Contributions to fMRI signal change: Monte Carlo modeling and diffusion-weighted studies. Magn Reson Med 34:4–10

Cohen M, Weisskoff R (1991) Ultra-fast imaging. J Magn Reson Imaging 9:1–37

Cohen MS (1996) Rapid MRI and functional applications. In: Toga AW, Mazziotta JC (eds) Brain mapping: the methods. Academic, San Diego, p 250–251

Cox RW (1996) AFNI: software for analysis and visualization of functional magnetic resonance neuroimages. Comput Biomed Res 29:162–173

Dale A, Sereno M (1993) Improved localization of cortical activity by combining EEG and MEG with MRI cortical surface reconstruction: a linear approach. J Cogn Neurosci 5:162–176

Eddy WF, Fitzgerald M, Genovese CR, Mockus A, Noll DC (1996) Functional imaging analysis software – Computational olio. In: Prat A (ed) Proceedings in computational statistics. Physica, Heidelberg, pp 39–49

Eddy WF, Fitzgerald M, Noll DC (1996) Improved image registration by using Fourier interpolation. Magn Reson Med 36:923–931

Friston KJ, Holmes AP, Worsley KJ, Poline JP, Frith CD, Frackowiak RSJ (1995) Statistical parametric maps in functional imaging: a general linear approach. Hum Brain Mapping 2:189–210

Friston KJ, Williams S, Howard R, Frackowiak RSJ, Turner R (1996) Movement-related effects in fMRI time-series. Magn Reson Med 35:346–355

Genovese CR, Noll DC, Eddy WF (1997) Estimating test-retest reliability in functional MR imaging I: statistical methodology. Magn Reson Med 38:497–507

Gold S, Christian B, Arndt S, Zeien G, Cizadlo T, Johnson DL, Fiaum M, Andreasen NC (1998) Functional MRI statistical software packages: A comparative analysis. Hum Brain Mapping 6:73–84

Guimaraes AR, Melcher JR, Talavage TM, Baker JR, Rosen BR, Weisskoff RM (1996) Detection of inferior colliculus activity during auditory stimulation using cardiac gated functional MRI with T1 correction. Neuro Image 3: S9

Hu X, Le TH, Parrish T, Erhard P (1995) Retrospective estimation and correction of physiological fluctuation in functional MRI. Magn Reson Med 34:201–212

Just MA, Carpenter PA, Keller TA, Eddy WF, Thulborn KR (1996) Brain activation modulated by sentence comprehension. Science 274:114–116

Kwong KK, Belliveau JW, Chesler DA, Goldberg IE, Weisskoff RM, Poncelet BP, Kennedy DN, Hoppel BE, Cohen MS, Turner R, Cheng H-M, Brady TJ, Rosen BR (1992) Dynamic magnetic resonance imaging of human brain activity during primary sensory stimulation. Proc Natl Acad Sci USA 89:5675–5679

Lee CC, Jack CR, Grimm RC, Rossman PJ, Felmlee JP, Ehman RL, Riederer SJ (1996) Real-time adaptive motion correction in functional MRI. Magn Reson Med 36:436–444

Lee CC, Grimm RC, Manduca A, Felmlee JP, Ehman RL, Riederer SJ, Jack CR (1998) A prospective approach to correct for inter-image head rotation in fMRI. Magn Reson Med 39:234–243

Luna B, Thulborn KR, Strojwas MH, McCurtain BJ, Berman RA, Genovese CR, Sweeney JA (1998) Dorsal cortical regions subserving visually-guided saccades in humans: a fMRI study. Cereb Cortex 8:40–47

Maas LC, Frederick BD, Renshaw PF (1997) Decoupled automated rotational and translational registration for functional MRI time series data: the DART registration algorithm. Magn Reson Med 37:131–139

Ogawa S, Lee TM, Nayak AS, Glynn P (1990) Oxygenation-sensitive contrast in magnetic resonance image of rodent brain at high fields. Magn Reson Med 14:68–78

Ogawa S, Tank DW, Menon RS, Ellermann JM, Kim S-G, Merkle H, Ugurbil K (1992) Intrinsic signal changes accompanying sensory stimulation: functional brain mapping using MRI. Proc Natl Acad Sci U S A 89:5951–5955

Rademacher J, Galaburda AM, Kennedy DN, Filipek PA, Caviness VS (1992) Human cerebral cortex: localization, parcellation, and morphometry with magnetic resonance imaging. J Cogn Neurosci 4:352–374

Reese T, Davis T, Weisskoff R (1995) Automated shimming at 1.5 T using echo planar image frequency maps. J Magn Reson Imaging 5:739–745

Rosenberg DR, Sweeney JA, Gillen JS, Chang SY, Varanelli MJ, O'Hearn K, Erb PA, Davis D, Thulborn KR (1997) Magnetic resonance imaging of children without sedation: preparation with simulation. J Am Acad Child Adolesc Psychiatry 36:853–859

Strupp JP (1996) Stimulate: a GUI based fMRI analysis software package. NeuroImage 3:S607

Talairach J, Tournoux P (1988) Co-planar stereotaxic atlas of the human brain: 3D proportional system: an approach to cerebral imaging, Georg Thieme, New York

Thulborn KR, Davis D, Erb P, Strojwas M, Sweeney JA (1996a) Clinical fMRI: Implementation and experience. NeuroImage 4:S101-S107

Thulborn KR, Gillen JS, McCurtain B, Betancourt C, Sweeney JA (1996b) Functional magnetic resonance imaging of the human brain. Bull Magn Reson 18:37–42

Thulborn KR, McCurtain B, Voyvodic J, Chang S, Gillen J, Sweeney JA (1996c) Functional MRI: the environment and technology for clinical application. In: Pavone P, Rossi P (eds) Functional MRI. Springer, Berlin Heidelberg New York, p 15–19

Thulborn KR, Talagala SL, Chang SY, Pitcher EE, Voyvodic JT, Shen GX, Sweeney JA (1996d) High field clinical fMRI. In: Scotti G, LeBihan D (eds) Functional neuroanatomy of motion and vision. Edizioni del Centauro, Udine, pp 53–62

Thulborn KR, Voyvodic J, McCurtain B, Gillen J, Chang S, Just MA, Carpenter P, Sweeney JA (1996e) High field functional MRI in humans: applications to cognitive function. In: Pavolone P, Rossi P (eds) Functional MRI. Springer, Berlin Heidelberg New York, pp 91–96

Thulborn KR, Chang SY, Shen GX, Voyvodic JT (1997a) High resolution echo planar fMRI of human visual cortex at 3.0 Tesla. NMR Biomed 10:183–190

Thulborn KR, Uttecht S, Betancourt C, Talagala SL, Boada FE, Shen GX (1997b) A functional, physiological and metabolic toolbox for clinical magnetic resonance imaging: integration of acquisition and analysis strategies. Int J Imaging Syst Technol 8:572–581

Thulborn KR, Martin C, Shen GX (1998a) An integrated head immobilization system for fMRI of visual paradigms at 1.5 T. In: Proceedings Sixth Scientific Meeting International Society of Magnetic Resonance in Medicine. Sydney, Australia, April, p. 2134

Thulborn KR, Voyvodic J, Chang S, Strojwas M, Sweeney JA (1998b) New approaches to cognitive function by high field functional MRI. In: Yuasa T, Prichard JW, Ogawa S (eds) Current progress in functional brain mapping: science and applications. Smith-Gordon, London, pp 15–23

Thulborn KR, Boada FE, Shen GX, Christensen JD, Reese TG (1998c) Correction of B1 inhomogeneities using echo planar imaging of water. Magn Reson Med 39:369–375

Van Essen DC, Drury HA (1997) Structural and functional analyses of human cerebral cortex using a surface-based atlas. J Neurosci 17:7079–7102

Weisskoff RM (1996) Simple measurement of scanner stability for functional NMR imaging of activation of the brain. Magn Reson Med 36:643–645

Woods RP, Mazziotta JC, Cherry SR (1993) MRI-PET registration with automated algorithm. J Comput Assist Tomogr 17:536–546

29 The Psychophysiological Laboratory in the Magnet: Stimulus Delivery, Response Recording, and Safety

R.L. Savoy, M.E. Ravicz, R. Gollub

CONTENTS

29.1
Introduction

The first reported use of MRI for detecting neural activity changes in the human brain was based on changes in visual system during the presentation of light via a set of "Grass goggles" that used light-emitting diodes (BELLIVEAU et al. 1991). This was (literally) the same apparatus that was used by Fox and

R. L. SAVOY, PhD; The Rowland Institute for Science, 100 Edwin Land Boulevard, Cambridge, MA 02142-1297, USA
M. E. RAVICZ, MS; Eaton-Peabody Laboratory, Massachusetts Eye and Ear Infirmary, 243 Charles Street, Boston, MA 02114, USA
R. GOLLUB, PhD; Department of Psychiatry, Massachusetts General Hospital, Psychiatric Neuroimaging, Room 9109, Building 149, 13th Street, Charlestown, MA 02129, USA

Raichle, in their classic positron emission tomography (PET) study of the visual system (Fox and RAICHLE 1984). These goggles were manually turned on and off by an experimenter in the MR room who watched a clock while the subject was being scanned. Given the explosion of fMRI-based research, it is not surprising that many improvements have been made in the technology of conducting psychological experiments in the MR environment.

The term "psychophysiological laboratory in the magnet" (PLM) will be used in the present chapter to denote issues relating to the practical considerations of interacting with human subjects in fMRI experiments. This includes technology for stimulus presentation, behavioral response recording, physiological monitoring, and some safety issues specific to fMRI.

29.1.1
Challenges of the Psychophysiological Laboratory in the Magnet

People who study perception would like to be able to present stimuli that match the natural world as closely as possible, but they also want to be able to control and manipulate those stimuli. To accomplish this goal requires a host of technologies, even in a conventional psychophysiological laboratory. Each sensory process (e.g., vision, audition, olfaction, taste, touch, proprioception) requires a different technology for the presentation of controlled stimuli. For a discussion of the basic information processing requirements (stimulus representation, data storage, data transmission rates, and physical transduction) in the context of vision and audition, see SAVOY (1986).

The challenge is made significantly more difficult when the stimuli must be presented in the MRI environment. The bore of the magnet is small enough that it introduces many practical problems for the PLM. The high levels of acoustic noise in the MR environment – both from standard equipment like the magnet coolant pump and from special pulse sequences for high speed imaging – make presentation of auditory stimuli especially difficult. Finally, the electromagnetic environment in the MRI room precludes the use of many conventional pieces of equipment. Special devices must be built that are nonmagnetic (so they do not interact with the main magnet), that are immune to rapidly changing electromagnetic fields (both from the rapidly switching gradient magnets used for imaging and the rapidly oscillating radiofrequency (RF) fields used to generate the NMR signal), and that do not, themselves, generate significant RF energy which would interfere with the quality of the MR images.

These challenges have been addressed in unique and creative ways by individual laboratories. They are also increasingly addressed by commercial vendors who appreciate the growth of fMRI and its potential for the future.

29.1.2
Research, Vendors, and the World Wide Web

Functional MRI is a technique that is undergoing rapid development in all areas: pulse sequences, data analysis, experimental design, and the present topic of the PLM. In the years since fMRI started, each laboratory that was actively interested in this technology had to develop their own methods for stimulus presentation and response recording – there were no off-the-shelf commercial products available. This situation has changed, but many unique procedures continue to be developed in different laboratories.

Because these technologies are being developed in a research setting, there are several practical and safety-related questions that arise. How can one find out about these devices? Are they safe? How well do they work?

In the context of auditory and visual stimulus presentation, the situation has changed the most from early days. At least two vendors now offer integrated systems for presentation of visual and auditory stimuli. Also, there are at least two other vendors who offer physiological monitoring equipment that is MR-compatible.

Because the pace of development in the technologies associated with fMRI is so rapid, it is difficult to be fair in describing or comparing currently available devices from different vendors. It is difficult to do a complete evaluation of the devices; new vendors

appear regularly; existing vendors improve their equipment on a time scale that is rapid with respect to book publication. Keeping those caveats in mind, we will provide information about some of the vendors who have developed equipment specifically relevant to the PLM.

One of the most important places to seek information about new developments for the PLM is on the World Wide Web. Vendors in this high-tech field almost universally present their wares on the Web. In contrast, there are relatively few papers devoted exclusively to the description of equipment for the PLM in refereed research journals. (Of course, the "Methods" sections of specific papers often supply useful information.)

29.1.3
A Few Words on Stimulus Generation

The topic of stimulus generation will not be covered in detail in the present chapter. There are many software packages for visual and auditory stimulus generation. Some are specific to individual computer platforms (e.g., Macintosh, PC, SGI), and some are specific to custom hardware (e.g., LabVIEW, National Instruments, Austin, TX, USA). However, the issues associated with a choice of these packages are largely independent of issues specific to functional MRI. That is, almost all of these packages (e.g., PsyScope, PsychLab) were developed in the context of general psychology laboratories and can be readily adapted to the requirements of stimulus generation for fMRI-based experiments. A few (MacStim, for example, by David Darby, Melbourne, Australia) were developed specifically for fMRI, but they are still basically general purpose software systems for stimulus presentation and response recording.

There is, perhaps, one issue that should be mentioned in this regard. Many software systems from the psychological laboratory treat the temporal duration of individual stimuli as the crucial variable and are more casual about the precision of the intertrial interval, and the total amount of time taken for a collection of stimulus presentations. This can be a problem in fMRI-based experiments. Because almost all data analysis procedures require knowledge of the precise timing of stimulus presentation over a period of several minutes, small drifts due to individual variations on specific trials can create significant time differences when many trials are included in a run. It is, therefore, important that whatever software tools are used for stimulus generation, they give the user the ability to control the absolute timing of trials throughout a session, rather than just the relative timing between trials.

Finally, it should be mentioned that some vendors are moving toward incorporating many aspects of stimulus generation and stimulus presentation in a single package for fMRI. For example, Neuroscan is a company that has developed a software system for visual stimulus generation (STIM) which it bundles with a hardware system for visual and auditory stimulus presentation (from Avotec, mentioned below). Further information on this system is available at http://www.neuro.com/neuroscanstimfmri.htm, including a list of some purchasers of the system. Analogous systems from other vendors are likely to be available by the time this book is published.

29.2
Stimulus Presentation

This section will deal with the technology for presenting various kinds of stimuli to the subject in the magnet. In the case of vision and audition, a great deal of effort has been expended in development. In the case of other sensory modalities, the developments have been more idiosyncratic at individual laboratories.

In the context of piloting new studies, which may require novel technology for stimulus presentation, it should be remembered that (as in the first human fMRI study) it is often possible for an experimenter to be in the room with the subject and to present stimuli using very simple means (such as hand-held cards for visual stimuli). It is difficult to be precise in the timing and other aspects of such stimulus presentation procedures, but they can help get one started.

29.2.1
Visual Display Systems

The greatest efforts, initially, went into the presentation of visual stimuli. This was driven by two forces. First, the visual system was a natural domain of interest. A great deal was known about its neurophysiology; there were PET studies to which the data could be compared; and the retinotopic delineation of many different visual areas in the cortex was a natural challenge. Second, the ability to present visual stimuli (including words and pictures) is sufficient to conduct a host of cognitive and language studies.

The source of the visual image is almost always a computer. There are some exceptions. Video tape or a "live" camera can be used to generate a video signal; 35 mm or larger transparencies can be projected to create the visual signal; reflection prints can be used. However, the computer generated stimuli are far more flexible and the timing of their presentation is easier to control precisely.

Given a computer generated signal (typically in RGB format with a spatial resolution of 640×480 pixels or better) or a standard NTSC video signal (with less spatial, temporal, and intensity resolution than RGB, but still adequate for most experiments), the next questions are: How is that signal transduced into light? And how is that light transferred into the subject's eye?

The usual way to create the light is with some version of a liquid crystal display (LCD). Because the display is not affected by the MRI system, it can be placed in the MR room near the subject. Subjects can view the LCD screen directly, or through a variety of optical systems. Most computer and video projection systems use LCDs as their light source. An alternative light source is the conventional computer monitor (cathode ray tube display, CRT), placed outside the MR room or mounted securely within the MR room.

There are three common methods for conveying the light to the subjects' eyes. One method is to have subjects view the display apparatus (LCD or CRT) through a fiber optic cable. A second method is to have the subjects view the display apparatus through lenses that serve as a set of binoculars. The purpose of both the fiber optic cable and the binoculars is to increase the visual angle subtended by the stimulus at the eye of the subject. A third method is to have subjects view an image focused on a rear-projection screen. If the screen is outside the bore of the magnet, the visual angle subtended is necessarily small. If the screen can be placed near to the subjects' eyes, then it can subtend a much larger visual angle.

Various combinations of these devices are in use, as will be discussed below. In evaluating these systems, it is important to keep in mind the image quality characteristics to which the human visual system is sensitive. These are discussed in the next section.

29.2.1.1
Spatial, Temporal, Intensity and Color Resolution

As discussed in Savoy (1986), visual stimuli can be thought of as having six and one half dimensions. There are three intensity dimensions, due to the different spectral sensitivities of the three cone classes in the retina; there are two spatial dimensions, corresponding to the two dimensional surface of the retinal and its projected visual angle in the real world; there is one temporal dimension, as visual stimuli vary with time, and there is a "half" dimension, corresponding to the fact of having two eyes that can be independently stimulated.

To create reasonably realistic, continuous tone images, it is sufficient to have intensity resolution that encompasses at least 100 levels of long-wave, middle-wave, and short-wave light (i.e., red, green and blue). Modern computer systems that permit "millions of colors" (i.e., typically 256 levels of red, green, and blue phosphor in a CRT or LCD) are adequate for this level of intensity resolution. More limited systems (such as the standard North American television conventions embodied in NTSC) are adequate for many purposes. Other technologies (such as color transparencies) also achieve something like the desired intensity resolution range. Color photographs and other reflection prints have a more limited intensity range, but are still adequate for most purposes.

There are some contexts in which greater intensity resolution is needed. For example, measuring absolute intensity thresholds or contrast thresholds can require as much as 1000 luminous intensity levels. There are a collection of optical and digital tricks (Savoy 1986; Pelli and Zhang 1991; Tyler 1997) for increasing the effective intensity resolution in those special cases.

Ideally, the spatial resolution should match the finest resolution of the human visual system, which is about 1 min of visual angle ($1/60°$) in the central fovea. The spatial extent of the visual stimulus should encompass the entire visual field (more than 180° horizontally, for the visual field of the two combined eyes, and more than 90° vertically). These goals are not met by any existing system (even outside the magnet!), but some technologies come much closer than others.

The temporal resolution of the visual system is more difficult to specify. Some experiments in visual psychophysics require temporal variations of a few milliseconds. However, the presentation rates of most modern computers (50–70 Hz) are adequate for the vast majority of experiments in visual perception, including those involving motion processing. Even the compromise rate employed in NTSC standard television (30 full frames per second, interleaved with alternate horizontal lines every 1/60-th seconds) is adequate for most purposes. However, if one is using a specialized task that requires finer temporal resolution (as is sometimes needed in visual back-masking experiments), the temporal resolution limits of your display technology must be kept in mind.

Finally, it is necessary to present different stimuli to the two eyes for certain visual experiments, notably those involving stereopsis.

29.2.1.2
LCD Projectors and Rear Projection Screens

Liquid crystal display projectors are designed to create a large image (for example, 3 m wide by 2 m high) at a modest distance from the projector (for example, 5 m away). With many projectors, there is a variable zoom lens so that smaller (but still large) images can be displayed at closer distances. Such projectors have been used in the MR environment to create images on a large (1×1.5 m) screen that is placed outside the bore of the magnet. Subjects must look up into a mirror or else use prism glasses to see the screen.

The advantages of this system are that a suitable projector can be purchased without modification and that the screen can be easily set in place by the experimenter. The disadvantages are that the visual angle subtended by the screen is relatively small (unless the subject uses special optics), and the projector must be either in the MR room (which can be dangerous and can generate RF noise), or must project through a window (which, if screened with RF shielding wire mesh, will generate a poor quality visual image). This system is better suited to MRI machines in which the rear is open, optically, and the screen can be mounted just behind the magnet.

An alternative is to modify the projector by getting a custom built projection lens that will create a smaller image at the desired distance for the particular MR installation. If this is done, the rear projection screen can be much smaller, and can be mounted within the bore of the magnet. The point of this exercise is to get the image closer to the eyes of the subject, so that it subtends a much larger visual angle (for a schematic figure, see Savoy 1998).

The advantages of such a system are the greater visual angle subtended, and the ability to project through a screened window (by having the projector outside the MR room, and the custom made lens in the MR room on the other side of the window). The disadvantages of this system are that the rear projection screen must be mounted inside the bore of the magnet after the subject is in place (which can be awkward with patients), and that the addition of a custom projection lens adds cost (typically $2000–$3,000). Some of the awkwardness of placing the screen can be ameliorated by having it mounted on the head coil. However, use of the head coil generally limits the size of the screen (and therefore the size of the image). For cognitive experiments involving the presentation of pictures or words, this is not a serious problem. For studies of the visual system it is a problem, and surface coils (which permit the use of wider visual field displays in the magnet. as well as greater sensitivity in imaging the occipital cortex) are often used, and the subject places the screen and adjusts the viewing mirror to obtain as large a field of view as possible.

The image quality in any of these systems is subject to several sources of degradation. First, the subjects typically see the rear projection screen by looking up at a mirror tilted at 45°. A conventional silvered mirror cannot be used because the silver supports eddy currents that will distort the MR images. Therefore plastic mirrors with a mylar reflecting surface are used. However, these are rear surface mirrors. That is, the reflecting surface is behind the plastic. This means that there will, to some extent, be a double image because the front surface of the plastic also creates a reflection (albeit of much lower intensity). It is possible to purchase dichroic front surface mirrors, which should solve this problem, though the 25×10 cm size would make them expensive.

Another source of image degradation is the rear projection screen. When mounted externally, it is usually a light, flexible material that is difficult to keep perfectly flat. When mounted within the bore it is rigid, but the quality of the image depends upon the material. A plastic screen (e.g., Daplex, Crimson Tech, Cambridge, MA, USA) is adequate; a ground glass screen is more expensive but better.

In general, these systems are reasonable to use. The cost (for high-quality projector, custom lens, and rear projection screen) is about $15,000; an adequate system can be obtained for substantially less. The image quality is good. The image size is adequate, though not sufficient to create anything like a "virtual reality" for the subject.

29.2.1.3
LCD or CRT Displays and Fiber Optics

While LCD displays can be placed in the MR room near the subject, they cannot easily be operated immediately in front of the subjects' eyes as they lie in a head coil. CRTs can give better spatial, temporal and intensity resolution than LCDs, but they must be outside the MR room (or be carefully mounted within the room). In any of these situations, the images that are created subtend an unacceptably small angle for the subject. One natural way to address this problem is with the use of collimated fiber optic cables. Such cables, in effect, can move the image to a location closer to the subjects' eye. Suitable optics must also be included to allow the subject to be able to focus.

This use of fiber optics has appeared in at least two places. One is a commercial product called "Silent Vision" (Avotec, Jensen Beach, FL, USA), and is part of a combined visual and auditory stimulus display system. This system uses fiber optics and one or two LCD displays (depending upon whether the purchaser wants a true stereo system, or is content to have the same visual stimulus presented to both eyes). The advantages of this system are the reasonably large visual angle subtended (30°×23°), an adjustable focus and adjustable inter-pupillary distance, and its design for use with conventional head coils. The disadvantages are its cost ($20,000-$30,000 depending upon options) and the problems inherent with fiber optic cables, which will be mentioned below.

A second system that uses fiber optics does so in conjunction with a conventional CRT outside the MR room (Cornelissen et al. 1997). This system takes advantage of the greater resolution of a CRT than an LCD display. The article also describes the choice of eyepieces that can be used to increase the visual angle (at the expense of the image quality). The lens that was normally used gave a visual field of 35°×28°.

Both of the above systems suffer from one problem with fiber optics. A collimated fiber optic cable, such as the one described in Cornelissen et al. (1997) is composed of a regular array of 1000×800 fibers. In the manufacture of these cables, some small fraction of the 800,000 fibers break. These breaks appear as small black dots in the image. It may be possible, but very expensive, to obtain such cables with no breaks. The cables with breaks cost about $8000 at the time Cornelissen et al. (1997) was written. That article also includes a reproduction of the image as seen through the fiber optic cable, including the effects of the broken fibers. The authors point out that these broken fibers do not tend to increase over time. That is, the breaks one gets with the manufactured cable are stable. This is especially important in the context of fMRI experiments, in which the brain response to two different conditions is typically being examined. Having some visual noise in the stimulus is not likely to be a significant problem for such studies if it is stable across conditions. Furthermore, in the context of cognitive experiments, in which the primary stimuli are complex pictures or words, the small black dots apparently do not interfere with the easy recognition of the stimuli.

Notwithstanding the image quality problem that fiber optics can introduce, there is much to be said for these systems. In conjunction with a good auditory stimulus package, they can be used to create a virtual reality, wherein enough of the subjects' visual field is filled with the experimenters images (and the remaining portion of the visual field is blocked by the eyepiece) to significantly distract the subject from awareness of the MR environment. The commercial system from Avotec has been used successfully in a number of laboratories.

29.2.1.4
LCD or CRT Displays and Binoculars

Both LCD and CRT displays have also been presented to subjects using conventional optics. In effect, a custom set of binoculars is developed in order to have the displays subtend a large visual angle.

In one installation, a CRT monitor is mounted on the ceiling several meters away from the subject. The subject looks through a set of lenses that serve as binoculars to have the CRT display fill a large portion of the field of view. Obviously, considerable care must be taken in mounting (for safety) and shielding the monitor (for RF noise reduction and proper CRT function).

A commercial system (Resonance Technology, Northridge, CA, USA) uses an LCD placed very close to the subject (e.g., resting on the subject's chest) with conventional optics to present the image. This system comes with NTSC video resolution. It is part of an integrated visual and auditory system costing about $35,000. The advantage of this system is the image quality. A disadvantage of the system is the limited NTSC resolution. Various improvements to this system are underway.

The main advantage of the LCD or CRT with binoculars compared to the fiber optics systems is the improved image quality. The main disadvantage is cost.

29.2.1.5
Summary of Visual Display Systems

All of the systems described above have been used successfully in functional MRI. For virtually all cognitive and language experiments they are more than adequate. If high resolution visual stimuli are essential (as when mapping multiple visual areas), it is wise to obtain a high resolution system. When there are special subject considerations (such as working with patients, children, or elderly subjects), systems that are easiest to use (such as the commercial systems) are particularly valuable. It should be noted that none of these systems are likely to work perfectly "off-the-shelf." The substantial cost of the commercial systems includes installation, which can be nontrivial. The net result will be a visual stimulus that is acceptable for the vast majority of fMRI-based experiments.

It should be emphasized that there are other companies that are entering this market and that existing companies are upgrading their systems and integrating more features. Specifically, Avotec is developing a system that includes an eyetracker; Resonance Technology is developing higher resolution systems that will include an eyetracker and response devices; and a company called Psychology Software Tools (Pittsburgh, PA, USA) is developing an integrated stimulus presentation, response recording and data analysis package. This list is not exhaustive. Development of these innovations invariably takes longer than is initially suggested and problems with initial versions are common. "Caveat emptor" is the relevant phrase.

29.2.2
Auditory Stimulus Presentation

The first MR imagers had no provision for electronically modulated auditory communication with the person in the magnet. Modern imagers typically include a small speaker/microphone in the bore above a subject's head. The primary purpose of this communication system is patient ease and comfort, rather than high fidelity or psychophysical experiments. As the number and sophistication of auditorily based experiments using fMRI expands, the need for high-quality stimulus delivery increases. As with visual stimulation equipment, there has been considerable effort by commercial developers to provide reasonable quality auditory input to patients in conventional MRI and subjects in fMRI. The companies mentioned previously (Avotec, Resonance Technology) have incorporated sound systems with their products, and there are several other companies that have developed sound systems for the MR environment.

The MR environment is much more difficult for auditory stimulus presentation than it is for visual stimulus presentation. In the present section, we will discuss the issues associated with generating and presenting sound stimuli in an MRI environment, some techniques for obtaining high-quality sound stimuli within the constraints of magnet-compatible equipment, and methods to reduce the background noise from the imager that can interfere with a subject's perception of the stimulus. While some of these technical goals are much greater than is needed for the ordinary presentation of music or speech, the high-quality sound and noise reduction systems are essential for specialized studies of the auditory system.

29.2.2.1
Acoustic Transducers

In the MRI environment, acoustic transducers are the most problematic component of an auditory stimulus system, and their capabilities and limitations influence the design of the rest of the system. Acoustic transducers convert an electrical signal from a source (e.g., a compact disc player, tape recorder, or computer) to sound. The MRI environment places constraints on the type, location, and properties of acoustic transducers. The constraints include: the transducer must not be a hazard in the magnet; the strong magnetic fields must not affect the operation of the transducer or introduce spurious sounds; and the transducer and its connections to the rest of the system must not affect imaging (e.g., by introducing electromagnetic signals into the imager or distorting the imager's magnetic field).

These constraints affect the quality of sound the transducer produces. Therefore, the other components of the stimulus system are selected to compensate for these limitations. From the standpoint of acoustic fidelity, the transducer should be located as close to the subject's ears as possible, which requires that the amount of metal in the transducer be minimized. If the transducers cannot be located near the subject's ears, the stimulus must be conducted to the ears, usually through air-filled tubes. Such tubes frequently pass through an earmuff or earplug to deliver the stimulus to the subject's ears in a controlled and reproducible fashion while minimizing the influence of background imager noise. The tubes degrade the quality of the sound stimulus from the transducer.

Acoustic transducers generally fall into three types, based on the principles underlying their operation: (1) piezoelectric, in which a crystal deforms in response to a varying voltage across it; (2) electrostatic (condenser), in which a thin metallic diaphragm moves under the influence of a varying electric field; and (3) dynamic, in which variations in the current passing through a coil of wire attached to a diaphragm cause it to move in a magnetic field (Beranek 1986). Of these three types, piezoelectric and electrostatic transducers are compatible with the magnetic fields present in MRI. Their fundamental method of operation is not significantly affected by the magnetic fields, and they can be constructed mostly or totally from nonmagnetic materials. Dynamic transducers, the most common type in general use in home and public sound reproduction systems, are inherently ill-suited for the imaging environment because their means of operation involves varying magnetic fields and usually permanent magnets as well. Nonetheless, even dynamic transducers have been used successfully in some commercial MRI-compatible sound systems. Finally, a novel pneumatic amplifier that need not contain metallic parts may be useful for overcoming some of the limitations of piezoelectric or dynamic transducers by amplifying a stimulus near a subject's ears (Drzewiecki and Poindexter 1996).

29.2.2.1.1
Piezoelectric Transducers

Most commercially available transducers use piezoelectric drivers (e.g., Newmatics, Petaluma, CA, USA; Magnacoustics, Atlantic Beach, NY, USA), and patient intercoms are also generally piezoelectric. Their construction generally consists of a thin patch of piezoelectric material 2–3 cm on a side and ≤1 mm thick, driven in a bending mode and attached to a stiff plastic diaphragm several centimeters in diameter. The stiffness of the piezoelectric bender reduces the output at low frequencies, and waves in the diaphragm reduce the output at high frequencies. Distortion can become significant at high stimulus levels. Resonances in the piezoelectric bender and in the enclosure for the diaphragm generally cause the frequency response to include several peaks and nulls. Though the transducers themselves are nonmetallic except for the lead wires, in many commercial systems they are enclosed in metal boxes for electrical shielding; hence, they generally must be located at the foot of the magnet near the bore, whence sound is conducted to the subject's ears (or to earmuffs or earplugs) through 1–2 m-long rubber or plastic tubes (e.g., BINDER et al. 1995). The tubes have their own acoustic effects: Resonances in the tubes accentuate some frequencies and introduce nulls at others; the tubes attenuate high-frequency sound (attenuation increases as tube length increases and tube diameter decreases); the tubes cause dispersion (the speed of sound through the tube depends on frequency, so low-frequency sounds travel faster than high-frequency sounds, and the timing or phase relationship between different frequencies changes: for example, a "click" stimulus can get smeared in time to a "chirp" (KINSLER et al. 1982); and the tubes can pick up imager noise and transmit it to the subject's ears (especially if they touch the imager shroud or structure). Tubes are not strictly necessary: two systems developed for active noise reduction (see Sect. 29.2.2.3) use piezoelectric transducers in nonmetallic enclosures located near the subject's head to generate a sound field near the subject's ears. One group has developed a prototype headset that puts the transducers near the ears to minimize most of these effects (PALMER, personal communication to MER).

29.2.2.1.2
ELECTROSTATIC TRANSDUCERS

Electrostatic transducers are characterized by a very flat frequency response, broad frequency and dynamic range, and fairly low distortion. For this reason, they are frequently used in high-end stereo systems and headphones. If electrostatics are placed at the base of the magnet and tubes are used to transmit the stimulus to the subject's ears, the tubes will be subject to the problems described above. Electrostatics have a higher output than piezoelectric transducers and can be manufactured with only a small amount of metal for the diaphragm and backplane. This may allow electrostatics to be positioned in the bore near a subject's ears or incorporated into headphones. One group has developed a prototype headset (PALMER et al. 1998), and a similar headset is being developed commercially (Psychology Software Tools, Pittsburgh, PA, USA).

29.2.2.1.3
DYNAMIC TRANSDUCERS

Dynamic transducers include magnets and use magnetic fields. Hence, they must be either well shielded from the magnet or located outside the imager room to avoid becoming a hazard or being influenced by the imager's magnetic fields. This tends to negate their advantages in sound reproduction (high output, wide dynamic range, relatively wide frequency range and flat frequency response, very low distortion) relative to most other transducers. If they are sufficiently small and well shielded, they can be located at the base of the magnet (as in the Avotec system), but then their low-frequency output is limited by their small size. Tubes are still necessary, so the system is subject to the problems listed above. If the transducer is located outside the magnet room, larger transducers may be used (e.g., BINDER et al. 1994); but the high sound levels necessary to drive the long (several meters) tubes to conduct sound to the subject may introduce nonlinearities and distortion. It may be possible to use a well-shielded voice coil in the imager's own static magnetic field as a dynamic transducer.

29.2.2.3
Stimulus Generation and Transmission

The other components of an acoustic stimulus system have fewer requirements and more options than the acoustic transducers. They must transmit an appropriate input to the acoustic transducer without introducing noise; and they may compensate for deficiencies in the performance of the transducers, select between several stimulus sources, control stimulus level, provide a means to monitor stimulus level at the subject's ears, incorporate a patient intercom, or introduce an active noise control signal (see Sect. 29.5.1). Fine control over sound level and quality is generally not necessary for most fMRI-based experiments but is important in experiments that are specifically directed towards the details of auditory psychophysics.

The different transducers described in the previous section require different types of inputs: electrostatic and piezoelectric transducers require a relatively high voltage but need only low currents; and dynamic transducers are inductive devices that draw a high current but require relatively low voltage. Electrostatic transducers also require a bias voltage between the diaphragm and the backplate which can be as high as several hundred volts. The high-voltage, low-current inputs to electrostatic and piezoelectric transducers are less likely to pick up electrical noise in the magnet room than the low-voltage, high-current inputs to dynamic transducers. Shielding and grounding the transducer leads between the stimulus system and the transducer (e.g., shielded twisted pair or dual coax) is generally sufficient, though some groups use an optical link.

The frequency response of the transducer may be compensated to some extent by filtering the input signal appropriately. To develop such an inverse filter to equalize the transducer output, the frequency response of the transducer and the other components of the sound system must be known. If simple octave- or third-octave-band correction is sufficient, a commercial pro-audio equalizer may be adequate. Such equalizers may introduce phase distortion between different bands. Commercially-available digital filters (e.g., Tucker-Davis Technologies, Gainesville FL) can provide more flexibility in filter design, and digital finite-impulse-response (FIR) filters have a linear phase response (introduce only a simple delay) (e.g., OPPENHEIM and SHAFER 1989). The transducer frequency response may be sufficiently complex that a combination of filters is required for adequate compensation.

Acoustic stimuli may be produced from a variety of sources: commercial sound reproduction equipment such as radio, cassette tapes, or CDs; standard signal generators such as oscillators or click or noise generators; or a sound board in a computer. A pro-audio mixer provides the capability to switch between different stimulus sources, set their input levels independently, and control output levels as well as monitor stimulus levels in the control room. Most commercial sound systems for imagers include these capabilities. For auditory experiments or other applications in which output levels must be finely controlled and reproducible, a separate precision attenuator (e.g., Tucker-Davis Technologies, Gainesville, FL, USA) may be used. If the stimulus system includes a patient intercom, many mixers allow the control room microphone to override the acoustic stimulus automatically (e.g., Symetrix, Lynnwood, WA, USA).

Monitoring stimulus levels at the subject's ear or a two-way subject intercom system also requires a microphone(s) near the subject to facilitate communication with the control room. Small pro-audio condenser lavalier microphones or electret (a variety of electrostatic) hearing-aid microphones are well suited for the imaging environment. Pro-audio lavalier microphones are available with plastic cases (e.g., Shure, Evanston IL); and though most hearing-aid microphones have a stainless-steel case (e.g., Knowles Electronics, Elk Grove Village IL; Tibbetts, Camden ME), they are generally small enough not to disturb the magnetic field to an unacceptable degree. Both are relatively unaffected by the magnetic field (e.g., HURWITZ et al. 1989; RAVICZ et al. 1997) and may be incorporated into earmuffs or earplugs to monitor sound levels or to serve as an intercom. A throat microphone may be more appropriate for an intercom. A multizone mixer (e.g., Symetrix) can integrate two-way communication into the stimulus and monitoring system.

29.2.2.3
Minimizing the Effects of Background Noise

The acoustic noise present during image acquisition is a complicating factor in fMRI studies. The most intense noise is generated by the gradient coils and can reach levels of 103–134 dB SPL. (See Sect. 29.5.1 for a more comprehensive description of the imager noise and its sources.) At a global level, the noise causes brain activity unrelated to experimental stimulation (BANDETTINI et al. 1998; TALAVAGE and EDMISTER 1998a; TALAVAGE et al. 1998), and long exposures to imager noise levels without hearing protection can damage hearing (e.g., VON GIERKE and NIXON 1992; MELNICK 1992; SUTER 1996; see Sect. 29.5.1). More specifically for experiments involving sound stimuli, the noise can mask a stimulus (PELLI and ZHANG 1991), and brain activity due to the noise can hinder detection of brain activity due to the stimulus (BANDETTINI et al. 1998; TALAVAGE and EDMISTER 1998b; TALAVAGE et al. 1998). Ideally, experiments involving sound stimuli would be performed in quiet. For these reasons, an acoustic stimulus system should incorporate ear protection or noise reduction.

Most commercial acoustic systems currently available include a headset with earmuffs, earplugs, or some combination of the two. Well-fitting earmuffs will generally attenuate noise by 20–40 dB at 500 Hz and above, and properly inserted foam earplugs will provide 20–35 dB attenuation over the same range (BERGER et al. 1998; RAVICZ and MELCHER 1998a,b; RAVICZ et al., submitted). There are several factors that influence the choice of earmuffs or earplugs: Most people find earmuffs more comfortable to wear for an extended period than earplugs (ROYSTER and ROYSTER 1986). Wearing eyeglasses under earmuffs can reduce their comfort and attenuation by compromising the seal between the muff and the head (BERGER 1986), so subjects that need to use their eyeglasses during imaging may want to use earplugs. Estimating the effectiveness of earplugs is not a simple process. While the attenuation obtained in the field with earmuffs matches manufacturers' specifications fairly well, manufacturers' attenuation data for earplugs overestimate their performance significantly (BERGER 1983b, 1988; BERGER et al. 1996). There is a wide range of ear canal sizes in the general population, and it is unrealistic to expect one size of earplug to fit all subjects well (ROYSTER and ROYSTER 1986). Earplugs must be of the proper size and must be properly inserted in the ear canal to obtain their full effect (BERGER 1983a), and proper insertion requires instruction and practice (ROYSTER and ROYSTER 1986). Semi-aural (e.g., "cone-type") hearing protectors that fit only into the concha appear to provide attenuation comparable to foam earplugs (BERGER 1986).

A combination of earmuffs and earplugs provides only slightly more attenuation than earmuffs or earplugs alone, due to conduction of noise directly through the head and body into the ear (BERGER 1983b; RAVICZ and MELCHER 1998a ,b; RAVICZ et al., submitted). A "helmet" that protected a subject's entire head from sound provided 55–65 dB attenuation at 500 Hz and above (RAVICZ and MELCHER et al. 1998a, b; RAVICZ et al., submitted).

Active noise reduction (ANR or "cancellation") brings about a reduction in noise levels by introducing an inverted copy of the noise waveform to interfere destructively with the original noise. Currently, ANR systems are limited to frequencies below 500 Hz (e.g., CASALI and BERGER 1996). Three groups have developed ANR systems to reduce such low-frequency noise in the vicinity of an MRI subject's ear (GOLDMAN et al. 1989; PLA et al. 1995; CHEN et al. 1998). Currently available ANR headsets that incorporate the signal processing electronics in the headset are probably unusable in an imager. A magnet-tolerant ANR headset that reduces noise levels in the ear canal up to at least 2 kHz has been developed, but its effectiveness is limited by noise conduction through the head and body as described above (PALMER et al. 1998; RAVICZ and MELCHER 1998a, b; RAVICZ et al., submitted).

Though earplugs, earmuffs, a helmet, and/or ANR may protect a subject's ears from imager noise sufficiently to ensure subject safety, these methods alone are not adequate to eliminate the noise. Substantial reductions will require a combination of approaches in addition to those listed above (RAVICZ et al. 1997), including reducing the levels of noise produced by the imager (e.g., MANSFIELD et al. 1995) and reduc-

ing noise transmission from the imager's gradient coils to the subject (RAVICZ and MELCHER 1998a, b; RAVICZ et al., submitted).

29.2.2.4
Summary of Acoustic Stimulation Systems

The standard speaker and microphone that ordinarily come with an MRI system are not sufficient for conducting auditory experiments in fMRI. They are intended for use between scans, not during the loud noises created by echo planar imaging (EPI) and other pulse sequences, and the quality of their sound reproduction is just adequate for understanding speech (which is a minimal level of quality). In contrast, any of the commercially available acoustic stimulation systems for fMRI is sufficient for communicating with the subject and for presenting reasonably loud and clear sounds during the scans in a standard 1.5 Tesla system. With the additional noise of a higher field system, or if one is studying the details of auditory psychophysics, more specialized acoustic equipment may be necessary.

29.2.3
Tactile, Olfactory, Gustatory, Pain, Proprioceptive Stimulation

In contrast to vision and audition, the remainder of the body's sensory systems have not been systematically addressed in the context of fMRI. For several of these systems (e.g., somatosensory stimulation) a common form of stimulation is the same as that used in a non-MR environment: namely, the experimenter uses standard tools (e.g., von Frey hairs or acupuncture needles) to apply the stimulation directly to the subject. In studies of acupuncture and pain it is common for one or more of the experimenters to be in the MR room administering the stimulus.

However, abstracts at the Fourth International Conference on Functional Mapping of the Human Brain (Montreal, June, 1998) revealed a number of new approaches to these problems of stimulus delivery. Vibrating tactile stimulation was delivered using a piezoelectric buzzer (HARRINGTON et al. 1998). Subjects were tickled via a self-manipulated or experimenter-manipulated wooden robot (BLAKEMORE et al. 1998). Painful stimuli based on heat or cold were delivered via a modified peltier-type thermal stimulator (DAVIS et al. 1998). Painful stimuli based on transcutaneous electrical nerve stimulation were delivered via a commercial device previously used in a PET study (J.H. Downs et al. 1998). The point of this summary is that a number of laboratories have developed methods for administering somatosensory and painful stimuli, but these devices are limited to fairly specific experimental protocols, rather than the more general and programmable systems available for auditory and visual stimulation.

For taste and olfaction, precise control of the stimulation is essential, and pneumatic systems are used in psychophysical laboratories outside the magnet. Because the ultimate stimulus is a gas or liquid delivered through a plastic tube, such systems are relatively straightforward to adapt to the MR environment.

At least one laboratory has adapted such pneumatic devices for the application of somatosensory stimulation. Zacks (http://www.psych.stanford.edu:80/~zacks/somatosensory/fyp/FYP.html#RTFToC7) used an array of ten small nozzles attached to plastic tubing and a set of computer controlled valves at a safe distance from the MR scanner to deliver controlled sequences of stimulation to the arms of his subjects. Such equipment could presumably be adapted to the delivery of gases or liquids for studies of taste and olfaction.

29.3
Recording Voluntary Responses

In most fMRI-based experiments, it is necessary to record behavioral responses made by the subject. There are exceptions, such as experiments in which subjects are asked to "imagine" a particular set of stimuli, or in which the relevant variable is modulation of attention, but even in these cases, obtaining some objective measure of the subjects' voluntary responses is desirable. This section describes some systems for obtaining and recording voluntary behavioral responses.

29.3.1
Simple Choice Responses

There are many contexts in which it is sufficient to have a subject select one of n (e.g., $n=2$ or $n=4$) responses. Several approaches have been developed to address this situation. It is normally desired to have the results of these responses automatically re-

corded (electronically) via computer. How, in the context of the MR environment, can this be accomplished?

There are at least three approaches to this problem. The most "low-tech" approach is to have the subject squeeze one of two rubber bulbs that have partially inflated, different color balloons hanging down. Each squeeze causes one balloon to rise, and this can easily be seen from outside the MR room. (If the observing experimenter is inside the MR room, the balloons are unnecessary and the subject can simply lift a finger.) This system is limited to two responses; it requires someone else to watch the balloons (or fingers); and it does not supply response data directly to the computer. Its virtues are simplicity and low cost and should be used only until a more sophisticated system can be implemented.

Both other systems require the subject to push some form of button. These buttons can be in one box (set, for example, in a horizontal row) or divided across boxes (so left and right hands hold separate response boxes). The buttons cause either an electronic or optical change.

In the case of an electronic change, the basic idea is to simulate a keyboard button press remotely in the magnet. This can be done using commercially available circuitry and software for entering data through a serial port or special board (e.g., LabVIEW, National Instruments, Austin, TX, USA). Alternatively, a simple circuit can be used to emulate an actual keyboard keypress remotely. A sample circuit is shown in Fig. 29.1. This is circuit was designed for a Macintosh keyboard, in which the keys are simple momentary contact switches. A spare keyboard is cannibalized for switches that are used in the MR room. The ribbon cable passes through the MR room penetration panel. The "Interface Box" receives wires from the two sides of the keyboard keys, and simulates the joining of those wires via the PVA3324 chip, which detects the remote button press. The reason for the circuit on the left is to permit operation over long distances (e.g., 20 m) that

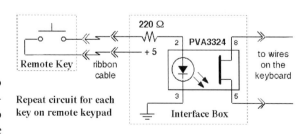

Fig. 29.1. The remote key for Macintosh keyboard

would not be possible if the wires from the keyboard were connected directly to the remote key. Note that the keys on a Macintosh keyboard are multiplexed, so two wires for each key must go to the Interface Box, while only one wire per key (plus the +5 Volt power) need go to the remote keys. This circuit can be repeated for as many keys as necessary, and has been used to create a remote keyboard in the magnet at modest cost (device designed by Winfield Hill at the Rowland Institute, Cambridge, MA, USA; see Kraft et al. 1998 for one application of this device).

While at least one laboratory has found this system to be reliable and not a source of RF noise, there are potential problems with such a design. Every time a button push is made, some current flows and RF are generated. While this has not been a problem in practice, there are ways to avoid this problem completely. Instead of using electronic switches, the alternative is to use fiber optic cable and optical switches. The optical signal can then be transduced to create an electrical signal that a computer can use. At least one commercial vendor offers such a system (Lightwave Medical, Vancouver, British Columbia, Canada) at a cost of approximately $1,350 for a 4-button optical box that feeds the serial port or a TTL port of a computer.

29.3.2
Complex Movements

The measurement of complex movements in the MR environment is difficult. The movements themselves can cause artifacts in the MR images. Movements as apparently benign as talking, typing, and supination/pronation of the wrist can cause severe artifacts. This occurs for at least three reasons. First, complex movements of the arms or legs are likely to result in movement of the rest of the body, including the head and brain, thus degrading the image. Second, some movements, such as those associated with speech, can cause changes in the size of the air cavity in the mouth, and hence near the base of the brain. These cause changes in the susceptibility artifacts. Third, movements of some muscles in the shoulder, upper arm and back, can cause a significant change in the coupling between a nearby receiver head coil and the body. In all of these cases, the changes are usually correlated with the experimental paradigm, making interpretation of the resulting data difficult or impossible.

In order to study complex movements such as eye-hand coordination, response sensing devices must be adapted to the MR environment. Some of the systems ordinarily used in the psychophysical laboratory (such as electronic tablets) are difficult or impossible to modify appropriately. Other systems (e.g., trackballs, joysticks) can be more easily adapted. At least one vendor (Resonance Technology) is developing an integrated response device of that sort in the next version of their visual display system.

Force and acceleration sensors can be adapted to the MR environment and have been used to monitor head movements (Slifer et al. 1993). However, virtually all of these systems are developed by individual laboratories, and are not yet commercially available fMRI devices. By way of contrast, this is a context in which the environment of PET is much more hospitable. In a recent PET study of motor learning (Krebs et al. 1998), a sophisticated robot was used to manipulate, sense, and give force feedback to limbs of the human subject – this would be a difficult system to make MR-compatible.

29.4
Monitoring Systemic Responses

There are a number of physiological measures that can be used to guide the acquisition and/or interpretation of fMRI data. In the context of the present chapter, these may be thought of as "involuntary responses." Physiological fluctuations (e.g., breathing, heart rate) are critically important in some experiments. Electrical brain activity (as measured by EEG) can be monitored in the magnet, even during fMRI. Eye movements (which can be both voluntary and involuntary) are often critical components of cognitive processing. Gaining access to information about these processes is discussed below.

29.4.1
Physiological Monitoring

Physiological monitoring in the MRI environment is of interest to those investigators who wish to study the interfaces between systemic physiology, cerebrovascular physiology, focal brain activation and fMRI signaling. Physiologic monitoring in the MRI environment is a necessity when conducting experiments in medically unstable subjects (e.g., acute stroke) or when utilizing pharmacological probes that effect the cardiorespiratory system (e.g., acute cocaine administration). Physiologic parameters of interest include heart rate (HR), with or without the electrocardiogram (ECG) trace, blood pressure, oxygen saturation (O_2Sat), respiratory rate (RR) and end tidal carbon dioxide ($ETCO_2$) concentration. Most scanners are equipped with the ability to monitor the HR and ECG as this is needed to perform cardiac gated imaging. Similarly, many scanners are equipped to monitor respiratory rate in order perform respiratory gated image acquisition.

The specific problems inherent to the need for clinical monitoring, required to assure subject safety, have been largely overcome by vendors who have modified existing tools for this purpose. For example, both Invivo Research, Inc. (Orlando, FL) and Magnetic Resonance Equipment Corporation (Bay Shore, NY) sell FDA-approved, MRI-compatible subject monitoring equipment. These units are generally safe, reliable and accurate to the degree necessary for clinical monitoring. Investigators can choose from very basic units (still quite expensive) which allow continuous measurement of HR, ECG, O_2 Sat, and noninvasive blood pressure (NIBP) or add components which measure $ETCO_2$, RR and invasive blood pressure. Because of magnetohydrodynamic effects on the ECG, which cause aberrations in the tracing, a baseline rhythm strip should be obtained at the start of each study to which all subsequent tracings can be compared. The temporal resolution of these systems for sampling NIBP is typically 2 min; each of the other parameters are sampled once per second. Pediatric monitoring capabilities are built into most units. The newest technology allows for monitoring in magnet anesthesia.

Additional problems, not addressed by the vendors, arise when the physiological measures are to be used in the context of studying the correlation between these measures and fMRI data. Foremost is that the precision of the measures obtained by these instruments, while suitable for clinical management, has low temporal resolution and is inherently very noisy. Additional effort must be expended to filter and smooth the data. Another challenge is to set up a computer interface that allows physiologic data to be stored directly to a hard disk for later analysis.

These problems have been partially addressed in recent studies investigating the effects of acute cocaine administration to drug-dependent subjects (BREITER et al. 1997; GOLLUB et al. 1998). Physiologic monitoring was conducted using an InVivo OmniTrak 3100 patient monitoring system (Orlando, FL) custom modified to permit on-line computer acquisition of physiologic measurements.

Electrocardiogram, HR, $ETCO_2$, and noninvasive systemic mean blood pressure (MBP) were continuously measured. The physiologic parameters were ported to a Macintosh Power PC 7100 running a custom National Instruments LabVIEW data acquisition program. This program allowed simultaneous acquisition of: (1) digitized analog ECG trace, (2) the scanner trigger pulse which indicated when the gradient coils of the magnet were firing, and (3) physiologic measures from the InVivo system.

Figure 29.2 displays the continuous physiological data (HR, MBP, and the change in $ETCO_2$, $\Delta ETCO_2$) recorded from a representative subject during an fMRI study investigating the effects of acute cocaine administration. Note the stability of the measurements over the duration of the saline infusion scanning epoch as well as during the pre-infusion phase of the cocaine infusion scanning epoch. The HR began to increase within the first minute following cocaine infusion, MBP increased more slowly and less dramatically and the $ETCO_2$ dropped slightly after a delay. $ETCO_2$ measures do not reflect absolute measures of the partial pressure of CO_2 ($PaCO_2$); however, $ETCO_2$ provides a reliable estimate of true changes in $PaCO_2$. Because of this, the data are analyzed and displayed in terms of $\Delta ETCO_2$ from the baseline measure.

Precautions taken to ensure safe conduct of any imaging studies involving drug challenges or medically unstable subjects should include the use of advanced cardiac life support ACLS trained personnel, frequent running of mock codes, and the presence of a physician at the time of all studies whose sole responsibility is to monitor subject safety.

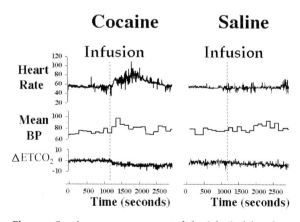

Fig. 29.2. Continuous measurement of physiological data during fMRI of cocaine and saline infusions

29.4.2
Multimodality Monitoring: Electro-oculogram, Electro-encephalogram

It has been demonstrated that electro-encephalo-gram (EEG) measurements can be safely made during fMRI experiments (IVES et al. 1993). This technology can be used to simultaneously detect EEG signals and monitor gross eye movements via similar electrodes placed near the eye to obtain an electro-oculogram (EOG), all during EPI (HUANG-HELLINGER et al. 1995). It is possible to use EEG signals to trigger the MR scanner based on the onset of an epileptic seizure (WARACH et al. 1996). In theory, EEG could also be used in the magnet to monitor the locus of spatial attention, as has been demonstrated outside the magnet (HILLYARD et al. 1995).

However, the electrical environment of the MR room makes detecting the much smaller signals used in evoked response potential (ERP) studies very difficult. The wiring in ERP is the same as in EEG, but instead of examining the raw electrical signal in the absence of overt stimulation, the idea with ERP is to repeatedly present a known, precisely timed stimulus and average the electrical signal over hundreds of repetitions. In this way, the average EEG signal is eliminated and the variations triggered by the stimulus remain. However, the amplitude of these signals is typically two orders of magnitude smaller than the raw EEG signals. Even the slightest movements of the subject's head will cause the wires to move, which, in the presence of the strong magnetic field of the magnet, causes signals much bigger than those being studied via ERP. This is true even when the MRI machine is not in operation; the problems get much worse when the RF and gradient fields used in imaging are active. These create noise in the EEG signals as well, but because those signals are not being repeatedly averaged, the artifacts can be filtered out after the fact.

29.4.3
Eye Movements

Eye movements, both voluntary and involuntary, are a natural subject for study. In addition to their intrinsic interest, they are a possible source of artifact and confound when interpreting functional MRI data. There are a number of technologies for monitoring eye movements with good precision outside the MR environment. Some of these use magnetic sensors and would be inappropriate in conjunction with MRI. However, several other technologies could, in principle, be adapted to the MR environment.

One approach to monitoring eye movements uses an infrared or visible light video camera focused on the eye. The circular boundary between the iris and the sclera is a high contrast contour that can be selected using image processing software. The movement of that circle can be used to compute eye movements. This system is used by ISCAN (Cambridge, MA, USA), and more than one group has attempted to adapt the ISCAN system to the MR environment. In addition, the two companies mentioned previously (Avotec, Resonance Technology) are developing systems that will be incorporated into their visual display systems. These systems may also use algorithms based on tracking the shape of the iris via camera and computer algorithms.

There is at least one article (O'CRAVEN et al. 1997) and abstract (BRANDT et al. 1997) reporting the use of a different eye tracking system in the magnet. These investigators used an Ober2 system (Permobil Meditech, Woburn, MA USA) that had been slightly modified for the MR environment. This device uses goggles with printed circuit boards shaped like rectangles with a rectangular hole cut in the middle. Subjects look through the hole, while infrared light-emitting diodes and photo sensors yield signals that can be interpreted to find the horizontal and vertical boundaries between the iris and sclera. This system has good accuracy, measures each eye independently, and has a high sampling rate. When it is used in conjunction with an MR surface coil receiver placed at the back of the head (to obtain MR images of the occipital cortex), the system works reasonably well, as reported (BRANDT et al. 1997; O'CRAVEN et al. 1997). The eye movement data contain artifacts due to the RF and gradient fields, but these can be filtered. More problematic, however, is the susceptibility artifact caused by this system when the anterior portions of the brain are being imaged in a head coil.

In summary, various attempts have been made to monitor eye movements while conducting fMRI experiments. EOG can be used to report gross movements. The Ober2 system can be used for studies of the occipital lobe. These and other systems are being developed, with the intent of including them in visual display systems (e.g., Avotec, Resonance Technology). However, there is, at the time of this writing, no completely satisfactory, operational system for measuring eye movements in the MR environment. Various groups and vendors have suggested that their problems will be solved shortly, but again, caveat emptor.

29.5
Safety

While this chapter is not primarily concerned with safety, the subject naturally arises here for two reasons. First, stimulus presentation and response recording naturally entail the design of novel equipment for the MR room. Second, high speed imaging pulse sequences such as EPI generate substantial acoustic noise, especially in higher field MR systems. This auditory noise makes presentation of high-quality auditory stimuli difficults and also raises a serious issue of possible hearing damage associated with long exposure to that noise. The present section will supply some references for general MRI safety issues. The subsequent section will discuss acoustic noise in detail. The last section will describe some anecdotal problems in the use of bite bars to help with subject stabilization.

The standard safety reference for conventional MRI is *Magnetic Resonance: Bioeffects, Safety, and Patient Management* (SHELLOCK and KANAL 1994). (A second edition of the book is now available, SHELLOCK and KANAL 1996.) This book was originally written in 1994 and did not address some of the special issues associated functional MRI, such as the loud noises associated with EPI and the long scanning sessions. There is an active web site, "International MR Safety Central Web Site" (*http://www.kanal.arad.upmc.edu/mrsafety.html*) that is maintained by Shellock and Kanal for these and other current issues. The web site includes some answers to more recent questions about acoustic noise levels in functional MRI, but Sect. 29.5.1 (below) has more specific information. Another web site of interest is: *http://www.gasbone.herston.uq.edu.au:8080/reference/bibliography/snacc/MRIList1.html*, which is a bibliography of articles related to MR safety.

29.5.1
Acoustic Noise

The imager produces acoustic noise every time an image is acquired. This noise is produced by the currents in the gradient coils that set up the magnetic gradients, which cause the coils to flex under inducted (Lorentz) forces (e.g., HURWITZ et al. 1989). The frequency and duration of the noise depend on the waveforms of the gradient currents (HEDEEN and EDELSTEIN 1997). For anatomical imaging, the noise generally has mostly low-frequency content and a "clunking" sound. For EPI, the noise can be noticeably tonal with a fundamental frequency between 600 and 1400 Hz and sounds like a loud "beep." Other ongoing noise is produced by the magnet coolant pump and the patient fan, and noise from the room air handling system is usually present. These sounds are of lower frequency and intensity (RAVICZ and MELCHER 1998b; RAVICZ et al., submitted).

Peak gradient noise levels (A-weighted) from published measurements taken during (normal) imaging in imagers with field strengths of 0.35–3.0 Tesla range from 86 (in a 1.0 T) to 109 dB SPL (in a different 1.0 T) and during EPI range from 101 (in a 1.5 T) to almost 140 dB SPL (in a 3 T) (HURWITZ et al. 1989; McJURY et al. 1994; SHELLOCK et al. 1994, 1998; McJURY 1995; COUNTER et al. 1997; RAVICZ and MELCHER 1998a; RAVICZ et al., submitted). The A-weighting matches the noise spectrum to the human audiogram and tends to de-emphasize frequencies below 1 kHz. Generally, the higher gradient currents associated with the higher gradients used with higher magnetic fields and with EPI cause greater flexure of the coils and more intense noise.

Noise in higher-strength imagers, especially during EPI, reaches levels that will damage an unprotected ear during a prolonged exposure (GIERKE et al. 1992; SUTER 1996). Current United States Food and Drug Administration (FDA) standards (FDA 1988) recommend that noise levels meet the requirements of the American Conference of Governmental Industrial Hygienists for exposure up to 1 h (99–100 dB SPL) or be within the United States Occupational Safety and Health Act (OSHA) peak and time-averaged noise exposure limits (105 dB SPL for 1 h; 115 dB maximum, 140 dB peak impulse; OSHA 1970; SHELLOCK et al. 1998). This recommendation is for patients who are generally not in the imager for long periods of time. For experimental subjects, who may remain in the imager for several hours, the noise exposure limits should be examined more closely. The duration of the noise from each image acquisition (50 to several hundred milliseconds; CHO et al. 1997; COUNTER et al. 1997; RAVICZ and MELCHER 1998a; RAVICZ et al., submitted) falls in an ill-defined area between impulsive and sustained noise, though during multislice imaging the noise becomes almost continuous. The OSHA level-exposure trading table mandates a halving of exposure time with each 5-dB increase in noise level, starting with a permitted 8-h exposure at 90 dB SPL (OSHA 1970), and is more liberal than most other military or foreign standards (SUTER 1996). An attempt to set limits on short-duration noise was undertaken by the Committee on Hearing, Bioacoustics, and Biomechanics (CHABA) in 1968 but not formally adopted (VON GIERKE et al. 1992); the limit on sounds in excess of 200 ms duration striking the ear at perpendicular incidence (as in an imager) is 138 dB SPL for 100 sounds per day, lower by 1.5 dB for each doubling of the number of sounds. The trend toward higher-field imagers that produce higher-intensity noise, coupled with the current lack of a noise standard tailored for the noise produced during imaging, argues strongly for a conservative approach to hearing protection and the use of noise reduction devices (such as those discussed in Sect. 29.2.2.3) as a matter of course during imaging.

29.5.2
Safety Considerations When Using Bite Bars

As indicated in other sections of this book, minimizing head movements is a constant challenge in conducting fMRI-based experiments. One of the techniques used in our laboratory is a bite bar, with mouth pieces custom made for each subject, and rigidly attached to the receiver coil or other structure attached to the patient table. This system has been effective and comfortable for many (though certainly not all) of our subjects. However, there are several safety issues associated with the use of a bite bar that should be emphasized.

First, the choice of dental impression material is important. The material normally used in psychophysical laboratories outside the magnet is chosen because it is inexpensive, has a low melting point, and solidifies reasonably quickly. These properties make it easy to work with. However, it is somewhat brittle; it does not develop very smooth edges; and some subjects complain about its taste. The brittleness is the most important concern. A brittle bite bar can chip, sending some material into a subject's mouth. If the subject is in a normal laboratory setting, seated in front of the experimental apparatus, this is not a serious problem: they can simply open their mouths and move back from the bite bar. However, in the MR, with the subject lying on their back and with no way to move away from the bite bar, a falling piece of bite bar material could be a choking hazard.

For this reason we use a material that is not brittle (Hydroplastic, TAK Systems, East Wareham, MA, USA). However, this material has a much higher melting point (near the boiling point of water), takes a long time to solidify completely (about 15 min) and is very solid once it has solidified. These properties lead to some potential problems. If too much material is used, and there is any irregularity in the teeth of the subject, then the material might go over a ridge that would make it very difficult to remove after the material solidified. Two steps are taken to minimize this danger. First, only a small amount of material is used – just enough to cover 2–3 mm of each tooth. Second, subjects are instructed to open their mouths after a few minutes – before the material has solidified completely, but after it has taken enough form to be stable when the subjects return their teeth to it.

There is one additional safety issue with respect to bite bars (and any other system that keeps heads particularly rigid). If there is an emergency in the MR room and a subject needs to be removed quickly, the standard procedure is to release the patient table and pull it rapidly from the bore of the magnet. This often results in a jarring stop as the table reaches the end of its guide, on the way out of the magnet. In normal situations, this is not important, but in a situation in which the subject is on a bite bar, this could lead to significant damage to the teeth or neck.

29.6
Conclusion

The study of human brain activity using functional MRI is an enterprise that started in 1991. The explosion of interest in this technique has led many individual investigators to develop their own unique psychophysiological laboratories for the MR environment. As the number of research centers using fMRI has grown, so has the development of commercial systems. These commercial systems are improving both in terms of the quality of the stimuli presented and in attempts to integrate more of the necessary features (e.g., visual and auditory stimuli; simple button and more complex trackball responses; eye movement detection) in a single package. As yet, however, there are no off-the-shelf systems that can do all that researchers might want in this domain, and there will continue to be developments in both the home-grown and commercial arenas for some time to come.

Acknowledgments. The authors wish to thank the many people who have helped develop the PLM at the MGH-NMR Center. Thanks to Terry Campbell of MGH and Mark S. Cohen of UCLA for early work on many of the systems. Special thanks go to Don Rogers, Winfield Hill, and Robert Newton at the Rowland Institute for Science for work on optical, mechanical, and electronic devices. Specific thanks are due to Mark P. Haggard, Douglas A.R. Kelley, Jennifer R. Melcher, Alan R. Palmer, Ishmael J. Stefanov-Wagner, and István L. Vér for helpful discussions regarding the issues of auditory stimulus presentation and management of acoustic noise. Thanks to John Baker of MGH for his help in the design of the physiological monitoring system. In addition, we wish to thank the various vendors (including Paul Bullwinkel of AVOTEC, Walter Schneider and Karen Jensen of Psychology Software Tools, Sol Aisenberg of International Technology Group) who have come to the MGH-NMR Center's Visiting Fellowship Program in Functional MRI to demonstrate their equipment.

References

Bandettini PA, Jesmanowicz A, Kylen JV, Birn RM, Hyde JS (1998) Functional MRI of brain activation induced by scanner acoustic noise. Magn Reson Med 39:410–416

Belliveau JW, Kennedy DN, McKinstry RC, Buchbinder BR, Weisskoff RM, Cohen MS, Vevea JM, Brady TJ, Rosen BR (1991). Functional mapping of the human visual cortex by magnetic resonance imaging. Science 254:716–719

Beranek LL (1986) Acoustics. American Institute of Physics, New York

Berger EH (1983a) Laboratory attenuation of earmuffs and earplugs both singly and in combination. Am Ind Hyg Assoc J 44:321–329

Berger EH (1983b) Using the NRR to estimate the real world performance of hearing protectors. Sound Vibrat 17(1):12–18

Berger EH (1986) Hearing protection devices. In: Berger EH, Morrill JC, Ward WD, Royster LH (ed) Noise and hearing conservation manual. American Industrial Hygiene Association, Akron, Ohio, pp 319–382

Berger EH (1988) Can real-world hearing protector attenuation be estimated using laboratory data? Sound Vibrat 22(12):26–31

Berger EH, Franks JR, Lingren F (1996) International review of field studies of hearing protector attenuation. In: Axelsson A, Borchgrevink HM, Hamernik RP, Hellstrom PA, Henderson D, Salvi RJ (eds) Scientific basis of noise-induced hearing loss. Thieme, New York, pp 361–377

Berger EH, Franks JR, Behar A, Casali JG, Dixon-Ernst C, Kieper RW, Merry CJ, Mozo BT, Nixon CW, Ohlin D, Royster JD, Royster LH (1998). Development of a new standard laboratory protocol for estimating the field attenuation of hearing protection devices. Part III. The validity of using subject-fit data. J Acoust Soc Am 103:665–672

Binder JR, Rao SM, Hammeke TA, Zetkin FZ, Jesmanowicz A, Bandettini PA, Wong EC, Estkowski LD, Goldstein MD, Haughton VM, Hyde JS (1994) Functional magnetic resonance imaging of human auditory cortex. Ann Neurol 35:662–672

Binder JR, Rao SM, Hammeke TA, Frost JA, Bandettini PA, Jesmanowicz A, Hyde JS (1995) Lateralized human brain language systems demonstrated by task subtraction functional magnetic resonance imaging. Arch Neurol 52:593–601

Blakemore S-J, Wolpert DM, Frith CD (1998) Why can't we tickle ourselves? An fMRI study. NeuroImage 7(4), (abstract) S418

Brandt SA, Reppas J, Dale A, Wenzel R, Savoy R, Tootell R, (1997) Simultaneous infra-red oculagraphy and fMRI. International Society for Magnetic Resonance in Medicine, Vancouver

Breiter HC, Gollub RL, Weisskoff RM, Kennedy DN, Makris N, Berke JD, Goodman JM, Kantor HL, Gastfriend DR, Riorden JP, Mathew RT, Rosen BR, Hyman SE (1997) Acute effects of cocaine on human brain activity and emotion. Neuron 19(9):591–611

Casali JG, Berger EH (1996) Technology advancements in hearing protection circa 1995: Active noise reduction, frequency/amplitude sensitivity, and uniform attenuation. Am Ind Hyg Assoc J 57:175–185

Chen C, Chiueh T-D, Chen J-H (1998) Real-time active noise cancellation system for MRI. 6th Sci Mtg Int Soc Magn Reson Med, Sydney, (abstract) 749

Cho ZH, Park SH, Kim JH, Chung SC, Chung ST, Chung JY, Moon CW, Yi JH, Sin CH, Wong EK (1997) Analysis of acoustic noise in MRI. Magn Reson Imaging 15:815–822

Cornelissen FW, Pelli DG, Farell B, Huckins SC, Szeverenyi NM (1997) A binocular fiberscope for presenting visual stimuli during fMRI. Spatial Vision 11(1):75–81

Counter A, Olofsson Å, Grahn HF, Borg E (1997) MRI acoustic noise: sound pressure and frequency analysis. J Magn Reson Imaging 7:606–611

Davis KD, Kwan CL, Crawley AP, Mikulis DJ (1998) fMRI of the anterior cingulate cortex during painful thermal and motor tasks in individual subjects. NeuroImage 7(4):(abstract) S426

Downs JHI, Crawford HJ, Plantec MB, Horton JE, Vendemia JMC, Harrington GC, Yung S, Shamro C (1998) Attention to painful somatosensory TENS stimuli: An fMRI study. NeuroImage 7(4):(abstract) S432

Drzewiecki TM, Poindexter JC (1996) Acousto-fluidic sound augmentation for orthodox Jewish worship spaces. J Acoust Soc Am 100 (abstract):2608

Food and Drug Administration (1988) Magnetic resonance diagnostic device: Panel recommendation and report on petitions for MR reclassification. Fed Reg 53:7575–7579

Fox PT, Raichle ME (1984) Stimulus rate dependence of regional cerebral blood flow in human striate cortex, demonstrated by positron emission tomography. J Neurophysiol 51(5):1109–1120

Goldman AM, Gossman WE, Friedlander PC (1989) Reduction of sound levels with antinoise in MR imaging. Radiology 171:549–550

Gollub RL, Breiter HC, Kantor H, Kennedy D, Gastfriend D, Mathew RT, Makris N, Guimaraes A, Riorden J, Campbell T, Foley M, Hyman SE, Rosen B, Weisskoff R (1998) Cocaine decreases cortical cerebral blood flow but does not obscure regional activation in functional magnetic resonance imaging in human subjects. J Cereb Blood Flow Metab 18:724–734

Harrington GS, Raman MP, Kassel NF, Downs JHI (1998) Somatosensory response to vibrotactile stimuli in fMRI. NeuroImage 7(4):(abstract) S401

Hedeen RA, Edelstein WA (1997) Characterization and prediction of gradient acoustic noise in MR Images. Magn Reson Med 37:7–10

Hillyard SA, Anllo-Vento L, Clark VP, Heinze H-J, Luck SJ, Mangun GR (1995) Neuroimaging approaches to the study of visual attention: A tutorial. In: Kramer AF, Coles MGH, Logan GD (eds) Converging operations in the study of visual selective attention). American Psychological Association, pp 107–138

Huang-Hellinger FR, Breiter HC, McCormack G, Cohen MS, Kwong KK, Sutton JP, Davis TL, Savoy RL, Weisskoff RM, Belliveau JW, Rosen BR (1995) Simultaneous functional magnetic resonance imaging and electrophysiological recording. Hum Brain Mapping 3(1):13–23

Hurwitz R, Lane SR, Bell RA, Brant-Zawadzki MN (1989) Acoustic analysis of gradient-coil nose in MR imaging. Radiology 173:545–548

Ives JR, Warach S, Schmitt F, Edelman RR, Schomer DL (1993) Monitoring the patient's EEG during echo planar MRI. Electroencephalogr Clin Neurophysiol 87:417–420

Kinsler LE, Frey AR, Coppens AB, Saunders JV (1982) Fundamentals of acoustics, 3rd edn. John Wiley and Sons, New York

Kraft E, Chen AJ-W,.Kwong KK, Rosen BR, Anderson M, Graybiel AM, Jenkins BG (1998) Basal ganglia activation induced during typing tasks. An fMRI study at 3 T. NeuroImage 7(4):(Abstract) S993

Krebs HI, Brashers-Krug T, Rauch SL, Savage CR, Hogan N, Rubin RH, Fischman AJ, Alpert NM (1998) Robot-aided functional imaging: Application to a motor learning study. Hum Brain Mapping 6:59–72

Mansfield P, Chapman BLW, Bowtell R, GLover P, Coxon R, Harvey PR (1995) Active acoustic screening: Reduction of noise in gradient coils by Lorentz force balancing. Magn Reson Med 33:276–281

McJury M, Blug A, Joerger C, Condon B, Wyper B (1994) Short communication: Acoustic noise levels during magnetic resonance imaging scanning at 1.5 T. Br J Radiol 67:413–415

McJury MJ (1995) Acoustic noise levels generated during high field MR imaging. Clin Radiol 50:331–334

Melnick W (1992) Occupational noise standards: Status and critical issues. In: Dancer AL, Henderson D, Salvi RJ, Hamernik RP(eds) Noise-induced hearing loss). Mosby, St. Louis, pp 521–530

Occupational Health and Safety Act (1970) Washington, DC, <http://www.osha-slc.gov/OshStd_toc/OSHA_Std_toc.html>

O'Craven KM, Rosen BR, Kwong KK, Treisman A, Savoy RL (1997) Voluntary attention modulates fMRI activity in human MT/MST. Neuron 18

Oppenheim AV, Shafer RW (1989) Discrete-time signal processing. Prentice Hall, Englewood Cliffs, NJ

Palmer AR, Bullock DC, Chambers JD (1998) A high-output, high-quality sound system for use in auditory fMRI. Neuroimage 7(4):(abstract) S359

Pelli DG, Zhang L (1991) Accurate control of contrast on microcomputer displays. Vision Res 31:1337–1350

Pla FG, Sommerfeldt SD, Hedeen RA (1995) Active control of noise in magnetic resonance imaging, Active 95. Noise Control Foundation, Poughkeepsie, NY, pp 573–582

Ravicz ME, Melcher JR (1998a) Imager noise and noise reduction during fMRI. NeuroImage 7(4):(abstract) 556

Ravicz ME, Melcher JR (1998b) Reducing imager-generated noise at the ear during functional magnetic resonance imaging: Passive attenuation, Twenty-first Midwinter Meeting of the Association for Research in Otolaryngology, Mount Royal, NJ, (abstract) pp 208

Ravicz ME, Melcher JR, Talavage TM, Benson RR, Rosen BR, Kiang NYS (1997) Characterization and reduction of imager-generated noise during functional magnetic resonance imaging (fMRI). Twentieth Midwinter Meeting of the Association for Research in Otolaryngology, Des Moines, IA, (abstract) pp 205

Ravicz ME, Melcher JR, Talavage TM, Rosen BR, Kiang NYS Charcterization and reduction of acoustic noise during functional magnetic resonance imaging (fMRI). Submitted to J Acoust Soc Am

Royster LH, Royster JD (1986) Hearing protection devices. In: Feldman AS, Grimes CT (eds) Hearing conservation in industry. Williams and Wilkins, Baltimore, pp 103–150

Savoy RL (1986) Making quantized images appear smooth: Tricks of the trade in vision research. Behav Res Methods Instrum Comput 18(6):507–517

Savoy RL (1998) Functional magnetic resonance imaging (fMRI). Encyclopedia of neuroscience, 2nd edn. Elsevier, Amsterdam

Shellock FG, Kanal E (1994) Magnetic resonance: Bioeffects, safety, and patient management. Raven, New York

Shellock FG, Kanal E (1996) Magnetic resonance: Bioeffects, safety, and patient management, 2nd edn. Lippincott-Raven, New York

Shellock FG, Morisoli SM, Ziarati M (1994) Measurement of acoustic noise during MR imaging: Evaluation of six "worst-case" pulse sequences. Radiology 191:91–93

Shellock FG, Ziarati M, Atkinson D, Chen DY (1998) Determination of acoustic noise MRI using echo planar and three dimensional fast spin echo techniques. J Magn Reson Imaging 8:1154–1157

Slifer KJ, Cataldo MF, Llorente AM, Gerson AC (1993) Behavior analysis of motion control for pediatric neuroimaging. J Appl Behav Anal 26(4):469–470

Suter AH (1996) Current standards for occupational exposure to noise. In: Axelsson A, Borchgrevink HM, Hamernik RP, Hellstrom PA, Henderson D, Salvi RJ (eds) Scientific basis of noise-induced hearing loss. Thieme, New York, pp 430–436

Talavage TM, Edmister WB (1998a) Measuring and reducing the impact of imaging noise on echo-planar functional magnetic resonance imaging (fMRI) of auditory cortex. Twenty-first Midwinter Meeting of the Association for Research in Otolaryngology, Mt. Royal, NJ, (abstract) pp 35

Talavage TM Edmister WB (1998b) Saturation and nonlinear fMRI responses in auditory cortex. NeuroImage 7(4):(abstract) S362

Talavage TM, Edmister WB, Ledden PJ, Weisskoff RM (1998) Measurement of signal changes induced by fMRI imaging noise. Neuroimage 7(4):(abstract) S360

Tyler CW (1997) Colour bit-stealing to enhance the luminance resolution of digital displays on a single pixel basis. Spatial Vision 10:369–377

von Gierke HE V, Nixon CW (1992) Damage risk criteria for hearing and human body vibration. In: Beranek LL, Vér IL (eds) Noise and vibration control engineering: Principles and applications. John Wiley, New York, pp 585–616

Warach S, Ives JR, Schlaug G, Patel MR, Darby DG, Thangaraj V, Edelman RR, Schomer DL (1996) EEG-triggered echo-planar functional MRI in epilepsy. Neurology 47:89–93

Research Applications

30 Experimental Design for Brain fMRI

G.K. Aguirre and M. D'Esposito

CONTENTS

30.1
Experimental Design for Brain fMRI

This section concerns the design of fMRI experiments. If there is any value to our writing (and your reading) a discourse on the subject, then it must be the case that there are such things as "better" and "worse" experimental designs for fMRI. Normative judgments, in turn, require criteria on which they can be based, and here we consider two. An fMRI experiment should: (1) be inferentially capable of rejecting a hypothesis of interest, (2) maximize sensitivity for a predicted effect. This section will consider a variety of experimental designs for fMRI with regard to these standards.

An fMRI experiment should be capable of rejecting a hypothesis of interest. In one sense this is a trivial point – if the design cannot be used to reject a hypothesis, it is not by definition an experiment (Platt 1964)! Beyond this glib statement, however, lies a fair bit of complexity. Different experimental designs for fMRI rely upon different sets of assumptions and are sensitive to different types of confounds. The possibility that assumptions are not met or confounds are present can render the interpretation of an experiment equivocal. While all of science

grapples with these challenges, certain fMRI designs are prone to rather plausible inferential failures. In this section, we will explore how some experimental designs reduce reliance upon untenable assumptions and discount the possibility of certain types of confounds.

Given inferential soundness, an experimental design should maximize sensitivity for the effect to be detected. Greater sensitivity allows one to infer with greater confidence that the absence of a significant statistical test is the result of the absence of an effect of a certain magnitude or larger. Because fMRI experiments that demonstrate localized responses to some task are often tacitly interpreted as showing the absence of a response at other locations, sensitivity is a particularly important issue to keep in mind when designing and interpreting neuroimaging studies. The search for optimally sensitive fMRI designs will require us to become acquainted with two properties of the BOLD fMRI system: the transfer function that maps neural activity onto BOLD hemodynamic signal and the temporal autocorrelation structure of the noise. With knowledge of these two characteristics of the system, we will be in a position to rate the relative power of different experimental designs. In considering these issues, reference will be made to the Fourier analysis of periodic time-series. While extensive knowledge of these concepts is not essential to understand the conclusions presented here, the explanations will require some familiarity.

We begin by considering salient aspects of BOLD fMRI data that will guide subsequent discussion. Next, we discuss several experimental designs with regard to their relative statistical power and inferential strength. Finally, we consider the limitations of neuroimaging experiments (including PET, fMRI, evoked-potentials, and electrophysiology) with regard to strong inference about the neural substrates of cognitive processes.

G.K. Aguirre, MD; M. D'Esposito, MD; Department of Neurology, Hospital of the University of Pennsylvania, 3400 Spruce Street, Philadelphia, PA 19104-4283, USA

30.2
The BOLD fMRI System and Its Output

As has been well described in previous chapters in this volume, BOLD fMRI data are time-series measurements produced by a nearly linear system. We will unpack this jargon-laden sentence over the next few paragraphs and consider how these features of BOLD fMRI impact experimental design.

First, the absolute level of BOLD fMRI signal values are not readily interpretable. Unlike PET, for example, where the signal measured can be expressed as a physical quantity (e.g., ml blood/100 g of tissue per minute), the BOLD fMRI signal has no absolute interpretation. (Recent developments in perfusion imaging, however, offer the possibility of an fMRI signal that can be interpreted in concrete physical units.) This is because the particular signal value obtained is not *exactly* a measure of deoxyhemoglobin concentration, but is instead a measure that is *weighted* by this concentration (i.e., is T2* weighted) and is also influenced by a number of other factors that can vary from voxel to voxel, scan to scan, and subject to subject. As a result, experiments conducted with BOLD fMRI generally test for differences in the magnitude of the signal between different conditions within a scan. One could not, for example, directly contrast the *mean* level of the BOLD fMRI signal obtained within the temporal lobe of Alzheimer's disease patients with that from controls with much hope of obtaining a reliable or unbiased statistical test regarding functional activity. Because the mechanism that mediates a *change* in signal level may be constant across subjects and groups, task x group interactions might be tested (but see Sect. 30.5 below).

Second, BOLD fMRI data can be treated as the output of a system that transforms neural activity

and is time-invariant and approximately linear (BOYNTON et al. 1996). A linear system can be completely characterized by its impulse response function: the output of the system to an infinitely brief and powerful input. In the context of BOLD fMRI, the change in hemodynamic fMRI signal that results from a brief (approximately <1 s) period of neural activity is an adequate stand-in for the impulse response function. The hemodynamic response function can also be represented as a frequency response (like those that characterize a resistance-capacitance circuit). The frequency representation of the hemodynamic response function can be termed the transfer function of the system. The transfer function shows how information at frequencies in the input (in this case neural activity) are scaled by the linear system. The (square of) an estimate of the BOLD transfer function (provided in Fig. 30.1B) shows that low frequencies are preferentially allowed to "pass" through the system. Hence, we call the BOLD system a "low-pass" system.

Low-pass filtering reduces temporal resolution. For instance, changes in fMRI signal corresponding to changes in neural activity every 2 s will be very difficult to detect. Indeed, the higher the paradigm frequency (and presumably the frequency of neural activity changes), the less efficiently the variance of the task will be passed into the fMRI signal. It should be noted that this limitation cannot be readily overcome by more rapid imaging. Even if BOLD fMRI data are collected every 100 ms, the filtering properties of the hemodynamic response (which are dictated by physiology and are not influenced by the scan-to-scan repetition time) will still make rapid alternations in neural activity nearly undetectable. As will be developed below, these limits of temporal resolution do not prevent fMRI experiments from detecting: (1) brief changes in neural activity, (2) dif-

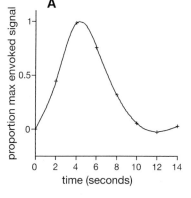
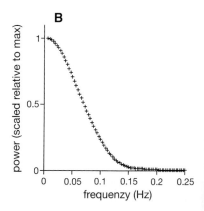

Fig. 30.1A,B. The hemodynamic response. A The change in fMRI signal that results from a brief period of neural activity (AGUIRRE et al. 1998b). B The power spectrum of the response shown in A

ferences in evoked neural activity of randomly ordered, closely spaced events, or (3) neural onset asynchronies on the order of hundreds of milliseconds between different trial types.

Finally, BOLD fMRI data are temporally autocorrelated, or "colored," under the null-hypothesis. That is to say, in fMRI data that are collected from human subjects in the absence of any experimental task or time varying stimuli, greater power is seen at some frequencies than at others. The shape of this distribution of power is well characterized by a 1/frequency (1/f) function (ZARAHN et al. 1997a), and is shown in Fig. 30.2. As can be seen, there is increasing power at ever lower frequencies. In addition to rendering traditional parametric (AGUIRRE et al. 1997; ZARAHN et al. 1997b) and nonparametric (AGUIRRE et al. 1998a) statistical tests invalid, this temporal autocorrelation causes relative reductions in sensitivity for some experimental designs. Specifically, experiments with fundamental frequencies in the lower range (e.g., a boxcar design with 60 s epochs) will have reduced sensitivity, due to the presence of greater noise at these lower frequencies. We noted just above that, because of the low-pass filtering properties of the hemodynamic transfer function, paradigms in which the variance is present at low frequencies will tend to have greater statistical sensitivity. Now we observe that, because of the presence of ever greater noise at lower frequencies, higher frequency paradigms will tend to have greater statistical sensitivity. This suggests a trade-off and the existence of an optimum.

The hemodynamic response function and the 1/f power structure of the noise can be considered the Scylla and Charybdis of fMRI experimental design: experimental variance must be present at sufficiently low frequencies to pass through the hemodynamic transfer function but at sufficiently high frequencies to avoid the elevated noise range. As a result, the sensitivity of fMRI experiments will be optimized when the design concentrates its power at frequencies in the mid-range. Throughout this chapter we will comment upon the relative statistical power of different designs by considering the frequency structure of the experimental paradigm in relation to these factors.

30.3
Categorical, Subtractive, Blocked Designs

The prototypical fMRI experimental design is shown in Fig. 30.3. This, the original boxcar approach in which two conditions alternate over the course of a scan, is a categorical, subtractive, blocked design. Categorical because the experiment examines two levels of a category, and blocked because, for most hypotheses of interest, these periods of time will not be utterly homogeneous but will consist of a block of several "trials" of some kind presented together. For example, a given block might present a series of faces to be passively perceived, or a sequence of words to be remembered, or a series of pictures to which the subject must make a living/non-living judgment and press a button to indicate his response. The block of trials is designed to evoke a particular cognitive process, such as face percep-

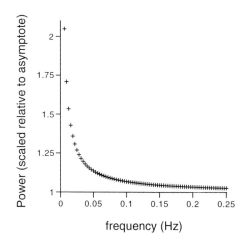

Fig. 30.2. Temporal autocorrelation under the null-hypothesis. Average power spectrum across subjects of fMRI data collected while the subjects rested quietly

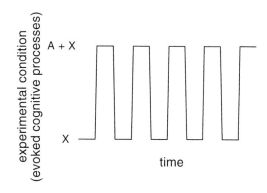

Fig. 30.3. Categorical, blocked, subtractive experimental design

tion, episodic encoding, or semantic recall. These "experimental" blocks alternate with "control" blocks that are designed to evoke all of the cognitive processes present in the experimental block except for the cognitive process of interest. Under the assumptions of "cognitive subtraction" (POSNER et al. 1988), differences in neural activity between the two conditions can be attributed to the cognitive process of interest.

One issue of some importance in the design of blocked experiments concerns the pacing of presentation of experimental trials. In many cases, the particular hypothesis to be tested will dictate the duration of presentation of stimuli and the duration of the inter-trial-interval. For example, the evocation of certain cognitive processes (e.g., semantic priming) requires the presentation of stimuli with a certain duration and minimal spacing. It should be noted, however, that sensitivity will be maximized by making each blocked period evoke the cognitive process of interest in as homogeneous a manner as possible. This may be facilitated by maximizing the period of time in which stimuli are presented and minimizing any inter-trial-interval. For example, a putative face-responsive region would generate a maximal change in fMRI signal given a series of face stimuli with no blank inter-face-interval. In those experiments in which the subject makes a response to each behavioral trial, "self-pacing" offers the ability to minimize the spacing between each trial. In a self-paced design, the rate of presentation of stimuli is dependent upon the reaction time of the subject. Perhaps surprisingly, the selection of self-paced or "fixed-paced" ordering of trials can have a nontrivial impact upon the inferences that may be drawn from a blocked imaging experiment. For details, the reader is referred to (D'ESPOSITO et al. 1997).

What types of assumptions are being made, and what sorts of confounds are present, in categorical, blocked fMRI designs? The discussion of these issues offered here is drawn from (ZARAHN et al, 1997b). Cognitive subtraction (in neuroimaging) generally relies upon two assumptions: "pure insertion" and linearity. Pure insertion is the idea that a cognitive process can be *added* to a pre-existing set of cognitive processes without affecting them. This assumption is difficult to prove because one would need an independent measure of the preexisting processes in the absence and presence of the new process. This problem exists in both chronometric psychological studies (STERNBERG 1969) and neuroimaging studies (FRISTON et al. 1996). If pure insertion fails as an assumption, a difference in neuroimaging signal between the two conditions might be observed not because of the evocation of the cognitive process of interest, but because of an interaction between the added component and preexisting components. For example, the act of pressing a button to signal a semantic judgment may be different from pressing a button in response to a visual cue. Effects upon the imaging signal that result from this difference would be erroneously attributed to semantic judgment per se.

A second assumption of cognitive subtraction is that the transformation of neural activity into fMRI signal is linear. While the BOLD fMRI system has been shown to exhibit behavior close to that of a linear system, there is some evidence for systematic departures (BOYNTON et al. 1996; DALE and BUCKNER 1997; VASQUEZ and NOLL 1996). What effects might the failure of linearity have? Consider a paradigmatic working memory experiment that presents the subject with a stimulus to be remembered, a brief delay, and then a choice stimulus. Multiple trials of this type are contrasted with a control condition in which the delay follows the choice condition, allowing the subject to make responses without relying upon working memory (JONIDES et al. 1993). Cognitive subtraction requires that the total fMRI signal evoked by neural events associated with the temporally separated presentation and choice stimuli and motor response of working memory trials be equivalent to the fMRI signal evoked by the neural event associated with the contemporaneous presentation and choice stimuli and motor response of the control condition. If there is a failure of linearity such that the response to the temporally adjacent stimuli is less than the total response to the separated stimuli, then the experimental design might lead to the erroneous inference that a region displayed delay-correlated increases in neural activity when it actually did not. In fact, failures of cognitive subtraction in these kinds of working memory studies have been empirically demonstrated (ZARAHN et al. 1997b).

Blocked designs also, by their very nature, do not allow the randomization of the order of stimuli and are constrained to grouping trials of the same type with each other in time. The consequent predictability of trial type may act as a confound in a blocked experiment. For example, many imaging studies of the neural substrates of recognition/novelty processing have involved presenting subjects with blocks of either all old (i.e., previously presented during an encoding condition) or all new (i.e., not presented during an encoding condition) stimuli together for judgments of recognition. Such a situation highlights the a priori undesirability of being constrained to blocked trial structures. The influence of trial order (i.e., blocked or random) on functional neuroimaging data can occur on at least two levels. First, the order of trial presentation may have an effect upon the cognitive processes engaged within the trials themselves (JOHNSON et al. 1997). Second, blocked or random presentation may affect the cognitive processes during the inter-trial interval. For example, changes in imaging signal may be the result of anticipatory behaviors in which the subject engages before the presentation of each stimulus. Another way of stating these observations is that every blocked experiment is confounded by behaviors that may be the result of groups of similar trials being presented together, as opposed to the effect of the individual trials themselves.

Because of these relatively untenable assumptions and plausible confounds, categorical, blocked fMRI experiments are not capable of strong inference. Although a particular instantiation of this design might have better or worse claims to satisfying the assumptions noted above, these failures exist as logical possibilities regardless of their credibility. In some cases, however, a categorical, blocked experimental design is acceptable. When an experiment is to address a purported cognitive process that: (1) is an all-or-none phenomena (i.e., cannot be subjected to parametric manipulation), (2) is homogeneous in its evocation (e.g., there are not correct or incorrect trials) and (3) cannot be separated by several seconds in time from other cognitive processes (i.e., is unlike the delay period of working memory trials) then many of the alternative designs described below offer no advantage.

One reason to actually favor blocked designs is their superior statistical power. The fundamental frequency of the boxcar can be positioned so that variance is maximally passed by the hemodynamic response function but avoids the elevated nose range at low frequencies. Simulations that have used the hemodynamic response function shown in Fig.

30.1A and the $1/f$ noise structure shown in Fig. 30.2 indicate that the optimal block length for a boxcar design is around 14–20 s (0.036–0.025 Hz) (ZARAHN et al. 1997b; Aguirre, unpublished observation). This value assumes a good estimate of the hemodynamic response function (perhaps obtained empirically from the subject; see AGUIRRE et al. 1998b). If this is not available, slightly longer block lengths (e.g., 30 s) become preferable.

When more than two conditions are included in a blocked experiment, the experimenter has several options for how those blocks are to be ordered during the scan (e.g., fixed: A-B-C-A-B-C-A-B-C; or random: A-C-C-B-A-B-C-B-A; see Fig. 30.4A,B). While randomizing the order of the blocks may have appeal from a psychological design standpoint, this randomization decreases sensitivity for differences between the conditions by distributing the variance of the task paradigm over multiple frequencies, including low frequencies that are in the high noise range. If the experiment is to be conducted in several subjects, then a desirable compromise is to fix the order of the blocks within a subject, but to vary (perhaps counterbalance) this order across subjects (see Sect. 30.5 for a discussion of the appropriate statistical model to use in group analyses).

A final application of blocked designs is as an initial experimental probe. Below we discuss several alternative experimental designs that, while providing for stronger inference, have reduced statistical power compared to blocked designs. A possible approach is to combine both the blocked design just described and other designs within a series of experiments. For example, one might use a blocked experiment initially to define regions of interest and then interrogate those regions in subsequent experiments with the designs described below (e.g., AGUIRRE et al. 1998c). The primary drawback of a combined design is that there may exist regions that, because of their response properties, are only detectable using one of the more sophisticated designs. In this case, the combined approach would not be able to detect these regions.

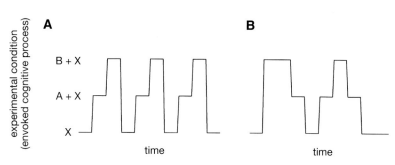

Fig. 30.4A,B. Three condition categorical, blocked experiment, showing **A** fixed and **B** randomized block orders

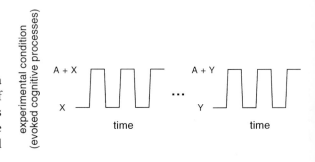

Fig. 30.6. Cognitive conjunction design

30.4
Factorial, Conjunction, and Parametric Designs

Several experimental designs have as their goal a reduction in the reliance upon the assumption of pure insertion. We will describe these approaches as they apply to blocked experiments, but it should be appreciated that these concepts can also be applied to the event-related designs described below.

Factorial experiments (FRISTON et al. 1996) are explicitly designed to examine the interactions of two different, candidate cognitive processes. The scheme of the design, illustrated in Fig. 30.5, involves (in the simplest case) four conditions, during which two different processes are evoked individually and then jointly. In essence, this amounts to a categorical, blocked design with four conditions. The proposed advantage of the design is that interactions between the two cognitive processes ("A" and "B" in this example) can be examined. The presence of an interaction is indicated if the difference in imaging signal between the presence and absence of cognitive process "A" is itself different when cognitive process "B" is present or absent (i.e., if [A+B+X]–[B+X] is different from [A+X]–[X]). While factorial designs do provide a compelling method for gaining greater insight into the neural implementation of cognitive processes, it is a mistake to claim that such designs obviate the need for the pure insertion assumption. Interpretation of the design requires the assumption that the two cognitive processes have, indeed, been isolated. The logic by which this isolation is to occur is the same as that outlined for cognitive subtraction above. That is, process "A" and process "B" must be purely inserted into the other cognitive components ("X") that allow the experiment to evoke these processes.

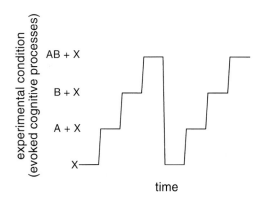

Fig. 30.5. Blocked factorial design

The "cognitive conjunction" design (PRICE and FRISTON 1997) has also been proposed to reduce reliance upon the assumption of pure insertion. The logic of the approach is that, if one wishes to discount the possibility of an interaction (i.e., a failure of pure insertion) between the cognitive component to be added and the set of preexisting processes, one should repeat the experiment with a different set of preexisting processes and replicating the result (Fig. 30.6). A rigorous implementation of this notion (PRICE and FRISTON 1997) involves conducting a series of categorical subtraction experiments that all aim to isolate the same cognitive process. The novel twist is that the subtractions need not be complete; that is, the experimental and control conditions can differ in several cognitive processes in addition to the one of interest. The imaging data are then analyzed to identify areas that have a significant, consistent response to the putatively isolated process (i.e., a significant main effect across subtractions in the absence of any significant interactions). Again, while this design reduces the plausibility of some failures of cognitive subtraction, it does not eliminate the possibility. In particular, some cognitive processes, by their very nature, require the evocation of an antecedent process. For example, can working memory be meaningfully present if not preceded by the presentation of a stimulus to be remembered? If not, then any cognitive conjunction design that attempts to demonstrate the presence of neural activity during a delay period will be susceptible to erroneous results due to interactions between the task manipulation and preexisting task components.

Finally, parametric designs, when applicable, offer the opportunity to truly obviate the assumption of pure insertion. In a parametric design, the experimenter presents a range of different levels of some parameter, and seeks to identify relationships (most simply, a linear one) between imaging signal and the values that the parameter assumes (Fig. 30.7A). This can be done to identify the neural correlates of

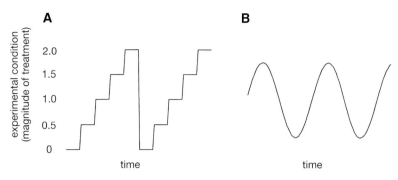

Fig. 30.7A,B. Parametric designs that are **A** blocked and **B** continuously varying

straightforward changes in stimulus properties (e.g., the chrominance of a stimulus, ENGEL et al. 1997) or manipulations of a cognitive process (e.g., working memory, BRAVER et al. 1997). The reason that a parametric design may eschew the pure insertion assumption is that only the magnitude of the process of interest is altered. While it is still possible to conceive of inferential failures using this design, this approach is able to avoid several of the questionable experimental assumptions considered above. It should be noted, however, that a parametric design has reduced sensitivity compared to a two-condition design of the same length (i.e., with the same number of observations) that only uses the extreme levels of the parameter. This is because the two-condition design maximizes the ratio of task-induced variance to noise.

The parametric design illustrated in Fig. 30.7A is blocked, but it should be noted that continuously varying parametric designs can also be conducted (Fig.30.7B). In this case, the parameter of interest is continuously varied over the course of the scan, and correlations between the imaging signal and this independent variable are sought (after accounting for the effects of the hemodynamic transfer function). A twist on the continuously varying parametric design is the so-called traveling wave stimulus, in which the subject is exposed to an expanding annulus of flickering light, or a continuously rotating wedge of flickering light. Interestingly, these designs, used to map early visual areas (ENGEL et al. 1994; SERENO et al. 1995) are parametric in *space*, but blocked in *time*.

30.5
Event-Related Designs

Continuously varying parametric designs serve as an appropriate segue to the discussion of event-related experimental design. An appealing aspect of

the continuously varying parametric design is that it avoids the possibility of behavioral confounds that are the result of blocking of stimuli together. An event-related design enjoys this advantage and others as well, including the ability to: (1) randomize trial presentations, and (2) test for functional changes between different measurable aspects of behavior (e.g., accuracy) or different characteristics of a trial (e.g., stimulus type). These advantages apply to all event-related designs and the reader is advised to consult the chapter by BUCKNER (this volume) and ZARAHN et al. (1997b) for a complete description. As we will discuss, a more refined advantage of a particular event-related fMRI design (ZARAHN et al. 1997b) is the ability to examine separately the neural substrates of components of behavior temporally dissociable on the order of a few seconds *within* a trial.

Event-related fMRI designs attempt to model signal changes associated with individual trials as opposed to a larger unit of time comprised of a block of trials (Fig. 30.8). Each individual trial may be composed of one behavioral event (such as the presentation of a single word) or several behavioral events (such as the presentation of a cue, a delay period, and a motor response in a delayed response task). In the simplest type of event-related experiment, the behavioral trials are distant enough in time from one another to allow the hemodynamic response that results from the hypothesized brief period of evoked neural activity to fully run its course (e.g., 16 s). A variety of analysis approaches are available that allow the statistical evaluation of these responses both with respect to the inter-trial-interval and with respect to one another (DALE and BUCKNER 1997; JOSEPHS et al. 1997; ZARAHN et al. 1997b). While this is properly the topic for a different review, we note here that when trials are spaced far enough apart in time to avoid any overlap in the hemodynamic response of one trial to the next, neither analysis nor inference (in one sense) requires the assumption of linearity. Additionally, analysis methods exist that require no a priori assumptions regarding the specific shape of the evoked response (JOSEPHS et al. 1997).

Because the analysis focuses upon individual trials, it is possible to ascribe changes in the neuroimaging signal to the effect of one particular trial type, regardless of when it is presented within the experiment. This feature of event-related designs allows for the randomization of stimuli, thus avoiding behavioral confounds that are the result of blocking trials, and allows the separate analysis of functional responses that are only identified in retrospect (e.g., trials on which the subject made a correct or incorrect response).

In the simple case in which an event-related design has only a single trial-type, presented at a regular interval, it is possible to determine what particular trial spacing will result in optimal sensitivity for evoked responses. Assuming the hemodynamic response and noise structure shown in Figs. 30.1 and 30.2, a trial spacing of about 16 s is optimal (Aguirre, unpublished observation). (Optimal meaning: "maximizes sensitivity for an effect over a fixed duration of scanning." If the duration of the scan is free to vary and the number of trials is held constant, ever greater separation between the trials leads to ever greater theoretical sensitivity in all cases, including those considered below.) If the design calls for different trial types to be intermixed, optimal spacing becomes a more complicated issue. If the trials are spaced more closely together, the hemodynamic response from one trial overlaps with the response of the adjacent trial. This closer spacing of trials decreases the sensitivity of the design for evoked changes relative to the inter-trial-interval, but increases sensitivity for differences between the trial types, *as long as they are in a random order*. Additionally, closer spacing of the trials increases the

stringency of the assumptions that must be satisfied for a successful analysis. Specifically, the analysis must now assume linearity for the system. Notably, failures of these assumptions can be expected to lead to *false negative* results (due to reductions in sensitivity), as opposed to the false positives that might result from the failures of assumptions in other experimental designs. In the limit, with the assumptions of linearity perfectly satisfied, the optimal spacing to detect a difference between two randomly ordered trial types approaches zero. Again, as this spacing decreases, the ability to detect the evoked response of either trial type relative to the inter-trial interval also approaches zero. Empirical tests conducted within the primary visual cortex are in broad agreement with these assertions (DALE and BUCKNER 1997).

Because the frequency structure of a train of impulses (the neural activity proposed to result from an event-related design) is itself a series of impulses, much of the variance in an event-related design is present at higher frequencies and is therefore lost after passing through the hemodynamic response function. As a result, event-related designs as a class are reduced in sensitivity relative to blocked designs, regardless of the spacing of trials and manipulations of the inter-trial-interval. However, one way to improve sensitivity in an event-related design is to introduce "jitter" into the inter-trial-interval (Fig. 30.9). Variability in the inter-trial-interval acts to distribute some of the variance of the design from higher frequencies to lower ones. Such jitter designs also have the advantage of reducing the ability of the subject to engage in anticipatory behaviors prior to the onset of each trial.

The discussion thus far regarding event-related designs has assumed an ability to randomize perfectly the order of presentation of different event types. There are certain types of behavioral paradigms, however, that do not permit a random ordering of the trial events. For example, the delay period of a working memory experiment always follows the presentation of a stimulus to be remembered. In this case, the different events of the trial cannot be placed arbitrarily close together without risking the possibility of false *positive* results that accrue from the hemodynamic response to one trial event (e.g., the stimulus presentation) being interpreted as resulting from neural activity in response to another event (e.g., the delay period). It turns out that, given the shape typically observed for hemodynamic responses, events within a trial as close together as 4 s can be reliably discriminated within the context of a

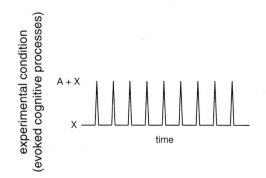

Fig. 30.8. Event-related design

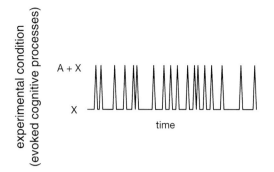

Fig. 30.9. Event-related design with variable inter-trial-intervals

least-squares analysis (ZARAHN et al. 1997b). Thus, event-related designs can be used to examine directly, for example, the hypothesis that certain cortical areas increase their activity during the delay period of a working memory paradigm without requiring the problematic assumptions traditionally employed in blocked, subtractive designs (ZARAHN et al. 1997b; see also the chapter by COHEN, this volume).

The transition to event-related design offers the opportunity to test many hypotheses in a principled, rigorous fashion that was simply not previously possible. As a final example of event-related design, consider an experiment that aims to identify a neural onset asynchrony. We have recently demonstrated that the hemodynamic response observed for a subject during a scanning session is highly reliable in its shape (AGUIRRE et al. 1998b). As a result, it might be possible to use fMRI to detect small neural onset asynchronies. Such a design might present one of two different behavioral trials (in a random order) every 16 s. Because of the reliability of the hemodynamic transformation, differences in the mean time-to-peak of the responses to the two different types of stimuli could be identified and ascribed to an asynchrony in onset of neural activity. Such a design might allow one, for example, to test the hypothesis that a cortical area that responds to pictures of faces responds with a slightly longer latency (on the order of 100 ms) to pictures of inverted faces.

30.6
Issues in Intergroup Comparisons

The discussion so far has focused upon experimental designs that attempt to address hypotheses regarding neural activity in individual subjects. Often,

it is of interest to test the hypothesis that either: (1) the *population* from which the subjects are drawn posses the hypothesized effect, or (2) that two different populations differ in the evocation of some effect. The movement from individual subject tests to studies of groups of subjects is accompanied by several complications.

The most immediate of these is that different subjects have brains that are shaped differently. If one wishes to test a hypothesis regarding a certain area of the brain, then it is first necessary to identify that same area of the brain across subjects. While there are a variety of sophisticated methods available for registering and aligning the brains of different subjects into a standard space, there are theoretical limits to what such an alignment can achieve. First, there may be inter-subject variability in anatomy that cannot be overcome by warping brains to a standard space. For example, the arrangement of the sulci in ventral occipitotemporal cortex is known to vary between subjects (ONO et al. 1990). Thus, while two subjects may have neural responses at the same "true" cyto-architectonic location, the position of this site with respect to other landmarks in the brain may differ between subjects, leading to spread of these locations when data are converted to a standard space (WOODS 1996). Second, even given rigid alignment of anatomy across subjects, there may be variability in the structure:function relationships between subjects. For example, two subjects may truly have distinct face selective neural regions, but these may be located in different sections of a cortical area as a consequence of differences in nature or nurture. Again, when normalized to a standard space, this variability in location will obscure functional dissociations.

An alternative to anatomical registration is functional identification. The approach here is to first identify a region across subjects by its functional responses. For example, one might identify a region that responds more to pictures of faces than to general objects. Then, hypotheses regarding the response of this functionally defined region to other types of stimuli (for example, faces compared to hands) can be independently tested across subjects within this area (KANWISHER et al. 1996). This powerful approach allows one to make inferences across subjects regarding the responses of some functional area (e.g., the fusiform face area) at the expense of making statements regarding some particular position in a standardized space.

The next issue is a statistical one. In virtually all group PET and fMRI studies reported to date in which repeated observations have been obtained from each subject, a fixed-effect statistical model has been employed. This type of model makes the assumption that observations from different subjects are the same as observations from within a single subject, i.e., that there are no subject x task interactions (HOLMES et al, 1998). If one wishes to make inferences regarding an effect that extends to the population from which the subjects were drawn (i.e., the population of neurologically intact young college and medical students for most studies!) then it is necessary to employ a statistical model that explicitly accounts for subject x task interactions in the data. Such a random effects model (as subject x task interactions imply that the effect of task in each subject is a random effect) is actually very simple to implement for fMRI. All that is needed is a single value from each subject (from each anatomical location that is to be compared) that reflects the effect of the task for that subject. Within the context of the general linear model, this value should be the parameter estimate (or its corresponding t value) obtained for the predictor that models the hypothesized effect. These values across subjects are then tested using a simple t test against the null-hypothesis that their mean is zero. There is no need to correct for any kind of autocorrelation in the data, as these values are independent. The alert reader may have noted one downside of this statistical approach: the degrees of freedom of the test are only equal to the number of subjects involved in the study (minus 1)! As a result, hypotheses that attempt to demonstrate consistent effects across subjects using fMRI are far less powerful (in the statistical sense) than identical hypotheses that seek this effect only in individual subjects. While this is unfortunate, it is also unavoidable if appropriate inference is to be drawn. Furthermore, if population inference is desired, experimental resources should be devoted towards gathering data from more subjects as opposed to more data per subject.

This type of design can be extended to test hypotheses regarding differential responses of different populations to a task. For example, one might propose that within an anatomically specified area of the fusiform gyrus, copy editors have a greater fMRI signal response to the presentation of letters of the alphabet as compared to normal controls. Again, a mixed-effect model that compared the effect sizes between the two populations would appropriately test this idea. These tests seem straightforward when both populations are healthy, neurologically intact subjects who differ only in their job experience. They

become inferentially more challenging, however, when one population is composed of patients with neurological or psychiatric impairments, the elderly, or the recipients of a pharmacological agent. In these cases, the experimenter must be concerned about a confounding change in physiology or metabolism that might create artifactual results. For example, if elderly subjects have altered *vascular* responses as compared to young controls, then the observation of a decreased fMRI response to certain cognitive tasks cannot necessarily be interpreted as a difference in *neural* response. Ideally, one would also perform a control task that is not hypothesized to have any task x group interactions, thus disputing the possibility of this confound.

30.7
Involvement and Implementation Hypotheses

So far, our discussion of experimental design has not considered the specific question regarding the relationship between the brain and cognition that is under study. Regardless of the particular type of fMRI design selected, there are two broad categories of question that might be addressed using neuroimaging techniques. We would like to suggest here that neuroimaging can provide for stronger inference regarding one compared to the other. The logical framework from which this discussion is drawn can be found in (ZARAHN 1998).

One class of hypotheses that are frequently tested using neuroimaging methods might be termed "involvement" hypotheses. These are proposals of the kind that a region is causally involved in the production of a particular cognitive process. It turns out that neuroimaging experiments do not allow for strong inference regarding these types of hypotheses, such as interpreting a positive result as a demonstration that the region is involved in the putatively isolated cognitive process. The primary cause of this state of affairs is the observational, correlative nature of neuroimaging (SARTER et al. 1996). Although we make inferences regarding cognitive processes, these processes are not themselves directly subject to experimental manipulations. Instead, the investigator controls the presentation of stimuli and instructions, with the hope that these circumstances will provoke the subject to enter a certain cognitive state and *no other*. Careful consideration reveals how this assumption might fail. For instance, although cooperative, the subject may unwittingly engage in confounding cognitive processes in addition to that intended by the experimenter, or alternatively, may fail to differentially engage the process (i.e., it may already be on). It is therefore not possible to know if observed changes in neural activity in a brain region are the result of the evocation of the cognitive process of interest or an unintended, confounding process. Negative results (even in the face of arbitrarily high statistical power) are also not conclusive, both because of the failure of cognitive control and because of the possibility that the neuroimaging method employed might not be sensitive to the critical change in metabolic activity (e.g., pattern of neuronal firing as opposed to bulk, integrated synaptic activity) (PUCE et al. 1997).

Alternatively, neuroimaging techniques can provide inferentially strong tests regarding *implementation* hypotheses. This improvement in inference derives from a shift in the structure of the hypothesis. An implementation hypothesis *begins* with the assumption that a cortical region is involved in a particular cognitive process. The experiment then examines the activity in that area during different experimental conditions to: (1) characterize the nature of the computation that underlies the involvement of the region, or (2) learn something about a behavioral state. For example, the first type of implementation study might ask if the bulk rate of neuronal activity in area MT is monotonically related to a behavioral measure of motion perception. In the second type of implementation experiment, one might use activity in area MT as an index of motion perception, and then test hypotheses regarding how unrelated distractor tasks affect motion perception (REES et al. 1997). Neuroimaging can provide for stronger inference for these types of hypotheses because there is an isomorphic relationship between the independent variables that the experimenter manipulates and the subject of inference. Of course, the value of these types of experiments is itself dependent upon the veracity of the assumptions employed.

References

Aguirre GK, Zarahn E, D'Esposito M (1997) Empirical analyses of BOLD fMRI statistics. II. Spatially smoothed data collected under null-hypothesis and experimental conditions. NeuroImage 2:199–212
Aguirre GK, Zarahn E, D'Esposito M (1998a) A critique of the use of the Kolmogorov-Smirnov statistic for the analysis of BOLD fMRI. Magn Reson Med 39:500–505
Aguirre GK, Zarahn E, D'Esposito M (1998b) The variability of human BOLD hemodynamic responses. NeuroImage 8:360–369
Aguirre GK, Zarahn E, D'Esposito M (1998c) An area within human ventral cortex sensitive to "building" stimuli: evidence and implications. Neuron 21:373–383
Boynton G, Engel S, Glover G, Heeger D (1996) Linear systems analysis of functional magnetic resonance imaging in human V1. J Neurosci 16:4207–4221
Braver TS, Cohen JD, Nystrom LE, Jonides J, Smith EE, Noll DC (1997) A parametric study of prefrontal cortex involvement in human working memory. NeuroImage 5:49–62
Dale AM, Buckner RL (1997) Selective averaging of rapidly presented individual trials using fMRI. Hum Brain Mapping 5:329–340
D'Esposito M, Zarahn E, Aguirre GK, Shin RK, Auerbach P, Alsop DC, Detre JA (1997) The effect of pacing of experimental stimuli on observed functional MRI activity. NeuroImage 6:113–121
Engel S, Zhang X, Wandell B (1997) Colour tuning in human visual cortex measured with functional magnetic resonance imaging. Nature 388:68–71
Engel SA, Rumelhart DE, Wandell BA, Lee AT, Glover GH, Chichilnisky EJ, Shadlen MN (1994) fMRI of human visual cortex [letter] [published erratum appears in Nature 1994 Jul 14;370(6485):106]. Nature 369:525
Friston KJ, Price CJ, Fletcher P, Moore C, Frackowiak RSJ, Dolan RJ (1996) The trouble with cognitive subtraction. NeuroImage 4:97–104
Holmes AP, Friston KJ (1998) Generalisability, random effects and population inference. NeuroImage 7:S754
Johnson MK, Nolde SF, Mather M, Kounios J et al. (1997) The similarity of brain activity associated with true and false recognition memory depends on test format. Psychol Sci 8:250–257
Jonides J, Smith EE, Koeppe RA, Awh E, Minoshima S, Mintun MA (1993) Spatial working memory in humans as revealed by PET. Nature 363:623–625
Josephs O, Turner R, Friston KJ (1997) Event-related fMRI. Hum Brain Mapping 5:243–248
Kanwisher N, Chun MM, McDermott J, Ledden PJ (1996) Functional imagining of human visual recognition. Cogn Brain Res 5:55–67
Ono M, Kubik S, Abernathey CD (1990) Atlas of cerebral sulci. Thieme, New York
Platt JR (1964) Strong inference. Science 146:347–353
Posner MI, Petersen SE, Fox PT, Raichle ME (1988) Localization of cognitive operations in the human brain. Science 24:1627–1631
Price CJ, Friston KJ (1997) Cognitive conjunctions: a new experimental design for fMRI. NeuroImage 5:261–270
Puce A, Allison T, Spencer SS, Spencer DD, McCarthy G (1997) Comparison of cortical activation evoked by faces measured by intracranial field potentials and functional MRI: Two case studies. Hum Brain Mapping 5:298–305
Rees G, Frith CD, Lavie N (1997) Modulating irrelevant motion perception by varying attentional load in an unrelated task. Science 278:1616–1619
Sarter M, Berntson G, Cacioppo J (1996) Brain imaging and cognitive neuroscience: toward strong inference in attributing function to structure. Am Psychol 51:13–21
Sereno MI, Dale AM, Reppas JB, Kwong KK, Belliveau JW, Brady TJ, Rosen BR et al. (1995) Borders of multiple visual

areas in humans revealed by functional magnetic resonance imaging. Science 268:889–893

Sternberg S (1969) The discovery of processing stages: extensions of Donder's method. Acta Psychol 30:276–315

Vasquez AL, Noll DC. Non-linear temporal aspects of the
BOLD response in fMRI. Proc Int Soc Magn Reson Med,
New York, NY, 1996, pp 1765

Woods RP (1996) Modeling for intergroup comparisons of
imaging data. NeuroImage 4:S84-S94

Zarahn E (1998) The neural correlates of spatial mnemonic
processing. PhD dissertation., University of Pennsylvania

Zarahn E, Aguirre GK, D'Esposito M (1997a) Empirical analyses of BOLD fMRI statistics. I. Spatially unsmoothed data
collected under null-hypothesis conditions. NeuroImage
5:179–197

Zarahn E, Aguirre GK, D'Esposito M (1997b) A trial-based
experimental design for fMRI. NeuroImage 6:122–138

31 Functional MRI of the Sensorimotor System

M. Hallett, N. Sadato, M. Honda, K. Ishii, D. Waldvogel, K. Bushara

CONTENTS

31.1
Brain Activation with Simple Movement

To determine how specific brain areas contribute to the selection of particular muscle patterns that underlie a coordinated movement is an important issue for movement control. In the human motor pathways, the neurons that regulate the activity of individual body parts are topographically arranged (somatotopy). Initially these maps were obtained using electrical stimulation of the cortex (Penfield and Boldrey 1937). More recently, PET has been utilized for mapping the somatotopic organization in the primary and nonprimary motor cortex (Fox et al. 1985; Colebatch et al. 1991; Grafton et al. 1991, 1993), but its limited spatial resolution and signal-to-noise ratio did not allow individual analysis.

M. Hallett, MD; K. Ishii, MD; D. Waldvogel, MD; K. Bushara, MD; NINDS, Human Motor Control Section, NINDS, NIH, Building 10, Room 5N226, 10 Center Dr., MSC 1428, Bethesda, MA 20892-1428, USA
N. Sadato, MD, PhD; Biomedical Imaging Research Center, Fukui Medical University, 23 Shimoaizuki, Matsuoka, Yoshida, Fukui 910-1104, Japan
M. Honda, MD, PhD; Department of Brain Pathophysiology, Kyoto University School of Medicine, 54 Shogoin, Sakyo, Kyoto 606-8507, Japan

Functional MRI done during simple motor tasks could provide a useful way to map the somatotopy (Le Bihan et al. 1995). The location of the hand representation is in an omega-shaped region of the central sulcus (Fig. 31.1) (Yousry et al. 1997). Using fMRI and voluntary movements of the hand, arm, and foot, Rao et al. (1995) confirmed the somatotopy of the primary sensorimotor cortex in individual subjects. With higher spatial resolution, fMRI enabled mapping of representation of each finger movement. Within the hand, individual finger movements are controlled by networks of neurons that occupy overlapping areas within the primary motor cortex (Sanes et al. 1995). This finding is consistent with an electrical stimulation study suggesting the territories controlling different fingers overlap (Schieber and Hibbard 1993). Using functional MRI during saccadic eye movement, and simple repetitive movement of wrist, ankle and tongue, Nitschke et al. (1996) and Honda et al. (1997) confirmed a somatotopic representation in the cerebellum. Functional MRI has also been successfully applied to the presurgical mapping of the motor representation of the face and hand to avoid postsurgical deficit (Jack et al. 1994; Yousry et al. 1995). With its higher spatial and temporal resolution, mapping somatotopy with fMRI is useful for scientific investigation of human motor control and for clinical applications.

It is important to keep in mind that statistically significant activation in PET or fMRI does not necessarily mean that the area is truly functionally "relevant" for the condition. Thus, the fMRI study combined with other modalities of physiological techniques such as electroencephalogram (EEG), magnetoencephalogram (MEG), and transcranial magnetic stimulation (TMS) will be helpful for evaluating the physiological significance of the results.

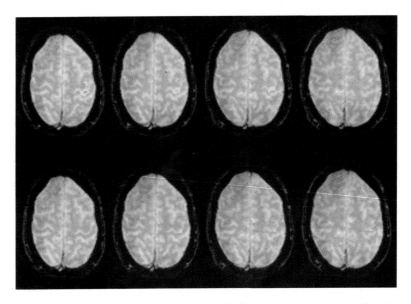

Fig. 31.1. Examples of fMRI scans from the same normal subject with finger tapping (*top row*) and tactile stimulation (*bottom row*). For the motor task, the subject tapped the little finger at a frequency of 2 Hz, and for the sensory task the little finger was passively tapped at the same frequency. The four images in each row are successive axial slices of the same study, from higher to lower going from *left to right*. Sulci are *white*. The motor task produced prominent activation in an omega-shaped portion of the central sulcus. There is activation of the supplementary motor area (SMA) as well. With the pure tactile task, there is weaker activation in the central sulcus as well as an inferior and slightly lateral shift of the activation maximum. Activation is also seen in the post-central sulcus and cingulate motor area. The images were acquired with a 3D fMRI sequence using large magnetic susceptibility weighting based on the echo-shifting principle combined with multiple gradient echoes per excitation (VAN GELDEREN et al. 1995) with a 3.75 mm isotropic resolution (64×51×24 voxels/volume). TE was 39 ms, TR 26 ms, time/volume 2000 ms. The images were analyzed with SPM95, the maximal Z-score for the activation in the sensorimotor cortex was 8.18 for the motor and 5.52 for the sensory task. The functional images were superimposed on anatomical images acquired with the same 3D sequence but with double resolution, giving identical distortions and therefore allowing superimposition without misregistration

31.1.1
Dependence of Activation on Movement Rate

A direct relation between the repetition rate of a stimulus and the metabolic rate of glucose utilization has been established in the peripheral nervous system (YAROWSKY et al. 1983), and for subcortical structures in the central nervous system (TOGA and COLLINS 1981). Assuming that energy-dependent changes in neuronal function and regional cerebral blood flow (rCBF) are coupled and that neuronal discharge rate is a measure of energy-dependent neuronal function (RAICHLE 1987), studies in humans with PET and O-15 water have explored the effect of stimulus rate on the central nervous system. The rCBF change in the striate cortex is proportional to the repetition rate of photic stimulation between 0 and 7.8 Hz (FOX and RAICHLE 1984). A linear rate response function was also observed in the primary auditory cortex (WISE et al. 1991; PRICE et al. 1992). These studies underscore the significance of the stimulus rate as a determinant of rCBF response.

The quantitative relationship between MR signal intensity change and blood flow is not well understood. It has been hypothesized that MR signal intensity change in the T2* weighted gradient echo sequence is proportional to changes in the total deoxyhemoglobin concentration in the voxel, which is affected by changes in cerebral blood volume (CBV) and hematocrit as well as by changes in percent saturation of oxygen (JEZZARD et al. 1994). As CBF (and oxygen delivery) changes exceed changes in CBV by two- to four-fold and oxygen extraction increases only slightly with neuronal activation (FOX et al. 1988a), total deoxyhemoglobin decreases; hence, less intravoxel dephasing and increased MR signal occur (KWONG et al. 1992). DETRE et al. (1992) proposed a one-compartment model with the longitudinal magnetization and blood flow effect, showing that flow change was proportional to change of the inverse of T1. Using inversion recovery echo planar imaging (EPI), which was a T1-sensitive sequence, KWONG et al. (1992) showed that percent change of MR signal by a T2*-sensitive sequence was identical to that of a T1-sensitive sequence in the activation of the primary visual cortex with photic stimulation of different frequencies, which in turn correlated well with PET results by Fox and Raichle (1984). This implies that the signal intensity change observed with the blood oxygen level-dependent (BOLD) method is proportional to rCBF changes elicited by increased neuronal activity.

The effect of the movement repetition rate on rCBF has been studied by several groups. Using PET with group analysis, Sadato et al. (1996b) found that the rCBF increased in the primary sensorimotor cortex (SM1) with the repetition rate of simple, repetitive finger movements, with saturation of CBF at rates faster than 2 Hz. To minimize the partial volume effect due to the limited resolution of PET, which precludes dissociation of volume from magnitude (Fox et al. 1985), they also used fMRI with the BOLD method, which has better spatial resolution and allows individual analysis. They evaluated the effect of repetition rate of a simple movement on the magnitude as well as area of recruitment separately in SM1 using correlational analysis in the Fourier domain (Sadato et al. 1997). Percent change in signal intensity of the left SM1 linearly increased from 1 to 4 Hz. Area of activation increased up to 2 Hz and showed a tendency to decrease at higher frequencies. The combination of progressively increasing signal intensity with an area that increases to 2 Hz and declines at faster frequencies explains the PET finding of a plateau of rCBF at the faster frequencies. A linear relationship in SM1 between MR BOLD signal intensity change and movement rate has also been reported by other authors (Rao et al. 1996; Schlaug et al. 1996).

In contrast to SM1, the supplementary motor area (SMA) did not show a linear effect of movement rate by PET (Blinkenberg et al. 1996; Sadato et al. 1996b) or by fMRI (Schlaug et al. 1996). Using PET, Sadato et al. (1996b) measured rCBF in eight normal volunteers during auditory-cued, repetitive flexion movement of the right index finger against the thumb, performed at very slow (0.25 and 0.5 Hz), slow (0.75 and 1 Hz), fast (2 and 2.5 Hz), and very fast (3 and 4 Hz) rates. The SMA showed its highest activation at the very slow rates but no significant activation at the very fast rates. The authors suggested that the decreases in CBF may reflect a progressive change in performance from reactive to predictive, as only the slow rate conditions are really reaction time tasks. Maximal activation in the SMA different from that in the SM1 could be explained by a trade-off between preparatory activity and execution

(Sadato et al. 1996b). Preparatory activity includes motor set and perceptual set (Evarts et al. 1984). Motor set is the covert biasing of downstream motor systems with respect to some specific aspect of the subsequent movement. Perceptual set is related to the expectation of target appearance. With a long interstimulus interval, there is more time for activity related to motor set and perceptual set. As the SMA has a greater ratio of preparatory to execution activity than does the primary motor cortex (Alexander and Crutcher 1990), it will be relatively more active with slow rates.

31.2
Brain Activation with Complex Movement and Other Motor Features

More complex movement has also been studied using fMRI. Activation of nonprimary motor cortex was first reported by Rao et al. (1993). While their subjects performed self-paced, complex finger movements consisting of a repeating fixed sequence, more widespread activation was observed in the contralateral (and occasionally ipsilateral) primary motor cortex (M1), SMA, the premotor cortex of both hemispheres, and the contralateral somatosensory cortex (S1) compared with the performance of simple repetitive movement without a sequence. On the other hand, Boecker et al. (1994) showed that the SMA was activated by simple repetitive movement and argued that it is involved in self-paced finger tapping and not exclusively reserved for more complex motor control. The question on its role in self-initiated vs externally triggered movement as well as simple vs complex movements has been recently studied by Deiber et al. (unpublished data). In that study, different parameters of movement (i.e., length of motor sequence, movement rate, self-paced or visually triggered), which had made the interpretation of the previous studies difficult, were systematically controlled. More extended and consistent activation during self-initiated movement than during visually triggered movement was observed in the anterior SMA, the rostral part of the cingulate motor zone (RCZ) and the caudal part of the cingulate motor area (CCZ), whereas more complex movement was associated with more extensive activation than simple movement in the posterior part of the SMA (SMA proper) and the CCZ. These findings suggest an aspect of functional dissociation in the nonprimary motor areas in the medial wall of the hemisphere.

Preparatory aspects of movement can be studied by using more recently developed techniques with better temporal resolution, called event-related or time-resolved fMRI. These techniques permit detection of transient signal changes that occur with single cognitive or motor events as opposed to conventional functional imaging paradigms using repetitive task performance to generate sustained functional signal changes. Using such a technique, RICHTER et al. (1997) reported activity in the human M1, the premotor cortex and the SMA during a delayed cued finger movement task. All three areas were active during both movement preparation and movement execution. Activity in the primary motor cortex was considerably weaker during movement preparation than during movement execution; in the premotor cortex and the SMA, activity was of similar intensity during both periods. HUMBERSTONE et al. (1997) successfully demonstrated a functional subdivision of the medial premotor cortex by measuring temporal activation patterns during a go/no-go motor paradigm. They showed that the anterior SMA was involved in movement decision making and the posterior SMA was directly involved in motor execution.

Motor ideation or imagination is an interesting aspect of motor function. TYSZKA et al. (1994) reported that activity in the medial premotor areas was decreased in magnitude during motor ideation compared to the execution of the same movement. However, they observed a differential change between the anterior and posterior subdivision of the medial premotor areas; namely, response in the anterior part was consistently greater than the activity in the posterior region, suggesting that the more anteriorly located area plays a greater role in ideation of movement than the posteriorly located area. LEONARDO et al. (1995) showed that two of their five subjects had significant activation in the left SM1 during ideation of right finger tapping, but to a lesser degree than execution of the same movement, whereas the left premotor area showed comparable activation with both actual and imagined performance in three subjects. PORRO et al. (1996) also reported significant increases of activity, compared to the control (visual imagery) tasks, in a region including the anterior bank and crown of the central sulcus, the presumed site of M1, during both motor performance and motor imagery, but approximately three times greater during motor performance than motor imagination. However, these findings are not consistent with the report by STEPHAN et al. (1995) using PET, reporting a lack of activation in the primary motor area during motor imagery. One of the most important criticisms of these studies on motor imagery is that subjects' performance is difficult to evaluate objectively.

HIKOSAKA et al. (1996) studied the neural correlates of procedural learning of motor sequences. During the test scans the subjects learned a new sequence (position or color) of button presses; during the control scans they pressed the buttons in any order. They found that the anterior SMA was particularly active for learning new sequential procedures (either position or color sequences), not movements per se. In contrast, the posterior SMA was active for the performance of sequential movements, not learning. More recently, the same group (SAKAI et al. 1998) reported the time course of activity in the different brain regions along the learning curve using the same task and wider coverage of the brain. Their studies revealed four brain areas specifically related to learning: the dorsolateral prefrontal cortex (DLPFC), the anterior SMA, the precuneus, and the intraparietal sulcus (IPS). They also observed that the DLPFC and anterior SMA were activated in the earlier stages of learning, whereas the two parietal areas, precuneus and IPS, were activated in the later stages. They interpreted these findings to mean that the shift of activation might reflect the transition from the declarative to the procedural stage of learning. KARNI et al. (1995) studied the long-term aspect of motor skill learning. Before training, a comparable extent of M1 was activated by two different sequences. Subjects performed daily training of one of the two sequences extensively. By week 4 of training, the extent of cortex activated by the practiced sequence enlarged compared with the unpracticed sequence regardless of the fact that the rate of movement during fMRI scan was the same between practiced and unpracticed sequences. These changes persisted for several months. Their findings suggest that long-term reorganization of M1 may play a role in the acquisition of the motor skill.

31.3
Motor Control from the Ipsilateral Hemisphere

It has long been known that the motor cortex has some influence on the muscles of the ipsilateral side. There is anatomical evidence that 10%–15% of fibers in the lateral cortical spinal tracts of humans are uncrossed (NYBERG-HANSEN and RINVIK 1963).

Another possible pathway, which could be involved in ipsilateral motor control, is a transcallosal pathway innervating homologous corticospinal neurons in the contralateral hemisphere (MEYER et al. 1995). TANJI et al. (1988) has shown that the majority of M1 neurons in the monkey brain are related to contralateral movement, while 7%–8% of the neurons are related to ipsilateral distal limb movement but not to contralateral movement. KIM et al. (1993a), using a functional MRI imaging technique in humans, described that the M1 signal related to distal ipsilateral hand movements was 20 times smaller than the contralateral signal. Ipsilateral cortical connections may play a subsidiary role or be involved in the control of ipsilateral movements in a more subtle way. Lesion studies have suggested that ipsilateral control is particularly important in proximal movements (COLEBATCH and GANDEVIA 1989) and skilled fine movements (BRODAL 1973; JONES et al. 1989).

The ipsilateral corticospinal projection of M1 neurons in monkeys goes predominantly to the proximal limb (KUYPERS and BRINKMAN 1970). Ipsilateral control of upper limb innervation has been shown to be strongest for axial and proximal limb innervation and weakest for individual finger movements (EVARTS 1966; GAZZANIGA et al. 1967). Correspondingly, PET has shown considerable bilateral M1 activation in relation to unilateral shoulder movements, but not to finger movements (COLEBATCH et al. 1991). The ipsilateral activation described in the PET studies of GRAFTON et al. (1993) also could have resulted from proximal arm and shoulder movements that were necessary in performing their studies.

Impairment of complex movements on the ipsilateral side has been reported in patients with hemiplegia (BRODAL 1973; JONES et al. 1989). CHEN et al. (1997a, b) showed that repetitive rTMS over ipsilateral M1 induced timing errors of ipsilateral sequential finger movements. Neuroimaging studies with fMRI (KIM et al. 1993a; RAO et al. 1993; LI et al. 1996) and PET (SHIBASAKI et al. 1993; SADATO et al. 1996a) have described ipsilateral activation during complex finger movements, but not during simple movements.

Both anatomical and functional asymmetries in the human brain have been known for many years. Several studies have shown that the ipsilateral motor control has also some interhemispheric difference. Functional neuroimaging studies with PET (KAWASHIMA et al. 1993) and fMRI (KIM et al. 1993b; LI et al. 1996) demonstrated asymmetric activation of the ipsilateral motor area with finger movements related to the handedness. KAWASHIMA et al. (1993) and LI et al. (1996) found greater ipsilateral activation during the performance of a left-hand task than during a right-hand task in right handers. These findings are consistent with the rTMS results by CHEN et al. (1997a, b) showing that more timing errors were induced by left-sided than by right-sided ipsilateral M1 stimulation during performance of complex sequences. These results suggests that the left hemisphere plays a greater role in controlling ipsilateral complex sequential movements than the right hemisphere and may be more involved in the processing of complex motor programs.

WASSERMANN et al. (1994) found with TMS that the ipsilateral hand representation is more lateral than the representation of the contralateral hand. SADATO et al. (1996a) described in a PET study that the activation of the ipsilateral sensorimotor area is more anterior than the activation of the contralateral one. These results suggest that the ipsilateral hand representation in the motor cortex might not be identical to the contralateral hand representation. The better spatial resolution of the fMRI technique will enable us to explore the ipsilateral motor representation in comparison with the contralateral representation in single subjects.

Little is known about the role of the premotor areas in ipsilateral motor control. The right dorsal premotor area has been shown to have a linear increase in activation when the complexity of right finger movements increased (SADATO et al. 1996a), suggesting that it might be an area storing motor sequences.

31.4.
Brain Activation with Somatosensory Stimulation

The discussion of activation studies of the somatosensory system will focus on the primary somatosensory cortex, S1. Compared to the reliable activation of M1 seen with motor tasks, activation of S1 is more difficult. This phenomenon has been already appreciated by PET researchers (PAULESU et al. 1997). In PET imaging, vibratory stimuli consistently activate S1 (FOX et al. 1987, 1988b; SEITZ and ROLAND 1992; TEMPEL and PERLMUTTER 1992), while pain and pure tactile stimuli do not.

The question whether pain per se activates S1 or not is still a controversial issue since some workers could not find significant activation of S1 applying noxious stimuli (JONES et al. 1991; DERBYSHIRE et al. 1994; XU et al. 1997) while others could (TALBOT et al. 1991; CASEY et al. 1994; RAINVILLE et al. 1997) and even reported somatotopic organization (ANDERSSON et al. 1997).

For tactile stimuli, the reported PET results are even more divergent. An example of tactile activation is illustrated in Fig. 31.1. One group (PAULESU et al. 1997) reported that they found a decrease in blood flow in S1 when they applied light tactile stimuli of short duration. However, reliable activation of S1 was found when subjects had to distinguish between different textures (BURTON et al. 1997). The conclusion might be that S1 is either more involved in the precise differentiation of incoming tactile signals and/or that its activation is dependent on the attention that is given to the incoming signal.

For fMRI studies, vibration is a difficult stimulus to apply. Therefore, researchers have used methods like scratching of the palm with the hand of the investigator (HAMMEKE et al. 1994; YETKIN et al. 1995), brushing the fingers (SAKAI et al. 1995), rubbing the fingers across a textured surface (LIN et al. 1996), attaching an airdriven balloon diaphragm to the fingers (ROBERTS and ROWLEY 1997) or electrical stimuli (KURTH et al. 1998), even at painful intensities (DAVIS et al. 1995). In one study, three sensory tasks were compared in three volunteers (PUCE et al. 1995): electrical stimulation of the median nerve with 5–30 Hz, continuous brushing of the palm and compressed air blowing continuously over the palm. The study concluded that median nerve stimulation did not produce reliable activation, while brushing and air blowing did. Even when median nerve stimulation was applied with frequencies up to 30 Hz, activation was seen in only one of three volunteers, which seems to highlight one of the interesting differences between fMRI and PET, where reliable activation was reported with median nerve stimulation with frequencies of 2 Hz and more (IBAÑEZ et al. 1995).

In two studies (PUCE et al. 1995; YETKIN et al. 1995), the sensory activation patterns were compared to the result of a motor activation task, and considerable overlap was seen. Several explanations can be offered for the finding that sensory and motor tasks seem to give similar results. It might be that the subjects studied moved their hands when the stimuli were applied; for example, simply holding the hands still when being brushed or scratched. Another reason might be that the maximal BOLD effect is picked up millimeters away from the neuronal activity, mainly in postcapillary vessels, and, therefore, it is difficult to distinguish between the adjacent anterior and poste-

rior wall of the central sulcus even with high resolution fMRI (ROBERTS and ROWLEY 1997). An additional explanation might be that sensory and motor areas are not strictly separated. In one of Penfield's original articles (PENFIELD and BOLDREY 1937), he notes that of the 102 points evoking finger movements, 77 were pre- and 25 post-central, while sensation in the fingers was evoked from 28 pre- and 130 post-central points. More recent authors also challenged the notion of a strict separation between pre-central motor and post-central sensory areas (UEMATSU et al. 1992a, b; NII et al. 1996). It might therefore very well be that activation picked up in the central sulcus might indeed have contributions from the precentral area even for a pure somatosensory paradigm (see below).

Somatotopy of S1 was delineated in some studies. Different representations for the hand and the sole were reported using a 3–5 Hz pressure stimulation (MOORE et al. 1996). Another study found a medial-to-lateral organization of the representations for foot, hand and tongue using a scrubbing stimulus at about 3 Hz (SAKAI et al. 1995). To study finger somatotopy (KURTH et al. 1998), investigators used ring electrodes to stimulate the second and the fifth fingers with a stimulation frequency of 8.1 Hz and an intensity twice the threshold plus 1 mA. In five of 20 subjects, the activation was reported to be separated; in three it was overlapping; in six activation could only be seen with stimulation of one finger; in six no activation was detected at all. In four of the five subjects in whom different representation could be detected, the little finger was located more medial and more superior than the index finger, corresponding to earlier mapping reports with MEG or EEG (BAUMGARTNER et al. 1991, 1993). A more recent study by GELNAR et al. (1998) tried to differentiate the subdivisions of SI. The authors used a newly developed MR-friendly vibration device to apply the sensory stimulus to the fingertips of digits I, II and V separately. Using a surface coil, they could detect activation mostly in areas 1 and 2. Of eight volunteers, six showed activation for all fingers tested in area 2, 4 in area 1 but none in either area 3b or 3a, a surprising finding that was not expected and that was ascribed to the spatiotemporal characteristics of the stimulus used. The distance between the center-of-mass of digits I and V was measured to be 9.5 mm, the fifth finger representation being more medial, corresponding to the findings mentioned above.

As seen in somatotopic studies of the motor cortex (SANES et al. 1995), the study by KURTH et al (1998) showed overlapping areas of activation for the fingers in three of eight volunteers. This raises the question whether this is due to the limited spatial resolution or whether it represents a true physiological finding, which would be in contrast to the findings from electrocorticography from subdural grids (SUTHERLING et al. 1992), where the sensory representation of the fingers was found to be separate. In addition, this study as well as the one by GELNAR et al. (1998), highlighted once more that activation of the post-central area with a simple somatosensory stimulus proves to be inconsistent. The question whether attentional or discrimination tasks are critical factors for the activation of SI with tactile stimuli is one of the many interesting areas for further research.

31.5
Pathology

In addition to the great potential of fMRI in research, the noninvasiveness of the technique, its repeatabilty, and the wide availability of 1.5 Tesla MR scanners also make fMRI a suitable clinical diagnostic tool (CAO et al. 1993; THULBORN et al. 1996). Several reports have already demonstrated that fMRI is a reliable technique for pre-surgical functional mapping of the sensorimotor cortex to identify eloquent brain tissue and to assess the risk of post-operative neurological deficits (JACK et al. 1994; MUELLER et al. 1996, 1997; YETKIN et al. 1997). Functional cortical maps obtained by fMRI correlated well with those obtained by standard functional mapping techniques such as direct electrocortical stimulation or sensory evoked potential recordings acquired intra-operatively or after subdural grid placement (JACK et al. 1994; MUELLER et al. 1996, 1997; YETKIN et al. 1997). Indeed, fMRI may have the advantage of identifying deep functional tissue inaccessible to surface cortical stimulation or recordings. In 87% of 28 patients undergoing craniotomy, the location of cortical function determined by fMRI was within 1 cm from that obtained by intra-operative electrocortical stimulation (YETKIN et al. 1997). In some studies, activation of the sensorimotor cortex could be achieved by passive tactile stimulation of the palm (MUELLER et al. 1996). Passive tactile stimulation may be a particularly useful paradigm in patients who are too weak to perform motor tasks; however, this remains to be confirmed.

Functional MRI was also used to investigate the cortical and subcortical pathophysiology in several neurological disorders. In patients who partially recovered from hemiparetic cortical infarction, increased activation was seen in the unaffected ipsilateral sensorimotor cortex during paretic hand movement (CAO et al. 1994, 1998; CRAMER et al. 1997). Increased activation was also seen in the ipsilateral dorsolateral prefrontal cortex, the posterior parietal cortex, the SMA and the contralateral cerebellum (CAO et al. 1994, 1998; CRAMER et al. 1997). These findings are in agreement with previous PET studies of patients with subcortical infarcts and suggest that motor recovery relies on reorganization of the cortico-spinal pathways with recruitment of the undamaged cortical areas especially the ipsilateral sensorimotor cortex (CHOLLET et al. 1991; WEILLER et al. 1992). Similar patterns were also seen in hemiparetic patients with brain tumors and in patients with congenital mirror movements (LEINSINGER et al. 1997; YOSHIURA et al. 1997).

In amyotrophic lateral sclerosis (ALS), a larger volume of activation was seen in the sensorimotor cortex during motor task performance when compared to controls (HERSHBERGER et al. 1996; BUSHARA et al. 1997). The results were in agreement with previous PET activation studies (KEW et al. 1993, 1994). The enlarged cortical motor output zones in ALS are believed to represent functional reorganization of the motor cortex in response to pyramidal cell loss or corticospinal tract dysfunction. Cortical hyperexcitability and loss of local inhibitory circuits have also been hypothesized as a possible underlying mechanism (EISEN 1995). This is supported by the results of TMS studies and may lend further support to the hypothesis that glutamate-induced excitotoxicity plays a role in the etiopathogenesis of ALS (EISEN 1995; KOHARA et al. 1996; ENTERZARI et al. 1997; MILLS and NITHI 1997; ZIEMANN et al. 1997).

Due to the relatively small task-related change in BOLD MR signal (approximately 5%), fMRI at 1.5 Tesla may not be sensitive enough to reveal abnormalities secondary to altered cortical physiology. However, comparing the location and/or the volume of significantly activated voxels at a fixed statistical threshold among patient and control groups may still provide insight into disease related changes. The development of blood-flow sensitive quantitative fMRI techniques as well as the use of higher magnetic field scanners may provide more sensitive methods to detect these pathological changes (KIM et al. 1993a; DETRE et al. 1994; WONG et al. 1997; YE et al. 1997).

The use of fMRI to study patients with altered sensorimotor function in a clinical setting would require several modifications of the currently available techniques (THULBORN et al. 1996). Rapid automated post-acquisition data processing is necessary to provide the results in timely fashion (Cox et al. 1995; THULBORN et al. 1996). Also required is the development of MR compatible electrophysiological devices (such as electromyography and electrocutaneous stimulators) to improve standardization of the motor and sensory paradigms used.

References

Alexander GE, Crutcher MD (1990) Preparation for movement: Neural representations of intended direction in three motor areas of the monkey. J Neurophysiol 64:133–150

Andersson JL, Lilja A, Hartvig P, Langstrom B, Gordh T, Handwerker H et al (1997) Somatotopic organization along the central sulcus, for pain localization in humans, as revealed by positron emission tomography. Exp Brain Res 117:192–199

Baumgartner C, Doppelbauer A, Sutherling WW, Zeitlhofer J, Lindinger G, Lind C et al (1991) Human somatosensory cortical finger representation as studied by combined neuromagnetic and neuroelectric measurements. Neurosci Lett 134:103–108

Baumgartner C, Doppelbauer A, Sutherling WW, Lindinger G, Levesque MF, Aull S et al (1993) Somatotopy of human hand somatosensory cortex as studied in scalp EEG. Electroencephalogr Clin Neurophysiol 88:271–279

Blinkenberg M, Bonde C, Holm S, Svarer C, Andersen J, Paulson OB et al (1996) Rate dependence of regional cerebral activation during performance of a repetitive motor task: a PET study. J Cereb Blood Flow Metab 16:794–803

Boecker H, Kleinschmidt A, Requardt M, Hanicke W, Merboldt KD, Frahm J (1994) Functional cooperativity of human cortical motor areas during self-paced simple finger movements. A high-resolution MRI study. Brain 117:1231–1239

Brodal A (1973) Self-observations and neuro-anatomical considerations after stroke. Brain 96:675–694

Burton H, MacLeod AM, Videen TO, Raichle ME (1997) Multiple foci in parietal and frontal cortex activated by rubbing embossed grating patterns across fingerpads: a positron emission tomography study in humans. Cereb Cortex 7:3–17

Bushara K, Wheat J, Mock BJ, Sorenson J, Lowe MJ, Brooks BR (1997) Decreased cortical activation to sensory stimulation in amyotrophic lateral sclerosis; a functional magnetic resonance imaging study. Neurology 47:A507

Cao Y, Towle VL, Levin DN, Balter JM (1993) Functional mapping of human motor cortical activation with conventional MR imaging at 1.5 T. J Magn Reson Imaging 3:869–875

Cao Y, Vikingstad EM, Huttenlocher PR, Towle VL, Levin DN (1994) Functional magnetic resonance studies of the reorganization of the human hand sensorimotor area after

unilateral brain injury in the perinatal period. Proc Natl Acad Sci USA 91:9612–9616

Cao Y, D'Olhaberriague L, Vikingstad EM, Levine SR, Welch KM (1998) Pilot study of functional MRI to assess cerebral activation of motor function after poststroke hemiparesis. Stroke 29:112–122

Casey KL, Minoshima S, Berger KL, Koeppe RA, Morrow TJ, Frey KA (1994) Positron emission tomographic analysis of cerebral structures activated specifically by repetitive noxious heat stimuli. J Neurophysiol 71:802–807

Chen R, Cohen LG, Hallett M (1997a) Role of the ipsilateral motor cortex in voluntary movement. Can J Neurol Sci 24:284–291

Chen R, Gerloff C, Hallett M, Cohen LG (1997b) Involvement of the ipsilateral motor cortex in finger movements of different complexities. Ann Neurol 41:247–254

Chollet F, DiPiero V, Wise RJ, Brooks DJ, Dolan RJ, Frackowiak RSJ (1991) The functional anatomy of motor recovery after stroke in humans: a study with positron emission tomography. Ann Neurol 29:63–71

Colebatch JG, Gandevia SC (1989) The distribution of muscular weakness in upper motor neuron lesions affecting the arm. Brain 112:749–763

Colebatch JG, Deiber M-P, Passingham RE, Friston KJ, Frackowiak RSJ (1991) Regional cerebral blood flow during voluntary arm and hand movements in human subjects. J Neurophysiol 65:1392–1401

Cox RW, Jesmanowicz A, Hyde JS (1995) Real-time functional magnetic resonance imaging. Magn Reson Med 33:230–236

Cramer SC, Nelles G, Benson RR, Kaplan JD, Parker RA, Kwong KK et al (1997) A functional MRI study of subjects recovered from hemiparetic stroke. Stroke 28:2518–2527

Davis KD, Wood ML, Crawley AP, Mikulis DJ (1995) fMRI of human somatosensory and cingulate cortex during painful electrical nerve stimulation. NeuroReport 7:321–325

Derbyshire SW, Jones AK, Devani P, Friston KJ, Feinmann C, Harris M et al (1994) Cerebral responses to pain in patients with atypical facial pain measured by positron emission tomography. J Neurol Neurosurg Psychiatry 57:1166–1172

Detre JA, Leigh JS, Williams DS, Koretsky AP (1992) Perfusion imaging. Magn Reson Med 23:37–45

Detre JA, Zhang W, Roberts DA, Silva AC, Williams DS, Grandis DJ et al (1994) Tissue specific perfusion imaging using arterial spin labeling. NMR Biomed 7:75–82

Eisen A (1995) Amyotrophic lateral sclerosis is a multifactorial disease. Muscle Nerve 18:741–752

Enterzari TM, Eisen A, Stewart H, Nakajima M (1997) Abnormalities of cortical inhibitory neurons in amyotrophic lateral sclerosis. Muscle Nerve 20:65–71

Evarts EV (1966) Pyramidal tract neuron activity associated with a conditional hand movement in the monkey. J Neurophysiol 29:1011–1027

Evarts EV, Shinoda Y, Wise SP (1984) Neurophysiological approaches to higher brain functions. Wiley, New York

Fox PT, Raichle ME (1984) Stimulus rate dependence of regional cerebral blood flow in human striate cortex, demonstrated by positron. J Neurophysiol 51:1109–1120

Fox PT, Fox JM, Raichle ME, Burde RM (1985) The role of cerebral cortex in the generation of voluntary saccades: a positron emission tomographic study. J Neurophysiol 54:348–369

Fox PT, Burton H, Raichle ME (1987) Mapping human somatosensory cortex with positron emission tomography. J Neurosurg 67:34–43

Fox PT, Raichle ME, Mintun MA, Dence C (1988a) Nonoxidative glucose consumption during focal physiologic neural activity. Science 241:462–464

Fox PT, Mintun MA, Reiman EM, Raichle ME (1988b) Enhanced detection of focal brain responses using intersubject averaging and change-distribution analysis of subtracted PET images. J Cereb Blood Flow Metab 8:642–653

Gazzaniga MS, Bogen JE, Sperry RW (1967) Dyspraxia following division of the cerebral commissures. Arch Neurol 16:606–612

Gelnar PA, Krauss BR, Szeverenyi NM, Apkarian AV (1998) Fingertip representation in the human somatosensory cortex: an fMRI study. NeuroImage 7:261–283

Grafton ST, Woods RP, Mazziotta JC, Phelps ME (1991) Somatotopic mapping of the primary motor cortex in humans: activation studies with cerebral blood flow and positron emission tomography. J Neurophysiol 66:735–743

Grafton ST, Woods RP, Mazziotta JC (1993) Within-arm somatotopy in human motor areas determined by positron emission tomography imaging of cerebral blood flow. Exp Brain Res 95:172–176

Hammeke TA, Yetkin FZ, Mueller WM, Morris GL, Haughton VM, Rao SM et al (1994) Functional magnetic resonance imaging of somatosensory stimulation. Neurosurgery 35:677–681

Hershberger J, Brooks BR, Lowe MJ et al (1996) Evaluation of upper motor neuron physiologic tests for functional magnetic resonance imaging assessment of cortical activation patterns in amyotrophic lateral sclerosis: development of test paradigm for longitudinal studies. Neurology 46:A207

Hikosaka O, Sakai K, Miyauchi S, Takino R, Sasaki Y, Putz B (1996) Activation of human presupplementary motor area in learning of sequential procedures: a functional MRI study. J Neurophysiol 76:617–621

Honda M, Zee DS, Hallett M (1997) Cerebellar control of voluntary saccadic eye movement in humans: fMRI study. Soc Neurosci Abstr 23:18

Humberstone M, Sawle GV, Clare S, Hykin J, Coxon R, Bowtell R et al (1997) Functional magnetic resonance imaging of single motor events reveals human presupplementary motor area. Ann Neurol 42:632–637

Ibañez V, Deiber MP, Sadato N, Toro C, Grissom J, Woods RP et al (1995) Effects of stimulus rate on regional cerebral blood flow after median nerve stimulation. Brain 118:1339–1351

Jack CR Jr, Thompson RM, Butts RK, Sharbrough FW, Kelly PJ, Hanson DP et al (1994) Sensory motor cortex: correlation of presurgical mapping with functional MR imaging and invasive cortical mapping. Radiology 190:85–92

Jezzard P, Heineman F, Taylor J, DesPres D, Wen H, Balaban RS et al (1994) Comparison of EPI gradient-echo contrast changes in cat brain caused by respiratory challenges with direct simultaneous evaluation of cerebral oxygenation via a cranial window. NMR Biomed 7:35–44

Jones AK, Brown WD, Friston KJ, Qi LY, Frackowiak RSJ (1991) Cortical and subcortical localization of response to pain in man using positron emission tomography. Proc R Soc Lond B Biol Sci 244:39–44

Jones RD, Donaldson IM, Prakin PJ (1989) Impairment and recovery of ipsilateral sensory-motor function following unilateral cerebral infarction. Brain 112:113–132

Karni A, Meyer G, Jezzard P, Adams MM, Turner R, Ungerleider LG (1995) Functional MRI evidence for adult motor cortex plasticity during motor skill learning. Nature 377:155–158

Kawashima R, Yamada K, Kinomura S, Yamaguchi T, Matsuik Y, Yoshioka S et al (1993) Regional cerebral blood flow changes of cortical motor areas and prefrontal areas in humans related to ipsilateral and contralateral hand movement. Brain Res 623:33–40

Kew JJ, Leigh PN, Playford ED, Passingham RE, Goldstein LH, Frackowiak RSJ et al (1993) Cortical function in amyotrophic lateral sclerosis. A positron emission tomography study. Brain 116: 655–680

Kew JJ, Brooks DJ, Passingham RE, Rothwell JC, Frackowiak RS, Leigh PN (1994) Cortical function in progressive lower motor neuron disorders and amyotrophic lateral sclerosis: a comparative PET study. Neurology 44:1101–1110

Kim SG, Ashe J, Georgopoulos AP, Merkle H, Ellermann JM, Menon RS et al (1993a) Functional imaging of human motor cortex at high magnetic field. J Neurophysiol 69:297–302

Kim SG, Ashe J, Hendrich K, Ellermann JM, Merkle H, Ugurbil K et al (1993b) Functional magnetic resonance imaging of motor cortex: hemispheric asymmetry and handedness. Science 261:615–617

Kohara N, Kaji R, Kojima Y, Mills KR, Fujii H, Hamano T et al (1996) Abnormal excitability of the corticospinal pathway in patients with amyotrophic lateral sclerosis: a single motor unit study using transcranial magnetic stimulation. Electroencephalogr Clin Neurophysiol 101:32–41

Kurth R, Villringer K, Mackert B-M, Schwiemann J, Braun J, Curio G et al (1998) fMRI assessment of somatotopy in human area 3b by electrical finger stimulation. NeuroReport 9:207–212

Kuypers HGJM, Brinkman J (1970) Precentral projections of different parts of the spinal intermediate zone in the rhesus monkey. Brain Res 24:29–48

Kwong KK, Belliveau JW, Chesler DA, Goldberg IE, Weisskoff RM, Poncelet BP et al (1992) Dynamic magnetic resonance imaging of human brain activity during primary sensory stimulation. Proc Natl Acad Sci USA 89:5675–5679

Le Bihan D, Jezzard P, Haxby J, Sadato N, Rueckert L, Mattay V (1995) Functional magnetic resonance imaging of the brain. Ann Int Med 122:296–303

Leinsinger GL, Heiss DT, Jassoy AG, Pfluger T, Hahn K, Danek A (1997) Persistent mirror movements: functional MR imaging of the hand motor cortex. Radiology 203:545–552

Leonardo M, Fieldman J, Sadato N, Campbell G, Ibañez V, Cohen LG et al (1995) A functional magnetic resonance imaging study of cortical regions associated with motor task execution and motor ideation in humans. Hum Brain Mapping 3:83–92

Li A, Yetkin FZ, Cox R, Haughton VM (1996) Ipsilateral hemisphere activation during motor and sensory tasks. Am J Neuroradiol 17:651–655

Lin W, Kuppusamy K, Haacke EM, Burton H (1996) Functional MRI in human somatosensory cortex activated by touching textured surfaces. J Magn Reson Imaging 6:565–572

Meyer BU, Röricht S, Gräfin von Einsiedel H, Kruggel F, Weindl A (1995) Inhibitory and excitatory interhemispheric transfers between motor cortical areas in normal humans and patients with abnormalities of the corpus callosum. Brain 118:429–440

Mills KR, Nithi KA (1997) Corticomotor threshold is reduced in early sporadic amyotrophic lateral sclerosis. Muscle Nerve 20:1137–1141

Moore CI, Gehi A, Guimeras AR, Corkin S, Rosen BR, Stern CE (1996) Somatotopic mapping of cortical areas SI and SII using fMRI. Neuroimage 3:S333

Mueller WM, Yetkin FZ, Hammeke TA, Morris GL III, Swanson SJ, Reichert K et al (1996) Functional magnetic resonance imaging mapping of the motor cortex in patients with cerebral tumors. Neurosurgery 39:515–520; discussion 520–511

Mueller WM, Yetkin FZ, Haughton VM (1997) Functional magnetic resonance imaging of the somatosensory cortex. Neurosurg Clin North Am 8:373–381

Nii Y, Uematsu S, Lesser RP, Gordon B (1996) Does the central sulcus divide motor and sensory functions? Cortical mapping of human hand areas as revealed by electrical stimulation through subdural grid electrodes. Neurology 46:360–367

Nitschke MF, Kleinschmidt A, Wessel K, Frahm J (1996) Somatotopic motor representation in the human anterior cerebellum. A high-resolution functional MRI study. Brain 119:1023–1029

Nyberg-Hansen R, Rinvik E (1963) Some comments on the pyramidal tract, with special reference to its individual variations in man. Acta Neurol Scand 39:1–30

Paulesu E, Frackowiak RSJ, Bottini G (1997) Maps of somatosensory systems. In: Frackowiak RSJ, Friston K, Frith C, Dolan R, Mazziotta JC (eds) Human brain function. Academic, San Diego, pp 183–242

Penfield W, Boldrey E (1937) Somatic motor and sensory representation in the cerebral cortex of man as studied by electrical stimulation. Brain 60:389–443

Porro CA, Francescato MP, Cettolo V, Diamond ME, Baraldi P, Zuiani C et al (1996) Primary motor and sensory cortex activation during motor performance and motor imagery: a functional magnetic resonance imaging study. J Neurosci 16:7688–7698

Price C, Wise R, Ramsay S, Friston K, Howard D, Patterson K et al (1992) Regional response differences within the human auditory cortex when listening to words. Neurosci Lett 146:179–182

Puce A, Constable RT, Luby ML, McCarthy G, Nobre AC, Spencer DD et al (1995) Functional magnetic resonance imaging of sensory and motor cortex: comparison with electrophysiological localization. J Neurosurg 83:262–270

Raichle ME (1987) Circulatory and metabolic correlates of brain function in normal humans. In: Mountcastle VB, Plum F, Geiger SR (eds) Handbook of physiology, section 1: the nervous system, vol V: higher functions of the brain. American Physiological Society, Bethesda, pp 643–674

Rainville P, Duncan GH, Price DD, Carrier B, Bushnell MC (1997) Pain affect encoded in human anterior cingulate but not somatosensory cortex. Science 277:968–971

Rao SM, Binder JR, Bandettini PA, Hammeke TA, Yetkin FZ, Jesmanowicz A et al (1993) Functional magnetic resonance imaging of complex human movements. Neurology 43:2311–2318

Rao SM, Binder JR, Hammeke TA, Bandettini PA, Bobholz JA, Frost JA et al (1995) Somatotopic mapping of the human primary motor cortex with functional magnetic resonance imaging. Neurology 45:919–924

Rao SM, Bandettini PA, Binder JR, Bobholz JA, Hammeke TA, Stein EA et al (1996) Relationship between finger movement rate and functional magnetic resonance signal change in human primary motor cortex. J Cereb Blood Flow Metab 16:1250–1254

Richter W, Andersen PM, Georgopoulos AP, Kim SG (1997) Sequential activity in human motor areas during a delayed cued finger movement task studied by time-resolved fMRI. NeuroReport 8:1257–1261

Roberts TP, Rowley HA (1997) Mapping of the sensorimotor cortex: functional MR and magnetic source imaging. Am J Neuroradiol 18:871–880

Sadato N, Campbell G, Ibañez V, Deiber M-P, Hallett M (1996a) Complexity affects regional cerebral blood flow change during sequential finger movements. J Neurosci 16:2693–2700

Sadato N, Ibañez V, Deiber M-P, Campbell G, Leonardo M, Hallett M (1996b) Frequency-dependent changes of regional cerebral blood flow during finger movements. J Cereb Blood Flow Metab 16:23–33

Sadato N, Ibañez V, Campbell G, Deiber M-P, Le Bihan D, Hallett M (1997) Frequency dependent changes of regional cerebral blood flow during finger movements:functional MRI compared with PET. J Cereb Blood Flow Metab 17:670–679

Sakai K, Watanabe E, Onodera Y, Yamamoto E, Koizumi H et al (1995) Functional mapping of the human somatosensory cortex with echo-planar MRI. Magn Reson Med 33:736–743

Sakai K, Hikosaka O, Miyauchi S, Takino R, Sasaki Y, Putz B (1998) Transition of brain activation from frontal to parietal areas in visuomotor sequence learning. J Neurosci 18:1827–1840

Sanes JN, Donoghue JP, Thangaraj V, Edelman RR, Warach S (1995) Shared neural substrates controlling hand movements in human motor cortex. Science 268:1775–1777

Schieber MH, Hibbard LS (1993) How somatotopic is the motor cortex hand area? Science 261:489–492

Schlaug G, Sanes JN, Thangaraj V, Darby DG, Jancke L, Edelman RR et al (1996) Cerebral activation covaries with movement rate. Neuroreport 7:879–883

Seitz RJ, Roland PE (1992) Vibratory stimulation increases and decreases the regional cerebral blood flow and oxidative metabolism: a positron emission tomography (PET) study. Acta Neurol Scand 86:60–67

Shibasaki H, Sadato N, Lyshkow H, Yonekura Y, Honda M, Nagamine T et al (1993) Both primary motor cortex and supplementary motor area play an important role in complex finger movement. Brain 116:1387–1398

Stephan KM, Fink GR, Passingham RE, Silbersweig D, Ceballos-Baumann AO, Frith CD et al (1995) Functional anatomy of the mental representation of upper extremity movements in healthy subjects. J Neurophysiol 73:373–386

Sutherling WW, Levesque MF, Baumgartner C (1992) Cortical sensory representation of the human hand: size of finger regions and nonoverlapping digit somatotopy. Neurology 42:1020–1028

Talbot JD, Marrett S, Evans AC, Meyer E, Bushnell MC,

Duncan GH (1991) Multiple representations of pain in human cerebral cortex. Science 251:1355–1358

Tanji J, Okano K, Sato KC (1988) Neuronal activity in cortical motor areas related to ipsilatral, contralateral, and bilateral digit movements of the monkey. J Neurophysiol 60:325–434

Tempel LW, Perlmutter JS (1992) Vibration-induced regional cerebral blood flow responses in normal aging. J Cereb Blood Flow Metab 12:554–561

Thulborn KR, Davis D, Erb P, Strojwas M, Sweeney JA (1996) Clinical fMRI: implementation and experience. NeuroImage 4:S101–S107

Toga AW, Collins RC (1981) Metabolic response of optic centers to visual stimuli in the albino rat: anatomical and physiological considerations. J Comp Neurol 199:443–464

Tyszka JM, Grafton ST, Chew W, Woods RP, Colletti PM (1994) Parceling of mesial frontal motor areas during ideation and movement using functional magnetic resonance imaging at 1.5 tesla. Ann Neurol 35:746–749

Uematsu S, Lesser R, Fisher RS, Gordon B, Hara K, Krauss GL et al (1992a) Motor and sensory cortex in humans: topography studied with chronic subdural stimulation. Neurosurgery 31:59–71

Uematsu S, Lesser RP, Gordon B (1992b) Localization of sensorimotor cortex: the influence of Sherrington and Cushing on the modern concept. Neurosurgery 30:904–912

van Gelderen P, Ramsey NF, Liu G, Duyn JH, Frank JA, Weinberger DR et al (1995) Three-dimensional functional magnetic resonance imaging of human brain on a clinical 1.5-T scanner. Proc Natl Acad Sci USA 92:6906–6910

Wassermann EM, Pascual-Leone A, Hallett M (1994) Cortical motor representation of the ipsilateral hand and arm. Exp Brain Res 100:121–132

Weiller C, Chollet F, Friston KJ, Wise RJ, Frackowiak RSJ (1992) Functional reorganization of the brain in recovery from striatocapsular infarction in man. Ann Neurol 31:463–472

Wise RJ, Chollet F, Hadar U, Friston KJ, Hoffner E, Frackowiak RSJ (1991) Distribution of cortical neural networks involved in word comprehension and word retrieval. Brain 114:1803–1817

Wong EC, Buxton RB, Frank LR (1997) Implementation of quantitative perfusion imaging techniques for functional brain mapping using pulsed arterial spin labeling. NMR Biomed 10:237–249

Xu X, Fukuyama H, Yazawa S, Mima T, Hanakawa T, Magata Y et al (1997) Functional localization of pain perception in the human brain studied by PET. Neuroreport 8:555–559

Yarowsky P, Kadekaro M, Sokoloff L (1983) Frequency-dependent activation of glucose utilization in the superior cervical ganglion by electrical stimulation of cervical sympathetic trunk. Proc Natl Acad Sci U S A 80:4179–4183

Ye FQ, Smith AM, Yang Y, Duyn J, Mattay VS, Ruttimann UE et al (1997) Quantitation of regional cerebral blood flow increases during motor activation: a steady-state arterial spin tagging study. NeuroImage 6:104–112

Yetkin FZ, Mueller WM, Hammeke TA, Morris GL III, Haughton VM (1995) Functional magnetic resonance imaging mapping of the sensorimotor cortex with tactile stimulation. Neurosurgery 36:921–925

Yetkin FZ, Mueller WM, Morris GL, McAuliffe TL, Ulmer JL, Cox RW et al (1997) Functional MR activation correlated with intraoperative cortical mapping. Am J Neuroradiol 18:1311–1315

Yoshiura T, Hasuo K, Mihara F, Masuda K, Morioka T, Fukui M (1997) Increased activity of the ipsilateral motor cortex during a hand motor task in patients with brain tumor and paresis. Am J Neuroradiol 18:865–869

Yousry TA, Schmid UD, Jassoy AG, Schmidt D, Eisner WE, Reulen HJ et al (1995) Topography of the cortical motor hand area: prospective study with functional MR imaging and direct motor mapping at surgery. Radiology 195:23–29

Yousry TA, Schmid UD, Alkadhi H, Schmidt D, Peraud A, Buettner A et al (1997) Localization of the motor hand area to a knob on the precentral gyrus. A new landmark. Brain 120:141–157

Ziemann U, Winter M, Reimers CD, Reimers K, Tergau F, Paulus W (1997) Impaired motor cortex inhibition in patients with amyotrophic lateral sclerosis. Evidence from paired transcranial magnetic stimulation. Neurology 49:1292–1298

32 Functional MRI of the Auditory System

J.R. Melcher, T.M. Talavage, M.P. Harms

CONTENTS

J.R. Melcher, PhD; Harvard Medical School, Eaton-Peabody Laboratory, Massachusetts Eye and Ear Infirmary, 243 Charles Street, Boston, MA 02114, USA
T.M. Talavage, PhD; Purdue University, 1285 Electrical Engineering Building, West Lafayette, IN 47907, USA
M.P. Harms, PhD; Speech and Hearing Sciences Program, Harvard-Massachusetts Institute of Technology Division of Health Sciences and Technology, NMR-Center, Massachusetts General Hospital, 149 Thirteenth St., Charlestown, MA 02129, USA

Binder et al. 1994a, b; Guimaraes et al. 1998). By enabling sites of brain activation to be mapped throughout the auditory pathway in individual subjects (Fig. 32.1), fMRI provides a powerful capability not provided by other noninvasive methods. Thus, fMRI has the potential to provide considerable new information concerning auditory neurophysiological processes.

At this time, the application of fMRI to the auditory system is at an early stage. Much of the work in the field has taken a preliminary, rather than an exhaustive, look at particular auditory neuroscientific issues or has focused on overcoming technical difficulties confronted in auditory fMRI experiments. Nevertheless, new information concerning central auditory function and dysfunction has emerged from these efforts. We anticipate that this initial work represents the beginning of an important role for fMRI in auditory neuroscience.

In this chapter, we review the state of the field of auditory fMRI, describing both neuroscientific findings and relevant technical developments. We par-

32.1
Introduction

Blood oxygenation level-dependent (BOLD) fMRI (Bandettini et al. 1992; Kwong et al. 1992; Ogawa et al. 1992) can be used to study auditory processing, from brainstem to cortex, in human listeners (e.g.,

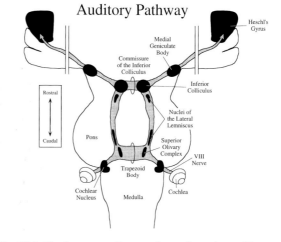

Fig. 32.1. The human auditory pathway, from the cochlea to Heschl's gyrus, which includes primary auditory cortex (e.g., Rademacher et al. 1993). Shown are major nuclei (*black*) and connecting fiber tracts (*gray*)

ticularly emphasize nonlinguistic issues because fMRI studies of speech and language are the subject of Chap. 33 in this volume. To begin, we discuss the effects of scanner-generated acoustic noise, a technical problem for auditory fMRI, as well as approaches for handling this problem (Sect. 32.2). We then review data illustrating that auditory activity can be studied down to the lowest levels of the central auditory pathway (i.e., the cochlear nucleus, Fig. 32.1), and describe the technical advances that have made functional imaging of brainstem auditory structures possible (Sect. 32.3). Most auditory fMRI data pertain to the cortex, and this work is reviewed in Sect. 32.4. In Sect. 32.5, we describe several investigations that have demonstrated the applicability of fMRI to subjects with auditory disorders.

32.2
Scanner-Generated Acoustic Noise and Auditory fMRI Experiments

The imaging environment includes several sources of acoustic noise which can interfere with fMRI experiments (RAVICZ and MELCHER 1998; SHELLOCK et al., in press; SAVOY et al., this volume). The compressor for cooling the magnet and the air-handling system in the imager room produce ongoing noise, while the imager gradient coils produce noise each time an image is acquired. During echo-planar imaging, the readout gradients produce the most intense noise, a "beep" with a primary frequency at the gradient-current switching frequency and levels as high as 118–134 dB SPL (RAVICZ and MELCHER 1998; SAVOY et al., this volume). In this section, we describe the effects of acoustic noise on auditory fMRI experiments and review two strategies for reducing these effects.

Imager-generated acoustic noise poses difficulties for auditory fMRI experiments from both perceptual and physiological perspectives. For example, the noise can mask sound stimuli presented during an fMRI paradigm, making it difficult for subjects to hear the stimuli or perform stimulus-dependent tasks (e.g., EDMISTER et al. 1998; VAN DE MOORTELE et al. 1998). In addition, the noise evokes activity in the auditory pathway, so the baseline level of activity during fMRI is elevated compared with quiet conditions and the dynamic range of auditory system responsiveness is reduced (SCHEFFLER et al. 1997; SHAH et al. 1997; BANDETTINI et al. 1998; EDMISTER et al. 1998; ROBSON et al. 1998; TALAVAGE et al. 1998;

ULMER et al. 1998). The fact that the auditory system responds to imager noise is illustrated by measurements of cortical activation in response to taped imager noise (ULMER et al. 1998), and in response to actual beeps (BANDETTINI et al. 1998; TALAVAGE et al. 1998). Demonstrations that sound-evoked fMRI activation in auditory cortex decreases with increasing image acquisition rate (i.e., increasing beep rate) indicate that the background imager beeps reduce the dynamic range of auditory system responsiveness (SHAH et al. 1997; EDMISTER et al. 1998; ROBSON et al. 1998). This reduction may be a consequence of saturating auditory neuronal responses, which would be consistent with electrophysiolological data concerning neuronal responses in the auditory periphery; e.g., it is well-known that auditory nerve fiber discharge rates increase, then saturate, with increasing stimulus level (e.g., SACHS and ABBAS 1974). Alternatively, the reduction in dynamic range may be a consequence of hemodynamic saturation or a combination of neuronal and hemodynamic saturation.

One strategy for reducing the perceptual and physiological effects of imager beeps during auditory fMRI experiments involves imaging a volume of slices in a "cluster" and leaving a "beep-free" interval between clusters (BELIN et al. 1998; EDMISTER et al. 1998; HALL et al. 1998a, b; ROBSON et al. 1998; SCHEFFLER et al. 1998; TALAVAGE et al. 1998; VAN DE MOORTELE et al. 1998). With this paradigm, the masking effects of the beeps can be avoided by presenting stimuli during the beep-free interval. In addition, the suppressive effect of imager beeps on auditory activation can be avoided by: (1) making the duration of the beep cluster shorter than the onset time of the fMRI response to the first beep in the cluster, and (2) making the time between clusters (TR) longer than the fMRI response to a cluster. As illustrated in Fig. 32.2, clustered volume acquisition using a long TR (8 s) can yield substantial increases in detected auditory cortical activation over paradigms in which image acquisitions are evenly distributed in time (i.e., distributed volume acquisition; EDMISTER et al. 1998). Although leaving a long interval between clusters suggests that the temporal resolution of response measurements must be sacrificed, there is a strategy for getting around this problem: The response to a sound stimulus can be accumulated over multiple stimulus presentations such that a different time-point in the response is sampled with each presentation (BELIN et al. 1998; ROBSON et al. 1998). Thus, there are demonstrated approaches that can be used to measure auditory activation

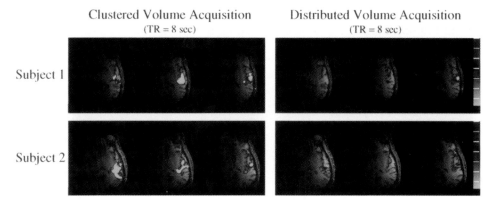

Fig. 32.2. Activation in response to music measured using clustered vs distributed volume acquisition. For each condition and subject, activation maps (*color scale*) are shown superimposed on anatomical images (*gray scale*) of three slices oriented parallel to the Sylvian fissure. A total of eight slices were imaged using a surface coil positioned over the left temporal lobe. During functional imaging, instrumental music was repeatedly turned on for 24 s and off for 24 s. The same segment of music was played at a comfortable listening level during each "on" period. Activation maps were derived by comparing images acquired during the "on" and "off" periods using an unpaired t test. Color scale for activation maps indicates the results of this test with *blue* and *yellow* corresponding to $p=0.01$ and $p=4.5\times10^{-5}$, respectively. In this and all subsequent figures (unless indicated otherwise): (1) functional images were acquired using an asymmetric spin echo sequence (TE=70 ms; offset=25 ms) and had an in-plane resolution of 3.1×3.1 mm, (2) activation maps have been interpolated and superimposed on T1-weighted anatomical images acquired during the same imaging session (in-plane resolution 1.5×1.5 mm), and (3) images are displayed using radiological convention (i.e., subject's left is displayed on the right). (Adapted from EDMISTER et al., in press)

while reducing contamination by background imager beeps. However, they do require compromises in either temporal resolution or the efficiency with which data are obtained.

A second strategy for reducing the impact of imager noise is to reduce the noise reaching the subject (RAVICZ and MELCHER 1998; SAVOY et al., this volume). Blocking noise transmission through the ear canal using earplugs or earmuffs is standard procedure in fMRI experiments. However, it is important to recognize that imager noise can be heard as a consequence of noise transmission through the head and body as well as the ear canal (BERGER 1983; RAVICZ and MELCHER 1998). A recently demonstrated approach involves enclosing a subject wearing earplugs or earmuffs in an acoustic shield to further reduce noise transmission through the ear canal and to reduce transmission through the head and body. With: (1) passive reduction of noise to the ear canal, head and body, (2) modifications to the imager to reduce the noise produced and, (3) active noise reduction, it should be possible to achieve substantial reductions in imager noise (RAVICZ and MELCHER 1998). However, in the interim, auditory fMRI experiments can still be performed and are already yielding new information about the human central auditory system, as described in the subsequent sections.

32.3
Auditory Subcortical Activity

Until recently, published fMRI data on the auditory system were limited to cortex, primarily because of the particular technical difficulties associated with brainstem imaging (PONCELET et al. 1992; GUIMARAES et al. 1998; see Sect. 32.3.1 below). This left substantial portions of the auditory pathway unstudied with fMRI, as can be appreciated from Fig. 32.1. The ability to image brainstem structures using fMRI is particularly important because other noninvasive methods have limitations in showing brainstem activity: (1) evoked potentials reflect activity in only a subset of auditory brainstem neurons (MELCHER and KIANG 1996), (2) evoked magnetic fields generated by brainstem activity approach the practical limits of detectability (ERNÉ and HOKE 1990) and, (3) definitive images of individual brainstem auditory structures have not been reported with positron emission tomography (PET). In the following sections, we review a fMRI method for imaging brainstem function and summarize two studies that investigated low levels of the auditory pathway in which the early stages of auditory processing take place.

32.3.1
Cardiac Gating with T1 Correction

The technical difficulties associated with functionally imaging the brainstem arise because there is considerable cardiac-related, pulsatile brainstem motion (PONCELET et al. 1992; GUIMARAES et al. 1998). GUIMARAES et al. (1998) developed an approach that avoids this problem and tested it by imaging sound-evoked activity in a particular auditory brainstem structure, the inferior colliculus. The approach involved synchronizing image acquisitions to the cardiac cycle, then correcting image signal strength to account for the variability in interimage interval (TR) that resulted from fluctuations in heart rate. When this "gating" method was compared with standard fMRI technique in which images are acquired at regular intervals, the gating method resulted in significantly lower signal variability in the inferior colliculus, and therefore improved activation detectability. This is illustrated in Fig. 32.3,

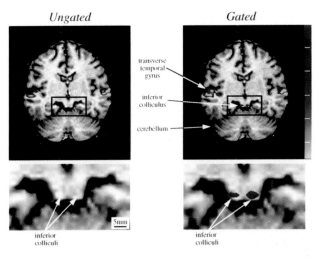

Fig. 32.3. Activation in response to orchestral music obtained with (*right*) and without (*left*) cardiac gating and correction. The same subject and slice were imaged in both conditions. The slice intersected the transverse temporal gyri (which includes auditory cortex) and the inferior colliculi. Functional images were acquired every other heart beat (*right*) or every 2 s (*left*) while the music was repeatedly turned on for 30 s and off for 30 s. The same segment of music was played at a comfortable listening level during each "on" period. Activation maps were derived by comparing images acquired during music "on" vs "off" periods using a *t test*. The maps are shown in color with *blue* and *yellow* corresponding to the lowest (*p*=0.001) and highest (*p*=2×10^{-9}) significance levels, respectively. Each map is based on data acquired over 9 min. Areas of enlargements at *bottom* are indicated by *rectangles* in the upper images. Slice thickness: 7 mm. (From GUIMARAES et al. 1998; copyright: John Wiley & Sons Inc., 1998)

which shows sound-evoked activation in a slice passing through the inferior colliculi and auditory cortices measured with and without cardiac gating.

32.3.2
Responses to Binaural vs Monaural Sound

One initial investigation into the functional organization of the auditory pathway using the gating technique has mapped responses to binaural and monaural sound (MELCHER et al. 1997). Four structures were targeted in this investigation: the cochlear nucleus, the inferior colliculus, the medial geniculate body, and Heschl's gyrus. These structures were chosen because they lie at different levels of the pathway (Fig. 32.1) and because their approximate dimensions are well within the resolution of standard fMRI technique (e.g., cochlear nucleus: 3×3×7 mm, inferior colliculus 6×6×4 mm, medial geniculate body 5×5×7 mm; KIANG et al. 1984; PENHUNE et al. 1996). Two stimuli were used to investigate the relationship between auditory activity and the side of acoustic stimulation: music, because it proved to be a particularly effective activator in preliminary experiments, and noise bursts, because these are used routinely in auditory neurophysiological experiments. Binaural stimulation produced clear activation on both the right and left in the cochlear nucleus, inferior colliculus, and medial geniculate body (Fig. 32.4, left), as well as on Heschl's gyrus (not shown). Monaural stimulation produced greater activation in the cochlear nucleus ipsilateral, rather than contralateral to the stimulus (Fig. 32.4, right). In contrast, activation was greater contralaterally in the inferior colliculus and medial geniculate body. Activation was also greater contralaterally on Heschl's gyrus (not shown; see also WOLDORFF et al. 1997 and SCHEFFLER et al. 1998). These differences in ipsilateral vs contralateral activation were seen consistently across subjects, as demonstrated in quantitative, structure-by-structure comparisons of activation extent and percent signal change ipsilaterally vs contralaterally (MELCHER et al. 1997).

The findings for monaural stimulation indicate that, from a functional standpoint, the auditory pathway crosses from the ipsilateral to the contralateral side below the level of the inferior colliculus. These findings are consistent with animal single unit and 2-deoxyglucose data showing a similar contralateral functional bias at and above the level of the inferior colliculus (e.g., MASTERTON et al. 1981;

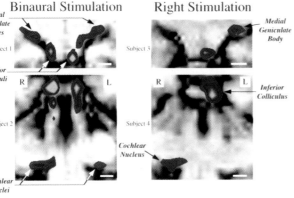

Binaural Stimulation   **Right Stimulation**

Fig. 32.4. Activation in the medial geniculate body, inferior colliculus, and cochlear nucleus in response to binaural (*left*) and monaural (*right*) stimulation. Each panel shows an anatomical image and superimposed activation map for a slice passing through the medial geniculate bodies and inferior colliculi (*top*) or the inferior colliculi and cochlear nuclei (*bottom*). Functional images of one slice were acquired every other heart beat and were corrected for fluctuations in interimage interval (GUIMARAES et al. 1998). A single slice, rather than multiple slices, was functionally imaged to reduce the effect of acoustic scanner noise on activation. The stimulus was orchestral music repeatedly turned on for 30 s and off for 30 s. Activation maps are as described in the caption for Fig. 32.3, except that they are based on between 13.5 and 18 min of data. *Scale bar at lower right* in each panel corresponds to 5 mm. Slice thickness: 7 mm (subjects 1–3) or 5 mm (subject 4)

SEMPLE and KITZES 1985; CAIRD et al. 1991). Nevertheless, this direct demonstration in humans is important because there are known, substantial differences between the human and animal auditory pathways; e.g., brainstem structures such as the lateral superior olive, medial nucleus of the trapezoid body, and ventral nucleus of the lateral lemniscus are represented quite differently in animals than in humans (e.g., IRVING and HARRISON 1967; MOORE and MOORE 1971; RICHTER et al. 1983). Hence, the applicability of animal data to humans cannot be assumed.

32.3.3
Response Dependence on Stimulus Presentation Rate

In a second investigation using the gating technique, HARMS et al. (1998) examined the dependence of activation on noise burst presentation rate in both subcortical and cortical structures (the inferior colliculus, medial geniculate body, Heschl's gyrus and superior temporal gyrus). The four structures studied exhibited clear differences in activation,

quantified in terms of extent and percent signal change (calculated from signal levels averaged over 30 s stimulus "on" and "off" periods). For example, activation in the inferior colliculus increased monotonically with increasing rate, while activation in the superior temporal gyrus varied nonmonotonically, first increasing, then decreasing, with increasing rate. Overall, the rate of maximum activation decreased with ascending level in the auditory pathway (inferior colliculus: 35 and 20/s ; medial geniculate body: 20/s; Heschl's gyrus: 10 and 2/s; superior temporal gyrus: 2/s). Additional differences between structures were evident in signal time courses (Fig. 32.5). For example, the inferior colliculus showed a sustained signal elevation during stimulus "on" periods for high presentation rates (e.g., 35/s). In contrast, Heschl's gyrus and the superior temporal gy-

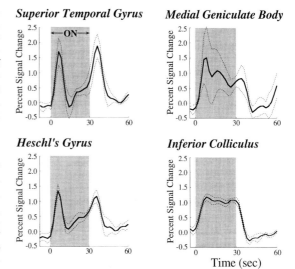

Fig. 32.5. Percent signal change time courses in response to 35/s noise bursts for four auditory structures: the superior temporal gyrus, Heschl's gyrus, the medial geniculate body, and the inferior colliculus. *Solid lines* are mean time courses; *dotted lines* are the mean±one standard error. Functional imaging was performed as described in the caption for Fig. 32.4. The imaged slice intersected either: (1) the inferior colliculi, the posterior aspect of Heschl's gyri, and the posterior aspect of the superior temporal gyri (lateral to Heschl's gyri), or (2) the inferior colliculi and medial geniculate bodies . The time course shown for the inferior colliculus is based on data taken in the latter plane. Image signal vs time was resampled to a consistent interval of 2 s, low-pass filtered, and averaged across "on"/"off" epochs (8–12/subject) and voxels (2, 2, 8 and 8 in the two inferior colliculi, medial geniculate bodies, Heschl's gyri, and superior temporal gyri, respectively). Signal time courses were then averaged across subjects, yielding the mean and standard errors shown (*N*=4 for the medial geniculate body, *N*=5 for the other structures). Noise burst duration and rise/fall time were 25 ms and 2.5 ms, respectively

rus showed transient "onset" and "offset" signal elevations at the beginning and after the end of the "on" periods. These findings demonstrate that auditory structures can be functionally distinguished based on rate dependencies of fMRI activation.

32.4
Auditory Cortical Activity

It is now well-established that cortical responses to acoustic stimuli can be measured reliably using fMRI (e.g., Binder et al. 1994a, b; Berry et al. 1995; Millen et al. 1995; Strainer et al. 1997; Huckins et al. 1998), so a growing number of fMRI studies are investigating sound-evoked activity in auditory cortex.

32.4.1
Parametric Studies of
Auditory Cortical Activation

The dependence of auditory-cortical activation on basic stimulus parameters remains largely unexplored, although some data are available. Dependencies on side of stimulation have been examined in several studies, as summarized in Sects. 32.3.2 and 32.5.1 (Melcher et al. 1997; Woldorff et al. 1997; Scheffler et al. 1998). Data concerning dependencies on stimulus intensity or interaural stimulus differences are sparse but some have been reported (Millen et al. 1995; Wang et al. 1996; Freeman et al. 1997; Jäncke et al. 1997b; Strainer et al. 1997; Woldorff et al. 1997). Activation dependencies on stimulus presentation rate have been examined fairly extensively, and are therefore described next (Binder et al. 1994b; Dhankhar et al. 1997; Rees et al. 1997; Harms et al. 1998).

Most studies examining the dependence of auditory-cortical activation on stimulus presentation rate have reported monotonic dependencies, rather than nonmonotonic dependencies such as those described by Harms et al. (1998) (see Sect. 32.3.3). For example, using consonant-vowel stimuli or nouns presented at rates ranging from 0.17 to 2.5/s, Binder et al. (1994b) and Rees et al. (1997) reported monotonically increasing activation with increasing presentation rate, a trend consistent with PET work using comparable rates and stimuli (Price et al. 1992; Rees et al. 1997). Some of the data reported by Dhankar et al. (1997) for single-syllable nouns sug-

gest a fall-off in activation at the highest rate studied (2.17/s), but the main trend is an increase in activation with increasing rate. The findings of Harms et al. (1998) for noise burst stimuli presented at low rates (≤2/s) are consistent with the monotonic dependencies seen in the other studies just described. However, Harms and coworkers observed a marked decrease in cortical activation at higher rates (≥10/s). These rates were not achievable in the other studies because of the long duration of the stimuli. This fall-off in activation was largely attributable to the prominent signal "dip" seen within the "on" period at high presentation rates in cortical areas (Fig. 32.5). The complexities of the time courses for high rates indicate a rich underlying physiology that can be probed in future studies. These complexities highlight the fact that fMRI has more to offer than just steady state pictures of brain function (Gaschler-Markefski et al. 1997).

32.4.2
Frequency Organization of Auditory Cortex

Electrophysiological work in experimental animals has demonstrated an orderly relationship between the frequency of maximum neuronal sensitivity and position over the cortical surface (e.g., Imig et al. 1977; Reale and Imig 1980). This tonotopic organization has been the focus of several fMRI studies that have investigated whether different parts of human auditory cortex are differentially activated by higher vs lower acoustic stimulus frequencies.

Several fMRI studies have reported data consistent with a single tonotopically organized area, with higher frequencies represented medially and lower frequencies represented laterally in the transverse temporal gyri (which includes primary auditory cortex; Galaburda and Sanides 1980; Rademacher et al. 1993). For example, Wessinger et al. (1997) reported data compatible with this trend when they examined responses to binaural stimuli with primary frequencies of 55 and 880 Hz. In the left transverse temporal gyri, the focus of activation for the higher frequency stimulus was located posteromedial to the focus of activation for the lower frequency stimulus in most subjects. However, a consistent spatial relationship between higher and lower frequency activation foci was not seen in the right hemisphere. In a separate study, Lantos et al. (1997) reported that the "center of mass" of activation produced by binaural tone pips with frequencies of 100,

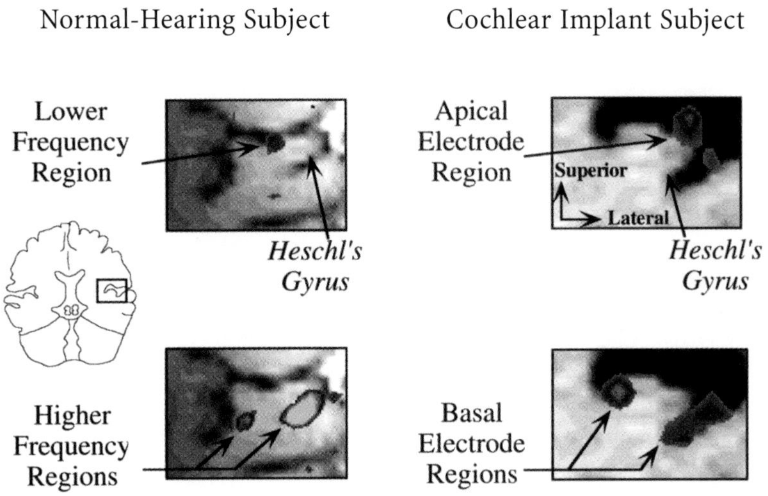

Normal-Hearing Subject   Cochlear Implant Subject

Fig. 32.6. Activation on Heschl's gyrus for lower vs higher frequency stimulation in a normal-hearing subject (*left*) and for apical vs basal electrical stimulation in a cochlear implant subject (*right*). The region shown in each panel corresponds to the rectangle on the diagrammatic slice (*far left*) and includes the left Heschl's gyrus. *Left:* A lower frequency region is located on the superior aspect of Heschl's gyrus (*top*), while higher frequency regions are located on the medial and lateral aspects of Heschl's gyrus (*bottom*). The stimuli were low- and high-pass filtered music. For functional imaging, lower frequency music and higher frequency music were alternately presented for 40 s, with an intervening 20 s "off" period. A total of five slices were functionally imaged using a distributed volume acquisition (TR=4 s). Activation maps were derived by comparing images acquired during periods of lower vs higher frequency stimulation (*top*) or vice versa (*bottom*) using a *t* test. *Blue* and *yellow* in the activation maps correspond to $p=0.01$ and $p=3\times10^{-7}$, respectively. Both ears were stimulated. Lower and higher frequency stimuli were comparable in loudness; the lower frequency stimulus was presented 30 dB relative to threshold. Low-frequency passband: 20–100 Hz. High-frequency passband: 7–8 kHz. Functional image in-plane resolution: 1.5×1.5 mm. Slice thickness: 4 mm (Adapted from Talavage et al. 1996). *Right:* Stimulation of an apical electrode resulted in activation on the superior aspect of Heschl's gyrus (*top*) while stimulation of a basal electrode resulted in activation on the medial and lateral edges of Heschl's gyrus (*bottom*). For functional imaging, the electrical current stimulus (a gated 1 kHz sinusoid) was repeatedly turned on for 30 s and off for 30 s. A total of six slices were functionally imaged using a distributed volume acquisition (TR=2 s). Activation maps were derived by comparing images acquired during "on" vs "off" periods. *Blue* and *yellow* in the activation maps correspond to $p=0.001$ and $p=2\times10^{-9}$, respectively. The subject's implant was on the right. Functional image in-plane resolution: 3.1×3.1 mm. Slice thickness: 7 mm. (Adapted from Melcher et al. 1998)

800, and 6400 Hz was located progressively more posteromedially in the left transverse temporal gyri for stimuli of progressively higher frequency. This result is compatible with that of Strainer et al. (1997), who reported that 1000 Hz tones (presented to the right ear) produced more extensive activation laterally in the transverse temporal gyri and 4000 Hz tones produced more extensive activation medially. These fMRI results are in general agreement with the PET work of Lauter et al. (1985), wherein lower frequency regions were localized to more lateral portions of the transverse temporal gyri than higher frequency regions, and with reports based on evoked magnetic field recordings (e.g., Romani et al. 1982).

One fMRI study of frequency organization identified multiple lower and higher frequency sensitive regions distributed over the superior temporal lobe (Talavage et al. 1996, 1997). This study examined left temporal lobe responses to several types of binaural stimuli (e.g., tone bursts, amplitude modulated

bandpass filtered noise). Four regions showing greater signal levels during lower rather than higher frequency stimulation were identified, as were four regions showing greater signal levels during higher frequency stimulation. Three of these regions were located on Heschl's gyrus (i.e., the first transverse temporal gyrus), and are shown in a near-coronal plane in Fig. 32.6 (left) where one lower frequency region on the superior aspect of Heschl's gyrus is flanked by two higher frequency regions. In three dimensions, the focus of activation for the medial higher frequency region was located posteromedial to the focus for the lower frequency region. The relative positions of these higher and lower frequency foci are consistent with, and therefore support, the picture provided by the other fMRI studies of frequency organization. However, the findings of Talavage and coworkers also provide substantial additional information concerning human cortical frequency organization.

Because they identified multiple regions sensitive to lower and higher frequencies, TALAVAGE and co-workers (1996, 1997) suggested that human auditory cortex includes multiple tonotopically organized areas. For example, two tonotopically organized areas on Heschl's gyrus were proposed, one located anteromedially and one located posterolaterally, with their low frequency regions abutting on the superior aspect of Heschl's gyrus. In the context of Fig. 32.6 (left), the anteromedial area corresponds to a decreasing frequency progression beginning with the medial higher frequency region and ending with the more lateral lower frequency region; the postero-lateral tonotopic area is the mirror image, corresponding to an increasing frequency progression beginning with the lower frequency region and ending with the lateral higher frequency region. Experiments using frequency-swept stimuli support this view and indicate that the other identified lower and higher frequency regions on the superior temporal lobe correspond to additional tonotopically organized areas (TALAVAGE et al. 1997). These findings indicate that humans, like animals, have multiple frequency-to-place mappings in auditory cortex.

A possibility suggested by electrophysiological work in animals is that different tonotopically organized cortical areas in humans are functionally distinguishable based on their responsiveness to different acoustic stimuli (e.g., RAUSCHECKER et al. 1995). fMRI and PET studies in humans have demonstrated that different cortical regions can exhibit varying degrees of responsiveness to simple (e.g., noise) vs complex (e.g., word) stimuli (ZATORRE et al. 1992; DÉMONET et al. 1992; BINDER et al. 1994a, 1996; BERRY et al. 1995; STEVENS et al. 1998; WESSINGER et al. 1998). However, experiments comparing this differential responsiveness to the pattern of frequency organization in human auditory cortex have yet to be performed.

32.4.3
Event-Related Responses to Acoustic Stimuli

Although most auditory fMRI studies have used experimental paradigms in which stimuli are presented in long (e.g., 30 s) time-blocks, several have demonstrated the feasibility of recording event-related responses to brief acoustic stimuli (e.g., see BUCKNER, this volume). HICKOK et al. (1997) measured the time course of MR signal change on the superior temporal lobe in response to single words and non-words of comparable duration (~536 ms).

ROBSON et al. (1998) and BELIN et al. (1998) measured responses to 100 ms tone bursts and to single phonemes, respectively. The event-related responses measured in these studies were comparable to those reported for nonacoustic stimuli in that they reached a peak 4–6 s following stimulus onset and returned to baseline within approximately 12 s post-stimulus. Event-related responses to individual acoustic stimuli, appropriately shifted in time and summed, have been used to model the response to multiple stimuli closely spaced in time. ROBSON et al. (1998) found this linear model inadequate in that long tone burst trains produced smaller percent signal changes than predicted by the superposition of responses to short tone burst trains (see also FRISTON et al. 1998). The capability of recording event-related auditory responses expands the range of possible fMRI experiments of the auditory system to include, for example, studies of responses to unexpected stimuli such as the deviant stimuli in a classic "oddball paradigm" (e.g., McCARTHY et al. 1997).

32.4.4
Effects of Subject State on Activation in Auditory Cortex

The effects of subject state on activation in auditory cortex have been examined explicitly in several fMRI studies. For example, GRADY et al. (1997) examined cortical activation in subjects counting targets in an aurally presented word list vs passively listening to the word list and reported greater activation in Heschl's gyrus and surrounding areas during the counting task. JÄNCKE et al. (1997a) also reported greater activation in auditory cortex during active, as compared with passive listening. In a study of selective attention, WOODRUFF et al. (1996) used a task that required switching attention between simultaneously presented auditory and visual stimuli (numbers presented aurally and visually) and reported greater activation in primary and association auditory cortices during the "auditory attend" condition than during the "visual attend" condition, a finding compatible with previous PET work (ROLAND 1982). The modulatory influence of selective attention on auditory cortical activity has also been demonstrated in the fMRI study of PUGH et al. (1996), who examined activation during binaural and dichotic listening conditions.

32.4.5
Activity in Auditory Cortex in the Absence of Acoustic Stimulation

Some fMRI studies have suggested that auditory cortical activity can be elevated even in the absence of external acoustic stimulation. For example, CALVERT et al. (1997) reported activation in auditory cortex during silent lipreading, a finding compatible with observations that auditory perception can be altered by simultaneous lipreading (McGURK and MacDONALD 1976). In addition, it has been reported that schizophrenic patients exhibit lower levels of acoustically evoked activation in auditory association cortex when they are experiencing auditory hallucinations (voices) than when they are hallucination-free (DAVID et al. 1996; WOODRUFF et al. 1997). The lower levels during hallucination were attributed to a reduced dynamic range of response in auditory cortex due to an abnormal elevation in baseline activity associated with the hallucinations. Interestingly, a similar explanation can account for activation abnormalities seen in patients with tinnitus, a condition in which simple sounds (e.g., tones) are perceived in the absence of an external stimulus (see Sect. 32.5.3 below and MELCHER et al., submitted). Thus, abnormally elevated levels of activity in the auditory pathway potentially underlie a wide range of phantom auditory sensations.

32.5
fMRI in Subjects with Auditory Disorders

The accumulating body of fMRI data concerning auditory function in normal subjects lays a groundwork for studying subjects with auditory disorders, so naturally efforts applying fMRI to clinical populations have been initiated. In this section, we describe studies directed at three groups: unilaterally deaf subjects, deaf subjects with cochlear implants, and tinnitus subjects.

32.5.1
Unilaterally Deaf Subjects

SCHEFFLER et al. (1998) compared auditory cortical responses in unilaterally deaf patients with those in normal-hearing subjects. Normal-hearing subjects stimulated monaurally with gated 1 kHz tones showed more extensive cortical activation contralat-

eral, rather than ipsilateral, to the stimulated ear. Unilaterally deaf subjects stimulated in the functioning ear also generally showed more extensive activation contralaterally, but the disparity in the extent of contralateral vs ipsilateral activation was, on average, less than in normal-hearing subjects. This is consistent with evidence that the upper auditory pathway may be less contralaterally biased than normal in animals with unilateral hearing loss induced at a young age. For example, in animals with a deafened ear, the number of neurons projecting from the cochlear nucleus ipsilateral to the normal ear to the ipsilateral inferior colliculus is abnormally large (e.g., MOORE and KOWALCHUK 1988), and single units in the inferior colliculus ipsilateral to the normal ear have abnormally high maximum discharge rates in response to ipsilateral stimulation (KITZES and SEMPLE 1985). Comparable anatomical and physiological abnormalities may underlie the abnormally low contralateral bias in cortical activation seen in unilaterally deaf humans.

The SCHEFFLER et al. study represents a first step in using fMRI to study brain function in patients with partial hearing loss. Future investigations could include examinations of patients with frequency-specific hearing loss to determine, for example, whether cortical frequency reorganization as demonstrated by electrophysiological recordings in hearing-impaired animals also occurs in humans (e.g., ROBERTSON and IRVINE 1989; RAJAN et al. 1993). Such investigations could also address whether abnormalities in brain function depend on factors such as the subject's age at the time of loss or the elapsed time since loss. These lines of investigation should provide fundamental insights into how the human central auditory system is functionally altered when deprived of sensory inputs.

32.5.2
Cochlear Implant Subjects

Cochlear implantation has become a standard approach for restoring hearing in deaf subjects. It involves stimulating surviving neurons in the auditory periphery via implanted, intracochlear electrodes (i.e., a cochlear implant). Implantees exhibit a wide range of auditory capabilities (e.g., some are conversationally fluent without lip reading, but others are not) which are likely related to differences in brain activity. Although there have been evoked potential (e.g., STYPULKOWSKI et al. 1986; GROENEN et al. 1997), evoked magnetic field (e.g., PELIZZONE et al.

1986; HARI 1997), and PET (e.g., HERZOG et al. 1991; OKAZAWA et al. 1996) studies on implantees, the relationship between brain activity and performance is largely unknown. There has been little application of fMRI to this issue because of the safety concerns associated with imaging implantees. However, a fMRI study performed on subjects prior to implantation has examined cortical activity in response to electrical stimulation delivered by a temporary electrode inserted near the round window of the cochlea (BERTHEZENE et al. 1997). In addition, a recent fMRI study demonstrated that a particular subset of implant patients can be imaged safely, even though MRI is contraindicated in most implantees (MELCHER et al. 1998).

In the fMRI study of implantees: (1) an implant with a magnet-compatible design was identified (Ineraid), (2) currents induced in the implant during imaging were measured and found to be safe, and (3) as a demonstration of feasibility, brain activation in response to electrical stimulation of the cochlea was mapped in three deaf volunteers with a unilateral Ineraid implant (MELCHER et al. 1998). When the cochlea was electrically stimulated in a standard "on"/"off" paradigm, there was clear activation on the superior temporal lobe, including Heschl's gyrus, in all three subjects. In one subject, two different electrodes were stimulated, one located basally in the cochlea (the cochlear region tuned to higher sound frequencies) and the other located apically (tuned to lower frequencies). Posteriorly on Heschl's gyrus, basal stimulation produced activation on the medial and lateral edges of Heschl's gyrus, while apical stimulation produced activation on the superior aspect of Heschl's gyrus (Fig. 32.6, right). These patterns for basal vs apical electrical stimulation are comparable to patterns in normal-hearing subjects stimulated with high vs low frequency sound (Fig. 32.6, left; TALAVAGE et al. 1996). The subject showing this "normal" pattern performs quite well with his implant. An important question is whether poorer performers show similarly normal patterns of activation.

32.5.3
Tinnitus Subjects

Tinnitus, the perception of sound when no external sound is present, is common. Almost everyone experiences transient episodes of tinnitus. In addition, many individuals experience chronic tinnitus which can be so bothersome that it interferes with normal daily function (e.g., COLES 1984). Although chronic tinnitus is often associated with sensorineural hearing loss, this is not always the case (e.g., LEVINE, submitted). Progress toward treatments of tinnitus has been slow, in part because the physiological mechanisms underlying tinnitus are poorly understood. However, recent developments in functional imaging have begun to change this situation by demonstrating that fMRI and PET can provide a physiological measure of tinnitus. In this section, we summarize these developments focusing particularly on fMRI findings.

Most experimental paradigms used in functional imaging studies of tinnitus have involved modulating tinnitus loudness and imaging subjects in two different loudness conditions. In most subjects, tinnitus loudness is decreased with acoustic stimula-

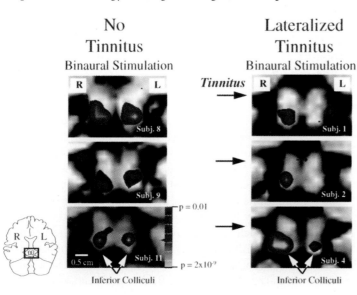

Fig. 32.7. Inferior colliculus activation in response to binaural noise in three control subjects without tinnitus (*left*) and in three subjects with tinnitus lateralized to the right ear (*right*). Functional imaging was performed as described in the legend for Fig. 32.4, except that the stimulus was continuous, binaural noise. Activation maps are based on a *t* test comparison of images during stimulus "on" vs "off" periods. Each map is based on data acquired over either 13.5 or 18 mins. Area of each panel corresponds to the *rectangle* on the schematic image at *left*. Slice thickness: 7 mm (Adapted from MELCHER et al., submitted)

tion (e.g., with continuous broadband noise), so several functional imaging studies have used acoustic stimulation to modulate tinnitus (LEVINE et al. 1997; MIRZ et al. 1998; MELCHER et al., submitted). In some tinnitus subjects, loudness can be modulated by nonacoustic methods (e.g., by shifting eye position, through orofacial movements, or with cutaneous stimulation), and these approaches have also been used in imaging studies of tinnitus (CACACE et al. 1995; LOCKWOOD et al. 1998; GIRAUD et al. 1998). An additional approach has been to compare the level of cortical metabolic activity in unstimulated subjects with vs without tinnitus (ARNOLD et al. 1996). Functional imaging data reported to date are generally consistent with the hypothesis that increases and decreases in tinnitus loudness correspond to increases and decreases in brain activity (MELCHER et al., submitted).

To illustrate that tinnitus-related brain activation can be detected using fMRI, we describe here a recent study of inferior colliculus activation in normal-hearing subjects: (1) without tinnitus and, (2) with lateralized tinnitus (i.e., tinnitus largely or completely in one ear) (MELCHER et al., submitted). In response to binaural noise, subjects without tinnitus showed comparable activation in the two inferior colliculi. In contrast, subjects with lateralized tinnitus showed abnormally asymmetric activation in the colliculi (Fig. 32.7). Thus, fMRI can provide a physiological measure of lateralized tinnitus. The extent to which this approach can be generalized to other types of tinnitus remains to be seen.

32.6 Summary

The studies described in this chapter demonstrate that a groundwork is being established for addressing a wide range of auditory neuroscientific issues, both basic and clinical, using fMRI in human subjects. On a technical front, strategies for reducing the physiological and psychophysical effects of scanner-generated acoustic noise have been demonstrated and more are under development. The capability of imaging activity down to the lowest levels of the auditory pathway has also been demonstrated, opening the possibility of using fMRI to investigate the early, as well as the later, stages of auditory processing. fMRI studies have already revealed functional distinctions between structures at different levels of the auditory pathway and between cortical areas. Future work can further probe the functional simi-

larities and differences between structures, and at the cortical level, relate functionally distinguishable areas to the emerging picture of cortical frequency organization. These lines of investigation should provide information needed to assign neurophysiological interpretations to fMRI findings in subjects performing psychophysical tasks (e.g., speech perception, sound localization). As the body of data in normal listeners grows, it will provide an important baseline for comparison with data from clinical populations (e.g., with hearing loss, cochlear implants, or tinnitus). As described in this chapter, fMRI studies of such populations have begun to reveal functional abnormalities and provide a launching point for continued, systematic investigations of subjects with auditory disorders. With the work conducted thus far and the numerous anticipated future directions, the field of auditory fMRI is poised to dramatically advance our understanding of human auditory function and dysfunction.

Acknowledgments. We wish to thank our collaborators at the Eaton-Peabody Laboratory (MEEI), Cochlear Implant Research Laboratory (MEEI), and the NMR-Center (MGH), especially Irina Sigalovsky, Robert Levine, Donald Eddington, Nico Garcia, and Whitney Edmister. We also wish to thank John Guinan Jr., Michael Ravicz, Robert Levine and Alex Guimaraes for their comments on earlier versions of this manuscript. We are grateful to Barbara Norris for her assistance with figure preparation and manuscript formatting and to Barbara Fullerton for designing the original layout for Fig. 32.1. Support was provided by NIH/NIDCD PO1DC00119, RO3DC03122, T32DC00038, R21DC03255.

References

Arnold W, Bartenstein P, Oestreicher E, Römer W, Schwaiger M (1996) Focal metabolic activation in the predominant left auditory cortex in patients suffering from tinnitus: a PET study with [18F]deoxyglucose. ORL 58:195–199

Bandettini PA, Wong EC, Hinks RS, Tikofsky RS, Hyde JS (1992) Time course EPI of human brain function during task activation. Mag Res Med 25:390–397

Bandettini PA, Jesmanowicz A, Van Kylen J, Birn RM, Hyde JS (1998) Functional MRI of brain activation induced by scanner acoustic noise. Mag Res Med 39:410–416

Belin P, Zatorre RJ, Hoge R, Pike B, Evans AC (1998) Event-related fMRI of the auditory cortex. Neuroimage 7:S369

Berger EH (1983) Laboratory attenuation of earmuffs and earplugs both singly and in combination. Am Hyg Assoc J 44:321–329

Berry I, Démonet J-F, Warach S et al (1995) Activation of association auditory cortex demonstrated with functional MRI. Neuroimage 2:215–219

Berthezene Y, Truy E, Morgon A et al (1997) Auditory cortex activation in deaf subjects during cochlear electrical stimulation. Evaluation by functional magnetic resonance imaging. Invest Radiol 32:297–301

Binder JR, Rao SM, Hammeke TA et al (1994a) Functional magnetic resonance imaging of human auditory cortex. Ann Neurol 35:662–672

Binder JR, Rao SM, Hammeke TA, Frost JA, Bandettini PA, Hyde JS (1994b) Effects of stimulus rate on signal response during functional magnetic resonance imaging of auditory cortex. Cog Brain Res 2:31–38

Binder JR, Frost JA, Hammeke TA, Rao SM, Cox RW (1996) Function of the left planum temporale in auditory and linguistic processing. Brain 119:1239–1247

Cacace AT, Cousins JP, Moonen CTW et al. (1995) In-vivo localization of phantom auditory perceptions during functional magnetic resonance imaging of the human brain. Proc 5th Int Tinnitus Semin 5:397–401

Caird D, Scheich H, Klinke R (1991) Functional organization of auditory cortical fields in the Mongolian gerbil (Meriones unguiculatus): binaural 2-deoxyglucose patterns. J Comp Physiol A 168:13–26

Calvert GA, Bullmore ET, Brammer MJ et al (1997) Activation of auditory cortex during silent lipreading. Science 276:593–596

Coles RRA (1984) Epidemiology of tinnitus: (2) demographic and clinical features. J Laryngol Otol [Suppl] 9:195–202

David AS, Woodruff PWR, Howard R et al (1996) Auditory hallucinations inhibit exogenous activation of auditory association cortex. Neuroreport 7:932–936

Démonet J-F, Chollet F, Ramsay S et al (1992) The anatomy of phonological and semantic processing in normal subjects. Brain 115:1753–1768

Dhankhar A, Wexler BE, Fulbright RK, Halwes T, Blamire AM, Shulman RG (1997) Functional magnetic resonance imaging assessment of the human brain auditory cortex response to increasing word presentation rates. J Neurophysiol 77:476–483

Edmister WB, Talavage TM, Ledden PJ, Weisskoff RM (1998) Auditory cortical activation affected by temporal organization of noise. Neuroimage 7:S367

Edmister WB, Talavage TM, Ledden PJ Weisskoff RM Improved auditory cortex imaging using clustered volume acquisitions Hum. Brain Mapping (in press)

Erné SN, Hoke M (1990) Short-latency evoked magnetic fields from the human auditory brainstem. Adv Neurol 54:167–176

Freeman AJ, Mohr CM, King WM, Briggs RM, Leonard CM (1997) Effect of stimulus intensity on the volume of activated cortex in auditory fMRI. Proc Int Soc Magn Res Med 5:710

Friston KJ, Josephs O, Rees G, Turner R (1998) Nonlinear event-related responses in fMRI. Magn Reson Med 39:41–52

Galaburda A, Sanides F (1980) Cytoarchitectonic organization of the human auditory cortex. J Comp Neurol 190:597–610

Gaschler-Markefski B, Baumgart F, Tempelmann C, Schindler F, Stiller D, Heinze H-J, Scheich H (1997) Statistical methods in functional magnetic resonance imaging with respect to nonstationary time-series: auditory cortex activity. Magn Reson Med 38:811–820

Giraud AL, Chery-Croze S, Fischer G, Fischer C, Gregoire M-C, Lavenne F, Collet L (1998) Bilateral activation of auditory association areas in gaze-evoked phantom auditory sensation. Neuroimage 7:S587

Grady CL, Van Meter JW, Maisog JM, Pietrini P, Krasuski J, Rauschecher JP (1997) Attention-related modulation of activity in primary and secondary auditory cortex. Neuroreport 8:2511–2516

Groenen P, Snik A, van den Broek P (1997) Electrically evoked auditory middle latency responses versus perception abilities in cochlear implant users. Audiology 36:83–97

Guimaraes AR, Melcher JR, Talavage TM et al (1998) Imaging subcortical auditory activity in humans. Hum Brain Mapping 6:33–41

Hall DA, Akeroyd MA, Palmer AR et al (1998a) Optimal sampling of haemodynamic changes in auditory cortex for functional magnetic resonance imaging (fMRI). Neuroimage 7:S576

Hall DA, Elliott MR, Bowtell RW, Gurney E, Haggard MP (1998b) "Sparse" temporal sampling in fMRI enhances detection of activation by sound for both magnetic and acoustic reasons. Neuroimage 7:S551

Hari R (1997) Neuromagnetic approach to human auditory cortical functions, with emphasis on subjects with cochlear implants. Adv Otorhinolaryngol 52:15–18

Harms MP, Melcher JR, Weisskoff RM (1998) Time courses of fMRI signals in the inferior colliculus, medial geniculate body, and auditory cortex show different dependencies on noise burst rate. Neuroimage 7:S365

Herzog H, Lamprecht, Kühn A, Roden W, Vosteen K-H, Feinendegen LE (1991) Cortical activation in profoundly deaf patients during cochlear implant stimulation demonstrated by $H_2^{15}O$ PET. J Comp Assist Tomogr 15:369–375

Hickok G, Love T, Swinney D, Wong EC, Buxton RB (1997) Functional MR imaging during auditory word perception: a single-trial presentation paradigm. Brain Lang 58:197–201

Huckins SC, Turner CW, Doherty KA, Fonte MM, Szeverenyi NM (1998) Functional magnetic resonance imaging measures of blood flow patterns in the human auditory cortex in response to sound. J Speech Lang Hearing Res 41:538–548

Irving R, Harrison JM (1967) The superior olivary complex and audition: a comparative study. J Comp Neurol 130:77–86

Imig TJ, Ruggero MA, Kitzes LM, Javel E, Brugge JF (1977) Organization of auditory cortex in the owl monkey (Aotus trivirgatus). J Comp Neurol 171:111–128

Jäncke L, Posse S, Shah NJ, Nosselt T, Schmitz N, Müller-Gärtner H-W (1997a) Attentional factors modify the BOLD-response in the human auditory cortex to auditory stimuli. Neuroimage 5:S191

Jäncke L, Posse S, Shah NJ, Müller-Gärtner H-W (1997b) Intensity of auditory stimuli determines the spatial extent of the BOLD-response in the human auditory cortex to auditory stimuli. Neuroimage 5:S192

Kiang NYS, Fullerton BC, Richter EA, Levine RA, Norris BE (1984) Artificial stimulation of the auditory system. Adv Audiol 1:6–17

Kitzes LM, Semple MN (1985) Single-unit responses in the inferior colliculus: effects of neonatal unilateral cochlear ablation. J Neurophysiol 53:1483–1500

Kwong KK, Belliveau JW, Chesler DA et al (1992) Dynamic magnetic resonance imaging of human brain activity during primary sensory stimulation. Proc Natl Acad Sci USA 89:5675–5679

Lantos G, Liu G, Shafer V, Knuth K, Vaughan H (1997) Tonotopic organization of primary auditory cortex: an fMRI study. Neuroimage 5:S174

Lauter JL, Herscovitch P, Formby C, Raichle ME (1985) Tonotopic organization in human auditory cortex revealed by positron emission tomography. Hear Res 20:199–205

Levine RA Somatic (craniocervical) tinnitus: clinical features and neurological basis (submitted)

Levine RA, Benson RR, Talavage TM, Melcher JR, Rosen BR (1997) Functional magnetic resonance imaging and tinnitus: preliminary results. Assoc Res Otolaryngol 20:65

Lockwood AH, Salvi RJ, Coad ML, Towsley ML, Wack DS, Murphy BW (1998) The functional neuroanatomy of tinnitus. Evidence for limbic system links and neural plasticity. Neurology 50:114–120

Masterton RB, Glendenning KK, Nudo RJ (1981) Anatomical-behavioral analyses of hindbrain sound localization mechanisms. In: Syka J, Aitkin L (eds) Neuronal mechanisms of hearing. Plenum, New York, pp 263–275

McCarthy G, Luby M, Gore J, Goldman-Rakic P (1997) Infrequent events transiently activate human prefrontal and parietal cortex as measured by functional MRI. J Neurophysiol 77:1630–1634

McGurk H, MacDonald J (1976) Hearing lips and seeing voices. Nature 264:746–748

Melcher JR, Kiang NYS (1996) Generators of the brainstem auditory evoked potential in cat III: identified cell populations. Hear Res 93:52–71

Melcher JR, Fullerton BC, Weisskoff RM (1997) Imaging human auditory function from brainstem to cortex. Neuroimage 5:S172

Melcher JR, Eddington DK, Garcia N, Qin M, Sroka J, Weisskoff RM (1998) Electrically-evoked cortical activity in cochlear implant subjects can be mapped using fMRI. Neuroimage 7:S385

Melcher JR, Sigalovsky I, Levine RA et al Abnormal brain activity in humans with lateralized tinnitus revealed using fMRI (submitted)

Millen SJ, Haughton VM, Yetkin Z (1995) Functional magnetic resonance imaging of the central auditory pathway following speech and pure-tone stimuli. Laryngoscope 105:1305–1310

Mirz F, Pedersen CB, Ovesen T, Madsen S, Gjedde A (1998) Brain mapping may reveal origins of tinnitus. Neuroimage 7:S386

Moore DR, Kowalchuk NE (1988) Auditory brainstem of the ferret: effects of unilateral cochlear lesions on cochlear nucleus volume and projections to the inferior colliculus. J Comp Neurol 272:503–515

Moore JK, Moore RY (1971) A comparative study of the superior olivary complex in the primate brain. Folia Primatol (Basel) 16:35–51

Ogawa S, Tank DW, Menon R, Ellermann JM, Kim S-G, Merkle H, Ugurbil K (1992) Intrinsic signal changes accompanying sensory stimulation: functional brain mapping with magnetic resonance imaging. Proc Natl Acad Sci USA 89:5951–5955

Okazawa H, Naito Y, Yonekura Y et al (1996) Cochlear implant efficiency in pre- and postlingually deaf subjects. A study with $H_2^{15}O$ and PET. Brain 119:1297–1306

Pelizzone M, Hari R, Mäkelä J, Kaukoranta E, Montandon P (1986) Activation of the auditory cortex by cochlear stimulation in a deaf patient. Neurosci Lett 68:192–196

Penhune VB, Zatorre RJ, MacDonald JD, Evans AC (1996) Interhemispheric anatomical differences in human primary auditory cortex: probabilistic mapping and volume measurement from magnetic resonance scans. Cereb Cortex 6:661–672

Poncelet BP, Wedeen VJ, Weisskoff RM, Cohen MS (1992) Brain parenchyma motion: measurement with cine echo-planar MR imaging. Radiology 185:645–651

Price C, Wise R, Ramsay S, Friston K, Howard D, Patterson K, Frackowiak R (1992) Regional response differences within the human auditory cortex when listening to words. Neurosci Lett 146:179–182

Pugh KR, Shaywitz BA, Shaywitz SE et al (1996) Auditory selective attention: an fMRI investigation. Neuroimage 4:159–173

Rademacher J, Caviness VS Jr, Steinmetz H Galaburda AM (1993) Topographical variation of the human primary cortices: implications for neuroimaging, brain mapping, and neurobiology. Cereb Cortex 3:313–329

Rajan R, Irvine DRF, Wise LZ, Heil P (1993) Effect of unilateral partial cochlear lesions in adult cats on the representation of lesioned and unlesioned cochleas in primary auditory cortex. J Comp Neurol 338:17–49

Rauschecker JP, Tian B, Hauser M (1995) Processing of complex sounds in the macaque nonprimary auditory cortex. Science 268:111–114

Ravicz ME, Melcher JR (1998) Imager noise and noise attenuation during fMRI. Neuroimage 7:S556

Reale RA, Imig TJ (1980) Tonotopic organization in auditory cortex of the cat. J Comp Neurol 192:265–291

Rees G, Howseman A, Josephs O, Frith CD, Friston KJ, Frackowiak RSJ, Turner R (1997) Characterizing the relationship between BOLD contrast and regional cerebral blood flow measurements by varying the stimulus presentation rate. Neuroimage 6:270–278

Richter EA, Norris BE, Fullerton BC, Levine RA, Kiang NYS (1983) Is there a medial nucleus of the trapezoid body in humans? Am J Anat 168:157–166

Robertson D, Irvine DRF (1989) Plasticity of frequency organization in auditory cortex of guinea pigs with partial unilateral deafness. J Comp Neurol 282:456–471

Robson MD, Dorosz JL, Gore JC (1998) Measurements of the temporal fMRI response of the human auditory cortex to trains of tones. Neuroimage 7:185–198

Roland PE (1982) Cortical regulation of selective attention in man. a regional cerebral blood flow study. J Neurophysiol 48:1059–1078

Romani GL, Williamson SJ, Kaufman L (1982) Tonotopic organization of the human auditory cortex. Science 216:1339–1340

Sachs MB, Abbas PJ (1974) Rate versus level functions for auditory nerve fibers in cats: tone-burst stimuli. J Acoust Soc Am 56:1835–1847

Scheffler K, Bilecen D, Seelig J (1997) Functional imaging of the auditive system. auditory stimulation of defined frequency with B_0-gradients. Proc Int Soc Mag Res Med 5:1689

Scheffler K, Bilecen D, Schmid N, Tschopp K, Seelig J (1998) Auditory cortical responses in hearing subjects and unilateral deaf patients as detected by functional magnetic resonance imaging. Cereb Cortex 8:156–163

Semple MN, Kitzes LM (1985) Single-unit responses in the inferior colliculus: different consequences of contralateral and ipsilateral auditory stimulation. J Neurophysiol 53:1467–1482

Shah NJ, Jäncke L, Grosse-Ruyken M-L, Posse S, Müller-Gärtner H-W (1997) On the influence of acoustic masking noise in fMRI of the auditory cortex during phonetic discrimination. Proc Int Soc Mag Res Med 5:350

Shellock FG, Ziarati M, Atkinson D, Chen D-Y Determination of gradient magnetic field-induced acoustic noise associated with the use of echo planar and three dimensional, fast spin echo techniques. J Magn Reson Imaging (in press)

Stevens AA, Whalen DH, Liberman AM, Gore JC (1998) FMRI analysis of auditory processing in the temporal lobe. Neuroimage 7:S166

Strainer JC, Ulmer JL, Yetkin FZ, Haughton VM, Daniels DL, Millen SJ (1997) Functional MR of the primary auditory cortex: an analysis of pure tone activation and tone discrimination. Am J Neuroradiol 18:601–610

Stypulkowski PH, van den Honert C, Kvistad SD (1986) Electrophysiologic evaluation of the cochlear implant patient. Otolaryngol Clin North Am 19:249–257

Talavage TM, Benson RR, Galaburda AM, Rosen BR (1996) Evidence of multiple tonotopic fields in human auditory cortex. Proc Int Soc Magn Reson Med 4:1842

Talavage TM, Ledden PJ, Sereno MI, Rosen BR, Dale AM (1997) Multiple phase-encoded tonotopic maps in human auditory cortex. Neuroimage 5:S8

Talavage TM, Edmister WB, Ledden PJ, Weiskoff RM (1998) Measurement of signal changes induced by fMRI Imaging noise. Neuroimage 7:S360

Ulmer JL, Biswal BB, Yetkin FZ et al (1998) Cortical activation response to acoustic echo planar scanner noise. J Comput Assist Tomogr 22:111–119

Van de Moortele PF, Le Clec'H G, Dehaene S, Le Bihan D (1998) Improving auditory comprehension in fMRI: insertion of silent intervals in multi-slice EPI. Neuroimage 7:S554

Wang J, Cohen MS, Bookheimer SY, Dapretto M (1996) Functional MRI of human auditory cortex during auditory image lateralization. Neuroimage 3:S320

Wessinger CM, Buonocore MH, Kussmaul CL, Mangun GR (1997) Tonotopy in human auditory cortex examined with functional magnetic resonance imaging. Hum Brain Mapping 5:18–25

Wessinger CM, Tian B, VanMeter JW, Platenberg RC, Pekar JJ, Rauschecker JP (1998) Processing of complex sounds in human auditory cortex examined with functional magnetic resonance imaging. Proc Int Soc Magn Reson Med 6:1530

Woldorff M, Tempelmann C, Fell J et al (1997) Lateralized auditory spatial perception and cortical processing contralaterality as studied with fMRI and MEG. Neuroimage 5:S173

Woodruff PWR, Benson RR, Bandettini PA et al (1996) Modulation of auditory and visual cortex by selective attention is modality-dependent. Neuroreport 7:1909–1913

Woodruff PWR, Wright IC, Bullmore ET et al (1997) Auditory hallucinations and the temporal cortical response to speech in schizophrenia: a functional magnetic resonance imaging study. Am J Psychiatry 154:1676–1682

Zatorre RJ, Evans AC, Meyer E, Gjedde A (1992) Lateralization of phonetic and pitch discrimination in speech processing. Science 256:846–849

33 Functional MRI of the Language System

J.R. Binder

CONTENTS

33.1
Introduction

Many animal species have developed systems for simple communication, but the human language capacity is relatively unique. Like no other species, humans convey information using arbitrary symbols and gestures (spoken and written) to represent things in the world, combining these tokens to produce a virtually infinite number of possible expressions. Language-related functions were among the first to be ascribed a specific location in the brain (BROCA 1861) and have been the subject of intense research for well over a century. A "classical model" of language organization, based on data from aphasic patients with brain lesions, was popularized during the late nineteenth century and remains in common use (LICHTHEIM 1885; GESCHWIND 1971). In its most general form, this model proposes a frontal, "expressive," area for planning and executing speech and writing movements, named after BROCA (1861), and a posterior, "receptive," area for analysis and identification of linguistic sensory stimuli, named after WERNICKE (1874). While many neuroscientists would accept this basic scheme, a more detailed ac-

J.R. Binder, MD; Department of Neurology, Medical College of Wisconsin, 9200 W. Wisconsin Ave., Milwaukee, WI 53226, USA

count of language organization in the brain has not yet gained widespread approval. There is not universal agreement, for example, on such issues as which cortical areas comprise the receptive language system (BOGEN and BOGEN 1976), or on the specific linguistic role of Broca's area (MARIE 1906; MOHR 1976).

Noninvasive functional imaging methods are a potential source of new data for addressing these problems. Because accidental lesions provide only approximate information about cortical localization, one goal of activation imaging is to obtain more precise and more detailed information about the location of functional systems. The lesion method reveals areas that are necessary for a particular function, but other, less essential, areas may also contribute to normal proficiency. Within the limits of sensitivity, functional imaging methods reveal all brain areas that normally participate in a function, regardless of whether this participation is critically necessary. Thus, another role for these techniques is to provide a more complete picture of intact brain function than is possible from studying the behavior of damaged brains. A number of fMRI language processing experiments have been reported. Although a complete survey is beyond the scope of this chapter, an attempt will be made to illustrate several notable areas of developing consensus and continued controversy.

33.2
Theoretical and
Methodological Considerations

Attempts to detect brain activity related to language processing are best preceded by a consideration of two general theoretical questions: What processes are linguistic? More importantly, if linguistic processes can be carried out autonomously ("internally" or "covertly") by humans, when can it be said that these processes are not occurring?

Language processes are those that enable communication. Although seemingly satisfactory, this definition is overly inclusive, in that many general supportive processes (e.g., cardiac, pulmonary, general arousal, and sustained attention functions) are necessary for communication to occur but are not linguistic in nature. Many linguistic and non-linguistic tasks require neural systems that process auditory or visual sensory information, hold such information in a short-term store, direct attention to specific features or aspects of the information, perform comparative and other operations on the information, select a response based on such operations, and carry out the response. The extent to which any of these systems is specialized for language-related functions (as in, for example, specialized speech perceptual systems or "verbal working memory" systems) is still a matter of debate. Careful consideration of these "general purpose" functions is especially relevant for interpreting and designing language studies, which often employ relatively complex tasks involving motor, sensory, attentional, memory, and "central executive" functions in addition to language. Should these other components be considered part of the language system because they are so necessary for adequate task performance, or should they be delineated from language processes per se? In choosing a control task against which a language task is to be contrasted, investigators tacitly establish which components of the task are not, by their definition, part of the language process in which they are interested. These implicit definitions can vary even among investigators studying the same language process, leading to a profusion of apparently conflicting results (PETERSEN et al. 1988; WISE et al. 1991; DÉMONET et al. 1992).

Clinicians working with aphasic patients historically have focused on the distinction between expressive and receptive language functions, but a more useful taxonomy of processing subcomponents is available from the field of linguistics. The major functional subdivisions include: (1) phonetics, the processes governing production and perception of speech sounds; (2) phonology, the language-specific rules by which speech sounds are represented and manipulated; (3) semantics, the processing of word meanings, names, and other declarative knowledge about the world; and (4) syntax, the processes by which words are combined to make sentences and sentences analyzed to reveal underlying relationships between words. Although conceptually distinct, these components act together during everyday language behaviors. The extent to which each

component can be examined in isolation remains a major methodological issue, as it is not yet clear to what extent the systems responsible for these processes become active "automatically" or in parallel when presented with familiar linguistic stimuli. Take as a hypothetical example a task in which subjects must compare the meaning of two sentences. In the "semantic" condition, the sentences are syntactically identical but differ by one word. In the "syntactic" condition, the sentences have identical words but differ in syntactic structure. Although accurate task performance requires semantic analysis in the first case and syntactic analysis in the second, it is almost certain that both processing components would be engaged in both of these conditions. A direct subtraction between conditions might show relative differences in some areas, but these selectively activated areas would be but a small extent of the entire semantic or syntactic system, the undetected parts having been activated during both conditions.

Converging evidence suggests that single words also provoke a considerable amount of automatic processing (CARR et al. 1982; MARCEL 1983; VAN ORDEN 1987; MACLEOD 1991; PRICE et al. 1996b). One familiar example is the Stroop effect, in which semantic processing of printed words occurs even when subjects are instructed to attend to the color of the print, and even when this processing interferes with task performance (MACLEOD 1991). PRICE et al. (1996b) demonstrated this general phenomenon in an important PET study. Subjects were required to detect vertical lines in printed text stimuli. This task remained constant while the stimuli varied in terms of linguistic value. Compared to activation produced by nonsense characters and consonant strings, pronounceable (i.e., orthographically legal) non-words and real words produced additional activation in widespread, left-lateralized cortical areas, even though the task was identical across all conditions.

If linguistic stimuli such as words and pictures evoke uncontrolled, automatic language processing, these effects need to be considered in the design and interpretation of language activation experiments. Use of such stimuli in a baseline condition could result in undesirable subtraction (or partial subtraction) of language-related activation. Because investigators frequently try to match stimuli in control and language tasks very closely, such inadvertent subtraction may be relatively commonplace in functional imaging studies of language processing. One notable example is the widely employed "word generation" task, which is frequently paired with a control task involving repetition or reading of words

(PETERSEN et al. 1988; RAICHLE et al. 1994; BUCKNER et al. 1995). In most of these studies, which were aimed at detecting activation related to semantic processing, there has been relatively little activation in temporal and temporoparietal structures that are known, on the basis of lesion studies, to be involved in semantic processing. In contrast, subtractions involving control tasks that use non-linguistic stimuli generally reveal a much more extensive network of left hemisphere temporal, parietal, and frontal language processing areas (DÉMONET et al. 1992; BOOKHEIMER et al. 1995; DAMASIO et al. 1996; PRICE et al. 1996b; BINDER et al. 1997).

Evidence thus suggests that familiar stimuli evoke language processes that may not be requested by experimenters or needed for task completion, but there is also reason to believe that language processes occur independent of any sensory stimulation. This becomes obvious when contrasting human language capacity to the "speech" behavior of parrots and tape recorders. Although possessing complex mechanisms for encoding and reproducing speech sounds, these non-human talkers have no language facility, and their speech occurs entirely in response to external events. Humans, on the other hand, are capable of drawing on past experience to determine the meaning of words they hear, of pondering these meanings after the words themselves are gone, of imagining the sounds of words, and of silently preparing an entirely original utterance of their own. These kinds of internal processes that distinguish real language capacity are essentially independent of external stimuli, and thus may not always (ever?) be under complete experimental control. Until these internal processes and the conditions under which they occur are better understood, the question of when language processing stops will remain largely a matter of speculation. Preliminary information regarding this issue (BINDER et al., in press) will be discussed in a later section of this chapter.

33.3
Studies of Normal Language Systems

33.3.1
Speech Perception and Reading

WERNICKE (1874) first drew attention to the superior temporal gyrus (STG), which he believed played a pivotal role in comprehension of both spoken and written linguistic tokens. Subsequent interest was focused particularly on the posterior STG and its dorsal surface, or planum temporale (PT; GESCHWIND 1971). This region shows interhemispheric, morphological and cytoarchitectural asymmetries that roughly parallel language lateralization, suggesting that it plays a key role in language function (GALABURDA et al. 1978). Consistent with this hypothesis, PET and fMRI studies consistently demonstrate activation of this region when subjects listen to speech sounds (WISE et al. 1991; MAZOYER et al. 1993; BINDER et al. 1994; FIEZ et al. 1996).

Recent research, however, has led to other interpretations of this region. Several investigators, for example, have been interested to know whether STG and PT activation resulting from speech sounds reflects processing of the acoustic content (i.e., physical features such as frequency and amplitude information) or the linguistic content (phonemic, lexical, and semantic associations) of the stimuli. These researchers compared activation with words or speech syllables to activation with simpler, non-speech sounds like noise and pure tones. The consistent finding from these PET and fMRI studies is that speech and non-speech sounds produce roughly equivalent activation of the dorsal STG, including the PT, in both hemispheres (DÉMONET et al. 1992; ZATORRE et al. 1992; BINDER et al. 1996, 1997). In contrast, more ventral areas of the STG within and surrounding the superior temporal sulcus (STS) are preferentially activated by speech sounds (Fig. 33.1). Although these findings support a specialized role for this more ventral area in speech perception, the exact nature of this role is still not clear, since the speech and non-speech stimuli in these studies differed drastically on a number of physical variables. For example, speech sounds contain complex frequency and amplitude modulations that are not present in the comparison sounds that were used, again suggesting the possibility that areas activated preferentially by speech sounds might be responding primarily to these physical features rather than to linguistic information. One method of settling this issue is to compare speech stimuli that differ in linguistic content but are closely matched in terms of physical features. Several research groups, for example, compared activation with words to activation with non-words, foreign words, non-word syllables, backwards speech, or complex environmental sounds (WISE et al. 1991; DÉMONET et al. 1992; MAZOYER et al. 1993; BINDER et al. 1994; O'LEARY et al. 1996; PRICE et al. 1996b, c). In nearly all of these comparisons there has been no difference in STG activation between real words and these other sounds,

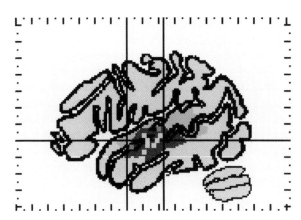

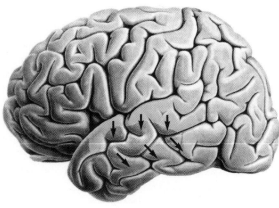

Fig. 33.1. Left hemisphere superior temporal areas activated in three auditory studies. *Blue* indicates regions activated equally by tones and words (Binder et al. 1996). Areas activated more by speech than by non-speech sounds are indicated by *red shading* (Binder et al. 1996), *orange squares* (Zatorre et al. 1992), and *yellow squares* (Démonet et al. 1992). All data are aligned in standard stereotaxic space at $x=-51$

Fig. 33.2. Hypothetical model of speech recognition areas in the left temporal lobe. Information flows in a dorsal-to-ventral direction from early auditory processing regions in the superior temporal gyrus (STG; *blue*) to phonemic pattern recognition systems near the superior temporal sulcus (STS; *red*) and finally to ventrolateral lexical-semantic processing areas (*yellow*)

although differences were sometimes observed in regions ventral to the STG, for example in the left middle and inferior temporal gyri.

The model of temporal lobe speech processing that emerges from these data is one based on a primarily dorsal-to-ventral hierarchical organization and includes at least three relatively distinct processing stages (Fig. 33.2). In accord with anatomical and neurophysiological studies of the auditory cortex, the earliest stage comprises sensory processors located in primary and belt auditory regions on the superior temporal plane, including the PT, that respond to relatively simple aspects of the auditory signal (Merzenich and Brugge 1973; Mesulam and Pandya 1973; Phillips and Irvine 1981; Galaburda and Pandya 1983; Mendelson and Cynader 1985; Morel et al. 1993; Rauschecker et al. 1997). Further ventrally, on the lateral surface of the STG and within the STS, are areas that appear to respond to more complex auditory phenomena, such as frequency and amplitude modulations, and to encode sequences of these phenomena as recognizable patterns (Rauschecker et al. 1995). Still further ventrally, beyond the STS, are large cortical regions that appear to process lexical and semantic (i.e., non-physical) information associated with stimuli. This new model thus differs from the traditional view in placing much less emphasis on the STG and PT as "language centers." While these regions undoubtedly play a critical role in auditory perception, information processing of a specifically linguistic nature appears to depend primarily on cortical areas

outside the STG. This model is in good agreement with a wealth of lesion data, which suggest primarily auditory perceptual deficits following isolated STG injury (Barrett 1910; Henschen 1920–1922; Tanaka et al. 1987), and naming and semantic deficits from lesions located outside the STG (Henschen 1920–1922; Warrington and Shallice 1984; Alexander et al. 1989; Damasio et al. 1996).

Several fMRI studies using visual stimuli provide additional insights into the function of these temporal lobe areas. Calvert et al. (1997) studied brain areas involved in lip-reading. In the lip-reading condition subjects watched a video of a face silently mouthing numbers and were asked to silently repeat the numbers to themselves. In the control condition a static face was presented, and subjects were asked to silently repeat the number "one" to themselves. The moving face condition produced activation in widespread extrastriate regions, but also in the vicinity of the STS bilaterally. The authors concluded that these areas, which were also activated by listening to speech, may be sites where polymodal integration of auditory and visual information occurs during speech perception. Several investigators have also demonstrated STS activation when subjects silently read printed words in comparison to reading meaningless letter strings (Bavelier et al. 1997; Indefrey et al. 1997). These activations were much stronger in the left than the right STS and were more prominent in the posterior half of the sulcus. Taken together, these data suggest that cortical areas in the STS receive inputs from both auditory and visual sensory cortices and thus may be important sites for early polymodal sensory integration, a conclusion that gains considerable support from anatomical and physiological studies of the STS in monkeys (DESIMONE and GROSS 1979; BAYLIS et al. 1987; HIKOSAWA et al. 1988; SELTZER and PANDYA 1994).

33.3.2
Lexical and Semantic Processing

Semantic processes are those concerned with storing, retrieving, and using knowledge about the world, and are a key component of such ubiquitous behaviors as naming, comprehending and formulating language, problem-solving, planning, and thinking. A general consensus regarding the brain localization of such processes has recently begun to emerge from functional imaging and aphasia studies. The latter have made it increasingly clear that deficits involving naming and knowledge retrieval are associated with lesions in a variety of dominant hemisphere temporal and parietal locations (WARRINGTON and SHALLICE 1984; ALEXANDER et al. 1989; HART and GORDON 1990; HILLIS and CARAMAZZA 1991; DAMASIO et al. 1996). Recent

functional imaging studies provide converging evidence, demonstrating that lexical-semantic processes engage a number of temporal, parietal, and prefrontal regions encompassing a large extent of the language dominant hemisphere. Given the complexity and the sheer amount of semantic information learned by a typical person – including, for example, all defining characteristics of all conceptual categories and all category exemplars, all relationships between these entities, and all linguistic representations of these concepts and relationships – it seems hardly surprising that a large proportion of the brain would be devoted to managing this information.

Functional imaging studies of semantic systems seek to distinguish brain areas involved in processing stored knowledge about stimuli from sensory and attentional areas involved in processing physical aspects of the stimuli. A typical strategy for making this distinction is to contrast tasks requiring knowledge retrieval (naming or semantic tasks) with tasks that do not (e.g., perceptual analysis tasks), using similar stimuli in both conditions to control for sensory processing. Binder and colleagues used fMRI to localize activation during a semantic task in comparison to a non-semantic task (BINDER et al. 1997).

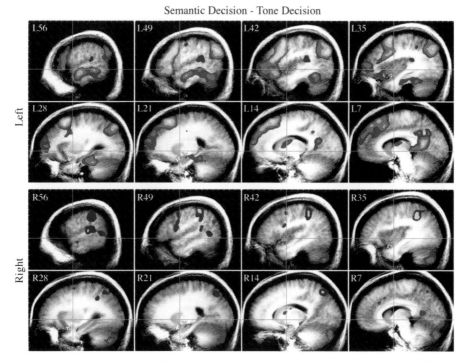

Fig. 33.3. Serial sagittal sections showing significantly activated areas in the semantic processing study of BINDER et al. (1997). Semantic processing areas, indicated in *red-yellow*, are strongly lateralized to the left cerebral hemisphere and right cerebellum. *Blue shading* indicates regions that are more active during the control (tone decision) task. (Adapted with permission from BINDER et al. 1997, copyright 1996 Society for Neuroscience)

In contrast to several prior studies (PETERSEN et al. 1988), non-linguistic stimuli were used during the control condition to minimize activation of language systems (CARR et al. 1982; MARCEL 1983; MACLEOD 1991; PRICE et al. 1996b). In the semantic task (semantic decision), subjects heard names of animals and were instructed to press a button for animals within a specified category ("native to the United States and used by people"). In addition to semantic processing, this task engages arousal and sustained attention systems, working memory functions for maintaining the task instructions and stimuli, sensory processing, and motor response systems. As a control for these non-semantic aspects of the task, subjects performed a perceptual control task (tone decision) in which short sequences of low-pitch and high-pitch tones were presented, and a button press was required for any sequence containing two high tones. The semantic and tone tasks both engage early auditory, attentional, working memory, and motor response systems. Whereas the tone task emphasizes perceptual processing of non-verbal stimuli, the language task emphasizes access and retrieval of knowledge associated with linguistic symbols.

The protocol included whole-brain fMRI in 30 right-handed subjects, spatial normalization, intersubject averaging, and reliability testing. The results provide a relatively detailed and highly reliable (reliability coefficient=0.92) average map of the brain areas differentially activated by the two tasks (Fig. 33.3). Relative to the tone task, the semantic task activated a distributed set of cortical areas in the left hemisphere and right cerebellum (red-yellow areas in Fig. 33.3). Semantic areas in the left temporal lobe include portions of the middle and inferior temporal gyri (Brodmann areas 21 and 37), fusiform gyrus (areas 37 and 20), and parahippocampal gyrus (area 36). Other left hemisphere regions activated by the semantic task included the angular gyrus (area 39);

cortex surrounding the splenium of the corpus callosum, including portions of the posterior cingulate gyrus, retrosplenial cortex, and precuneus (areas 23, 29, 31); inferior prefrontal cortex, including pars opercularis, pars triangularis, pars orbitalis, and cortex along the inferior frontal sulcus (areas 44–47); rostral portions of the middle frontal gyrus (area 10); much of the superior frontal gyrus and pre-supplementary motor area (areas 8–10 medially); anterior cingulate cortex (area 32); and parts of the caudate nucleus, anterior internal capsule, and anterior thalamus. In contrast to these areas, several others responded more strongly to the tone task (blue areas in Fig. 33.3), including the PT bilaterally, the posterior middle temporal gyrus in the right hemisphere (area 21), the supramarginal gyrus bilaterally (area 40), and premotor cortex bilaterally (area 6).

These results are in close agreement with a similar study by Démonet and colleagues (1992) using PET and with a PET study by Price et al. (1994) contrasting visual semantic and non-semantic tasks. Together these studies implicate four distinct left hemisphere cortical areas in semantic processing: (1) a posterior ventral temporal lobe region that includes parts of middle temporal, inferior temporal, fusiform, and parahippocampal gyri; (2) a large prefrontal region that includes inferior and superior frontal gyri, portions of the middle frontal gyrus, and part of the anterior cingulate; (3) angular gyrus; and (4) a perisplenial region including posterior cingulate cortex and ventral precuneus (Fig. 33.4). A number of other PET and fMRI studies demonstrated activation in these areas during semantic or word retrieval tasks, although the precise activation patterns were somewhat variable, probably owing to differences in control stimuli, task requirements, and imaging and analysis procedures (FRITH et al. 1991; HOWARD et al. 1992; BOTTINI et al. 1994; RAICHLE et al. 1994; BOOKHEIMER et al. 1995; DAMASIO et al. 1996; FIEZ

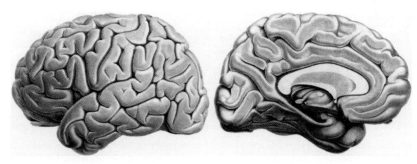

Fig. 33.4. Summary of left hemisphere brain regions implicated in semantic processing, including ventrolateral temporal lobe, angular gyrus, prefrontal cortex and anterior cingulate, and perisplenial cortex

et al. 1996; PRICE et al. 1996b; SMITH et al. 1996; VANDENBERGHE et al. 1996; BAVELIER et al. 1997).

Although the specific role of each of these regions in complex semantic tasks is not yet clear, a few general speculations can be offered based largely on lesion studies. For example, focal lesions in posterior and ventral temporal cortex occasionally cause very selective knowledge deficits, affecting only a particular semantic category or word class (WARRINGTON and SHALLICE 1984; HART and GORDON 1990; HILLIS and CARAMAZZA 1991; DAMASIO and TRANEL 1993; DAMASIO et al. 1996). The selective nature of the deficits suggests direct damage to stored knowledge related to these categories or classes, and hence that the posterior and ventral temporal regions observed by functional imaging may represent sites of information storage. Indeed, several PET studies have demonstrated that activation in this general region depends partly on the semantic category of presented stimuli (DAMASIO et al. 1996; MARTIN et al. 1996). In contrast, the prefrontal activation observed with functional imaging may represent processes involved in accessing, holding on-line, and using information from the posterior store. Patients with lesions in these regions typically demonstrate intact semantic knowledge in the presence of strongly directing cues (e.g., intact comprehension of words) but impaired access to this knowledge in the absence of constraining cues (e.g., impaired ability to produce lists of related words; RUBENS 1976; ALEXANDER and SCHMITT 1980; FREEDMAN et al. 1984; STUSS and BENSON 1986; COSTELLO and WARRINGTON 1989; RAPCSAK and RUBENS 1994). Several imaging groups working with word production tasks have also presented evidence for functional subdivision of the left inferior prefrontal cortex. Although a consistent model has yet to emerge, there is some evidence that the posterior left

inferior frontal gyrus (i.e., pars opercularis) plays a relatively greater role in phonological operations, while more anterior regions (i.e., rostral inferior frontal sulcus and middle frontal gyrus) may be relatively specialized for semantic processing (BUCKNER et al. 1995; PAULESU et al. 1997). Other studies comparing semantic and phonological tasks, however, did not support a specific role for rostral middle frontal gyrus in semantic processing (DÉMONET et al. 1992; SHAYWITZ et al. 1995a). Much of the inferior frontal gyrus, particularly pars opercularis and pars triangularis, shows activation across a very wide variety of language tasks (DÉMONET et al. 1992; BOTTINI et al. 1994; PRICE et al. 1994; BOOKHEIMER et al. 1995; BUCKNER et al. 1995; DEMB et al. 1995; SHAYWITZ et al. 1995a; PRICE et al. 1996b; SMITH et al. 1996; WARBURTON et al. 1996; BAVELIER et al. 1997; BINDER et al. 1997; KIM et al. 1997). Thus, this region may be involved in very general processes engaged during language task performance, such as maintaining representations of task instructions and performance strategies, or formulating relevant relationships between this "task set" information and information acquired from task stimuli and/or long-term memory.

33.3.3
Semantic Processing During Rest

The constructs "semantic processing" and "thinking" share important functional features. In contrast to perceptual systems driven primarily by external sensory information, semantic processing and thinking rely on internal sources of information such as episodic and semantic memory stores. Semantic processing and thinking both involve complex mechanisms for accessing information from

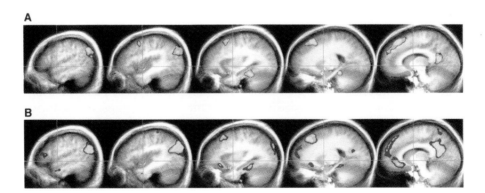

Fig. 33.5A, B. Left hemisphere areas associated with non-stimulus semantic processing (BINDER et al., in press). Areas with higher signal during a semantic decision task compared to a phonemic decision task (A) are virtually identical to areas with higher signal during rest compared to a tone decision task (B)

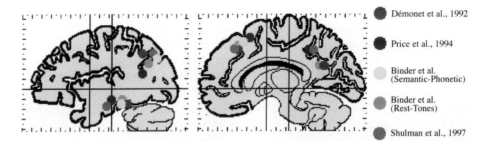

Fig. 33.6. Convergence of results across four studies comparing either semantic to non-semantic tasks (DÉMONET et al. 1992; PRICE et al. 1994; BINDER et al., in press) or resting to non-semantic tasks (SHULMAN et al. 1997; BINDER et al., in press)

these stores and manipulating this information to reach an intended goal, such as planning an action or making a decision. To the extent that semantic processing is defined by these operations involving storage, retrieval, and manipulation of internal sources of information, the conscious thinking state could also be said to involve semantic processing. In support of this view, Binder et al. (in press) recently presented evidence that many of the areas implicated in semantic processing – specifically the angular gyrus, dorsal prefrontal cortex, posterior cingulate, and ventral temporal lobe – are also active during a resting state compared to a non-semantic task.

In an extension of the previously described semantic processing study (BINDER et al. 1997), the same auditory semantic decision task (see Fig. 33.3) was compared to an auditory phoneme decision task similar to that described originally by DÉMONET et al. (1992). In the phoneme task, subjects heard non-words comprised of three syllables (e.g., /bakodu/) and pressed a button for stimuli containing both consonants /b/ and /d/. The intent of pairing this control task with the semantic decision task was to subtract any activation related to speech sound processing, thereby identifying brain areas specifically involved in processing non-stimulus information retrieved from semantic memory. The results, illustrated in Fig. 33.5A, very closely replicate those of DÉMONET et al. Activated regions were fewer and smaller in extent than in the semantic tones comparison (Fig. 33.3), reflecting subtraction of brain regions involved in speech sound perception and other non-semantic language task performance processes. The activated areas, which were all in the left hemisphere, included the angular gyrus, perisplenial cortex, dorsal prefrontal cortex (i.e., the medial aspect of areas 8, 9, and 10 in the superior frontal gyrus), and parahippocampus.

To determine whether these non-sensory semantic processing areas are also active during rest, a resting state (subjects were instructed only to relax and

remain still) was compared to the tone decision task described earlier. Areas that were more active during rest, illustrated in Fig. 33.5B, were nearly identical to those identified in the semantic-phonemic subtraction. Centers-of-mass in the two comparisons lay within 1 cm of each other for all four main activation areas. Finally, when the resting state was compared to the semantic decision task, these areas showed little or no difference in activation, consistent with the hypothesis that these regions are engaged in semantic processing during both of these conditions (BINDER et al., in press). These cortical areas, which are relatively distant (as measured by cortico-cortical connections) from primary sensory areas (JONES and POWELL 1970; MESULAM 1985; FELLEMAN and VAN ESSEN 1991), thus appear to comprise a distributed network for storing, retrieving, and manipulating internal sources of information independent of external sensory input.

The hypothesis that stimulus-independent semantic processing occurs in these brain areas during rest accounts for several puzzling findings from functional activation studies. The first of these is that studies comparing semantic tasks to a resting or rest-like (e.g., passive stimulation) baseline have not shown activation in these areas (WISE et al. 1991; KAWASHIMA et al. 1993; MAZOYER et al. 1993; TAMAS et al. 1993; EULITZ et al. 1994; HERHOLZ et al. 1994; YETKIN et al. 1995; WARBURTON et al. 1996). This outcome is readily explained by the hypothesis, which states that these areas are active during both rest and semantic task conditions. In contrast, comparisons between semantic tasks and attentionally demanding non-semantic tasks typically show activation in some or all of these areas (DÉMONET et al. 1992; BOTTINI et al. 1994; PRICE et al. 1994, 1996b; DAMASIO et al. 1996; VANDENBERGHE et al. 1996; BINDER et al. 1997). Activation contrast in these areas thus appears to depend on the degree to which spontaneous semantic processing is suppressed during the baseline state, which may in turn depend on a number of task variables that determine attentional allocation, and on the amount of automatic semantic processing elicited by control stimuli (PRICE et al. 1996b).

Spontaneous semantic processing during rest could also account for many instances of task-induced deactivation (SHULMAN et al. 1997). Interruption of spontaneous semantic processes by attentionally demanding non-semantic tasks would result in decreased neural activity in brain regions where these processes are localized. This model predicts that brain areas demonstrating deactivation during non-semantic tasks relative to rest should be the same as areas implicated in semantic processing. This is precisely what was demonstrated in Fig. 33.5, in which areas demonstrating deactivation during the tones task were described alternatively as "more active during rest." This convergence is also demonstrated by several PET studies of semantic processing and task-induced deactivation. For example, DÉMONET et al. (1992) and PRICE et al. (1994) contrasted semantic tasks with attentionally demanding non-semantic tasks. Although different in many ways, these contrasts identified the same left hemisphere regions shown in Fig. 33.5: angular gyrus, dorsal prefrontal cortex, perisplenial cortex, and ventral temporal cortex. These four areas also consistently demonstrated task-induced deactivation across a variety of visual tasks in a meta-analysis by SHULMAN et al. (1997). This unusual convergence of results, illustrated in Fig. 33.6, is remarkable given the considerable differences in methodology across the four studies. The hypothesis that task-induced deactivation results from interruption of spontaneous semantic processing provides one parsimonious explanation for this pattern of results.

33.4
Developmental Influences on Language Organization

The common practice of presenting averaged activation maps from a group of subjects (e.g., Fig. 33.3) obscures the fact that there is considerable variability among subjects in the precise spatial location, spatial extent, and magnitude of these activations (BINDER et al. 1994; BAVELIER et al. 1997; KIM et al. 1997; SPRINGER et al. 1997). This variation could conceivably arise from genetic or environmental sources, or from complex interactions between ge-

nome and environment. Two developmental factors that have received some attention in neuroimaging studies of language organization are the age of acquisition of languages learned by the subject (an almost purely environmental variable) and the sex of the subject (a genetic factor strongly associated with various environmental variables).

Available evidence suggests that brain activation during a language task depends on the subject's proficiency with the language, which in turn depends roughly on the age at which the language was acquired. YETKIN et al. (1996) studied five adult multilingual subjects using fMRI. In the language activation condition, subjects were asked to silently generate words in either their native language, a second fluent language, or a third nonfluent language known to the subject for less than 5 years. The baseline condition was a resting state in which subjects "refrained from thinking of words." Significantly more voxels in the frontal lobe showed activation in the nonfluent condition, while the native and second fluent languages produced equal activation. These results are consistent with the idea that, in general, tasks that are less practiced require more neural activity (HAIER et al. 1992; RAICHLE et al. 1994). Because this extra neural activity could be related to attentional rather than linguistic processes, however, the data of YETKIN et al. do not address the issue of whether different languages are actually represented in different brain areas.

A report by KIM et al. (1997) provides some initial evidence on this question. The authors studied 12 adult bilingual subjects who acquired a second fluent language either simultaneously with a first ("early bilingual") or during young adulthood ("late bilingual"). In the language activation condition, subjects were asked to "mentally describe" events that had occurred the previous day, using a specified language. The baseline condition was a resting state in which subjects looked at a fixation point. In late bilinguals, the left inferior frontal activation foci associated with task performance in the native and second languages were spatially separated by an average distance of 6.4 mm (range 4.5 mm to 9.0 mm). Of note, the relative location of these native and second language foci were highly variable across subjects, with the native language focus lateral to the second language focus in some subjects and medial or posterior in other subjects. This fact alone could explain why a previous PET study using averaged group activation maps showed no differences in cortical activation associated with native and second languages (KLEIN et al. 1995). Because KIM et al. did not report the relative language proficiency of these subjects or overall levels of activation as a function of language used, it is not clear whether the spatial separation of activation foci could be related to familiarity and attentional (i.e., workload) effects rather than to differences in the location of linguistic representations, although this seems unlikely given the reported lack of spatial overlap between the native language and second language activation foci. Nevertheless, early bilinguals showed no differences in the location of activation foci associated with different languages, suggesting that when two languages are learned equally well early in life, these languages typically are represented in the same brain areas.

Numerous studies report that women, on average, have slightly better verbal skills than men. Most of this evidence pertains to speech production tasks, whereas sex differences in higher-order language abilities like semantic processing are equivocal (see HALPERN 1992 for a review). Efforts to uncover the neurophysiological basis for these sex differences have so far met with limited success. Inferential techniques, such as deficit-lesion correlation, structural morphometry, and behavioral measures of lateralization (dichotic listening, divided visual field processing) have yielded very discrepant results. Compared to these other methods, functional imaging techniques provide a more direct measure of brain function, yet application of these methods has also generated inconsistent findings.

Using fMRI, SHAYWITZ et al. (1995b) found that frontal lobe activation was more left lateralized in men than in women during a visual phonological task in which subjects judged whether two printed non-words rhyme (e.g., lete and jeat). In a later description of the same study (PUGH et al. 1996), sex effects on functional lateralization were also reported during semantic processing (semantic categorization) of visually presented words. Compared with the phonological condition, the semantic task resulted in a larger volume of activation in men but not in women. This result was observed in the total area scanned, in medial extrastriate cortex, and in the middle and superior temporal gyri bilaterally. Based on this result, the authors suggested that there may be greater overlap between the semantic and phonological systems in women and, thus, more focal organization of language in women. Activations in men were also significantly more left lateralized than in women across the total area imaged and in the inferior frontal gyrus during both phonologic and semantic tasks. Of note, no sex differences in

performance were observed on these tasks; these data thus suggest that men and women carry out identical language processes with the same degree of proficiency using very differently organized brain systems.

In contrast, several other functional imaging studies have not found significant sex differences during language processing. PRICE et al. (1996a) used PET to examine activation during phonologic and semantic reading tasks that engaged many of the same processing components studied by SHAYWITZ et al. Large, statistically significant effects of task, task order, and type of baseline task were found, but sex effects were small and insignificant. In another PET study, BUCKNER et al. (1995) found no sex differences in activation during word-stem completion and verb generation tasks, speech production measures similar to those on which men and women typically show subtle performance differences (HALPERN 1992). Thus, no significant sex differences in large-scale activation patterns were found even on tasks for which there is some evidence of sex-related differences in processing capacity. Finally, FROST et al. (1997) used fMRI to study a large subject cohort (50 women and 50 men) during the semantic decision task described above (see Fig. 33.3). Men and women showed identical, strongly left-lateralized activation patterns. No sex differences in the degree of lateralization were observed for the brain as a whole or for any region of interest.

In summary, functional imaging research on developmental factors that influence language organization in the brain is still at a preliminary stage. Brain activation during language processing clearly depends on language proficiency, but whether this effect reflects changes in language organization as proficiency is acquired or merely the additional effort associated with an unfamiliar task is not yet clear. Available data suggest that two languages learned equally well early in life typically are represented in the same brain areas (KIM et al. 1997). Although sex effects on language organization in the brain have been extensively investigated and debated, there remains considerable controversy on this topic. Functional imaging data have so far not resolved this issue, and more studies are needed using larger subject samples and a wider variety of processing tasks.

33.5
Conclusion

fMRI is unquestionably a powerful tool for studying the neurophysiology of language processing in the intact brain. The large number and variety of language-related experiments reported in recent years (not all of which could be reviewed in this brief article) attests to the stimulating effect this new technique will certainly have on the study of language and language development. Although many of the published studies are somewhat preliminary, already there is evidence that new information from fMRI could significantly alter current concepts of normal language processing in the brain. fMRI and other functional activation data will be most meaningful if interpreted within the context of existing information about language processing acquired from neuropsychological, behavioral, and electrophysiological investigations.

References

Alexander MP, Schmitt MA (1980) The aphasia syndrome of stroke in the left anterior cerebral artery territory. Arch Neurol 37:97–100

Alexander MP, Hiltbrunner B, Fischer RS (1989) Distributed anatomy of transcortical sensory aphasia. Arch Neurol 46:885–892

Barrett AM (1910) A case of pure word-deafness with autopsy. J Nerv Ment Dis 37:73–92

Bavelier D, Corina D, Jezzard P et al (1997) Sentence reading: a functional MRI study at 4 tesla. J Cogn Neurosci 9:664–686

Baylis GC, Rolls ET, Leonard CM (1987) Functional subdivisions of the temporal lobe neocortex. J Neurosci 7:330–342

Binder JR, Rao SM, Hammeke TA et al (1994) Functional magnetic resonance imaging of human auditory cortex. Ann Neurol 35:662–672

Binder JR, Frost JA, Hammeke TA, Rao SM, Cox RW (1996) Function of the left planum temporale in auditory and linguistic processing. Brain 119:1239–1247

Binder JR, Frost JA, Hammeke TA, Cox RW, Rao SM, Prieto T (1997) Human brain language areas identified by functional MRI. J Neurosci 17:353–362

Binder JR, Frost JA, Hammeke TA, Bellgowan PSF, Rao SM, Cox RW Conceptual processing during the conscious resting state: a functional MRI study. J Cogn Neurosci (in press)

Bogen JE, Bogen GM (1976) Wernicke's region – where is it? Ann NY Acad Sci 290:834–843

Bookheimer SY, Zeffiro TA, Blaxton T, Gaillard T, Theodore W (1995) Regional cerebral blood flow during object naming and word reading. Human Brain Map 3:93–106

Bottini G, Corcoran R, Sterzi R, Paulesu E, Schenone P, Scarpa P, Frackowiak RSJ (1994) The role of the right hemisphere in the interpretation of figurative aspects of language. A positron emission tomography activation study. Brain 117:1241–1253

Broca P (1861) Remarques sur le siège de la faculté du langage articulé; suivies d'une observation d'aphemie. Bull Soc Anat Paris 6:330–357

Buckner RL, Raichle ME, Petersen SE (1995) Dissociation of human prefrontal cortical areas across different speech production tasks and gender groups. J Neurosci 74:2163–2173

Calvert GA, Bullmore ET, Brammer MJ et al (1997) Activation of auditory cortex during silent lipreading. Science 276:593–596

Carr TH, McCauley C, Sperber RD, Parmalee CM (1982) Words, pictures, and priming: On semantic activation, conscious identification, and the automaticity of information processing. J Exp Psychol (Human Percept Perf) 8:757–777

Costello AL, Warrington EK (1989) Dynamic aphasia: the selective impairment of verbal planning. Cortex 25:103–114

Damasio AR, Tranel D (1993) Nouns and verbs are retrieved with differently distributed neural systems. Proc Natl Acad Sci USA 90:4957–4960

Damasio H, Grabowski TJ, Tranel D, Hichwa RD, Damasio AR (1996) A neural basis for lexical retrieval. Nature 380:499–505

Demb JB, Desmond JE, Wagner AD, Vaidya CJ, Glover GH, Gabrieli JDE (1995) Semantic encoding and retrieval in the left inferior prefrontal cortex: a functional MRI study of task difficulty and process specificity. J Neurosci 15:5870–5878

Démonet J-F, Chollet F, Ramsay S et al (1992) The anatomy of phonological and semantic processing in normal subjects. Brain 115:1753–1768

Desimone R, Gross CG (1979) Visual areas in the temporal cortex of the macaque. Brain Res 178:363–380

Eulitz C, Elbert T, Bartenstein P, Weiller C, Müller SP, Pantev C (1994) Comparison of magnetic and metabolic brain activity during a verb generation task. Neuroreport 6:97–100

Felleman DJ, Van Essen DC (1991) Distributed hierarchical processing in the primate cerebral cortex. Cereb Cortex 1:1–47

Fiez JA, Raichle ME, Balota DA, Tallal P, Petersen SE (1996) PET activation of posterior temporal regions during auditory word presentation and verb generation. Cereb Cortex 6:1–10

Freedman M, Alexander MP, Naeser MA (1984) Anatomic basis of transcortical motor aphasia. Neurology 40:409–417

Frith CD, Friston KJ, Liddle PF, Frackowiak RSJ (1991) A PET study of word finding. Neuropsychologia 29:1137–1148

Frost JA, Springer JA, Binder JR, Hammeke TA, Bellgowan PSF, Rao SM, Cox RW (1997) Sex does not determine functional lateralization of semantic processing: evidence from fMRI. Neuroimage 5:S564

Galaburda AM, Pandya DN (1983) The intrinsic architectonic and connectional organization of the superior temporal region of the rhesus monkey. J Comp Neurol 221:169–184

Galaburda AM, LeMay M, Kemper T, Geschwind N (1978) Right-left asymmetries in the brain. Structural differences between the hemispheres may underlie cerebral dominance. Science 199:852–856

Geschwind N (1971) Aphasia. N Engl J Med 284:654–656

Haier RG, Siegel BV, MacLachlan A et al (1992) Regional glucose metabolic changes after learning a complex visuospatial/motor task: a positron emission tomographic study. Brain Res 570:134–143

Halpern DF (1992) Sex differences in cognitive abilities, 2nd edn. Erlbaum, Hillsdale.

Hart J, Gordon B (1990) Delineation of single-word semantic comprehension deficits in aphasia, with anatomic correlation. Ann Neurol 27:226–231

Henschen SE (1920–1922) Klinische und Anatomische Beitrage zur Pathologie des Gehirns. Nordiska Bokhandeln, Stockholm

Herholz K, Peitrzyk U, Karbe H, Würker M, Wienhard K, Heiss W-D (1994) Individual metabolic anatomy of repeating words demonstrated by MRI-guided positron emission tomography. Neurosci Lett 182:47–50

Hikosawa K, Iwai E, Saito H-A, Tanaka K (1988) Polysensory properties of neurons in the anterior bank of the caudal superior temporal sulcus of the macaque monkey. J Neurophysiol 60:1615–1637

Hillis AE, Caramazza A (1991) Category-specific naming and comprehension impairment: a double dissociation. Brain 114:2081–2094

Howard D, Patterson K, Wise R, Brown WD, Friston K, Weiller C, Frackowiak R (1992) The cortical localization of the lexicons. Brain 115:1769–1782

Indefrey P, Kleinschmidt A, Merboldt K-D, Krüger G, Brown C, Hagoort P, Frahm J (1997) Equivalent responses to lexical and nonlexical visual stimuli in occipital cortex: a functional magnetic resonance imaging study. Neuroimage 5:78–81

Jones EG, Powell TSP (1970) An anatomical study of converging sensory pathways within the cerebral cortex of the monkey. Brain 93:793–820

Kawashima R, Itoh M, Hatazawa J, Miyazawa H, Yamada K, Matsuzawa T, Fukuda H (1993) Chnages of regional cerebral blood flow during listening to an unfamiliar spoken language. Neurosci Lett 161:69–72

Kim KHS, Relkin NR, Lee K-M, Hirsch J (1997) Distinct cortical areas associated with native and second languages. Nature 388:171–174

Klein D, Milner B, Zatorre RJ et al (1995) The neural substrates underlying word generation: a bilingual functional imaging study. Proc Natl Acad Sci USA 92:2899–2903

Lichtheim L (1885) On aphasia. Brain 7:433–484

Macleod CM (1991) Half a century of research on the Stroop effect: an integrative review. Psychol Bull 109:163–203

Marcel AJ (1983) Conscious and unconscious perception: experiments on visual masking and word recognition. Cogn Psychol 15:197–237

Marie P (1906) Revision de la question de l'aphasie: la troisième circonvolution frontale gauche ne joue aucun rôle spécial dans la fonction du langage. Sem Med 26:241–247

Martin A, Wiggs CL, Ungerleider LG, Haxby JV (1996) Neural correlates of category-specific knowledge. Nature 379:649–652

Mazoyer BM, Tzourio N, Frak V et al (1993) The cortical representation of speech. J Cogn Neurosci 5:467–479

Mendelson JR, Cynader MS (1985) Sensitivity of cat primary auditory cortex (AI) to the direction and rate of frequency modulation. Brain Res 327:331–335

Merzenich MM, Brugge JF (1973) Representation of the cochlear partition on the superior temporal plane of the macaque monkey. Brain Res 60:315–333

Mesulam M (1985) Patterns in behavioral neuroanatomy: association areas, the limbic system, and hemispheric specialization. In: Mesulam M (ed) Principles of behavioral neurology. Davis, Philadelphia, pp 1–70

Mesulam M-M, Pandya DN (1973) The projections of the medial geniculate complex within the Sylvian fissure of the rhesus monkey. Brain Res 60:315–333

Mohr JP (1976) Broca's area and Broca's aphasia. In: Whitaker H (ed) Studies in neurolinguistics. Academic, New York, pp 201–236

Morel A, Garraghty PE, Kaas JH (1993) Tonotopic organization, architectonic fields, and connections of auditory cortex in Macaque monkeys. J Comp Neurol 335:437–459

O'Leary DS, Andreasen NC, Hurtig RR et al (1996) A positron emission tomography study of binaurally and dichotically presented stimuli: effects of level of language and directed attention. Brain Lang 53:20–39

Paulesu E, Goldacre B, Scifo P et al (1997) Functional heterogeneity of left inferior frontal cortex as revealed by fMRI. Neuroreport 8:2011–2016

Petersen SE, Fox PT, Posner MI, Mintun M, Raichle ME (1988) Positron emission tomographic studies of the cortical anatomy of single-word processing. Nature 331:585–589

Phillips DP, Irvine DRF (1981) Responses of single neurons in physiologically defined primary auditory cortex (AI) of the cat: frequency tuning and responses to intensity. J Neurophysiol 45:48–58

Price CJ, Wise RJS, Watson JDG, Patterson K, Howard D, Frackowiak RSJ (1994) Brain activity during reading. The effects of exposure duration and task. Brain 117:1255–1269

Price CJ, Moore CJ, Friston KJ (1996a) Getting sex into perspective. Neuroimage 3:S586

Price CJ, Wise RSJ, Frackowiak RSJ (1996b) Demonstrating the implicit processing of visually presented words and pseudowords. Cereb Cortex 6:62–70

Price CJ, Wise RJS, Warburton EA et al (1996c) Hearing and saying. The functional neuro-anatomy of auditory word processing. Brain 119:919–931

Pugh KR, Shaywitz BA, Shaywitz SE et al (1996) Cerebral organization of component processes in reading. Brain 119:1221–1238

Raichle ME, Fiez JA, Videen TO, MacLeod AM, Pardo JV, Fox PT, Petersen SE (1994) Practice-related changes in human brain functional anatomy during nonmotor learning. Cereb Cortex 4:8–26

Rapcsak SZ, Rubens AB (1994) Localization of lesions in transcortical aphasia. In: Kertesz A (ed) Localization and neuroimaging in neuropsychology. Academic, San Diego, pp 297–329

Rauschecker JP, Tian B, Hauser M (1995) Processing of complex sounds in the Macaque nonprimary auditory cortex. Science 268:111–114

Rauschecker JP, Tian B, Pons T, Mishkin M (1997) Serial and parallel processing in Rhesus monkey auditory cortex. J Comp Neurol 382:89–103

Rubens AB (1976) Transcortical motor aphasia. In: Whitaker H (ed) Studies in neurolinguistics. Academic, New York, pp 293–306

Seltzer B, Pandya DN (1994) Parietal, temporal, and occipital projections to cortex of the superior temporal sulcus in the rhesus monkey: a retrograde tracer study. J Comp Neurol 343:445–463

Shaywitz BA, Pugh KR, Constable T et al (1995a) Localization of semantic processing using functional magnetic resonance imaging. Human Brain Map 2:149–158

Shaywitz BA, Shaywitz SE, Pugh KR et al (1995b) Sex differences in the functional organization of the brain for language. Nature 373:607–609

Shulman GL, Fiez JA, Corbetta M, Buckner RL, Meizin FM, Raichle ME, Petersen SE (1997) Common blood flow changes across visual tasks: II. Decreases in cerebral cortex. J Cogn Neurosci 9:648–663

Smith CD, Andersen AH, Chen Q, Blonder LX, Kirsch JE, Avison MJ (1996) Cortical activation in confrontation naming. Neuroreport 7:781–785

Springer JA, Binder JR, Hammeke TA et al (1997) Variability of language lateralization in normal controls and epilepsy patients: an fMRI study. Neuroimage 5:S581

Stuss DT, Benson DF (1986) The frontal lobes. Raven, New York

Tamas LB, Shibasaki T, Horikoshi S, Ohye C (1993) General activation of cerebral metabolism with speech: a PET study. Int J Psychophysiol 14:199–208

Tanaka Y, Yamadori A, Mori E (1987) Pure word deafness following bilateral lesions: a psychophysical analysis. Brain 110:381–403

Van Orden GC (1987) A ROWS is a ROSE: Spelling, sound, and reading. Mem Cogn 15:181–198

Vandenberghe R, Price C, Wise R, Josephs O, Frackowiak RSJ (1996) Functional anatomy of a common semantic system for words and pictures. Nature 383:254–256

Warburton E, Wise RJS, Price CJ, Weiller C, Hadar U, Ramsay S, Frackowiak RSJ (1996) Noun and verb retrieval by normal subjects. Studies with PET. Brain 119:159–179

Warrington EK, Shallice T (1984) Category specific semantic impairments. Brain 107:829–854

Wernicke C (1874) Der aphasische Symptomenkomplex. Cohn and Weigert, Breslau

Wise R, Chollet F, Hadar U, Friston K, Hoffner E, Frackowiak R (1991) Distribution of cortical neural networks involved in word comprehension and word retrieval. Brain 114:1803–1817

Yetkin FZ, Hammeke TA, Swanson SJ, Morris GL, Mueller WM, McAuliffe TL, Haughton VM (1995) A comparison of functional MR activation patterns during silent and audible language tasks. Am J Neuroradiol 16:1087–1092

Yetkin O, Yetkin FZ, Haughton VM, Cox RW (1996) Use of functional MR to map language in multilingual volunteers. Am J Neuroradiol 17:473–477

Zatorre RJ, Evans AC, Meyer E, Gjedde A (1992) Lateralization of phonetic and pitch discrimination in speech processing. Science 256:846–849

34 Direct Comparison of Functional MRI and PET

N.F. Ramsey

CONTENTS

34.1
Introduction

34.1.1
Functional Imaging Techniques

Functional processes in the brain can be detected by direct measurement of electrical activity, i.e., electrical encephalography (EEG), or of magnetic fields induced by electric activity, i.e., magneto-encephalography (MEG), or by measurement of changes in blood dynamics. The latter can be achieved by recording radioactive tracers administered to the blood, which is done with positron emission tomography (PET) and single photon emission computed tomography (SPECT). With the advent of fast computers and high-sensitivity g-cameras, PET scanners have reached a high level of spatial and temporal resolution, i.e. on the order of 5 mm and 40 s (for a detailed overview see Aine 1995). These resolution variables form the basis of the application of any imaging method, in the sense that they determine the kind of brain process that can be measured. EEG and MEG, for instance, allow for very high sampling rates in time and can be used to distinguish short brain activity events from one another, but are limited in the accuracy of localization of such activity (typically on the order of centimeters). PET, on the other hand, measures relatively sustained brain processes, while generating fairly detailed maps of active foci. An important disadvantage of PET and SPECT is that these methods require use of radioactive compounds. Furthermore, PET scanning is quite costly, requiring not only a camera, but also a cyclotron and skilled personnel, and can only be done in a limited number of sites.

The demand for imaging techniques is growing fast, particularly in the fields of neuroscience, neurology and psychiatry. This growth is particularly noticeable in the explosive number of reports on functional magnetic resonance imaging (fMRI), the most promising new imaging technique. The widespread availability of MRI scanners, combined with their relatively low cost and absence of health hazards involved in their use, has prompted a multitude of research projects focused on mechanisms underlying cognitive processing in healthy subjects.

34.1.2
Blood Oxygen Level-Dependent
fMRI Techniques

For fMRI, several methods are currently available. The most widely used family of techniques makes use of the effect of deoxyhemoglobin on MRI signal, the so-called blood oxygen level-dependent (BOLD) signal change (Ogawa et al. 1992). Most of the BOLD pulse sequences use gradient-recalled echoes but

N.F. Ramsey, PhD; Dept. of Psychiatry, University Hospital of Utrecht, Room A.01.126, Heidelberglaan 100, 3584 CX, Utrecht, Netherlands

differ in the way that the image information is acquired, i.e., the way k-space is built up. In echo planar imaging (EPI) (Belliveau et al. 1992; Kwong et
al. 1992; Turner 1992) and in 2D spiral imaging
(Noll et al. 1995; Yang et al. 1996), information is
acquired per slice by reading all the k-space lines
within one excitation period, or TR. Multiple slices
are scanned in an interleaved sequence, resulting in
a stack of slices which constitute a volume. In fast
low-angle shot imaging (FLASH) (Frahm et al. 1992;
Menon et al. 1992) information is also acquired per
slice, but it requires multiple excitation periods, as
only one k-space line is acquired per TR. Again,
slices are scanned sequentially and form a volume
after stacking. One of the few techniques that acquire information in a 3D fashion, is PRESTO (principles of echo-shifting with a train of observations;
Liu et al. 1993; van Gelderen et al. 1995; Ramsey et
al. 1996b). This technique can be regarded as a special form of segmented EPI, in the sense that several
echoes are acquired per TR, but with two additional
features, namely, echo-shifting, which reduces scan
time by a factor of two, and 3D acquisition. The differences between the techniques are most obvious in
the images they generate. The important features
include: image stability, i.e., signal fluctuation across
repeated acquisitions, spatial integrity, i.e., correspondence of shape between the original object (the
brain) and the image, sensitivity to motion of the
scanned subject, and amount of "tissue loss" near
cranial cavities.

EPI and spiral are very fast (e.g., a 24-slice volume
in 2 s) and exhibit fair image stability (Duyn et al.
1996). Motion during acquisition, however, causes
distortion of the images and can result in misalign-
ment of the sequentially acquired slices. Tissue near
cranial cavities (tissue-air interface) is difficult to
image due to loss of signal. With FLASH, such tissue
loss is reduced, but scan speed is much lower.
PRESTO requires 6 s to acquire one volume with
conventional gradients. Due to the use of strong
"crusher gradients" (for echo-shifting), the images
are sensitive to motion and exhibit lower image stability than EPI or FLASH (Duyn et al. 1996). However, the latest version of the PRESTO pulse sequence
is greatly improved in this regard by incorporation
of a "navigator echo," which enables correction of
motion (Ramsey et al. 1998), and by the availability
of fast scanner gradient sets (van Gelderen et al.
1997). This version reduces scan time by a factor of 3
or 4.

34.1.3
Limitations of fMRI

The mechanisms underlying BOLD signal change
are not fully understood. For instance, whereas interpretation of positive task-related signal change is
fairly straightforward, that of negative changes is
not. Factors that are not directly related to neuronal
activity, such as inflow effects, draining vein signal,
stimulus-correlated motion and signal fluctuation
near cranial cavities and large blood vessels, have
been shown to cause signal change which is nearly
impossible to distinguish from the BOLD effect. Another complication in fMRI is the fact that detectability of BOLD signal change is not homogeneous
in the brain. Due to macroscopic susceptibility near
the cavities, signal intensity in tissue in the
orbitofrontal and inferior-temporal cortices is very
low, whereas signal variance in these regions is at
least as high as in the other parts of the brain. Signal
variance is increased in regions near moving tissue
such as the eyes and eye muscles, and near the circle
of Willis. These factors create inhomogeneity of signal variance, resulting in an uneven distribution of
sensitivity for BOLD signal change. In other words,
detection of neuronal activity with fMRI is easier in
some areas than in others.

For any new research tool, it is important to evaluate the advantages and disadvantages relative to preexisting tools. One way of gaining insight in the
properties of fMRI in this regard, is to perform experiments which allow for comparisons between
predicted and obtained results. In a general sense, an
imaging tool should meet at least three criteria: (1)
sensitivity, i.e., high contrast-to-noise ratio, (2) validity, i.e., selective detection of stimulus-related
brain activity combined with low sensitivity for nonspecific activity, and (3) reliability, i.e., good reproducibility of individual brain activity maps. Fundamental research into the mechanisms underlying the
BOLD effect is very important in determining the
quality of fMRI as a research tool, but in the end the
quality is judged by the results of experimental application. One way to assess the quality is by means
of cross-validation with a gold standard. The best
candidate for this is $H_2^{15}O$-PET, which is an established technique for imaging blood dynamics
coupled to neuronal activity. One of the most reliable
activation procedures is motor stimulation by movement of the fingers, which has been studied extensively with PET, with various other imaging methods
and with cortical stimulation during cerebral surgery. In this chapter, the results of a study that was

specifically designed to compare fMRI to $H_2^{15}O$-PET are summarized and explained.

34.2
Direct Quantitative Comparison of PET and 3D fMRI

34.2.1
Procedure

The most direct way to cross-validate fMRI with a gold standard is to apply both imaging methods to the same subjects with the same stimulation procedure. This experiment was done with 3D PRESTO and $H_2^{15}O$-PET, at the National Institute of Mental Health, with nine healthy volunteers (RAMSEY et al. 1996a). In this study, finger tapping was performed at a rate of 2 Hz, for a total of 8 min in the fMRI experiment, in runs of 30 s alternated with 30 s periods of rest. In the PET experiment, four runs of 4 min of finger tapping were alternated with 4-min rest runs. The PET procedure was divided into two PET sessions, spaced several weeks apart. The finger tap rate was verified at the bedside by one of the researchers.

34.2.2
Image Processing

Image registration was performed for each individual at two levels : (1) one functional volume (per imaging modality) to one and the same structural MRI scan, using surface matching, and (2) functional volumes to the MRI-registered functional volume (also per imaging modality), using the AIR program (WOODS et al. 1992) for the PET volumes and a special program for fMRI (THEVENAZ et al. 1995). For meaningful PET-fMRI comparison, the spatial resolution of both volume sets needed to be equal. For this purpose, the resolutions were calculated on the basis of scanner properties and were then modified with appropriate 3D Gaussian filters. The final computed resolution was 8.7 mm isotropic for both modalities. The voxel size of both modalities was also made equal and determined the number of voxels analyzed subsequently. The voxel size, based on the fMRI acquisition, was 3.75 mm isotropic and required regridding of the PET volumes.

Statistical analyses, applied to the functional data sets for each individual subject separately, entailed a Bonferroni-corrected z_t-statistic of the difference between the active state (finger tapping) and the rest state for each voxel in the superior part of the brain (VAN GELDEREN et al. 1995). This method is comparable to Worsley's approach (WORSLEY 1994), which is based on the theory of random Gaussian fields, but the Bonferroni-based threshold determination proved to be less conservative than his, due to the fact that the ratio of full width at half maximum (FWHM) and voxel size was less than three. On average, the critical z_t-score was 4.4, corresponding to a voxel-wise p-value of 4.5×10^{-6}, and to an omnibus p-value of 0.05 (one-sided). Subsequent analyses involved determination of the center-of-mass of activity in the contralateral primary sensorimotor cortex (PSM), mean percent signal change, distance of center-of-mass to the middle knee of the central sulcus, where the hand is represented, and distance between the PET and the fMRI center of mass.

34.2.3
Findings

After careful image registration and equalization of image smoothness (FWHM), the final step involved direct comparison of the statistical maps of both imaging methods within subjects. Significant activity was found in the contralateral PSM in all subjects and with both imaging techniques. The statistical maps were very selective in that only a small part of the analyzed brain volume was indicated as active (fMRI: 0.5%, PET: 0.3%). Of the total number of activated voxels, 78% were located in the PSM (equally for both methods), indicating selectivity for task related brain activity. Most of the remaining active voxels were located in the supplementary motor area (fMRI: 8%, PET: 14%), but this region was not activated in all subjects (fMRI: 5, PET: 6). Further comparisons were focused on the contralateral PSM, and involved several variables : size or extent (number of active voxels within PSM), magnitude (mean z_t-score of active PSM voxels), and location of PSM activity. Location was determined by calculating the center-of-mass of active PSM voxels, weighted by the z_t-scores, and was converted to Talairach coordinates. There was no difference in either extent or magnitude of PSM activity between PET and fMRI. On average, the z_t-score in activated PSM voxels was 5.5±0.8 for fMRI and 5.3±0.4 for PET. The actual percent signal change did differ (fMRI 0.99%, PET 30.4%), but the corresponding difference in standard deviation of the difference images within individuals results in an equal sensitivity for motor cortex activity. The mean size of the activated regions was 46 voxels for fMRI and 27 voxels with PET, but this was not significantly different, possibly due to a large variability in the fMRI data. The extent of activation was highly correlated between the imaging methods (r=0.87), suggesting that this variable is specific for individual subjects. With both PET and fMRI, the location of PSM activity, i.e., the center-of-mass, was very close to the middle knee of the central sulcus (on average: fMRI 2.2 mm, PET 3.5 mm). This indicates that both techniques are capable of accurately localizing the primary sensory and motor cortices responsible for finger movements. Between fMRI and PET, the location of PSM activity differed on average by 6.7 mm (Euclidian distance), but in Talairach coordinates the mean distance was less than 2 mm in either the x-, y- or z-direction. The activated areas with PET and fMRI overlapped in all subjects. In Fig. 34.1, the resulting z_t-maps for all subjects are displayed. For each subject the one slice closest to both the PET and the fMRI center-of-mass (in the PSM) is selected for presentation of the similarity of activity maps. In the fMRI z_t-maps, low frequency areas of sub-threshold signal change are apparent, whereas the PET z_t-maps exhibit patchy areas of sub-threshold signal change. The source of the low frequency patterns in the PRESTO fMRI maps appears to be related to respiration (NOLL and SCHNEIDER 1997). When correcting for this type of noise, as is done with the latest PRESTO technique in which navigator phase correction is applied (VAN DEN BRINK et al. 1997; RAMSEY et al. 1998), the low frequency signal fluctuations are reduced dramatically (Fig. 34.2). Navigator correction in PRESTO improves image stability by approximately 20%–50%, depending on image (in)stability, and therefore yields higher sensitivity to activity-related BOLD signal change than that of the pulse sequence used in the present study.

The findings indicate a high degree of agreement between the two imaging techniques. It is important to note that the results of this study rely very much on the functional modality, i.e., motor activity, and on the way the data were processed and statistically evaluated. Concerning the latter, careful measures were taken to meet criteria for comparing the data sets in terms of activation protocol, image smoothness and voxel size. Application of the Bonferroni correction method to statistical threshold determination may be perceived as conservative, but it is appropriate for the purpose of unbiased brain activity mapping. Mapping involves a search for active brain regions without a priori assumptions about either occurrence or location of activity, and as such requires testing against a null hypothesis which states that no activity is present. Under these circumstances, it is appropriate to adhere to the classic consensus of assuming a false positive rate of 0.05, i.e., an omnibus p-value of 0.05 per study (subject). Lower thresholds can of course be applied if selective regions are targeted a priori, but for the present study this was not the case, as determination of regional selectivity of detected activation was one of the objectives.

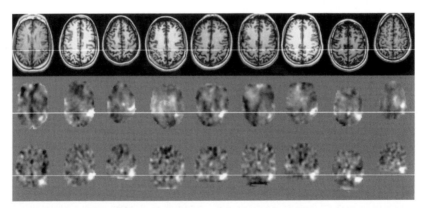

Fig.34.1. Summary of nine subjects, one anatomical slice per subject (*top row*), with corresponding z_t-map slice of the fMRI experiment (*middle row*) and PET experiment (*bottom row*). For each subject the slice nearest to (or on top of) the active primary sensorimotor cortex (PSM) foci of both techniques was selected. The location of the *white lines* in the bottom rows corresponds to the line on the anatomical slices

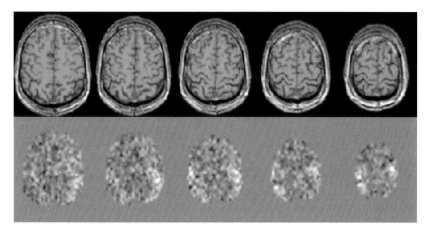

Fig. 34.2. Example of a bimanual finger tap (2 Hz) off-on experiment with fast navigated PRESTO (33 slices in 3 s; 72 scans). Five consecutive slices are shown of the statistical map (*bottom row*), with corresponding anatomy (*top row*), for one subject. Images are smoothed for comparison to Fig. 34.1

34.3
Properties of 3D PRESTO as an Imaging Tool

34.3.1
Sensitivity

The direct comparison results indicate that fMRI can equal PET in terms of sensitivity for sensorimotor cortex activity, as both extent and magnitude of signal change were roughly the same. For most motor studies, half the number of fMRI scans is generally sufficient to achieve near 100% detection rate across subjects (van Gelderen et al. 1995; Ramsey et al. 1996b). This may also be the case for PET, but the small number of PET scans would require another statistical approach for single-subject analysis. It could be argued that, in the PET procedure, only the first 60 s of each scan were relevant, as most of the signal is acquired in that period (implying that the results actually require only 4 min of finger tapping). Re-analysis of only the first half of each MRI data set (corresponding to a total of 4 min of finger tapping) yielded an average of 24 active voxels in the contralateral sensorimotor cortex, which is still comparable to the 27 voxels detected with PET. However, in some of the subjects, activity was no longer significant in this re-analysis, which was probably due to the smoothing operation. The same subjects had the smallest activations in the original, unsmoothed, analysis. Without smoothing, significant activity was present in all subject (mean 20 voxels in the PSM), which indicates that even moderate spatial smoothing can reduce sensitivity for focal

brain activity in fMRI. In general, the FWHM of any data set determines the size of activated regions for which subsequent analysis is most sensitive (Poline et al. 1997).

It is common practice to average PET maps across subjects before statistical evaluation (Friston et al. 1991), which requires a considerable degree of spatial smoothing to deal with intersubject anatomical variation. The recent trend toward applying this approach to fMRI data appears to be successful and suggests that the two imaging techniques are also comparable after group-wise map averaging (see below). It is noteworthy, however, that in fMRI sensitivity for activation of small brain structures is likely to get lost with substantial smoothing.

Good agreement has been reported between EPI and PET, with a graded motor activation procedure, in a qualitative comparison of activity maps in three subjects (Sadato et al. 1997). In a comparison study between single-slice FLASH and $H_2^{15}O$-PET, Dettmers et al. (1996) also found good agreement, with distances between activation peaks between 2 and 8 mm. Their FLASH results indicated a higher variability in the magnitude of motor activity related signal change (5.0%±0.9%) than with PET (13.7%±1.2%), whereas in our study the PRESTO results were less variable in comparison to PET (0.99%±0.09% vs 30.4%±6.5%). The difference in percent signal change with PET are probably related to the difference in activation paradigm (Dettmers et al. used a 1 Hz key press protocol with varying degrees of press-force). The PRESTO results do appear to be more consistent than the FLASH findings. In one study, the relationship between (auditory) stimulus presentation rate and BOLD signal change was compared to that of PET signal change (REES et al. 1997). In this carefully designed single-subject study, the BOLD effect proved to be nonlinear, tapering off towards higher stimulus rates, in contrast with PET.

An important question is whether the techniques perform equally with other stimulation procedures, such as those involving cognitive functions. This issue has been addressed in several papers, in an indirect way. PAULESU et al. (1995) compared activity patterns related to verbal working memory generated by single-slice FLASH and $H_2^{15}O$-PET in three subjects. They reported agreement in two of the three subjects, within the commonly imaged brain sections. Their comparison was, however, limited to qualitative evaluation and by differences in spatial resolutions. The authors suggested that better agreement may be achieved with 3D fMRI data sets, as motion correction and inflow effects were difficult to control for with FLASH. In a later paper, they reported that with multislice EPI, verbal fluency activity maps agreed, in a group-average analysis, with those obtained with PET (PAULESU et al. 1997). The advantage of fMRI was that the higher spatial resolution of fMRI enabled differentiation between closely located regions, resulting in detection of functionally separated regions within Broca's area. Spatial agreement has also been found with other frontal lobe activating paradigms, such as reading aloud (SMALL et al. 1996), verb generation (XIONG et al. 1998), verbal fluency (PHELPS et al. 1997) and externally cued finger tapping (HYDER et al. 1997). In the latter two studies the EPI results were compared to PET results from another study. The group-average maps were normalized in Talairach space, and specific activated regions were compared in terms of centers-of-mass in 3D coordinates. In spite of the fact that anatomic variability results in different average anatomic maps between groups of subjects, the compared centers of mass were located between 6 and 14 mm apart. One of the difficulties in using fMRI is underlined by these two studies (HYDER et al. 1997; PHELPS et al. 1997), in which almost half of the subjects were dropped from analyses due to motion artifacts.

34.3.2
Validity

The presence of non-task related activations in the statistical maps should be minimal for imaging purposes, particularly in studies aimed at functional topographical mapping. In the direct comparison study, 80% of all activated voxels were found within the primary sensorimotor cortex. The other 20% was not distributed in any consistent pattern in either imaging modality. Most of these voxels were, however, located in secondary motor areas (RAMSEY et al. 1996a). The combination of acquisition technique and post-processing thus yielded a high degree of validity (in terms of activation selectivity) in both fMRI and PET. It could be argued that lower statistical thresholds result in greater sensitivity for activity in less powerfully activated (secondary) regions, but the price for such an approach is that more activations will be found in arbitrary locations, thereby sacrificing topographical task selectivity. The tradeoff between sensitivity and selectivity can be decided upon on the basis of the objective of a particular study. Obviously, selectivity is essential for functional mapping applications, whereas sensitivity is more important when target regions are known a priori. Compared to PET, fMRI offers some freedom in this respect, as scanning can be prolonged to increase statistical power, and thereby sensitivity, while maintaining selectivity.

34.3.3
Reliability

fMRI has been tested for reproducibility by comparing test-retest results within subjects (RAMSEY et al. 1996b; ROMBOUTS et al. 1998). With PRESTO, repeating scan sessions with a finger opposition task yields nearly identical maps, using the same statistical procedure as described earlier (RAMSEY et al. 1996b). Although the activity patterns in the maps were reproducible, the numbers of activated voxels in motor areas was rather variable within subjects. This may be the result of varying image stability across scan sessions, or it may reflect an effect of learning. Reproducibility of activity maps generated by execution of cognitive tasks may not be as good as when generated by simple motor or visual stimulation, due to the fact that it is difficult to invoke all the functions of interest, which are thought to participate in networks, continually. Some cognitive functions are easier to detect than others, depending on the relative contribution of each to the execution of a given task.

34.4
Issues of Concern in fMRI

34.4.1
Draining Veins

The question whether fMRI brain activity maps reflect signal change in and around draining veins is of great importance for clinical applications such as presurgical planning. The comparison with $H_2{}^{15}O$-PET does not quite address this issue, because PET images may also contain signal in draining veins (AINE 1995). The results of the direct comparison study at least indicate that there is no systematic difference in location of PSM activity between the two imaging techniques. Subsequent investigation of the contribution of draining vein signal in PRESTO indicates that signal within veins with diameters greater than 4 mm is virtually absent, due to the use of strong magnetic gradients (crushers) in the pulse sequence (GRANDIN et al. 1997). The crushers induce a phase dispersion in these veins, where blood in the center travels at higher speeds than blood near the vessel walls. Currently, this effect is specific for the direction of the veins, but modifications of the pulse sequence may extend the effect to multiple directions. The effects of draining vein signal on surrounding tissue may still be a matter of concern, because voxels located near the surface of these veins may be affected by changes in deoxyhemoglobin concentration, and perhaps even by changes in vein diameter. As of yet it is not clear how strong these effects are. One way to investigate the functional-topographical accuracy of any fMRI technique is to make use of a neuronavigational tool. Currently, these computerized 3D localization tools are available which enable direct intraoperative integration of MRI image information with surgical stereotactic microscopes. The locations of motor or language areas, as determined by neural electrostimulation which is often done during surgery on epileptic patients, can thus be compared directly with 3D fMRI activation maps.

34.4.2
Image Resolution

Although fMRI has the potential for sub-millimeter spatial resolution, it is not clear whether such high resolutions are always desirable. Given the high sensitivity of fMRI techniques for motion, which in practice easily amounts to millimeters, it seems logical to adhere to voxel sizes in the order of 3–4 mm. Higher resolutions by definition increase scan time, hence increasing motion sensitivity, and reduce signal-to-noise ratio, requiring increased numbers of scans to avoid loss of sensitivity for BOLD effects. This is, however, more of a problem for unbiased mapping applications than for applications in which specific brain regions are targeted. In the latter case, scan time can be reduced by limiting the acquisition matrix size or field of view. On one hand, reduction of scan time results in lower signal-to-noise ratio, thereby reducing image stability, but on the other hand it improves stability by reducing motion sensitivity, as it reduces the amount of motion that is captured within one acquisition. Short scan times also increase the correlation between scans, because the physiological processes which contribute to fMRI signal, in particular hemodynamic responses to neuronal activity, are temporally smoothed (ZARAHN et al. 1997). Many fMRI researchers acknowledge this effect indirectly, by recognizing the fact that the BOLD effect requires approximately 6 s to develop fully. Although short activation episodes can be detected (AINE 1995; BUCKNER et al. 1996), discrimination between consecutive bursts of activity is rather limited due to the hemodynamic temporal smoothness (BANDETTINI et al. 1992; KWONG et al. 1992). High correlations in time series of images reduces statistical power, which can be compensated for by increasing the number of scans per experimental condition.

34.4.3
Regional Susceptibility Effects

As mentioned earlier, fMRI signal in tissue adjacent to cranial cavities is very low. As a result, BOLD signal change cannot be detected reliability (if at all) in orbitofrontal cortex and in parts of the inferior temporal cortices. Unfortunately, this limitation of fMRI techniques is rarely mentioned in the literature. To illustrate this phenomenon, brain coverage with PRESTO is displayed in Fig. 34.3, where the outline of an fMRI volume is projected onto the anatomical scan. The arrows indicate the regions near cranial cavities, i.e., inferior temporal cortex and orbitofrontal cortex, where tissue signal is lost. The volume was acquired with fast gradients (3 s for a 33-slice volume), with TE of 32–44 ms (acquisition window for 17 echoes). It should be noted that with longer TEs, as is often the case for single-shot EPI, loss of tissue signal is more extensive. At present, $H_2{}^{15}O$-

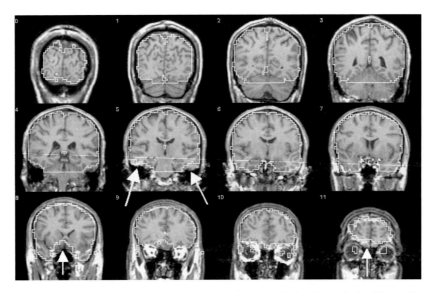

Fig. 34.3. PRESTO coverage of brain tissue. After registration with an anatomical volume obtained from the same subject, the outline of a PRESTO fMRI volume was projected onto the corresponding anatomical slices. Every third slice of the imaged volume is shown transaxially, bottom-to-top, in radiological orientation (left of each slice is right hemisphere and vice versa). The *arrows* indicate where the fMRI signal from brain-tissue is lost due to adjacent cranial cavities

PET is still the better technique for imaging of these cortices, even more so with the advent of 3D scanners with retractable septa, which require lower doses of radioactive tracer (i.e. 10 millicuries compared to 40 millicuries in 2D scanners) allowing for higher numbers of scans per experimental condition (see AINE 1995).

34.4.4
Regional Instability

In the majority of fMRI studies, analysis involves voxel-wise parametric or non-parametric statistics, in which the variance of signal in individual voxels directly affects the final variable (e.g. *t* value, cross-correlation). An important side-effect of this approach is that sensitivity for BOLD effects is not homogeneous across the brain, because the variance of signal is not homogeneous across voxels. Voxels near cranial cavities and near large pulsing arteries and veins generally exhibit very high variance. For those voxels, in order to detect a significant experimental effect, i.e., to exceed a globally determined *t* threshold, the (percent) signal change has to be accordingly high. There is however no reason why the BOLD signal change induced (indirectly) by neuronal activity would vary much across the brain. Use of *t* scores, or equivalents thereof, thus obscures the fact that fMRI is spatially biased. This appears to be

less dramatic in PET studies. To visualize this, two slices from standard deviation maps are shown in Fig. 34.4 for five techniques, i.e., one slice from the superior brain, and one from the inferior part near the cranial cavities and large blood vessels. For each technique, the two standard deviation slice-maps are scaled such that inhomogeneity of voxel variances is displayed optimally. For PET, the 2D technique used for the comparison study is shown (Fig. 34.4A), as well as a 3D PET technique with septa retracted (Fig. 34.4B). Both techniques yield relatively homogeneous distributions across the brain, with the exception of the midsagittal plane, where signal variance tends to be high. The unnavigated PRESTO map (Fig. 34.4C) shows increased variance near the base of the brain. The navigated PRESTO maps (Fig. 34.4D), obtained with fast gradients (van den Brink et al. 1997; van Gelderen et al. 1997), exhibit increased variance near the brainstem and circle of Willis. The EPI map (Fig. 34.4E) also exhibits increased variance in these areas, and sometimes (as in this case) along deeper sulci. The five maps differ in terms of spatial smoothness and numbers of scans from which they were derived, and can therefore not be compared directly. However, the point to be made is that image stability is generally not homogeneous across the brain, especially for fMRI, and particularly near large veins and near the brainstem.

Although voxel-wise standard deviation is not spatially homogeneous with PET (it is typically

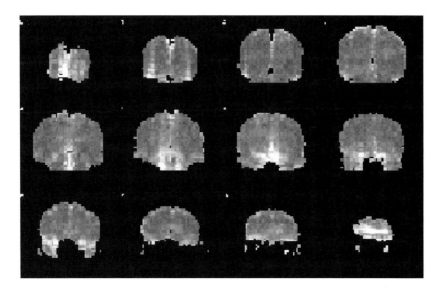

Fig. 34.5. Complete standard deviation map from a fast, navigated PRESTO experiment (TR 3 s, 33 slices). The slices correspond to the slices in Fig. 34.3. Brightness in this map reflects the standard deviation computed, per voxel, over repeated scans, as percent of signal intensity in the functional scans. Note high standard deviation near transverse sinus and around the brainstem

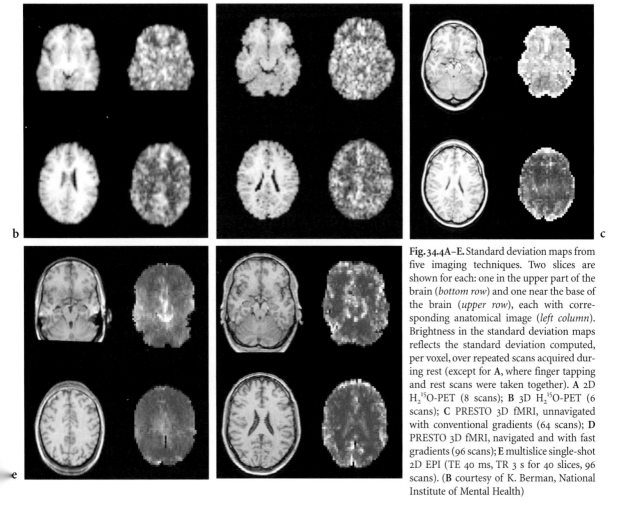

b

c

e

Fig. 34.4A–E. Standard deviation maps from five imaging techniques. Two slices are shown for each: one in the upper part of the brain (*bottom row*) and one near the base of the brain (*upper row*), each with corresponding anatomical image (*left column*). Brightness in the standard deviation maps reflects the standard deviation computed, per voxel, over repeated scans acquired during rest (except for **A**, where finger tapping and rest scans were taken together). **A** 2D $H_2^{15}O$-PET (8 scans); **B** 3D $H_2^{15}O$-PET (6 scans); **C** PRESTO 3D fMRI, unnavigated with conventional gradients (64 scans); **D** PRESTO 3D fMRI, navigated and with fast gradients (96 scans); **E** multislice single-shot 2D EPI (TE 40 ms, TR 3 s for 40 slices, 96 scans). (**B** courtesy of K. Berman, National Institute of Mental Health)

patchy as in Fig. 34.4A, B), it is pretty much the same across the brain, in contrast with fMRI. In Fig. 34.5, the standard deviation map is shown which corresponds to the volume presented in Fig. 34.3. The bright spots (representing high variance) in the first few slices are located near the sagittal and transverse sinuses, the spots in the middle part near the circle of Willis and the large veins which drain into the jugular veins, and the most anterior area (last slice) which borders the frontal cavity and the orbita. The main source of instability appears to be the larger draining veins, although signal from within these is below detection threshold, and to a lesser extent the eyes and eye muscles. For mapping applications, standard deviation maps such as these should be examined for each fMRI technique, to asses homogeneity of sensitivity for activation-related BOLD signal change. In fact, the distribution of instability is not only affected by the technique used, but also by orientation of the imaging plane, location and size of the volume within the brain, and voxel size. Given these factors, comparability of studies would be greatly improved if standard deviation maps as well as coverage maps were made available with publication. With the advent of Internet access to image databases, this should be quite feasible in the near future.

34.5
Summary

Direct, controlled comparison of PET and 3D fMRI has shown that fMRI is an attractive alternative to $H_2^{15}O$-PET, as its properties in terms of sensitivity, validity and reliability can equal those of PET. Other reports, in which PET and fMRI were compared in other ways, either indirectly or by means of group-averaging, extend this finding to other functional modalities, such as cognition. However, several disadvantages limit the application of fMRI, at least at this point in time. For one, BOLD fMRI techniques do not allow for adequate coverage of orbitofrontal and inferior temporal cortices, because signal in tissue adjacent to cranial cavities decays too fast. Furthermore, signal stability in tissue near these regions, as well as tissue near moving parts of the brain, is generally reduced relative to that in the superior part of the brain. This results in a non-homogeneous distribution of sensitivity for BOLD signal change across the brain. The effects of motion on fMRI remains to be a matter of concern, even when

image registration algorithms are applied. This is particularly the case in clinical studies in which patients and controls can be expected to exhibit different degrees of motion (CALLICOTT et al. 1998). If motion during scans is not corrected for adequately, the result may well be a systematic difference in imaging sensitivity, and a corresponding bias towards reduced brain activity in patients.

The BOLD fMRI techniques (FLASH, EPI, PRESTO, spiral and related) differ with regard to sensitivity and to the contribution of the various artifacts such as inflow, draining veins and motion. Generally speaking, 3D acquisition tends to be less sensitive (although with the advent of high-powered whole-body gradient sets and navigator phase correction technology this distinction becomes negligible) than 2D EPI and spiral. 3D has the advantage of whole-brain excitation (which essentially abolishes inflow effects), preservation of spatial integrity (i.e., minimal image warping), straightforward 3D image registration and putatively reduced sensitivity to draining veins (GRANDIN et al. 1997). FLASH appears to be better suited for imaging of tissue near cranial cavities, at least at relatively short echo times. The choice of any of these techniques should be guided by the particular objective of the study.

References

Aine CJ (1995) A conceptual overview and critique of functional neuroimaging techniques in humans: I. MRI/FMRI and PET. Crit Rev Neurobiol 9:229–309

Bandettini PA, Wong EC, Hinks MS, Tifofsky RS, Hyde JS (1992) Time course EPI of human brain function during task activation. Magn Reson Med 25:390–397

Belliveau JW, Kwong KK, Kennedy DN et al (1992) Magnetic resonance imaging mapping of brain function. Invest Radiol 27:S59–S65

Buckner RL, Bandettini PA, Ocraven KM, Savoy RL, Petersen SE, Raichle ME, Rosen BR (1996) Detection of cortical activation during averaged single trials of a cognitive task using functional magnetic resonance imaging. Proc Natl Acad Sci USA 93:14878–14883

Callicott JH, Ramsey NF, Tallent K et al (1998) Functional magnetic resonance imaging brain mapping in psychiatry: methodological issues illustrated in a study of working memory in schizophrenia. Neuropsychopharmacology 18:186–196

Dettmers C, Connelly A, Stephan KM et al (1996) Quantitative comparison of functional magnetic resonance imaging with positron emission tomography using a force- related paradigm. Neuroimage 4:201–209

Duyn JH, Yang YH, Frank JA, Mattay VS, Hou L (1996) Functional magnetic resonance neuroimaging data acquisition techniques. Neuroimage 4:S76–S83

Frahm J, Bruhn H, Merboldt KD, Hanicke W (1992) Dynamic MR imaging of human brain oxygenation during rest and photic stimulation. J Magn Reson Imaging 2:501–505

Friston KJ, Frith CD, Liddle PF, Frackowiak RSJ (1991) Comparing functional (PET) images: the assessment of significant change. J Cereb Blood Flow Metab 11:690–699

Grandin CB, Madio DP, Van Gelderen P, Moonen CTW (1997) Reduction of undesirable signal of large veins in functional MRI with PRESTO. In: Proceedings of the European Society for Magnetic Resonance in Medicine and Biology 14th annual Meeting, held in Brussels, Belgium, p. 54

Hyder F, Phelps EA, Wiggins CJ, Labar KS, Blamire AM, Shulman RG (1997) "Willed action": a functional MRI study of the human prefrontal cortex during a sensorimotor task. Proc Natl Acad Sci USA 94:6989–6994

Kwong KK, Belliveau JW, Chesler DA et al (1992) Dynamic magnetic resonance imaging of human brain activity during primary sensory stimulation. Proc Natl Acad Sci USA 89:5675–5679

Liu G, Sobering GS, Duyn JH, Moonen CTW (1993) A functional MRI technique combining Principles of Echo-shifting with a Train of Observations (PRESTO). Magn Reson Med 30:764–768

Menon RS, Ogawa S, Kim S, Ellermann J, Merkle H, Tank GW, Ugurbil K (1992) Functional brain mapping using magnetic resonance imaging: signal changes accompanying visual stimulation. Invest Radiol 27:S47–S53

Noll DC, Schneider W (1997) Respiration artifacts in functional brain imaging: sources of signal variation and compensation strategies. Proceedings of the Society for Magnetic Resonance in Medicine, Vancouver Canada, 1997, p. 647

Noll DC, Cohen JD, Meyer CH, Schneider W (1995) Spiral k-space MR imaging of cortical activation. J Magn Reson Imaging 5:49–56

Ogawa S, Tank DW, Menon RS, Ellermann J, Kim S, Merkle H, Ugurbil K (1992) Intrinsic signal changes accompanying sensory stimulation: functional brain mapping with magnetic resonance imaging. Proc Natl Acad Sci USA 89:5951–5955

Paulesu E, Connelly A, Frith CD et al (1995) Functional MR imaging correlations with positron emission tomography. Initial experience using a cognitive activation paradigm on verbal working memory. Neuroimaging Clin North Am 5:207–225

Paulesu E, Goldacre B, Scifo P et al (1997) Functional heterogeneity of left inferior frontal cortex as revealed by fMRI. Neuroreport 8:2011–2017

Phelps EA, Hyder F, Blamire AM, Shulman RG (1997) FMRI of the prefrontal cortex during overt verbal fluency. Neuroreport 8:561–565

Poline JB, Worsley KJ, Evans AC, Friston KJ (1997) Combining spatial extent and peak intensity to test for activations in functional imaging. Neuroimage 5:83–96

Ramsey NF, Kirkby BS, Vangelderen T et al (1996a) Functional mapping of human sensorimotor cortex with 3D bold fmri correlates highly with (H2O) O 15 Pet rCBF. J Cereb Blood Flow Metab 16:755–764

Ramsey NF, Tallent K, Van Gelderen P, Frank JA, Moonen CTW, Weinberger DR (1996b) Reproducibility of human3D fMRI brain maps acquired during a motor task. Hum Br Map 4:113–121

Ramsey NF, Van den Brink JS, Van Muiswinkel AMC, Folkers PJM, Moonen CTW, Jansma JM, Kahn RS (1998) Phase navigator correction in 3D fMRI improves detection of brain activation: quantitative assessment with a graded motor activation procedure. Neuroimage (in press)

Rees G, Howseman A, Josephs O, Frith CD, Friston KJ, Frackowiak RSJ, Turner R (1997) Characterizing the relationship between BOLD contrast and regional cerebral blood flow measurements by varying the stimulus presentation rate. Neuroimage 6:270–278

Rombouts SARB, Barkhof F, Hoogenraad FGC, Sprenger M, Scheltens P (1998) Within-subject reproducibility of visual activation patterns with functional magnetic resonance imaging using multislice echo planar imaging. Magn Reson Imaging 16:105–113

Sadato N, Ibanez V, Campbell G, Deiber MP, Le Bihan D, Hallett M (1997) Frequency-dependent changes of regional cerebral blood flow during finger movements: functional MRI compared to PET. J Cereb Blood Flow Metab 17:670–679

Small SL, Noll DC, Perfetti CA, Hlustik P, Wellington R, Schneider W (1996) Localizing the lexicon for reading aloud replication of a pet study using FMRI. Neuroreport 7:961–965

Thevenaz P, Ruttimann UE, Unser M (1995) Iterative multiscale registration without landmarks. In: Proceedings of the international conference on image processing, Washington DC (abstract)

Turner R (1992) Magnetic resonance imaging of brain function. Am J Physiol Imaging 3/4:136–145

Van den Brink JS, Ramsey NF, Van Muiswinkel AMC, Jansma JM, Folkers PJM (1997) Phase-navigated 3D shifted-echo FFE-EPI: assessment of assets for fMRI. In: Proceedings of the workshop on fast MRI, Monterey 1997 (abstract)

Van Gelderen P, Ramsey NF, Liu G, Duyn JH, Frank JA, Weinberger DR, Moonen CTW (1995) Three dimensional functional MRI of human brain on a clinical 1.5 T scanner. Proc Natl Acad Sci USA 92:6906–6910

Van Gelderen P, Van der Veen J, Moonen CTW (1997) PRESTO fMRI on a fast gradient system. Proc ISMRM 1997, Vancouver, p 1637

Woods RP, Cherry SR, Mazziotta JC (1992) Rapid automated algorithm for aligning and reslicing PET images. J Comput Assist Tomogr 16:620–633

Worsley KJ (1994) Local maxima and the expected Euler characteristic of excursion sets of Chi square, F and t fields. Adv Appl Prob 26:13–42

Xiong JH, Rao S, Gao JH, Woldorff M, Fox PT (1998) Evaluation of hemispheric dominance for language using functional MRI: a comparison with positron emission tomography. Hum Brain Mapp 6:42–58

Yang YH, Glover GH, Vangelderen P et al (1996) Fast 3D Functional Magnetic Resonance Imaging at 1.5 T with Spiral Acquisition. Magn Reson Med 36:620–626

Zarahn E, Aguirre GK, d'Esposito M (1997) Empirical analyses of BOLD fMRI statistics. I. Spatially unsmoothed data collected under null-hypothesis conditions. Neuroimage 5:179–197

35 Functional MRI and Hypercapnia

A. Kastrup, T.Q. Li, M.E. Moseley

35.1
Introduction

Functional magnetic resonance imaging (fMRI) techniques are rapidly moving away from the perceived role of solely mapping human cognitive functions such as vision, motor skills or language. These techniques are now capable of detecting and mapping regional hemodynamic responses to various stress tests, which involve the use of vasoactive substances such as acetazolamide or inhalation of carbon dioxide (CO$_2$), complementing the arsenal of functional brain investigations feasible with MRI. In this chapter we will review the mechanisms underlying the use of vasoactive stress tests in fMRI. Moreover we will illustrate their scientific and clinical applications in this setting for assessing cerebral hemodynamics and vascular reserve capacity.

35.2
Physiological Responses and Mechanisms of Action of CO$_2$

The effect of CO$_2$ on the cerebrovasculature is one of the most pronounced, most easily demonstrated and reproduced phenomena observed in the cerebral circulation. Numerous studies in humans and animals, involving the use of many different techniques, have shown that CO$_2$ exerts a profound influence on cerebral blood flow (CBF). Cerebral vascular vasodilatation to hypercapnia and vasoconstriction to hypocapnia are universal findings. In humans, 5% CO$_2$ inhalation raises CBF by approximately 50% and 7% CO$_2$ by 100% (Kety and Schmidt 1948).

Several mechanisms have been proposed to account for the effects of CO$_2$ on the cerebrovasculature: extracellular fluid [H$^+$] in the brain (Kontos et al. 1977a, b), prostaglandins (Pickard and MacKenzie 1973), nitric oxide (NO) (Iadecola 1992, Wang et al. 1992), and neural pathways (James et al. 1969). The main mechanism appears to be mediated by direct effects of the extracellular fluid [H$^+$] on cerebrovascular smooth muscle in the arterioles. The [H$^+$] in the area of the vascular smooth muscle depends on the bicarbonate concentration and the pCO$_2$ of the extracellular fluid at that site. In turn, the extracellular fluid pCO$_2$ depends on both arterial carbon dioxide tension (PaCO$_2$) and pCO$_2$ of the cerebrospinal fluid. While the blood-brain barrier is impermeable to bicarbonate and [H$^+$], it is freely permeable to CO$_2$, so that a rise of PaCO$_2$ will lead to an increase in local pCO$_2$ of vascular muscle, reduce extracellular fluid pH, and produce vasodilatation. The reverse occurs when PaCO$_2$ is decreased.

In phencyclidine-anaesthetized baboons, Pickard and MacKenzie (1973) first found that indomethacin, a cyclooxygenase inhibitor, attenuated the increase of CBF during hypercapnia, indicating that prostaglandins may be mediators of the CBF CO$_2$ response. Similar results have been reported since then in animals and humans; however, the prostaglandin mechanism of hypercapnic vasodilatation is species-dependent, being important in some species (baboons, rats, and gerbils), but not in others (cats and rabbits). Therefore, the role of prostaglandins in the mechanism of hypercapnic cerebrovasodilatation is somewhat unclear. Similarly, the importance of NO in

A. Kastrup, MD; T.Q. Li, PhD; M.E. Moseley, PhD; Department of Radiology, Lucas MRS Center, Stanford University School of Medicine, 1201 Welch Road, Stanford, CA 94305-5488, USA

the maintenance of resting cerebrovascular tone and perhaps in evoked vasodilatation is not well understood, since its effects have usually been inferred from studies of NO synthase activity or protocols which employed inhibitors of this enzyme. There may even be an interaction between the prostanoid system and NO production, with prostacyclin facilitating the release of NO.

In conclusion, several factors can influence both hyper- and hypocapnic CBF responses; however, there seems to be no doubt that the most important mechanism is related to the $[H^+]$ content of the extracellular fluid. This mechanism appears to occur across species, but could work in conjunction with other mechanisms such as prostanoids, NO, and neurogenic components.

The question of whether alterations in $PaCO_2$ change CBF equally in all brain regions is controversial (MADDEN 1993). Some investigators have shown no differences in CO_2 reactivity among brain regions and that blood flow to the hemispheres, brainstem, cerebellum, and medulla is altered by the same percentage per mm Hg $PaCO_2$. Others have shown that in both gray and white matter blood flow increases with hypercapnia; however, the white matter increase was less than the gray matter increase.

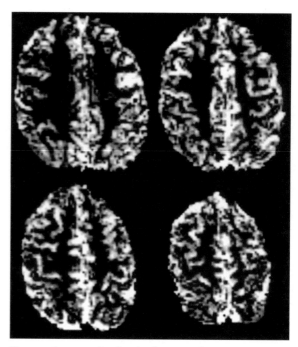

Fig. 35.1. An example of activation maps in response to a repeated challenge of breath holding of 40 s. The data were acquired using a single-shot gradient echo spiral readout with matrix size of 128×128 and TE/TR=50/2000

35.3
Functional MRI Methods To Map the Response to Vascular Challenges

Vasomotor responses of the cerebral vasculature to altered CO_2 tensions can easily be used for the study of CBF regulation and to determine the cerebrovascular reserve capacity. In a similar way, vasomotor responses are provoked by hypoxia, anoxia and acetazolamide. The latter is a potent, reversible inhibitor of carbonic anhydrase. Although the exact mechanism by which acetazolamide acts as a vasodilator agent and increases blood flow is controversial, the most commonly accepted mechanism is that inhibition of carbonic anhydrase causes a decrease of extracellular pH in the brain (BICKLER et al. 1988). Since increased CBF is not paralleled by functional or metabolic challenge, oxidative metabolism has been shown to remain unaffected (VORSTRUP et al. 1984).

In the past, cerebral hemodynamics and cerebrovascular reserve capacity have mainly been measured with positron emission tomography (PET) (GIBBS et al. 1984; POWERS et al. 1987), single photon

emission-computed tomography (SPECT) (VORSTRUP et al. 1984;), transcranial Doppler sonography (TCD; RINGELSTEIN et al. 1988; DAHL et al. 1992; WIDDER et al. 1994; KASTRUP et al. 1997), and dynamic or xenon computed tomography (STEIGER et al. 1993; ISAKA et al. 1994). These methods, however, suffer from disadvantages, e.g., use of radioisotopes, poor spatial and or temporal resolution, limited availability of the system and costly examinations. Recently, noninvasive MRI methods have been developed that are sensitive to "stimulus-induced" changes in blood flow and oxygenation (BELLIVEAU et al. 1991; BANDETTINI et al. 1992; DETRE et al. 1992; KWONG et al. 1992; OGAWA et al. 1992). In earlier studies exogenous contrast agents (such as Gd-DTPA) were used to investigate hemodynamic challenges (BELLIVEAU et al. 1991). The use of this technique, however, is limited because of the need for repeated injections of an exogenous contrast agent and the necessity to compare images acquired during two different administrations of the contrast agent bolus separated by several minutes. As discussed in earlier chapters of this book, the BOLD technique is based on the fact that deoxyhemoglobin acts as an endogenous contrast agent (BANDETTINI et al. 1992; KWONG et al. 1992; OGAWA et al. 1992;). As

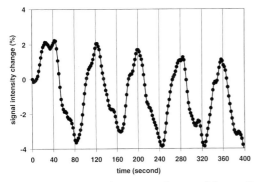

Fig. 35.2. The mean signal intensity change of the gradient echo in a representative region of interest (ROI; 5×5) of the activated areas measured as a function of the experimental time

shown in task activation studies, increases in CBF induced by acetazolamide or by CO_2 inhalation exceed the usual demands in oxidative metabolism. This uncoupling between CBF and cerebral metabolism causes a similar change in venous oxyhemoglobin concentration, as seen during brain stimulation. Thus, application of a reversible vasoactive stress can be visualized noninvasively with BOLD MRI. This is clearly demonstrated in Figs. 35.1 and 35.2. Figure 35.1 shows that the changes in gradient echo signal intensity (SI) in gray matter are significantly correlated with the repeated challenge of breath holding. Figure 35.2 shows the mean time course of the SI change from a representative activated region of interest (ROI) in the cortex. An average percent SI change of 2% was observed, whereas no significant SI change was observed in the white matter.

Despite the use of BOLD-based techniques in acetazolamide or CO_2 challenge studies, several methodological shortcomings have to be considered. MR signal changes induced by pharmacological as well as functional activation encompass signal originating from both brain microvasculature and large vessels. Therefore, signal originating in the microvasculature of the cerebral gray and white matter has to be separated from signal in the large veins. Using a maximum intensity projection (MIP) procedure, HEDERA et al. (1996) could partially distinguish MR signal originating from large draining veins from that generated at the level of the microvasculature. BOLD contrast images obtained under rapid radiofrequency (RF) pulsing conditions can have an inflow component from the large vessels that is dominated by fast flowing macrovascular blood in arteries and large veins (LAI et al. 1993; FRAHM et al. 1994). This confounding effect, however, can be eas-

ily eliminated by using longer TR or dual echo data acquisition.

As BOLD effects are related to multiple physiological parameters such as CBF and volume, and oxygen consumption, it is difficult to extract a single physiological parameter from the observed signal changes. This problem can partially be overcome using the arterial spin tagging techniques, which use magnetically tagged endogenous water as a tracer and are essentially CBF-based. A number of approaches based on this idea have been proposed, such as EPISTAR (signal targeting with alternating RF) (EDELMAN et al. 1994) and FAIR (flow-sensitive alternating inversion recovery) techniques (KWONG et al. 1992; KIM 1995). These are based on perturbing the magnetization of inflowing arterial blood and acquiring a flow-insensitive image and a flow-sensitive image. The CBF-based image is obtained by subtracting the flow-insensitive image from the flow-sensitive image to remove the signals from the static tissues. Arterial water can be labeled via either magnetic saturation or inversion (DETRE et al. 1992). Inversion is preferable because the observable signal change is larger.

The MR protocol then consists of acquiring a train of alternating selectively inverted and nonselectively inverted images during a perturbation with acetazolamide or CO_2 inhalation. An increase in the arterial delivery will produce a small increase (2%–5%) in image intensity depending on the TI, TR, slice thickness and placement of the inversion slab, B_0, CBF, and the blood-brain partition coefficient. Thus, application of a vasoactive perturbation can be "tracked" and quantitated noninvasively with CBF-based fMRI.

This is clearly depicted in Figs. 35.3 and 35.4, which show the correlation maps and the mean time course of the relative CBF change in response to a repeated challenge of 40 s breath holding. As shown in Fig. 35.3, the activated areas are dominantly confined within the gray matter as observed with the BOLD technique. Figure 35.4 shows the mean time course of the relative CBF change in the cortex. An average CBF increase of 40±20% was observed upon 40 s breath holding. An average CBF decrease of 20±10% was observed right after the breath holding task, due to a period of hyperventilation. Compared with the BOLD technique, the spin tagging technique can provide more quantitative data on CBF changes at the price of decreased signal-to-noise ratio and temporal resolution.

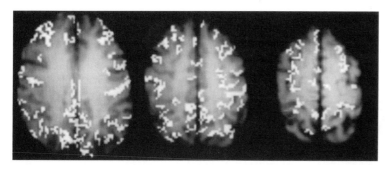

Fig. 35.3. An example of activation maps in response to a repeated challenge of breath holding of 40 s. The data were acquired using a single-shot FAIR spiral sequence. Since the data set for multislices were acquired in an inter-leaved fashion, the inversion time (TI) for the first slice was 1200 ms, while TI for the other slices were successively increased by about 90 ms. A bipolar gradient was employed prior to the spiral readout to attenuate the signals from large vessels

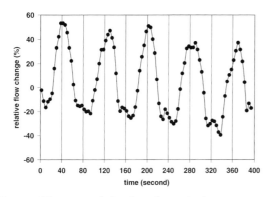

Fig. 35.4. The mean relative flow change in the cortex measured as a function of the experimental time

35.4
Current Applications

Due to the high spatial and temporal resolution, noninvasive fMRI techniques are increasingly used to study cerebral hemodynamics and cerebrovascular reserve. Several reports have successfully described investigation of the cerebrovascular reserve in healthy volunteers with acetazolamide (BRUHN et al. 1994; HEDERA et al. 1996), during breath holding (STILLMAN et al. 1995), during hyperventilation (TOFT et al. 1995; POSSE et al. 1997), and during CO_2 inhalation (ROSTRUP et al. 1994, 1996). KLEINSCHMIDT et al. (1995) demonstrated exhaustion of the autoregulatory reserve capacity in four patients with unilateral occlusion of the internal carotid artery, while monitoring cerebral blood oxygenation changes during vasodilatory stress. Moreover, several investigators have used the BOLD approach in the study of cerebral hemodynamics in rats (GRAHAM et al. 1994; ONO et al. 1997), cats (MOSELEY et al. 1992; PRINSTER et al. 1997), and dogs (RIGHINI et al. 1995).

Besides determination of cerebrovascular reserve, fMRI techniques have been applied to the study of human tumors (GRIFFITHS et al. 1997), trauma (FORBES et al. 1997), and stroke (ONO et al. 1997). In a

fascinating demonstration of tumor functional mapping, KARCZMAR et al. (1994) found that tumors in the rat could be distinguished from normal tissues by the increased response of the tumor to mild bouts of hyperoxia or hypercarbia.

Recently, the combination of task activation and global hypercapnic stress has been used to study the interactions between physiologic and pharmacological manipulations (SCHMITZ et al. 1996; BANDETTINI and WONG 1997, BOCK et al. 1998). In the landmark studies of BANDETTINI and WONG (1997), regional signal differences due to differences in vessel architecture were removed from neurofunctional MR images by normalization to a mask created by global hypercapnic stress. This hypercapnia-based normalization method led to markedly improved spatial localization of activation-induced flow changes. Moreover, the authors demonstrated that BOLD contrast-enhanced signal changes were strongly weighted by blood volume in each voxel. This suggests that pharmacological stress tests can increase functional resolution of fMRI and may be useful for noninvasive mapping of cerebral blood volume.

SCHMITZ et al. (1996) observed that brief episodes of hypercapnia produced a marked up-regulation of somatosensory activation of blood flow in five adult male Sprague-Dawley rats. This enhancement outlasted the CO_2 exposure by at least 60 min, although all blood variables had promptly returned to normal after termination of hypercapnia. Under control conditions, contralateral forepaw stimulation caused an increase of blood flow (as determined with laser-Doppler flowmetry, LDF) by 39%±11%. Some 25 min after CO_2 ventilation, somatosensory stimulation increased LDF by 86%±18%, and even after 60 min by 96%±26%. Using the same experimental model, BOCK et al. (1998) compared this up-regulation in perfusion- and T2*-sensitive imaging in a subsequent study. Under control conditions, stimulation of the forepaw led to an increase by 45%±48% of the perfusion-weighted signal intensity and by 6%±2% of the T2*-weighted image intensity. After transient hypercapnia, perfusion-weighted and T2*-weighted signal intensity increased during stimulation by 91%±62% and 7%±4%, respectively. This difference in behavior of the T2*-weighted and perfusion-weighted image signals can best be explained by a higher stimulus-induced oxygen metabolism after CO_2 ventilation. This will lead to a further increase in CBF. At the same time, however, the increased oxygen extraction results in a deoxyhemoglobin concentration in the blood that is similar to that before CO_2 breathing, thus leading to unchanged T2*-weighted signal intensity increase during stimulation. These data demonstrated that resetting of the functional-metabolic coupling after hypercapnia also resets the signal intensity changes of BOLD imaging during functional activation and, therefore, may lead to misinterpretations of the magnitude of the functional response. Although the underlying mechanism of the CO_2-induced conditioning is still unclear, further experiments will give new insights in the coupling between oxygen consumption and CBF during stimulation.

35.5
Conclusion

The physiological response of vasomotor tone to vasodilatory stress from either functional activation or pharmacological manipulation is one of the prime features of intact cerebral perfusion. The response of cerebral perfusion to vasodilatory stress is not merely of scientific interest, but also of potential clinical interest in patients with hemodynamicaly relevant atherosclerotic disease. For insufficiently collateralized occlusions of the internal carotid artery, it has been found that hemodynamic compromise, as evidenced by exhausted vasomotor reserve capacity, presents a considerable risk for subsequent ischemic stroke (KLEISER and WIDDER 1992). Although PET is considered the gold standard for assessing cerebral perfusion, due to its potential to separately quantify CBF, cerebral blood volume, and fractional oxygen extraction, fMRI has several advantages: fMRI has, in principle, considerably higher spatial and temporal resolution; fMRI procedures are completely noninvasive and can be repeated in a single subject without concern about exposure to ionizing radiation; since anatomic and functional images can be acquired during the same imaging session, functional maps can be compared directly with anatomic images without any misregistration. Repeated testing of a single patient with fMRI will allow clinicians to follow changes of cerebrovascular reactivity over the course of a progressive disease, during recovery from injury or stroke, and in response to treatment.

Besides determination of cerebrovascular reserve, fMRI imaging will prove useful to monitor the response of a tumor to acetazolamide or CO_2, and to distinguish viable or reactive tumor from surrounding tissue. Moreover, noninvasive measurement of a tumor's response to oxygenation and blood flow modification will enable clinicians to optimize treatment protocols, such as carbogen breathing, for individual radiotherapy patients.

A hypercapnia-based normalization method can be used to further characterize BOLD MRI signal changes caused by neuronal activation, enhance the functional resolution of fMRI and may also be useful for noninvasive mapping of cerebral blood volume.

It is evident from the work presented in this chapter that, besides mapping of task activation, fMRI has rapidly evolved to include imaging of the response of several organs or tumors to vasoactive substances. It is hoped that this technique will have a major impact in the field of neuroscience and that it will enable researchers and clinicians to better understand the cerebral hemodynamics of the human brain.

Acknowledgments. Andreas Kastrup is supported by a research grant from the Deutsche Forschungsgemeinschaft (Ka 1419/1-1).

References

Bandettini PA, Wong EC (1997) A hypercapnia-based normalization method for improved spatial localization of human brain activation with fMRI. NMR Biomed 10:197–203

Bandettini PA, Wong EC, Hinks RS, Tikofsky RS, Hyde JS (1992) Time course EPI of human brain function during task activation. Magn Reson Med 25:390–398

Belliveau JW, Kennedy DN, McKinstry RC, Buchbinder BR, Weisskopf RM, Cohen MS, Vevea JM, Brady TJ, Rosen BR (1991) Functional mapping of the human visual cortex by magentic resonance imaging. Science 254:716–719

Bickler PE, Litt L, Banville DL, Severinghaus JW (1988) Effects of acetazolamide on cerebral acid-base balance. J Appl Physiol 65:422–427

Bock C, Schmitz B, Kerskens CM, Gyngell ML, Hossmann KA, Hoehn-Berlage M (1998) Functional MRI of somatosensory activation in rat: effect of hypercapnia up-regulation on perfusion- and BOLD-imaging. Magn Reson Med 39:457–461

Bruhn H, Kleinschmidt A, Boecker H, Merboldt KD, Hänicke W, Frahm J (1994) The effect of acetazolamide on regional cerebral blood oxygenation at rest and under stimulation as assessed by MRI. J Cereb Blood Flow Metab 14:742–748

Dahl A, Lindegaard KF, Russell D, Nyberg-Hansen R, Rootwelt K, Sorteberg W, Nornes H (1992) A comparison of transcranial Doppler and cerebral blood flow studies to assess cerebral vasoreactivity. Stroke 23:15–19

Detre JA, Leigh JS, William DS, Koretsky AP (1992) Perfusion imaging. Magn Reson Med 23:37–45

Edelman RE, Siewer B, Darby DG, Thangaraj V, Nobre AC, Mesulam MM, Warach S (1994) Qualitative mapping of cerebral blood flow and functional localization with echo-planar MR imaging and signal targeting with alternating radio frequency. Radiology 192:513–520

Forbes ML, Hendrich KS, Kochanek PM, Williams DS, Schiding JK, Wisniewski SR, Kelsey SF, DeKosky ST, Graham SH, Marion DW, Ho C (1997) Assessment of cerebral blood flow and CO_2 reactivity after controlled cortical impact by perfusion magnetic resonance imaging using arterial spin-labelling in rats. J Cereb Blood Flow Metab 17:865–874

Frahm J, Merboldt KD, Hanicke W, Kleinschmidt A, Boecker H (1994) Brain and vein -oxygenation or flow? On signal physiology in functional MRI of human brain activation. NMR Biomed 7:45–53

Gibbs JM, Wise RJS, Leenders KL, Jones T (1984) Evaluation of cerebral perfusion reserve in patients with carotid artery occlusion. Lancet 1:310–314

Graham GD, Zhong J, Petroff OAC, Constable RT, Prichard JW, Gore JC (1994) BOLD MRI monitoring of changes in cerebral perfusion induced by acetazolamide and hypercapnia in the rat. Magn Reson Med 31:557–560

Griffiths JR, Taylor NJ, Howe FA, Saunders MI, Robinson SP, Hoskin PJ, Powell ME, Thoumine M, Caine LA, Baddeley H (1997) The response of human tumors to carbogen breathing, monitored by gradient-recalled echo magnetic resonance imaging. Int J Radiat Oncol Biol Phys 39:697–701

Hedera P, Lai S, Lewin JS, Haacke EM, Wu D, Lerner AJ, Friedland RP (1996) Assessment of cerebral blood flow reserve using functional magnetic resonance imaging. JMRI 6:718–725

Iadecola C (1992) Does nitric oxide mediate the increases in cerebral blood flow elicited by hypercapnia? Proc Natl Acad Sci U S A 89:3913–3916

Isaka Y, Okamoto M, Ashida K, Imaizumi M (1994) Decreased cerebrovascular dilatory capacity in subjects with asymptomatic periventricular hyperintensity. Stroke 25:375–381

James IM, Millar RA, Purves MJ (1969) Observations on the extrinsic neural control of cerebral blood flow in the baboon. Circ Res 25:77–93

Karczmar G, River J, Vijayakumar S, Goldman Z, Lewis MZ (1994) Effects of hyperoxia on T2* and resonance frequency weighted MR images of rodent tumors. NMR Biomed 7:3–11

Kastrup A, Thomas C, Hartmann C, Schabet M (1997) Sex dependency of cerebrovascular CO_2 reactivity in normal subjects. Stroke 28:2353–2356

Kety SS, Schmidt CF (1948) The effects of altered arterial tensions of carbon dioxide and oxygen on cerebral blood flow and cerebral oxygen consumption of normal young men. J Clin Invest 27:484–492

Kim SG (1995) Quantification of relative blood flow change by flow-sensitive alternating inversion recovery (FAIR) technique: application to functional mapping. Magn Reson Med 34:293–301

Kleinschmidt A, Steinmetz H, Sitzer M, Merboldt KD, Frahm J (1995) Magnetic resonance imaging of regional cerebral blood oxygenation changes under acetazolamide in carotid occlusive disease. Stroke 26:106–110

Kleiser B, Widder B (1992) Course of carotid artery occlusions with impaired cerebrovascular reactivity. Stroke 23:171–174

Kontos HA, Wie EP, Raper AJ, Patterson JL (1977a) Local mechanisms of CO_2 action on cat pial arterioles. Stroke 8:226–229

Kontos HA, Raper AJ, Patterson JL (1977b) Analysis of vaso-activity of local pH, PCO_2 and bicarbonate on cerebral vessels. Stroke 8:358–360

Kwong KK, Belliveau JW, Chesler DA, Goldberg IE, Weisskopf RM, Poncelet RM, Kennedy DN, Hoppel BE, Cohen MS, Turner R, Cheng HM, Brady TJ, Rosen BR (1992) Dynamic magnetic resonance imaging of human brain activity during primary sensory stimulation. Proc Natl Acad Sci U S A 89:5675–5679

Lai S, Hopkins AL, Haacke EM, Li D, Wasserman BA, Buckley P, Friedman L, Meltzer H, Hedera P, Friedland R (1993) Identification of vascular structures as a major source of signal contrast in high resolution 2-D and 3-D functional activation imaging of the motor cortex at 1.5 T: preliminary results. Magn Reson Med 30:387–392

Madden JA (1993) The effect of carbon dioxide on cerebral arteries. Pharmacol Ther 59:229–250

Moseley ME, Chew WM, White DL, Kucharcyk J, Litt L, Derugin N, Dupon J, Brasch RC, Norman D (1992) Hypercapnia-induced changes in cerebral blood volume in the cat: A ^1H MRI and intravascular contrast agent study. Magn Reson Med 23:21–30

Ogawa S, Tank D, Menon R, Ellermann JM, Kim SG, Merkle K, Ugurbil K (1992) Intrinsic signal changes accompanying sensory stimulation:functional brain mapping using MRI. Proc Natl Acad Sci U S A 89:5951–5955

Ono Y, Morikawa S, Inubishi T, Shimizu H, Yoshimoto T (1997) T2*-weighted magnetic resonance imaging of cerebrovascular reactivity in rat reversible focal cerebral ischemia. Brain Res 744:207–215

Pickard JD, MacKenzie ET (1973) Inhibition of prostaglandin synthesis and the response of baboon cerebral circulation to carbon dioxide. Nature New Biol 245:187–188

Posse S, Olthoff U, Weckesser M, Jancke L, Muller-Gartner HW, Drager SR (1997) Regional dynamic signal changes during controlled hyperventilation assessed with blood oxygen level-dependent functional MR imaging. AJNR 18:1763–1770

Powers WJ, Press GA, Grubb RL, Gado M, Raichle ME (1987) The effect of hemodynamically significant carotid artery disease on the hemodynamic status of the cerebral circulation. Ann Intern Med 106:27–35

Prinster A, Pierpaoli C, Turner R, Jezzard P (1997) Simultaneous measurement of DeltaR2 and DeltaR2* in cat brain during hypoxia and hypercapnia. NeuroImage 6:191–200

Righini A, Pierpaoli C, Barnett AS, Waks E, Alger JR (1995) Blue blood or black blood: R1 effects in gradient-echo echo-planar functional neuroimaging. Magn Res Imaging 13:369–378

Ringelstein EB, Sievers C, Ecker S, Schneider PA, Otis SM (1988) Noninvasive assessment of CO2-induced cerebral vasomotor response in normal individuals and patients with internal carotid artery occlusions. Stroke 19:963–969

Rostrup E, Larsson HB, Toft PB, Garde K, Thomsen C, Ring P, Sondergaard L, Henriksen O (1994) Functional MRI of CO_2 induced increase in cerebral perfusion. NMR Biomed 7:29–34

Rostrup E, Larrson HB, Toft PB, Garde K, Ring PB, Henriksen O (1996) Susceptibility contrast imaging of CO_2-induced changes in the blood volume of the human brain. Acta Radiol 37:813–822

Schmitz B, Böttiger BW, Hossmann KA (1996) Brief hypercapnia enhances somatosensory activation of blood flow in rat. J Cereb Blood Flow Metab 16:1307–1311

Steiger HJ, Aaslid R, Stooss R (1993) Dynamic computed tomographic imaging of regional cerebral blood flow and blood volume. Stroke 24:591–597

Stillman AE, Hu X, Jerosch-Herold M (1995) Functional MRI of the brain during breath holding at 4 T. Magn Res Imaging 13:893–897

Toft PB, Leth H, Lou HC, Pryds O, Peitersen B, Henriksen O (1995) Local vascular CO_2 reactivity in the infant brain assessed by functional MRI. Pediatr Radiol 25:420–424

Vorstrup S, Henriksen L, Paulson OB (1984) Effect of acetazolamide on cerebral blood flow and cerebral metabolic rate for oxygen. J Clin Invest 74:1634–1639

Wang Q, Paulsen OB, Lassen NA (1992) Effect of nitric oxide blockade by N^G-nitro-L-arginine on cerebral blood flow response to changes in carbon dioxide tension. J Cereb Blood Flow Metab 12:947–953

Widder B, Kleiser B, Krapf H (1994) Course of cerebrovascular reactivity in patients with carotid artery occlusions. Stroke 25:1963–1967

36 Event-Related Functional MRI

R.L. Buckner, T.S. Braver

CONTENTS

36.1
Introduction

One of the most exciting areas in functional magnetic resonance imaging (fMRI) today involves the development and application of methods based on the transient neuronal changes associated with individual cognitive and sensory events. These methods, referred to as single trial or event-related fMRI, have broadly expanded the spectrum of task designs and analytical techniques that can be used in neuroimaging studies. In particular, event-related fMRI (ER-fMRI) allows paradigms to depart from "blocked" testing procedures, in which long periods of task performance are integrated, to paradigms that isolate individual trial events or subcomponents of trial events (Fig. 36.1). This provides much greater flexibility in experimental design, by allowing for selective averaging of stimulus events or task conditions which may be intermixed on a trial-by-trial basis. Moreover, by focusing on responses to single events rather than to extended blocks, ER-fMRI provides a means of examining questions regarding the dynamics and time-course of neural activity under various conditions. In this chapter, we provide an in-depth discussion of ER-fMRI, describing its basic principles, methodology, current applications, and future directions. Two important foci of the chapter are: (1) current methodological issues surrounding the use of ER-fMRI, and (2) how ER-fMRI methods have been (or could be) fruitfully applied to expand the range of questions that can be asked in clinical and cognitive neuroscience studies.

36.2
The Hemodynamic Response

The development of ER-fMRI has followed the development of our understanding of the basic principles of the blood oxygenation level-dependent (BOLD) hemodynamic response (Ogawa et al. 1990, 1992; Kwong et al. 1992). Specifically, there are two key characteristics of the hemodynamic response: (1) it

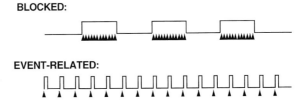

Fig. 36.1. The difference between blocked-trial and event-related paradigms. *Top,* In blocked-task paradigms, many events of the same type are presented in sequences (shown by the *closely spaced arrowheads*). Analysis proceeds by examining signal change averaged across the entire block. *Bottom,* Event-related paradigms attempt to isolate the individual trial events, or even the subcomponents of trial events. The simplest kind of event-related paradigm is illustrated, in which separate events (indicated by *arrows*) are spaced widely apart. As is discussed extensively, many kinds of event-related paradigm are possible, including those that space trials closely together (~2 s) and those that target subcomponents of individual events

R.L. Buckner, PhD; T.S. Braver, PhD; Department of Psychology, Washington University, Campus Box 1125, One Brookings Drive, St. Louis, MO 63130, USA

can be elicited following brief periods of neuronal activity, and (2) it can be characterized by a well-behaved and reliable impulse-response function.

The first characteristic of the BOLD hemodynamic response – that it can elicited by a brief period of neuronal activity – was observed soon after BOLD contrast became available for mapping brain function. BLAMIRE et al. (1992) presented subjects with brief visual stimuli (2 s), which presumably evoked correspondingly brief periods of neuronal activity. In response to each of the stimuli, the investigators observed transient positive changes in BOLD signal over visual cortex. Similarly, BANDETTINI (1993) demonstrated signal changes to even shorter task events, examining responses to finger movements for durations ranging from 0.5 s to 5 s. In all situations, including the brief 0.5 s movement duration, clear signal increases were detected in motor cortex. These early studies were followed by a number of similar investigations (HUMBERSTONE et al. 1995; SAVOY et al. 1995; BOULANOUAR et al. 1996; KONISHI et al. 1996). SAVOY et al. (1995), in an extreme demonstration of the temporal limits of these methods, showed that visual stimulation as brief as 34 ms in duration will elicit small, but clearly detectable, positive signal changes.

More recently, these observations have been carried over to the realm of cognitive task paradigms. In such paradigms, the evoked neural activity is less completely understood, and the responses are considerably more subtle than in most studies using sensory stimulation. Nonetheless, isolated trial events within cognitive task paradigms have been reliably shown to evoke transient hemodynamic responses. BUCKNER et al. (1996), for example, demonstrated that signal changes in visual and prefrontal brain areas can be detected during isolated trials of a word generation task. KIM et al. (1997) examined responses to tasks involving subject-initiated motor preparation. They detected hemodynamic responses in motor and visual cortex. MCCARTHY et al. (1997) noted transient responses in parietal cortex during infrequent presentation of target letter strings (see Sect. 36.5). Taken collectively, these and other observations make clear that fMRI can detect hemodynamic responses to extremely brief neuronal events, making it possible to be utilized in a truly event-related fashion (for review see ROSEN et al. 1998).

The second key characteristic of the BOLD hemodynamic response is the nature and reliability of the shape of the response to a given, brief, fixed interval of stimulation (often described as the impulse-response function). Early studies using sustained

stimulation (e.g., KWONG et al. 1992) noted that the BOLD response is delayed in onset from the time of presumed neural activity by about 2–6 s. The work of BLAMIRE et al. (1992) confirmed this finding for brief sensory events and further demonstrated that the hemodynamic response was prolonged in duration. Across a wide range of studies it has now been determined that, for a neural event that lasts a second, the robust positive deflection of the BOLD response will evolve over a 10–12 s period (see hemodynamic response for the "one-trial" condition in Fig. 36.2A). Certain, more subtle, components of the response may have considerably longer recovery periods. From this information, investigators began to

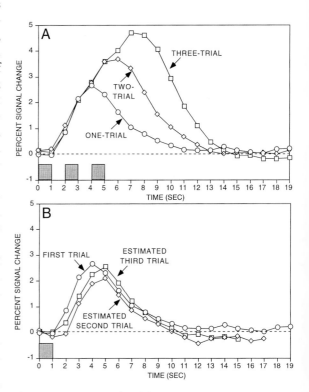

Fig. 36.2A, B. Event-related fMRI (ER-fMRI) data show approximately linear summation of the BOLD contrast signal for closely spaced (2 s apart) trials. A The raw fMRI signal intensity evoked when either one, two, or three sequential trials of a 1 s visual checkerboard stimulus are presented. The placement of each trial is indicated by *shaded bars* at the *bottom* of the graph. The response increases and is prolonged with the addition of multiple trials, indicating that the BOLD contrast signal does not saturate from one to three trials. B Estimates of the separate contributions of each trial are shown. To obtain these estimates, subtraction between trial conditions was employed. The one-trial condition was subtracted from the two-trial condition, and the two-from the three. The three estimated responses are roughly similar, although clear (but subtle) departures from linearity can be observed. These data come from early visual cortex. (Adapted from DALE and BUCKNER 1997)

incorporate explicit models of the hemodynamic impulse-response function into analyses of time-series data, in order to account better for the delayed onset and offset properties. An important step forward in this endeavor was provided by Boynton et al. (1996), who demonstrated that the shape of the hemodynamic response to a number of different stimuli could be modeled as a simple function within a linear system. In particular, a function of the form:

$$h(t) = \left(\frac{(t-\delta)}{\tau}\right)^2 e^{-\frac{(t-\delta)}{\tau}} \tag{36.1}$$

provides a good fit of activity profiles in primary visual cortex (V1) over a range of stimulus durations and intensities. h(t) refers to the signal intensity over time. Parameters d and t can be adjusted to modify the shape of the function. The advantage of having an analytical model of the BOLD response is that it provides a way of generating predictions regarding the idealized fMRI signal expected to a given neuronal event. As will be discussed below, these predictions can be incorporated into statistical procedures as reference functions in order to identify voxels responsive to specific patterns of stimulation or task-related events. Together, knowledge of the characteristics of the BOLD signal – its response to even very brief neuronal events and its shape and time-course – form the basis of ER-fMRI experimental design and data analysis.

36.3
Event-Related Functional MRI Data Analysis

Analytical methods have been developed in a number of laboratories to more specifically exploit the power and unique characteristics of ER-fMRI paradigms (Clark et al. 1998; Dale and Buckner 1997; Josephs et al. 1997; Zarahn et al. 1997; Friston et al. 1998). In general, procedures used in ER-fMRI data analysis are conceptually similar to those used in EEG and MEG data analysis, which also apply an event-related approach. At the most basic level, the primary characteristics of ER-fMRI analysis are: (1) determination of the onset of individual events, and (2) selective averaging and/or explicit modeling of responses for each different event-type based on these onsets. The extraction of event-related responses is first dependent upon the image acquisition procedure. That is, images should be acquired in

such a fashion that they could be aligned with the events of interest. This alignment or event-locking is most often done to the presentation of stimuli, but can also be locked to other events such as behavioral responses or even spontaneously occurring physiological events such as the beginning of seizure activity or hallucinations (see section 36.6).

Next, the full BOLD response should be extracted or modeled for each event. Of course, given that image acquisition typically occurs continuously across multiple repetitions of trials or stimulus events, this begs the question of what constitutes the appropriate time-course for a trial or stimulus event. In the evoked response potential (ERP) literature, the time-course extracted following an event is typically referred to as an epoch. The epoch chosen for a given event should encompass the duration expected for the full hemodynamic response. Based on previous studies, for transient neuronal events (i.e., less than 2 s) the duration of the hemodynamic response appears to be about 10–16 s. The duration of an epoch need not correspond to the duration between successive events. Indeed, as will be discussed below, some designs are now being explored in which trial or stimulus presentation rate is much shorter than the expected time-course of the hemodynamic response function and thus produces overlap in the epochs extracted for each event. Following extraction of the event-related response, the different event-types can be sorted into separate bins and/or modeled explicitly (including taking into account any overlap across event-types).

In the instance of selective averaging (e.g., Dale and Buckner 1997), the mean and variance of the fMRI time-course data can be computed separately, on a voxel-by-voxel basis, for each different trial type or task condition. Such averages yield a sufficient estimate of the central tendencies of the hemodynamic response and the associated variances for each event type. Statistical analysis procedures can then be applied to make inferences about the nature of the response. These procedures may test whether the response is significantly different from zero, or between one or more separate event types. There are a number of different approaches to this type of inferential analysis. The simplest approach is to determine whether there is a significant change in signal among the different images, which make up the epoch. This can be achieved using a one-way analysis of variance (ANOVA). A second approach is to assign fMRI images occurring with a certain delay after a trial to an "on" task state and temporally separate images to an "off" state. These two approaches, which were used in some initial ER-fMRI studies (e.g., BUCKNER et al. 1996; KONISHI et al. 1996; COHEN et al. 1997b), have the advantage of making few a priori assumptions about the event-related response. However, in situations in which a reasonable model of the hemodynamic response of interest is available, these approaches are likely to be less powerful than alternatives which make use of all known characteristics of the response, such as its shape and transition properties.

More recently, several analyses have been developed that compare the observed event-related response in each image with an idealized model of the expected hemodynamic response function or a range of possible responses (e.g., a basis set of hemodynamic responses). This comparison is typically achieved through a regression procedure that uses the idealized response(s) as a reference function and determines the statistical significance of the correlation at each tested voxel. Within a selective averaging (event-sorting) procedure, in which the mean timecourse of an event and the variance are the data of interest, statistical activation maps can be constructed via the covariance between the observed average signal and a normalized predicted impulse response function (DALE and BUCKNER 1997). For an extended time series which contains the full signal evolution of sequential events over time, the many separate events can be modeled using procedures more akin to typical blocked-design correlational analyses (KIM et al. 1997). Individual events can be thought of as extremely short task blocks. More recent approaches are now being explored that utilize full implementations of the general linear model (GLM) (e.g., JOSEPHS et al. 1997; ZARAHN et al. 1997; FRISTON et al. 1998; CLARK et al. 1998). Such methods promise the most flexibility because interactions of event-types with time and performance variables can be easily coded into the design matrix. Using any of these methods, voxels that best predicted by a particular response function in relation to the known onsets of the stimulus events will be identified.

36.4
Limits and Assumptions of Event-Related Functional MRI

A central question for effectively applying ER-fMRI methods is the boundary conditions for their use (e.g., how close in time can sequential events be

separated and what kinds of signal-to-noise tradeoffs can be expected). It is our current belief that extremely rapid presentation rates (<2 s between sequential events) are feasible and provide a powerful means of mapping brain function. Several distinct issues directly relate to this conclusion.

36.4.1
Stationarity and Linearity

The first issue concerns the stationarity and linearity of the BOLD impulse-response function. BOYNTON et al. (1996), relying on characterization of responses in visual cortex to controlled visual stimulation, suggested that, on first approximation, changes in intensity or duration of a visual stimulus have near linear and additive effects on the evoked BOLD response. These findings appear to hold for higher cognitive processes as well, in that similar results have been observed in prefrontal cortex activity through manipulations of intensity (load) and duration within working memory (COHEN et al. 1997a). Moreover, data from visual sensory responses suggest the hemodynamic response of one neural event will summate in a roughly linear manner on top of preceding events (DALE and BUCKNER 1997). Figure 36.2, for example, shows the approximately linear summation for multiple presentations of a 1 s visual stimulus.

The point that summation of the hemodynamic responses is only approximately linear should be seriously considered. Subtle departures from linear summation have been observed in nearly every study that has examined response summation and, in certain studies, the nonlinearities have been quite pronounced (FRISTON et al. 1997; VAZQUEZ and NOLL 1998). Fortunately, using parameters typical to many studies, the nonlinearities may be subtle enough to be considered approximately linear. It has been possible to assume linearity and carry out ER-fMRI studies using presentation rates (~1 event per 2 s or less) that are much faster than the time-course of the BOLD response, or even the repetition time (TR) being applied in a study. Directly relevant to this, DALE and BUCKNER (1997) showed that individual responses to simple sensory stimuli could be adequately separated and analyzed by using overlap correction methods. BUROCK et al. (1998) pushed this limit even farther, randomly intermixing varied sensory stimuli at a rate of one stimulus every 500 ms (250 ms stimulus duration, 250 ms gap between sequential stimuli). Recent rapid ER-fMRI studies of higher level cognitive processes, such as repetition priming (BUCKNER et al. 1998a) and face memory (CLARK et al. 1998), suggest the procedures can be effectively applied to cognitive tasks and higher-order brain regions (e.g., prefrontal cortex).

However, considerably more work must be done to define the precise limits of these "linear modeling" approaches to fMRI data analysis. One difficulty in resolving questions about how the hemodynamic signal summates over time is the fact that in many situations it is not known whether the underlying neuronal activity is itself linearly additive across time and trials. Put another way, when departures from linearity or stationarity are found, it is unclear whether they reflect an intrinsic nonlinear property of the hemodynamic response or of the underlying neuronal activity. For example, auditory word stimuli have been shown to exhibit roughly linear responses when stimuli were presented as frequently as one per 2 s or slower, but robust nonlinearities in the response are observed at higher stimulus presentation rates (FRISTON et al. 1997). It may be the case that the neuronal response to auditory words at such rapid rates is different to that of more widely spaced words; alternatively, the neuronal response to words may be constant across rates but hemodynamic response may saturate. The most parsimonious explanation is that the basic transformation between the summation of neuronal events and the BOLD response is approximately linear, at least with presentation rates typically used in fMRI studies. Instances where strong fMRI signal nonlinearities are observed, such as when very rapid stimuli are presented, may represent situations where there exist nonlinearities in the neuronal activity itself. Further investigation will clearly be needed to resolve this issue as well as develop analysis methods to take into account the nonlinearities, regardless of their origin.

36.4.2
Variability

A second central issue in analyzing ER-fMRI data is variability of the hemodynamic response (KIM et al. 1997). As would be expected in any real-world system, variability is present. Consequently, the relevant issues are: (1) the magnitude and practical implications of the variability; and (2) what the sources of variability can tell us about and/or do to limit our exploration of brain function. Preliminary analyses of these issues suggest the within-region hemodynamic response is reasonably stable across subjects (BUCKNER et al. 1998b), although individual subjects can clearly be shown to exhibit some variance in the timing of their response (KIM et al. 1997; RICHTER et al. 1997b). In one analysis, the hemodynamic response was examined across 13 subjects during a memory recognition task (BUCKNER et al. 1998b). Analyses were conducted separately for two different cortical regions (supplementary motor area, SMA, and extrastriate visual cortex). The response in each region was derived from many observations within a subject so that stable within-subject estimate of the responses could be obtained. The question then asked was: if the timing and shape of one subject's hemodynamic response was known for a given region, how well could it predict the other subjects' hemodynamic responses in that region? The answer was clear: the basic shape and timing of the hemodynamic response was stable across subjects (see Fig. 36.3). 72% of the variance of the shape of one subject's response could be predicted – on average – by any other subject. Moreover, the absolute range of the timing of the response was a few seconds, indicating that the standard error estimate of the mean response time was fractions of a second for the group of 13 subjects. As a further empirical dem-

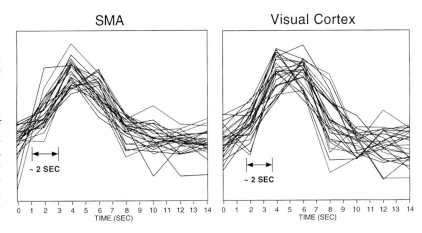

Fig. 36.3. The hemodynamic response from 13 separate subjects (two conditions per subject) are plotted in arbitrary unit for each of two brain regions: supplementary motor area (SMA) and visual cortex. As can be seen, variance of the timing of the response has a range of about 2 s for each region, suggesting strong central tendencies in the data and enabling signal averaging across subjects. (Adapted from BUCKNER et al. 1998b)

SMA

Visual Cortex

~ 2 SEC

~ 2 SEC

0 1 2 3 4 5 6 7 8 9 10 11 12 13 14
TIME (SEC)

0 1 2 3 4 5 6 7 8 9 10 11 12 13 14
TIME (SEC)

onstration, the response of one group of six subjects was compared to a second independent group of seven subjects. They nearly overlapped. Given this demonstration of the degree of reliability of the BOLD response within given regions, it should be possible to interpret changes in the onset or shape of the response to different event-types as reflecting changes in neural processing in that region (e.g., Luknowsky et al. 1998), even when central tendencies across averaged groups of subjects are considered.

Information about variation in the delay and shape of the hemodynamic response across brain regions has implications for questions regarding the latency and cascade of neural processing. In this regard, it is noteworthy that marked variations in the timing and shape of responses have been observed across regions even within the same subjects. For example, delays have been noted between visual and prefrontal regions on the order of 0.5–1 s during both word generation and memory retrieval tasks (BUCKNER et al. 1996; SCHACTER et al. 1997). In addition, more extreme delays between separate prefrontal regions (about 2–4 s) were noted during the memory retrieval task. While the source of this variation is currently unknown, several possibilities exist. One possible interpretation is that various delays result from differences in the underlying vasculature being sampled across regions (LEE et al. 1995). Vasculature explanations likely account for much of the pixel-by-pixel variance seen within a single functionally specialized region such as V1. However, this possibility seems unlikely to account for all of the broader regional findings observed so far, considering the longest delays have been noted in spatially averaged data and specifically in anterior prefrontal cortex, where large vasculature is minimal (SCHACTER et al. 1997). A second, more intriguing, possibility is that the observed regional differences in delay reflect delayed neuronal processing. While this possibility must currently be considered speculative, it will be fascinating to explore further the idea that certain neuronal responses are delayed and/or prolonged on the order of seconds following a task event (for a further discussion of this issue see ROSEN et al. 1998).

Aside from functional explanations, an important practical implication of hemodynamic variance across brain regions is that statistical methods used to identify areas of signal change will need to allow for variance in the timing and/or shape of the hemodynamic response to be sensitive to all forms of signal change. Several currently available statistical

methods either possess this feature (e.g., SCHACTER et al. 1997; FRISTON et al. 1998) or make no assumption about the shape (COHEN et al. 1997b).

36.4.3
Power

A nontrivial issue that confronts ER-fMRI is determining the relative tradeoffs in power when considering among several possible paradigm designs. For the purposes of this chapter, we reduce the issue of power to two separate questions: (1) What is the ideal mean rate of stimulus presentation? (2) What is the ideal temporal sequencing of the events about that mean rate? The two issues will interact and each has a large affect on the power of an ER-fMRI paradigm. It is perhaps easiest to start a discussion with the simplest example, in which the interstimulus interval is held constant. For purposes of this chapter, we also leave out discussion of interactions between paradigm design and colored noise properties of fMRI studies.

When the interstimulus interval is held constant (e.g., BUCKNER et al. 1996), the power of the design will begin to rapidly decrease as the intertrial interval becomes much less than the width of the hemodynamic response. It is easy to envision why this occurs: at fast rates, the hemodynamic response from a preceding event is decaying as the hemodynamic response of a subsequent is increasing. Within a linear model, the two will largely cancel each other and the observable response will diminish. Because sequential events are always positioned at a constant distance from each other in time, no deconvolution of the response is possible. Mathematical modeling (COX and BANDETTINI 1998) and empirical studies (BANDETTINI and COX 1998) suggest that, within a fixed interval design of this sort, the optimal rate for a typical hemodynamic response will be about one trial every 10–12 s. Fortunately, this particular kind of design likely represents the worst case scenario (Fig. 36.4).

A considerably more powerful design is to jitter the onset of the trials in time. For example, instead of having one trial appear every 8 s, trials could appear at random intervals either 6 or 10 s apart. The mean rate is held constant, but the timing is jittered. With such jitter, the underlying hemodynamic response can be appreciated through deconvolution (DALE and BUCKNER 1997). Considering the specific case in which the probability of an event occurring or not occurring is random and fixed, the obtainable power

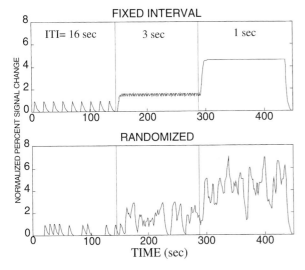

Fig. 36.4. Comparison of fixed interval spacing and randomized spacing of trials for three mean intertrial rates (16 s, 3 s, 1 s). A clear interaction between the kind of ER-fMRI paradigm and rate can be observed. *Top,* For fixed interval paradigms, as the rate of stimulus presentation is increased, the deflection from the mean decreases: sequential events cancel each other out (e.g., the signal goes flat in the 1 s condition). This behavior does not reflect saturation but rather the cumulative effect of summed responses within a linear system (see BUROCK et al., 1998 for more details). *Bottom,* For randomized paradigms, in which trial spacing is jittered in time, the deflection about the mean actually increases at faster rates. This deflection represents signal that can be deconvolved and used as the basis for time-course and statistical activation map generation. The increased mean deflection as stimulus presentation rate increases indicates increased power. For randomized designs, which are appropriate for a number of applications, extremely rapid presentation rates are possible. (Modified from BUROCK et al. 1998)

will increase as the interstimulus interval is decreased (BUROCK et al. 1998). Such behavior in statistical power is nearly opposite to that observed for the case of a fixed interval and considerably more amenable to cognitive and behavioral task design (Fig. 36.4). When the interval between separate events of the same type are jittered in time, short intertrial intervals (~2 s) typical of behavioral and ERP studies provide considerably more power than analogous designs with long intertrial intervals (see BUROCK et al. 1998 for a discussion of the nature of the distribution from which these random intervals can be best selected).

36.5
Implications for Human Brain Mapping

The observation that fMRI is sensitive to transient neuronal events has a number of important implications for cognitive neuroscientific and clinical applications. First, fMRI studies can now achieve the same flexibility in experimental design found in behavioral and ERP studies. In particular, these studies typically use paradigms in which individual trial events are elicited rapidly, with distinct event types randomly intermixed. Second, classification of events often cannot be determined a priori – such as when the subject's response to the event is a factor. Being able to isolate fMRI signals allows the BOLD response to be sorted by subject performance (e.g., by whether an event is performed correctly or not, or based on how long an event takes to complete). Third, certain kinds of neuronal responses may not be stable over time and are therefore best addressed through trial-by-trial measurements. Paradigms exploring novelty effects and learning provide prime examples. Fourth, rare and/or unpredictable events can be the target event of interest in which signal change from sequential or common events is the basis. Finally, ER-fMRI provides a means for resolving the activity and dynamics of within-trial events, which may aid many questions in attention and working memory that require the separation of cue- vs probe-related activity, or in examining the dynamics of activity during the delay period between these events.

Thus, the flexibility afforded to experimental design by ER-fMRI allows new classes of behavioral paradigms to be tested. However, as with any methodological advancement, the utility of ER-fMRI will be evaluated by the new scientific questions that are elucidated by their application. Below, we discuss several examples which both demonstrate the impact ER-fMRI is having on the field of cognitive neuroscience and illustrate how ER-fMRI already has, or could be, exploited along several of the dimensions described above.

36.5.1
Mixed Trial Designs

The most basic, and possibly most general, advance of ER-fMRI is the increased flexibility it affords to experimental design. In particular, the ability to separate out fMRI responses in an event-specific manner allows the possibility of intermixed event types. Mixed-trial designs provide a control for many of the strategic effects that can occur when conditions are blocked. For example, many findings in cognitive psychology will be influenced by practice, asymmetrical transfer between conditions, and/or fatigue. Mixed-trial designs avoid many of these effects by equally distributing conditions throughout the experimental session.

An additional issue associated with blocked-trial designs is that they may cause differences in the processing strategies adopted by subjects during task performance, which may result in differential patterns of neural activity. Subjects may anticipate or implicitly adjust performance when they are able to predict trials of a certain type. An illustration of this issue comes from blocked studies of recognition memory in which debate arose as to the role of certain prefrontal areas in memory retrieval (RUGG et al. 1996; BUCKNER et al. 1998b, c; WAGNER et al., 1998a). RUGG et al. (1996), in an influential study, suggested that certain prefrontal areas were most active during trials in which subjects successfully retrieved information. The manner in which this conclusion was derived, however, may have influenced the interpretation. In the aforementioned study and all those that proceeded, blocks of trials that had fewer or greater numbers of successfully retrieved items were the basis of exploration. RUGG and colleagues noted that blocks with the most successfully retrieved items activated the prefrontal areas to the greatest degree. However, by comparing an ER-fMRI study and a blocked-trial study similar to that of RUGG et al. (1996), BUCKNER et al. (1998b, c) were able to show that modulation of the prefrontal areas in relation to retrieval success was closely tied to the use of a blocked-trial procedure; ER-fMRI separation of successfully retrieved and correctly rejected items indicated equal levels of prefrontal signal change. The preliminary conclusion is that the blocked-trial paradigm, in which item events are predictable, may have encouraged subjects to adjust their strategy (implicitly or explicitly) and influenced prefrontal participation. ER-fMRI paradigms can circumvent this issue by presenting trials randomly and contrasting different trial types under conditions in which the specific upcoming event type cannot be predicted.

Another benefit of mixed-trial designs in fMRI studies occurs when experimental effects are necessitated upon the use of low probability events within trains of stimuli. Along these lines, McCARTHY et al. (1997) explored the ERP P300 (which is evoked by rare events) using ER-fMRI. They presented continuous strings of characters with a target string appearing unpredictably once every 20 or so trials – a procedure that can only be accomplished within randomly intermixed trial designs. By averaging data in a stimulus-locked manner to the onsets of the infrequent events, McCARTHY and colleagues observed that target events elicited transient increases in prefrontal and parietal cortex activity. Additional examples of the exploitation of ER-fMRI to examine neural activity to rare, randomly occurring, events can be seen in the work of KONISHI et al. (1997), involving response inhibition, and CARTER et al. (1998), examining response competition effects (discussed further below).

36.5.2
Post-hoc Sorting

Another dimension in which ER-fMRI increases the flexibility of functional neuroimaging studies is in the ability to sort trials on a post-hoc basis. The most practical aspect of this capability is in the area of artifact rejection. As is done in behavioral research, there are many instances in which it may be desirable to exclude responses on certain trials, based on performance measures such as outlier responses in terms of response time, incorrect responses, or instances in which subjects either do not fixate appropriately or have high motion-related artifact. ER-fMRI task designs make this possible by allowing the investigator to determine post-hoc which trials contain artifacts and exclude these from further analysis. One might even imagine situations in which the "good" trials are few and far between, such as in patients and children in whom motion is a serious issue. So long as enough artifact-free events can be collected, imaging protocols based on infrequently kept events can provide a powerful means of examining subject groups for whom data loss is considerable. In another example, BIRN et al. (in press) addressed the issue of speech-related motion artifact, which is a challenge to fMRI. They showed that modeling the hemodynamic response function to weight images occurring several seconds after the actual event of speaking allows movement artifacts occurring during speech to be minimized (remember, the hemodynamic response to an event is delayed by a few seconds). While not explicitly post-hoc, the study of BIRN et al. (in press) illustrates another instance in which throwing out, or more specifically in their instance, weighting, the inclusion of certain data differentially, may benefit data analysis.

A more substantive advantage conveyed by post-hoc sorting of fMRI data is for studies that ask questions regarding changes in brain activity associated with certain characteristics of subject performance. For example, in the recognition memory paradigm of BUCKNER et al. (1998b), discussed above, individual trial responses were sorted based on subjects' recognition judgments to previously studied items. ER-fMRI studies using performance-based sorting can also be applied to answer questions that link neural activity with subsequently measured behavioral effects, rather than behavioral effects acquired at the time of the activity. A prime example of such a procedure occurs when examining neural mechanisms underlying memory encoding. Signal change measured during the original presentation of an item can be later sorted according to whether subjects correctly remember or forget the item on a subsequent memory test. WAGNER et al. (1998b) used such a procedure to show that to-be-remembered words activate prefrontal and temporal regions more than to-be-forgotten words. In their study, words were presented rapidly, and subject performance after the imaging session dictated how the word items would be sorted. Such paradigm flexibility previously available to other modalities (e.g., ERP; PALLER et al. 1988) is now afforded to fMRI via event-locked sorting.

A third example of how ER-fMRI can be used to examine neural activity based on subject performance comes from a study by CARTER et al. (1998). In this study, correct vs error trials were sorted separately and compared during performance of a variant of a working memory task called the Continuous Performance Test. Anterior cingulate activity was found to be significantly increased during error trials, consistent with previous reports from the ERP literature of error-related activity stemming from a medial frontal generator (GEHRING et al. 1993; DEHAENE et al. 1994). In addition, CARTER et al. (1998) were also able to examine activity in this same anterior cingulate region during correct performance of low-frequency trials thought to produce differing degrees of response competition. This analysis found that anterior cingulate activity was increased in high-response competition trials relative to trials in which competition was low. These results were interpreted as suggesting that the region monitors the presence of processing conflict, rather than errors per se.

ER-fMRI can also be used in experimental designs in which it is desirable to sort trials based on other aspects of subject performance, such as reaction time (RT). For example, it may be of interest to compare activity in fast response vs slow response trials. An extension of this approach would be to identify regions whose activity correlated with RT on a trial-by-trial basis. This type of approach is complementary to the averaging procedures discussed in Sect. 36.3. In particular, averaging across trials allows the central tendencies in the modal hemodynamic response to be observed, while examination of single-trial hemodynamic responses may provide information about the variability in responses across individual events. Of course, this type of analysis is dependent upon having adequate signal-to-noise characteristics in the fMRI signal. RICHTER et al. (1997a) have recently provided evidence (using a high-field strength magnet) that a single trial of a mental rotation task is sufficient to detect parietal cortex activation. Such a demonstration underscores the kind of analysis that is possible; if individual trial events can provide detectable signals then we should be readily able to correlate with and sort between different item types in fMRI data analysis. As our understanding of the characteristics and limitations of event-related fMRI studies improves, it is likely that techniques will increasingly take advantage of this property in the future.

36.5.3
Within-Trial Components and Dynamics

Many clinical and cognitive neuroscientific questions involve resolving the activity and dynamics of the component neural events that may occur within a trial. For example, at the most basic level, in a sensorimotor task, sensory processing should occur in different neural regions and involve different dynamics than does motor processing. However, within a blocked-trial paradigm it would not be possible to dissociate these two components of processing. D'Esposito and colleagues (ZARAHN et al. 1997) recently examined whether ER-fMRI could be used to observe such dissociation. They had subjects make comparisons about the locations of pairs of objects either presented simultaneously (no-delay condition) or separated by 12 s delays (delay condition). Comparison of activation time-courses across the two conditions clearly showed temporal separation of the fMRI signal. The no-delay condition exhibited activation in regions of motor cortex well before similar activation in the delay condition. A similar pattern of results was found in a study by

KIM et al. (1997), which used a visual precuing procedure occurring at variable delays before sequential finger movement.

ER-fMRI can also be used to answer questions about the dynamics of higher level cognitive processes. COURTNEY et al. (1997) provided one of the earliest illustrations of this type of study. They explored a working memory paradigm and organized intermixed trials such that the event of encoding a stimulus could be temporally separated from the act of maintaining the stimulus in working memory. By using analysis procedures that separated the within-trial components related to encoding from those related to maintenance, they were able to show a pathway of brain areas active during both encoding and maintenance but showed differential participation between the two kinds of processes. Posterior visual areas contributed proportionately more to perceptual encoding operations, while prefrontal areas made their greatest contribution to maintenance operations. COHEN et al. (1997b) reported a similar finding by examining the within-trial time courses for a letter working memory task (called the n-back task). They looked for effects of time within the trials and its relation to a second factor, memory load. The logic was that load-sensitive sustained activity across the trial would indicate areas involved in maintenance or other sustained memory-related processes such as rehearsal. In contrast, transient activity (i.e., showing an effect of time) that was load-insensitive would not be related to memory processes. Consistent with the work of COURTNEY et al. (1997), they found effects of the latter type within certain prefrontal and parietal areas and effects of the former type within posterior visual areas and sensorimotor cortex.

These initial studies regarding the neural activity dynamics in working memory pave the way for more detailed explorations using ER-fMRI. In particular, it will now be possible to ask questions regarding how task factors affect multiple different aspects of the neural response such as its latency and duration, in addition to its amplitude. This aspect of ER-fMRI is critical because for many cognitive neuroscience questions the effect of task variables may be hypothesized not to affect the peak amplitude of response. An example of this type of question comes from the recent work of BRAVER et al. (1998) on interference effects in working memory. They presented interfering stimuli during the delay periods of a working memory task, a manipulation that was previously shown to produce maintenance-specific decrements in behavioral performance. Cue-related responses observed in dorsolateral prefrontal cortex were the same amplitude under both baseline and interference conditions. In contrast, the activity decayed more quickly during the delay period under interference, suggesting that the manipulation selectively affected the duration rather than the amplitude of the response in prefrontal cortex.

The advent of ER-fMRI has also paved the way for future studies asking related questions about the onset latency of neural responses under various task conditions. For example, it might be hypothesized that the response of a particular brain region would be delayed as a task increased in difficulty, or when an additional processing stage must occur prior to its activation. Methodological developments by Menon and colleagues (LUKNOWSKY et al. 1998) suggest onset latency differences of 125 ms or less may be possible to resolve.

36.6
Future Directions

Currently available ER-fMRI methods offer an array of benefits to human brain mapping research as outlined above. One broad area of growing interest is the integration of ER-fMRI with information from other imaging modalities. This interest arises because the ultimate limits of temporal resolution with fMRI will likely be imposed by the underlying changes in physiology that they measure, which are (for BOLD contrast) fairly indirect, temporally blurred, and affected by differences in regional vasculature (LEE et al. 1995). Transient coordination of neuronal activity occurring across segments of cortex on the time scale of tens to a few hundred milliseconds will likely remain the domain of other techniques (EEG, MEG, and perhaps certain optical imaging methods; GRATTON and FABIANI (in press). These techniques are capable of meaningful, rapid measurements of brain activity but provide relatively coarse spatial resolution. In order to overcome this limitation, methods for combining the temporal resolution of EEG and MEG with the spatial resolution of functional MRI are being developed (e.g., DALE et al. 1995, 1997). Using such methods, it is now becoming possible to study the precise spatiotemporal orchestration of neuronal activity associated with perceptual and cognitive events. Event-related fMRI allows a further refinement of such integration by affording the ability to study the same exact paradigms in fMRI settings and during EEG and MEG sessions.

Another direction of future research concerns the further evolution of statistical analyses for mapping event-related hemodynamic responses. Methods that make few or no assumptions about the shape of the hemodynamic response as well as those that consider the possibility of nonlinear summation of the hemodynamic response are on the horizon. Moreover, as new and more powerful analysis methods provide greater understanding of the true sensitivity and specificity of fMRI data, our ability to address increasingly sophisticated hypotheses about the underlying mechanisms of brain action will continue to improve. In addition, we have yet to come to fully understand the relative signal-to-noise tradeoffs between blocked-trial and event-related paradigms, and for event-related paradigms that space or position trials in fundamentally different ways. It has been empirically demonstrated that randomly intermixed trial events spaced just a few seconds apart can be used to generate activity maps as well as time-course information for the hemodynamic responses associated with these intermixed event types (DALE and BUCKNER 1997; BUCKNER et al. 1998a; CLARK et al.1998; WAGNER et al. 1998b). However, the limitations of this approach are still yet to be determined and may involve constraints imposed by cognitive and neuronal factors that may interact with trial spacing.

Along these lines, it may be important to examine how neural activity is modulated by the local sequential structure of trials even if these are spaced widely enough in time to resolve without overlap correction. Findings of modulation of brain activity by local sequential structure have already been observed in ERP research (SQUIRES et al. 1976), and this provides another arena in which ER-fMRI can provide both convergent and complementary information regarding an as yet unexplained neural phenomena. Another area of experimental design that should be explored in the future concerns pushing the definition of an event. Currently, almost all ER-fMRI studies treat the external presentation of a stimulus as the event of interest. Yet, here again, EEG and MEG research provide demonstration that measurements of brain activity can be aligned to other task-related events such as behavioral responses, eye movements, onset of seizure activity or other non-stimulus locked occurrences. Of course, there are methodological challenges that need to be faced before such techniques can be successfully incorporated, but the basic and clinical research applications of ER-fMRI make the avenues highly worth pursuing.

Acknowledgments. We thank Amy Sanders and Deanna Barch for thoughtful comments on an earlier version of this manuscript. Anders Dale, Marc Burock, and Peter Bandettini provided valuable discussion. Support for the work presented in this chapter comes from grants by the National Institute of Mental Health (MH57506-01), the National Institute on Deafness and Other Communication Disorders (DC03245-02), and the McDonnell Center for Higher Brain Function.

References

Bandettini PA (1993) MRI studies of brain activation: Dynamic characteristics. In: Functional MRI of the brain. Society of Magnetic Resonance in Medicine, Berkeley

Bandettini PA, Cox RW (1998) Contrast in single trial fMRI: Interstimulus interval dependency and comparison with blocked strategies. Proceedings of the International Society for Magnetic Resonance in Medicine, 6th meeting 1:161

Birn RM, Bandettini PA, Cox RW, Shaker R et al. (in press) Event-related fMRI of tasks involving brief motion. Hum Brain Map

Blamire AM, Ogawa S, Ugurbil K et al. (1992) Dynamic mapping of the human visual cortex by high-speed magnetic resonance imaging. Proc Natl Acad Sci USA 89:11069–11073

Boulanouar K, Demonet JF, Berry I, Chollet F, Manelfe C, Celsis P (1996) Study of the spatiotemporal dynamics of the motor system with fMRI using the evoked response of activated pixels: a deconvolutional approach. Proceedings of the International Society for Magnetic Resonance in Medicine, 4th meeting, 3

Boynton GM, Engel SA, Glover GH, Heeger DJ (1996) Linear systems analysis of functional magnetic resonance imaging in human V1. J Neurosci 16:4207–4221

Braver TS, Cohen JD, Barch DM, Noll DC et al. (1998) Effects of interference in working memory on prefrontal cortex activity: a test of a computational model. Neuroimage 7:515

Buckner RL, Bandettini PA, O'Craven KM, Savoy RL, Petersen SE, Raichle ME, Rosen BR et al. (1996) Detection of cortical activation during averaged single trials of a cognitive task using functional magnetic resonance imaging. Proc Natl Acad Sci USA 93:14878–14883

Buckner RL, Goodman J, Burock M et al. (1998a) Functional-anatomic correlates of object priming in humans revealed by rapid presentation event-related fMRI. Neuron 20:285–296

Buckner RL, Koutstaal W, Schacter DL, Dale AM, Rotte MR, Rosen BR (1998b) Functional-anatomic study of episodic retrieval: II. Selective averaging of event-related fMRI trials to test the retrieval success hypothesis. Neuroimage 7:163–175

Buckner RL, Koutstaal W, Schacter DL, Wagner AD, Rosen BR (1998c) Functional-anatomic study of episodic retrieval using fMRI: I. Retrieval effort versus retrieval success. Neuroimage 7: 151–162

Burock MA, Buckner RL, Woldorff MG, Rosen BR, Dale AM (1998) Randomized event-related experimental designs allow for extremely rapid presentation rates using functional MRI. NeuroReport 9:3735–3739

Carter CS, Braver TS, Barch DM et al. (1998) Anterior cingulate cortex, error detection, and the online monitoring of performance. Science 280:747–749

Clark VP, Maisog JM, Haxby JV An fMRI study of face perception and memory using random stimulus sequences. J Neurophysiol 79:3257–3265

Cohen JD, Nystrom LE, Sabb FW, Braver TS, Noll DC (1997a) Tracking the dynamics of FMRI activation in humans under manipulations of duration and intensity of working memory processes. Soc Neurosci Abstr 23:1678

Cohen JD, Perlstein WM, Braver TS, Nystrom LE, Noll DC, Jonides J, Smith EE (1997b) Temporal dynamics of brain activation during a working memory task. Nature 386:604–607

Courtney SM, Ungerleider LG, Keil K, Haxby JV (1997) Transient and sustained activity in a distributed neural system for human working memory. Nature 386:608–611

Cox RW, Bandettini PA (1998) Single trial fMRI: the optimal inter-stimulus interval. Proceedings of the International Society for Magnetic Resonance in Medicine, 6th meeting 1:244

Dale AM, Buckner RL (1997) Selective averaging of rapidly presented individual trials using fMRI. Hum Brain Map 5:329–340

Dale A, Ahlfors SP, Aronen H, et al. (1995) Spatiotemporal imaging of coherent motion selective areas in human cortex. Soc Neurosci Abstr 21:1275

Dale AM, Halgren E, Lewine JD, Buckner RL, Paulson K, Marinkovic K, Rosen BR (1997) Spatio-temporal localization of cortical word repetition-effects in a size judgement task using combined fMRI/MEG. Neuroimage 5: S592

Dehaene S, Posner MI, Tucker DM (1994) Localization of a neural system for error detection and compensation. Psychol Sci 5:303–306

Friston KJ, Josephs O, Rees G, Turner R (1997) Nonlinear event-related responses in fMRI. Magn Reson Med 39:41–52

Friston KJ, Fletcher P, Josephs O, Holmes A, Rugg MD, Turner R (1998) Event-related fMRI: characterizing differential responses. Neuroimage 7:30–40

Gehring WJ, Goss B, Coles MGH, Meyer DE, Donchin E (1993) A neural system for error detection and compensation. Psychol Sci 4:385–390

Gratton G, Fabiani M Dynamic brain imaging: the study of the time course of activity in localized brain areas. Psychonom Bull Rev (in press)

Humberstone M, Barlow M, Clare S et al. (1995) Functional magnetic resonance imaging of single motor events with echo planar imaging at 3 T, using a signal averaging technique. Proc Soc Magn Reson 3rd Sci Meet Exhib 2:858

Josephs O, Turner R, Friston K (1997) Event-related fMRI. Hum Brain Map 5:243–248

Kim SG, Richter W, Ugurbil K (1997) Limitations of temporal resolution in functional MRI. Magn Reson Med 37.631–636

Konishi S, Yoneyama R, Itagaki H et al. (1996) Transient brain activity used in magnetic resonance imaging to detect functional areas. Neuroreport 8:19–23

Konishi S, Nakajima K, Uchida I, Sekihara K, Miyashita Y (1997) Temporally resolved no-go dominant brain activity in the prefrontal cortex revealed by functional magnetic resonance imaging. Neuroimage 5:S120

Kwong KK, Belliveau JW, Chesler DA et al. (1992) Dynamic magnetic resonance imaging of human brain activity during primary sensory stimulation. Proc Natl Acad Sci USA 89:5675–5679

Lee AT, Glover GH, Meyer CH (1995) Discrimination of large venous vessels in time-course spiral blood-oxygen-level-dependent magnetic-resonance functional neuroimaging. Magn Reson Med 33:745–754

Luknowsky DC, Gati JS, Menon RS (1998) Mental chronometry using single trials and EPI at 4 T. Proc Int Soc Magn Reson Med 6th Meet 1:167

McCarthy G, Luby M, Gore J, Goldman-Rakic P (1997) Infrequent events transiently activate human prefrontal and parietal cortex as measured by functional MRI. J Neurophysiol 77:1630–1634

Ogawa S, Lee T, Nayak A, Glynn P (1990) Oxygenation-sensitive contrast in magnetic resonance image of rodent brain at high magnetic fields. Magn Reson Med 14:68–78

Ogawa S, Tank DW, Menon R, Ellerman JM, Kim SG, Merkle H, Ugurbil K (1992) Intrinsic signal changes accompanying sensory stimulation: functional brain mapping with magnetic resonance imaging. Proc Natl Acad Sci USA 89:5951–5955

Paller KA, McCarthy G, Wood CC (1988) ERPs predictive of subsequent recall and recognition performance. Biol Psychol 26:269–276

Richter W, Georgopoulos AP, Ugurbil K, Kim SG (1997a) Detection of brain activity during mental rotation in a single trial by fMRI. Neuroimage 5:S49

Richter W, Ugurbil K, Georgopolous A, Kim SG (1997b) Time-resolved fMRI of mental rotation. Neuroreport 8:3697–3702

Rosen BR, Buckner RL, Dale AM (1998) Event related fMRI: Past, present, and future. Proc Natl Acad Sci USA 95:773–780

Rugg MD, Fletcher PC, Frith CD, Frackowiak RSJ, Dolan RJ (1996) Differential response of the prefrontal cortex in successful and unsuccessful memory retrieval. Brain 119:2073–2083

Savoy RL, Bandettini PA, O'Craven KM et al. (1995) Pushing the temporal resolution of fMRI: studies of very brief visual stimuli, onset variability and asynchrony, and stimulus-correlated changes in noise. Proc Soc Magn Reson 3rd Sci Meet Exhib 2:450

Schacter DL, Buckner RL, Koutstaal W, Dale AM, Rosen BR (1997b) Late onset of anterior prefrontal activity during true and false recognition: an event-related fMRI study. Neuroimage 6:259–269

Squires KC, Wickens C, Squires NK, Donchin E (1976) The effect of stimulus sequence on the waveform of the cortical event-related potential. Science 193:1142–1146

Vazquez AL, Noll DC (1998) Nonlinear aspects of the BOLD response in functional MRI. Neuroimage 7:108–118

Wagner AD, Desmond JE, Glover GH, Gabrieli JDE (1998a)Prefrontal cortex and recognition memory: fMRI evidence for context-dependent retrieval processes. Brain 121:1985–2002

Wagner AD, Schacter DL, Rotte M et al. (1998b) Building memories: remembering and forgetting of verbal experiences as predicted by brain activity. Science 281:188–191

Zarahn E, Aguirre G, D'Esposito M (1997) A trial-based experimental design for fMRI. Neuroimage 6:122–138

37 Cortical Excitability and Connectivity Reflected in fMRI, MEG, EEG, and TMS

R.J. Ilmoniemi, H.J. Aronen

CONTENTS

37.1
Introduction

Functional brain imaging techniques reveal patterns of activation in the neuronal network – either directly as in magnetoencephalography (MEG), electroencephalography (EEG) and optical imaging of intrinsic signals, or indirectly as in functional MRI (fMRI), positron emission tomography (PET), near-infrared spectroscopy (NIRS) and other techniques that detect changes in blood flow or metabolism. Cortical activation is intimately tied with the neuronal connectivity, not only between the brain and the periphery but also and in particular between different brain areas. In fact, no less than 99%–99.9% of the axons in the white matter serve corticocortical and transcallosal communication.

R.J. Ilmoniemi, PhD; BioMag Laboratory, Medical Engineering Centre, Helsinki University Central Hospital, P.O. Box 508, FIN-00029 HYKS, Finland
H.J. Aronen, MD, PhD; Professor, Department of Clinical Radiology, Kuopio University Hospital, FIN-70100 Kuopio, Finland; Department of Radiology, Helsinki University Central Hospital, P.O. Box 380, FIN-00029 HYKS, Finland

In general, areas processing similar types of information tend to be connected with each other. For example, in the visual area V1, columns with similar orientation preference are interconnected. Speech areas in the temporal and frontal lobes are connected with each other; the motor system forms an exquisite network involving the sensorimotor cortex, basal ganglia, thalamus and cerebellum. About 45% of the cerebral volume is white matter, i.e., communication lines from the cortex and subcortical nuclei to other parts of the brain or to the periphery (Miller et al. 1980). There are striking differences between different tracts; e.g., the number of axons in each optic nerve is 1.3 million but only 28,000 in the auditory nerve. The strong interplay of the left and right side of the brain is reflected by the interhemispheric pathways, with about 20 million axons traversing the corpus callosum.

During this decade, we have witnessed tremendous progress with various imaging techniques that can characterize the in vivo function of the human brain (fMRI, MEG, EEG, PET, SPECT, and NIRS). However, each of these techniques used and interpreted in isolation has inherent limitations; to obtain a complete spatiotemporal picture of the functioning human brain, these methods must be integrated more tightly.

In this chapter, we emphasize that the combined use of different imaging techniques provides improved accuracy and reliability in the study of cerebral connectivity and excitability. Anatomical information from MRI is essential for providing a 3D map of the territory to be investigated, while the combination of information from functional MRI, MEG and EEG provide spatiotemporal information of the neuronal activity (Liu et al. 1998). Transcranial magnetic stimulation (TMS) combined with EEG (Ilmoniemi et al. 1997), PET (Paus et al. 1997) or fMRI (Bohning et al. 1998; Ives et al. 1998) provides direct evidence of functional connectivity, while fiber orientations can be obtained from diffusion-weighted MRI (Makris et al. 1997; Tuch et al. 1998a, b; Werring et al. 1998).

37.2
Cortical Excitability

Cortical excitability is a measure of how vigorously neurons react to input. In the case of epilepsy, cortical excitability is enhanced in the epileptogenic zone, whereas within areas affected by tumor or stroke it may be reduced. Attention, preparation for a task, the sensory environment or medication may alter the excitability. Repeated monotonous stimuli lead to habituation, i.e., to reduced responses to these stimuli; however, if a certain kind of sensory input is always accompanied by an event of great significance, the corresponding sensory mechanism may become sensitized.

Cortical excitability depends on the arousal level mediated by subcortical nuclei. It is also modulated via lateral inhibition and similar mechanisms from neighboring or otherwise related brain areas. The state of neurotransmitter systems affects the balance of inhibitory and excitatory mechanisms (ZIEMANN et al. 1996). On the whole, the overall balance of our neuronal network is governed by dynamic mechanisms; too high excitability may lead to epileptic seizures or other instabilities, too little excitability to diminished brain activation. The functional state of the system depends very much on the connectivity, as shown by the simulations reported by FRISTON (1997). We live at the borderline between derailment from balance and getting trapped into basins of attraction of the neuronal dynamic system.

Excitability can be defined as the increase of neuronal firing level when excitatory input, in one way or the other, is administered to an area of cortex. Quantification of the input is difficult, but well-controlled experiments can be done by comparing indices of neuronal activation between different experimental conditions. Electrophysiological measurements are widely used to diagnose changes in cortical excitability. The hemodynamic response provides another well-characterized measure of excitability.

37.3
Functional Connectivity

The interwoven patterns of activation in the cerebral cortex are to a large extent defined by neural connectivity. The brain is a web of multiple feedforward, feedback and lateral connections (FELLEMAN and VAN ESSEN 1991; VANDUFFEL et al. 1997). There is a general feedforward direction of information flow from the primary sensory to secondary to association and to motor areas. Feedforward connections tend to arise in superficial layers of the cortex and terminate in layer 4 in the target area, while feedback connections start in deep layers and end in both superficial and deep layers. Feedforward connections from one area to another are usually accompanied by feedback connections between the same areas (NOWAK et al. 1997). Both types of influence are mediated by pyramidal cells of which there are about 5 billion (NOBACK and DEMAREST 1981), i.e., more than 20,000 per square millimeter of cortex!

Local connections, typically on the order of millimeters in extent, are formed by fibers in the gray matter; here the signals travel at the low speed of under 1 m/s (NOWAK et al. 1997). In the white matter, functionally related cortical areas over long distances are coupled with each other directly (SCANNELL et al. 1995; ROUILLER et al. 1994) or indirectly (GUILLERY 1995), the transmission times being typically under or near 15 ms (MEYER et al. 1998), corresponding to speeds approaching 100 m/s.

While anatomical connectivity is easy to define (e.g., number of axons from region A to B per unit area of B) and can be characterized by means of diffusion-weighted MRI (Fig. 37.1; MAKRIS et al. 1997; TUCH et al. 1998a, b; WERRING et al. 1998), functional

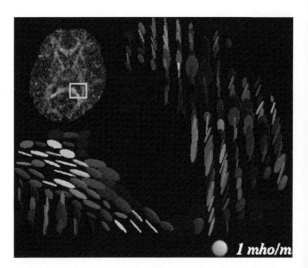

Fig. 37.1. Electrical conductivity tensor map of the region of interest (*inset*) derived from magnetic resonance diffusion tensor data (TUCH et al. 1998b). The tensor is depicted by an ellipsoid with each axis an eigenvector scaled by the corresponding eigenvalue. The color of the ellipsoid gives the orientation of the major eigenvector, with *red* indicating lateral, *green* anterior-posterior, and *blue* superior-inferior. The color is saturated by the degree of anisotropy. (Courtesy of David S. Tuch, MGH-NMR Center, Boston)

connectivity poses more difficult conceptual and experimental problems. For example, it depends critically on the excitability of the target structures, since a response at the target is required for connectivity to have an effect.

Functional connectivity (FRISTON 1994) has been "loosely defined as the correlation of activity among brain regions" (McINTOSH et al. 1997), but this definition is unfortunate since correlated activity does not imply connectivity between areas in question (see Fig. 37.2). This problem has been recognized and the term "effective connectivity" has been introduced; this is the influence an area has, directly or indirectly, on another area. Another suggestion is to speak of functional clustering or grouping – a cluster is formed of brain areas that interact among themselves much more than with other areas (GERSTEIN et al. 1978; FRISTON et al. 1996; TONINO et al. 1998).

There is functional connectivity from area A to area B provided that: (1) there is a connection from A to B either directly (Fig. 37.2a) or indirectly (Fig. 37.2b) and that (2) the connection is functional, i.e., capable of transmitting an influence. Functional connectivity can be measured by observing how activity at A affects activity at B, but one has to be able to rule out the possibility that a third area D is affecting both A and B (Fig. 37.2c). One has to bear in mind, however, that a large fraction of functional connections may be missed by macroscopic measurements that rely on correlated activity between areas. Hemodynamic measurements are blind to certain transient activation patterns or to activation where excitatory and inhibitory effects are in balance so that no overall hemodynamic changes take place. Macroscopic electrophysiological measures, on the other hand, are blind to activation patterns where the neurons do not fire synchronously.

For quantitative description of one aspect of functional connectivity, the term "path coefficient" has been suggested (McINTOSH and GONZALEZ-LIMA 1994). This measure indicates the expected change in the (macroscopically observed) activity in area B given a unit change of activity in area A, when all other regions are disregarded. Neuronal activity would be naturally described by the firing rate, but macroscopic imaging methods are limited to providing much coarser measures such as regional cerebral blood flow (rCBF) or estimates of source current density. Although the physiological interpretation of macroscopic path coefficients is problematic, these quantities have proven quite useful in the interpretation of measured activation patterns (McINTOSH et al. 1996).

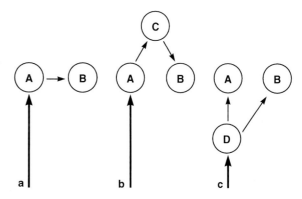

Fig. 37.2a–c. Basic types of connections that may lead to correlated activity between brain areas. **a** Direct connection from *A* to *B*. **b** Indirect connection via *C*. **c** Parallel activation. Input from *D* can result in correlated activity at areas *A* and *B* without any connection between them

Coherent activity in different parts of the brain in vivo have been studied by a number of investigators. GEVINS et al. (1989, 1995) used high-resolution EEG in order to establish correlations in brain activity between frontal and parietal areas during difficult motor tasks requiring intense concentration. Although useful information can be obtained from scalp-potential covariances, it will be more meaningful to estimate correlations directly between the neuronal sources on the basis of EEG or MEG (SMITH 1992).

BISWAL et al. (1995) obtained echo planar images from subjects in the resting state, observing correlated low-frequency (<0.1 Hz) fluctuations in several regions of cortex associated with motor functions and thereby concluding that fMRI is suitable for studies of functional connectivity. In a similar paradigm, LOWE et al. (1998) detected correlations between left- and right-hemisphere echo-planar imaging (EPI) signals, in particular between homologous areas in the motor and visual cortices and the left and right amygdalae. BUCHEL and FRISTON (1997) found that effective connectivity between the visual motion area V5 and posterior parietal cortex (PPC) is modulated by attention. Using a structural equation model, they concluded that the prefrontal cortex, which is connected to PPC, modulates the effect V5 afferents have on PPC.

We suggest that further improved measures of connectivity can be obtained by combining fMRI with EEG and MEG and by using TMS as a new direct neuronal activation tool. We discuss these issues in some detail below.

37.4
Magnetoencephalography and Electroencephalography

Both MEG and EEG measure directly the electrical source currents in the brain, allowing one to follow real-time activation patterns of the cerebral cortex. The technique requires sophisticated instrumentation and a thorough understanding of the intricacies of the forward and inverse problems (HÄMÄLÄINEN et al. 1993).

In 1853, Helmholtz showed that the electromagnetic inverse problem is nonunique, i.e., that even complete knowledge of the electric and magnetic fields surrounding a body does not enable one to determine uniquely the internal sources. It is necessary to apply supplementary information or assumptions to make the solution unique. Here lies the key to the benefits from integrating MEG/EEG with other brain imaging techniques such as fMRI (LIU et al. 1998).

MEG is most sensitive to postsynaptic pyramidal cell activity in fissural cortex, where the current flow along the cell structures is oriented tangentially, i.e., parallel to the skull, whereas it does not detect sources that are oriented exactly radially (perpendicular to the skull). By contrast, EEG complements MEG by being most sensitive to activity in the gyral cortex.

37.4.1
Conductivity Models of the Head

To make reliable deductions about brain activity on the basis of electromagnetic field measurements outside the skull, one must know accurately the relationship between electrical sources in the brain and the electromagnetic field produced. The computation of the electromagnetic field due to a given source (the forward problem) is complicated by the fact that sources produce volume or return currents in the tissue that in turn produce a magnetic field and modify the electric field. The return currents depend on the conductivity structure of the head; to take into account their contribution, one should know the conductivity distribution in detail. Unfortunately, this is typically not possible with high accuracy. Currently, most MEG data analysis relies on the spherical head model, in which the external magnetic field does not depend on the profile of conductivity along the radius of the sphere.

A significant improvement to the spherical model in MEG is the realistically shaped cranial cavity model (HÄMÄLÄINEN and SARVAS 1989), which is based on the idea that, because the skull is an insulator, volume currents are mostly confined into its interior (ILMONIEMI et al. 1985). Because the skull is a poor conductor of electricity, the electric potential distribution measured on the scalp with EEG depends very strongly on the local thickness and conductivity of the skull. Therefore, the cranial cavity model of the head is not suitable for EEG, which requires the use of much more elaborate models than MEG.

The cranial cavity model can be further refined by taking into account different compartments in the head that have different conductivities. This may be done on the basis on MR images, but a problem that remains is determination of the relative conductivities of the different compartments.

The anisotropy of the brain tissue affects current flow and thereby MEG and EEG signals, although again MEG appears to be less sensitive to details in the conductivity than EEG (ILMONIEMI 1995). The ultimate model would incorporate the complete anisotropic conductivity structure of the head, e.g., as obtained with diffusion-weighted MRI.

37.4.2
Source Models

The interpretation of neuroelectromagnetic fields generally involves solving, in one way or another, the inverse problem, i.e., the reconstruction of the distribution of sources in the brain on the basis of measured signals. The most straightforward solution to this problem is offered by the equivalent current dipole (ECD) model: one determines the source current element (dipole) that would most closely explain the registered field pattern.

Because of the complexity of the brain, however, MEG data cannot usually be satisfactorily explained by a single dipole, or for that matter, with a small number of discrete dipoles. If nothing is known a priori about the sources except for the region of space or the direction of source currents, minimum-norm estimates (HÄMÄLÄINEN and ILMONIEMI 1984, 1994) are optimal estimators of the currents.

According to estimation theory, the optimal solution of the inverse problem requires the use of all available information. In addition to anatomical constraints, physiological information can be used. For example, if one assumes that all source currents lie in the cortex and flow perpendicularly to it, the three-dimensional search for a vector field (source current density) is reduced to a two-dimensional search for a scalar (HARI and ILMONIEMI 1986; DALE and SERENO 1993).

37.5
Integration of fMRI with Magnetoencephalography and Electroencephalography

Although fMRI studies accurately show the sites of activation, they do not provide the exact temporal order of events and do not directly indicate the neuronal connectivities between the activated areas. Therefore, studies that allow the combination of information from fMRI and from MEG and EEG may help in identifying the connections between activated brain areas. This combination enables the mapping of the human brain with the spatial resolution of fMRI and the temporal resolution of EEG/MEG (BELLIVEAU et al. 1993).

During the last 5 years there have been considerable efforts to combine MEG with functional MRI (ILMONIEMI 1993; SIMPSON et al. 1993, 1995; GEORGE et al. 1995). Differences in the physiological response mechanisms suggest that optimal experimental designs for MEG, EEG and fMRI may differ. For example, the optimal interstimulus interval is generally different in fMRI and MEG experiments. A straightforward approach to combine the information from fMRI and MEG studies is to define the activation areas based on fMRI and to use these areas as constraints for ECDs (AHLFORS et al. 1996). This is illustrated in Fig. 37.3, where eight separate fMRI activation areas have been used to explain MEG data obtained in response to the electrical stimulation of the right median nerve.

It is also possible to combine fMRI data with distributed source models. The simulation results of LIU et al. (1998) have demonstrated that a priori anatomical and functional information from MRI can

be used to regularize the EEG/MEG inverse problem, giving an improved solution with high spatial and temporal resolution. They showed that fMRI weighting of approximately 90% provided the best compromise between separation of activity from correctly localized sources and minimization of errors due to sources missed by fMRI. The need for allowing electrophysiological sources outside the fMRI-detected areas was evident in the visual motion studies of AHLFORS et al. (1996) and DALE et al. (1995), where information from MEG, MRI and fMRI data was combined (Fig. 37.4). In occipital, parietal and temporal areas, fMRI and MEG localization was observed to match, but clear activity near the frontal eye field was observed only by MEG.

37.6
Transcranial Magnetic Stimulation

In TMS (BARKER et al. 1985; NILSSON et al. 1996; WALSH and COWEY 1998), cortical cells are stimulated noninvasively by strong magnetic field pulses that induce a flow of current in the tissue, leading to membrane depolarization and thereby to neuronal excitation. The magnetic field of up to 2–3 tesla needed in TMS is generated by discharging, in about 100 μs, a large capacitor from several kilovolts through a coil placed over the scalp; the induced electric field in the brain is of the order of 100 V/m.

TMS can be used in three quite different ways: (1) by studying the electrophysiological or hemodynamic local or conducted responses, (2) by observing the behavioral or electrophysiological consequences of disturbing ongoing neuronal signal pro-

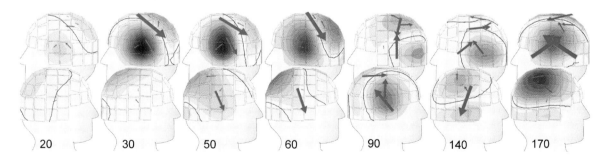

Fig. 37.3. Eight-dipole model of somatosensory evoked magnetic fields constrained with fMRI. The fMRI data were obtained with a Siemens Vision 1.5 T system and the MEG data with the Neuromag 122-channel magnetometer array at the BioMag Laboratory. *Red* and *blue* represent magnetic flux entering and exiting the head, respectively. The contour step is 30 fT. The *black lines* indicate the zero level of the radial field component. The *arrows* show the directions of the ECDs and are proportional to the dipole amplitudes. Although the dipoles were allowed to rotate, they retained their orientations during the analysis time (0–400 ms). (Courtesy of Antti Korvenoja, BioMag Laboratory, Helsinki)

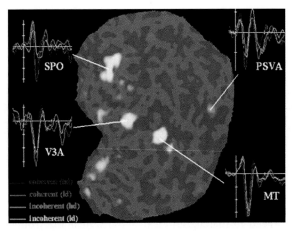

Fig. 37.4. Spatiotemporal activity displayed on flattened cortex, when subjects viewed two types of rotation/dilation random-dot flow-field stimuli. In the coherent-motion condition, each dot moved as part of the same flow-field, while in the incoherent-motion condition, each dot moved independently. MEG signal averaging was time-locked to the onset of motion. Time courses from MEG measurements were computed using fMRI and anatomically constrained linear estimation. The estimated activation amplitudes (0–500 ms) within several motion-sensitive cortical areas are plotted for both coherent and incoherent conditions. Early activity (70–80 ms) is observed in visual areas V1/V2, mediotemporal area (MT), and posterior sylvian visual area, also known as anterior motion area (PSVA, AMA). The amplitudes of the V1/V2 and MT activations do not appear to be strongly modulated by coherence. Area PSVA, on the other hand, shows stronger activation to coherent than to incoherent stimuli. The area most strongly modulated by motion coherence is the superior aspect of the parieto-occipital sulcus (SPO), showing a major peak in activation around 155–180 ms only in the coherent condition. (Courtesy of Anders Dale, MGH-NMR Center, Boston; MEG data from the BioMag Laboratory, Helsinki)

cessing, or (3) by treating patients with rapid-rate stimulation. TMS was pioneered by Barker et al. (1985), who found that stimulation of the motor cortex produced contralateral muscle movements. Initially, TMS was used to study neural conduction from the brain to the periphery. Amassian et al. (1989) showed that a subject's performance in a visual task was impaired when TMS pulses were delivered between 60 and 140 ms after the stimulus; a temporary functional lesion had been created.

In most present-day TMS studies, the stimulator coil is positioned manually until a muscular response such as a thumb twitch is generated. In stereotactic TMS, the coil is positioned over the target location on the basis of individual MRI (Ruohonen and Ilmoniemi 1998; Krings et al. 1997a, b; Paus et al. 1997). The selection of target areas in the brain can be based on anatomical structures seen in MRI

or on activation sites determined by fMRI, MEG/EEG or PET. When magnetic stimulation is combined with a functional imaging method capable of detecting brain activity evoked by TMS, cortical reactivity and connectivity can be measured directly.

Magnetic brain stimulation is the converse of MEG: the electric field induced in the tissue by TMS can be computed using the formulas that give the magnetic flux produced by a current dipole in the brain. This reciprocity (Plonsey 1972; Ilmoniemi et al. 1996) allows several results obtained in MEG to be used directly in magnetic stimulation, and vice versa. An analogous relationship exists between EEG and electrical stimulation.

Because of the strong dependence of the magnetic field on the distance from the coil, even millimeter level changes in coil position or small changes in its orientation may change the induced field considerably. Therefore, stimulation amplitudes are typically selected on the basis of muscle response thresholds, but this is not possible when other than motor areas are studied. An alternative is to use the EEG response to adjust the field. Stereotactic TMS, when made sufficiently precise, will allow one to select the level of the induced field instead of selecting the stimulus amplitude as a percentage of the maximum stimulator output or on the basis of the individual motor threshold.

37.7
Transcranial Magnetic Stimulation Combined with PET or fMRI

Paus et al. (1997) combined TMS and PET, introducing a new technique which permits the mapping of neural connections in the living human brain. While stimulating a selected cortical area, they simultaneously measured changes in cerebral blood flow. The exact location of the stimulation site was determined by frameless stereotaxy. They found significant correlations between cerebral blood flow and the number of TMS pulse trains, demonstrating functional connectivity from the left frontal eye field (FEF) to visual areas in the superior parietal and medial parieto-occipital cortex (Fig. 37.5).

Fox et al. (1997) stimulated the hand area of the left primary motor cortex (M1) with TMS while blood flow was recorded with PET. At the stimulated site, TMS increased blood flow by 12%–20%. Remote increases in blood flow were observed in ipsilateral primary and secondary somatosensory areas, in ip-

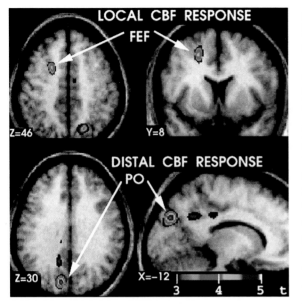

Fig. 37.5. Combination of TMS and PET. Areas where cerebral blood flow (CBF) correlated with the number of TMS pulse trains delivered to the frontal eye field (FEF) are shown color-coded. The *top row* shows activation at the stimulation site, the *bottom row* at the parieto-occipital (PO) cortex, indicating connectivity from FEF to PO. (Modified from PAUS et al. (1997); courtesy of Tômás Paus, McGill University, Montreal)

silateral ventral, lateral premotor cortex and in contralateral supplementary motor area. Reduced blood flow was observed in contralateral M1.

Very recently, BOHNING et al. (1998) and IVES et al. (1998) demonstrated that hemodynamic changes in response to TMS stimulation can be measured with fMRI. This technique appears to offer a new, powerful method for the study of connectivity using TMS.

37.8
Transcranial Magnetic Stimulation Combined with EEG

While the hemodynamic responses observed with PET and fMRI are an indirect and delayed reflection of neuronal activity, EEG provides direct and accurately timed information about TMS-evoked activity. High-resolution EEG (HR-EEG) makes it possible to locate the responses with an accuracy of 1–2 cm and to follow the spreading of activity with millisecond temporal resolution. The measurement of TMS-evoked EEG was first hampered by large artifacts (CRACCO et al. 1989; AMASSIAN et al. 1992), but now high-quality signals can be obtained when the

amplifier system is specifically designed to function in the presence of the strong TMS pulses (VIRTANEN et al. 1998).

We have used HR-EEG with 60 channels to monitor and locate the TMS-induced activity. By recording the cortical response just milliseconds after a TMS pulse, we can obtain an index of the local reactivity of the cortex. TMS-evoked EEG activity may last for up to 300 ms or more, presumably reflecting corticocortical connectivity and reverberating circuits (TIITINEN et al. 1998). In one set of experiments, we stimulated motor and visual cortices of volunteers (ILMONIEMI et al. 1997). The stimulation of the left sensorimotor hand area elicited an immediate strong response at the stimulated site. The activation spread to adjacent ipsilateral motor areas within 5–10 ms and to homologous regions in the opposite hemisphere within 20 ms (Fig. 37.6). Figure 37.7 shows the time sequence of the electric potential map as a function of time after left motor cortex stimulation, demonstrating the time evolution of the activation. Similar activation patterns were generated by magnetic stimulation of the visual cortex: after the immediate ipsilateral response, the contralateral response was observed at about 20 ms.

As the activation due to TMS is nonphysiological, quantitative measures of connectivity from TMS studies cannot be expected to be the same as when naturally occurring fluctuations or sensory input is causing the initial activation. We do not know what role the simultaneous activation of both excitatory and inhibitory neurons plays when TMS is applied. Also, TMS probably activates a large number of fibers antidromically, i.e., action potentials are transmitted along the axons toward rather than away from the soma. The effects of antidromic activation are poorly known. In any case, TMS offers a means for precise timing and localization of transmitted signals, although at present only mass action can be detected.

By means of TMS it is possible to study the excitability and the function of a relatively small area of cortex by careful selection of the target of the excitation pulse. A precondition for this kind of targeted pulses is the integration of anatomical and functional imaging modalities into the same coordinate system where the pulses can be planned in advance.

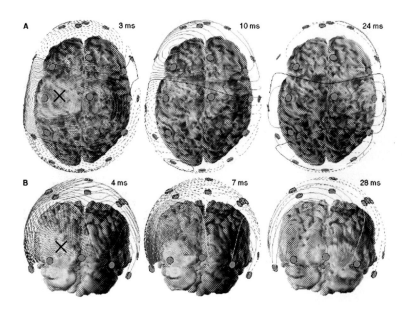

Fig. 37.6a, b. Activation maps based on TMS-evoked averaged EEG responses. Minimum-norm estimates of the cortical activity are shown as color maps drawn on 3D magnetic resonance images (MRIs) of the cortical surface. The MRIs were acquired with a Siemens Vision 1.5 T system using a set of 1 mm-thick sagittal MPRAGE images (TR 9.7 ms, TE 4 ms, TI 20 ms, flip angle 10°). Superimposed, the EEG is displayed as contour maps, with *red lines* indicating positive potential. The TMS coil position is indicated with a *cross*. **a** The response to left motor cortex stimulation. At latencies of 3 and 10 ms, the ipsilateral hemisphere shows prominent activation; at 24 ms, the contralateral activity dominates. The EEG contour spacing is 1 μV. **b** The response to visual cortex TMS at 4, 7, and 28 ms post-stimulus; the contour spacing is 2 μV. (From ILMONIEMI et al. 1997, with permission of Lippincot-Raven publishers)

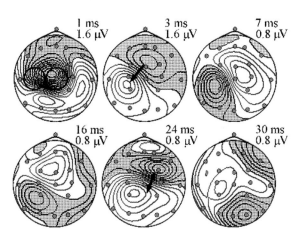

Fig. 37.7. The evolution of the EEG potential map during the first 30 ms after the stimulation of the hand area in the left hemisphere. The *dots* denote the recording electrodes. The *circles* in the *upper left panel* depict the two wings of the TMS coil. The contour spacing is indicated next to each map; the *red and blue lines* correspond to positive and negative potentials with respect to the average potential, respectively. The early ipsilateral (3 ms) and contralateral (24 ms) field patterns can be explained by equivalent current dipoles (ECDs) at the left and right sensorimotor areas, respectively. The ECD is the current dipole that best explains the measured electric potentials at a given time. The *arrows* show the locations and orientations of the ECDs. (From ILMONIEMI et al. 1997, with permission of Lippincot-Raven publishers)

37.9
Conclusion

Functional connectivity and excitability of neuronal tissue are key aspects in defining how the central nervous system works. Recent advances in multimodal imaging and stimulation will allow us to characterize these properties in the intact human brain. This will help us better understand how the brain is organized functionally in normal conditions and in various diseases. For example, changes in connectivity play a central role in many types of stroke, in schizophrenia and in demyelinating diseases such as multiple sclerosis. The possibility to study the recovery from stroke, consequences of trauma, altered excitability in epilepsies, dementias and coma may bring new tools for the diagnosis and follow-up of these diseases.

The use of MEG and EEG together with conventional and functional MRI allows for the spatiotemporal imaging of the working human brain. The effect of TMS pulses on the neuronal network can be registered by using EEG, PET or fMRI, allowing the characterization of functional connectivity and excitability.

Table 37.1. Comparison of functional brain imaging modalities

Method	Measures	Advantages	Limitations	Combination possibilities
EEG	Neuronal source currents	Temporal resolution	Sensitive to details in skull conductivity	fMRI, MEG, NIRS, TMS
		Deep sources	Inverse problem not unique	
MEG	Neuronal source currents	Temporal resolution Accurate spatial information	Blind to radial dipoles Inverse problem not unique	EEG, fMRI, NIRS
PET	Blood flow Metabolism	Measures physio-logical parameters	Radiation Low temporal resolution	TMS
	Receptor density		High cost	
fMRI	Blood oxygenation Blood flow	Excellent spatial resolution	Temporal resolution limited by hemodynamic response	EEG, MEG, TMS
	Blood volume			
NIRS	Blood oxygenation	Noninvasive, inexpensive	Limited to superficial cortex	EEG, MEG, TMS
SPECT	Blood flow Receptor density	Sensitive to picomole concentrations	Poor spatial and temporal resolution	EEG, fMRI, TMS
TMS	Behavioral, electrophysiological, hemodynamic, and muscular responses	Direct stimulation of the cortex noninvasively	Limited to superficial cortex	EEG, fMRI, NIRS, PET, SPECT

fMRI, functional magnetic resonance imaging; NIRS, near-infrared spectroscopy; TMS, transcranial magnetic stimulation; EEG, electroencephalography; PET, positron emission tomography; SPECT, single photon emission computerized tomography; MEG, magnetoencephalography.

Acknowledgments. The support of TEKES, the Foundation for Finnish Inventions, Runar Bäckström Foundation, Instrumentarium Science Foundation and the Academy of Finland is acknowledged. A research grant from the Helsinki University Central Hospital is acknowledged. We thank David Tuch for permission to use Fig. 37.1, Antti Korvenoja for Fig. 37.3, Dr. Anders Dale for Fig. 37.4, and Dr. Tômás Paus for Fig. 37.5. The valuable comments on the manuscript of Drs. Jack Belliveau and Jari Karhu are gratefully acknowledged.

References

Ahlfors SP, Aronen HJ, Belliveau JW et al (1996) Spatiotemporal imaging of human cortical areas selective to visual motion. In: Abstracts of the 10th international conference on biomagnetism, Santa Fe, New Mexico, p 39

Amassian VE, Cracco RQ, Maccabee PJ, Cracco JB, Rudell A, Eberle L (1989) Suppression of visual perception by magnetic coil stimulation of human occipital cortex. Electroencephalogr Clin Neurophysiol 74:458–462

Amassian VE, Cracco RQ, Maccabee PJ, Cracco JB (1992) Cerebello-frontal cortical projections in humans studied with the magnetic coil. Electroencephalogr Clin Neurophysiol 85:265–272

Barker AT, Jalinous R, Freeston IL (1985) Non-invasive magnetic stimulation of human motor cortex. Lancet 1:1106–1107

Biswal B, Yetkin FZ, Haughton VM, Hyde JS (1995) Functional connectivity in the motor cortex of resting human brain using echo-planar MRI. Magn Reson Med 34:537–541

Belliveau JW, Baker JR, Kwong KK et al (1993) Functional neuroimaging combining fMRI, MEG, and EEG. In: Proceedings of the 12th annual meeting of the Society of Magnetic Resonance in Medicine, SMRM, Berkeley, California, p 6

Bohning DE, Shastri A, Nahas Z et al (1998) Transcranial magnetic stimulation (TMS) during fMRI. NeuroImage 7(2):S685

Buchel C, Friston KJ (1997) Modulation of connectivity in visual pathways by attention: cortical interactions evaluated with structural equation modelling and fMRI. Cereb Cortex 7:768–778

Cracco RQ, Amassian VE, Maccabee PJ, Cracco JB (1989) Comparison of human transcallosal responses evoked by magnetic coil and electrical stimulation. Electro-encephalogr Clin Neurophysiol 74:417–424

Dale AM, Sereno MI (1993) Improved localization of cortical activity by combining EEG and MEG with MRI cortical surface reconstruction: a linear approach. J Cogn Neurosci 5:162–176

Dale AM, Ahlfors SP, Aronen HJ et al (1995) Spatiotemporal imaging of coherent motion selective areas in human cortex. Soc Neurosci Abstr 21:1275

Felleman DJ, Van Essen DC (1991) Distributed hierarchical processing in the primate cerebral cortex. Cereb Cortex 1:1–47

Fox P, Ingham R, George MS et al (1997) Imaging human intra-cerebral connectivity by PET during TMS. NeuroReport 8:787–2791

Friston KJ (1994) Functional and effective connectivity in neuroimaging: a synthesis. Hum Brain Mapping 2:56–78

Friston KJ (1997) Transients, metastability, and neuronal dynamics. NeuroImage 5:164–171

Friston KJ, Frith CD, Fletcher P, Liddle PF, Frackowiak RSJ (1996) Functional topography: multidimensional scaling and functional connectivity in the brain. Cereb Cortex 6:156–164

George JS, Aine CJ, Mosher JC et al (1995) Mapping function in the human brain with magnetoencephalography, anatomical magnetic resonance imaging, and functional magnetic resonance imaging. J Clin Neurophysiol 12:406–431

Gerstein GL, Perkel DH, Subramanian KN (1978) Identification of functionally related neuronal assemblies. Brain Res 140:43–62

Gevins AS, Bressler SL, Morgan NH, Cutillo BA, White RM, Greer DS, Illes J (1989) Event-related covariances during a bimanual visuomotor task. I. Methods and analysis of stimulus- and response-locked data. Electroencephalogr Clin Neurophysiol 74:58–75

Gevins A, Leong H, Smith ME, Le J, Du R (1995) Mapping cognitive brain function with modern high-resolution electro-encephalography. Trends Neurosci 18:429–436

Guillery RW (1995) Anatomical evidence concerning the role of the thalamus in corticocortical communication: a brief review. J Anat 187:583–592

Hämäläinen MS, Ilmoniemi RJ (1984) Interpreting measured magnetic fields of the brain: estimates of current distributions. Report TKK-F-A559, Helsinki University of Technology, Espoo, Finland

Hämäläinen MS, Ilmoniemi RJ (1994) Interpreting magnetic fields of the brain: minimum-norm estimates. Med Biol Eng Comput 32:35–42

Hämäläinen MS, Sarvas J (1989) Feasibility of the homogeneous head model in the interpretation of neuromagnetic fields. Phys Med Biol 32:91–97

Hämäläinen M, Hari R, Ilmoniemi RJ, Knuutila J, Lounasmaa OV (1993) Magnetoencephalography – theory, instrumentation, and applications to noninvasive studies of the working human brain. Rev Mod Phys 65:413–497

Hari R, Ilmoniemi RJ (1986) Cerebral magnetic fields. CRC Crit Rev Biomed Eng 14:93–126

Ilmoniemi RJ (1993) Improvement of brain source imaging by MRI, PET, electrical impedance tomography and other techniques. In Valdés S (ed) Book of abstracts. 4th inter-national symposium of the International Society for Brain Electromagnetic Topography, Society for Brain Electromagnetic Topography, Havana, pp 142–143

Ilmoniemi RJ (1995) Radial anisotropy added to a spherically symmetric conductor does not affect the external magnetic field due to internal sources. Europhys Lett 30:313–316

Ilmoniemi RJ, Hämäläinen MS, Knuutila JET (1985) The forward and inverse problems in the spherical model. In: Weinberg H, Stroink G, Katila T (eds) Biomagnetism: applications and theory. Pergamon, Amsterdam, pp 278–282

Ilmoniemi RJ, Ruohonen J, Virtanen J (1996) Relationships between magnetic stimulation and MEG/EEG. In: Nilsson J, Panizza M, Grandori F (eds) Advances in magnetic stimulation: mathematical modeling and clinical applications. Maugeri Foundation, Pavia, pp 65–72 (Advances in occupational medicine and rehabilitation, vol 2)

Ilmoniemi RJ, Virtanen J, Ruohonen J, Karhu J, Aronen HJ, Näätänen R, Katila T (1997) Neuronal responses to magnetic stimulation reveal cortical reactivity and connectivity. NeuroReport 8:3537–3540

Ives JR, Pascual-Leone A, Chen Q, Schlaug G, Keenan J, Edelman RR (1998) Experience and early findings using transcranial magnetic stimulation (TMS) during functional magnetic resonance imaging (fMRI) in humans. NeuroImage 7(2):S33

Krings T, Buchbinder BR, Butler WE, Chiappa KH, Jiang HJ, Cosgrove GR, Rosen BR (1997a) Functional magnetic resonance imaging and transcranial magnetic stimulation: complementary approaches in the evaluation of cortical motor function. Neurology 48:1406–1416

Krings T, Buchbinder BR, Butler WE, Chiappa KH, Jiang HJ, Rosen BR, Cosgrove GR (1997b) Stereotactic transcranial magnetic stimulation: correlation with direct electrical cortical stimulation. Neurosurgery 41:1319–1325

Liu AK, Belliveau JW, Dale AM (1998) Spatiotemporal imaging of human brain activity using fMRI constrained MEG data: Monte Carlo simulations. Proc Natl Acad Sci USA 95:8945–8950

Lowe MJ, Mock BJ, Sorenson JA (1998) Functional connectivity in single and multislice echoplanar imaging using resting-state fluctuations. NeuroImage 7:119–132

Makris N, Worth AJ, Sorensen AG et al (1997) Morphometry of in vivo human white matter association pathways with diffusion-weighted magnetic resonance imaging. Ann Neurol 42:951–962

McIntosh AR, Gonzalez-Lima F (1994) Structural equation modeling and its application to network analysis in functional brain imaging. Hum Brain Mapping 2:2–22

McIntosh AR, Grady CL, Haxby JV, Ungerleider LG, Horwitz B (1996) Changes in limbic and prefrontal functional interactions in a working memory task for faces. Cereb Cortex 6:571–584

McIntosh AR, Nyberg L, Bookstein FL, Tulving E (1997) Differential functional connectivity of prefrontal and medial temporal cortices during episodic memory retrieval. Hum Brain Mapping 5:323–327

Meyer B-U, Roricht S, Woiciechowsky C (1998) Topography of fibers in the human corpus callosum mediating interhemispheric inhibition between the motor cortices. Ann Neurol 43:360–369

Miller AK, Alston LR, Korcellis JA (1980) Variation with age in the volumes of grey and white matter in the cerebral hemispheres of man: measurements with an image analyser. Neuropathol Appl Neurobiol 6:119–132

Nilsson J, Panizza M, Grandori F (eds) (1996) Advances in magnetic stimulation: mathematical modeling and clinical applications. Maugeri Foundation, Pavia (Advances in occupational medicine and rehabilitation, vol 2)

Noback CR, Demarest RJ (1981) The human nervous system. McGraw-Hill, New York

Nowak LG, James AC, Bullier J (1997) Corticocortical connections between visual areas 17 and 18a of the rat studied in vitro: spatial and temporal organisation of functional synaptic responses. Exp Brain Res 117:219–241

Paus T, Jech R, Thompson CJ, Comeau R, Peters T, Evans AC (1997) Transcranial magnetic stimulation during positron emission tomography: a new method for studying connectivity of the human cerebral cortex. J Neurosci 17:3178–3184

Plonsey R (1972) Capability and limitations of electrocardiography and magnetocardiography. IEEE Trans Biomed Eng BME-19:239–244

Rouiller EM, Babalian A, Kazennikov O, Moret V, Yu X-H, Wiesendanger M (1994) Transcallosal connections of the distal forelimb representations of the primary and supplementary motor cortical areas in macaque monkeys. Exp Brain Res 102:227–243

Ruohonen J, Ilmoniemi RJ (1998) Focusing and targeting of magnetic brain stimulation using multiple coils. Med Biol Eng Comput 36:1–5

Scannell JW, Blakemore C, Young MP (1995) Analysis of connectivity in the cat cerebral cortex. J Neurosci 15:1463–1483

Simpson GV, Belliveau JW, Foxe JJ, Baker JR, Vaughan HG Jr (1993) Integration of ERP and fMRI measures yield spatial and temporal patterns of activation during visual processing. Brain Topogr 5:459

Simpson GV, Pflieger ME, Foxe JJ et al (1995) Dynamic neuroimaging of brain function. J Clin Neurophysiol 12:432–449

Smith WE (1992) Estimation of the spatio-temporal correlations of biological electrical sources from their magnetic fields. IEEE Trans Biomed Eng 39:997–1004

Tiitinen H, Virtanen J, Ilmoniemi RJ, Kamppuri J, Ollikainen M, Ruohonen J, Näätänen R (1999) Separation of contamination caused by coil click from responses elicited by transcranial magnetic stimulation. Electroencephalogr Clin Neurophysiol (in press)

Tonino G, McIntosh AR, Russell DP, Edelman GM (1998) Functional clustering: identifying strongly interactive brain regions in neuroimaging data. NeuroImage 7:133–149

Tuch DS, Belliveau JW, Reese TG, Wedeen VJ (1998a) Diffusion imaging at high angular resolution detects multiple fiber populations within a voxel. NeuroImage 7(2):S708

Tuch DS, Wedeen VJ, Dale AM, Belliveau JW (1998b) Electrical conductivity tensor map of the human brain using NMR diffusion imaging: an effective medium approach. Proceedings of the International Society for Magnetic Resonance in Medicine, Sydney, Australia, 6:572

Vanduffel W, Payne BR, Lomber SG, Orban GA (1997) Functional impact of cerebral connections. Proc Natl Acad Sci USA 94:7617–7620

Virtanen J, Ruohonen J, Näätänen R, Ilmoniemi RJ (1999) Instrumentation for the measurement of electric brain responses to transcranial magnetic stimulation. Med Biol Eng Comput (in press)

Walsh V, Cowey A (1998) Magnetic stimulation studies of visual cognition. Trends Neurosci 2:103–110

Werring DJ, Clark CA, Parker GJM et al (1998) Investigating the relationship between brain structure and function: combining diffusion tensor imaging with functional MRI in the visual system. NeuroImage 7(2):S34

Ziemann U, Lönnecker S, Steinhoff BJ, Paulus W (1996) The effect of lorazepam on the motor cortical excitability in man. Exp Brain Res 109:127–135

38 Combining Functional MRI with Neurochemical Mapping Obtained with PET and SPECT

B. Mazoyer

CONTENTS

38.1 Introduction

Over the past decade, human neuroimaging has become a major component of neuroscience, thanks to the advent of a panoply of new brain imaging techniques. In the mid-1980s, while magnetic resonance (MR) was establishing itself as the reference technique for in vivo structural imaging, positron emission tomography (PET) emerged as the functional imaging method of choice, superseding single photon emission computed tomography (SPECT), thanks to the availability of short-lived tracers and to technological advances that allows one to obtain quantitative maps of physiological parameters of interest. For 10 years, cognitive neuroimaging was thus preferentially, if not exclusively, performed using PET activation studies and has experienced a rapid development (Mazoyer 1996). Meanwhile, the sensitivity of the PET approach, coupled to the syn-

thesis of a variety of positron emitting radiolabeled ligands, also allowed the in vivo investigation of neurotransmission, providing density maps for several major neurotransmitter systems (Wagner Jr. 1986).

The advent of functional MR imaging (FMRI) in the mid-1990s (Turner 1995) has had a major impact on the respective roles of PET and MR in the neuroimaging domain, due to the superior spatial and temporal resolutions of BOLD FMRI, and the extensive availability of commercial MR scanners on which this technique can be implemented. In less than 3 years, FMRI has indeed replaced PET as the leading brain activation method, raising the issue of the future of the latter technique and of their synergistic use.

In this chapter, we will examine this question on the basis of two characteristics specific to PET, namely, its ability to provide absolute values of physiological parameters and its unique suitability, only shared in part with magnetic resonance spectroscopy, to investigate in vivo neurotransmission. Accordingly, provided that some technical challenges can be adequately addressed, it is anticipated that PET and FMRI could be jointly used to improve our knowledge of: (1) the mechanisms of neurovascular coupling during cognitive activity, (2) the modulation of cortical networks by pharmacological agents, (3) the relationships between neurotransmission parameter distribution and cognitive functions, (4) the mechanism of endogenous transmitter release during cognitive activities.

38.2 PET Methods

In this chapter, we will mainly focus on the PET method since SPECT can be merely understood as a degraded version of PET, having coarser spatial and temporal resolutions, reduced sensitivity and less quantification capability (Muehllehner and Karp

B. Mazoyer, PhD, MD; Groupe d'Imagerie Neurofonctionnelle, UPRES EA 2127, Université de Caen, LRC-CEA n 13 V, GIP Cyceron, BP 5229, 14074 Caen, France

1988). In addition, neurotransmission SPECT tracers are usually less numerous, less selective and more difficult to work with than their PET counterparts because single photon emitters such as ^{99m}Tc or^{123}I are heavy atoms with relatively long half-lives (6 and 13.2 h, respectively).

38.2.1
Basic Principles

PET is basically an in vivo autoradiographic technique in which molecules of biological interest are first labeled with cyclotron-produced, short-lived, positron-emitting nuclei before being intravenously injected to a human subject. A positron tomograph, surrounding the subject head, dynamically records coincident 511 keV antiparallel photon pairs that originate from positron emissions and local annihilations. A tomographic reconstruction algorithm applied to acquisition data provides, after correction for scatter and attenuation, the 3D distribution of positron emitter absolute concentration in the brain. Mathematical modeling is then used to convert time series of radiotracer concentration maps into physiological parameter maps (MAZOYER et al. 1986).

The most widely used positron emitters are oxygen-15, carbon-11 and fluorine-18, which have half-lives of 2, 20 and 110 min, respectively. The relative short half-life of positron emitters constitutes both an advantage and a limitation: multiple studies are possible at low subject radiation exposure but a cyclotron must be available in the vicinity of the tomograph. Because positron emitters are isotopes of natural components of biological molecules, tracers labeled with positron emitters will retain the same exact biochemical properties as their unlabeled equivalent (no isotopic effect).

Modern PET scanners are based on 15 cm long, axial cylindrical arrays of closely packed, high density scintillators and photomultiplier tubes and provide reconstructed image volume having a resolution around 6 mm in all directions, and being essentially free from artifacts apart from the most outer part of the field of view. 3D volumes can be collected as fast as one per second (MAZOYER et al. 1991).

38.2.2
Quantitative Maps of Local Hemodynamics and Metabolism

The tracer of choice for CBF mapping with PET is oxygen-15 labeled water (H$_2$^{15}O), a molecule that freely diffuses across the blood-brain barrier (HERSCOVITCH et al. 1983). In a typical study, 8–12 mCi of this tracer is intravenously injected after the task has started. Data collection is maintained during 40–80 s, requiring the cognitive task to be sustained by the subject over the entire data acquisition period. Either absolute (requiring arterial blood radioactive concentration assessment) or relative (to the global) CBF maps can be obtained in this manner. The delay between two such measurements in the same subject is 8–10 min to allow for near complete decay of the radioactivity present in the subject, a maximum of 12 injections being possible given radiation exposure regulations.

Cerebral blood volume (CBV) maps can be obtained with oxygen-15 labeled CO, a tracer that irreversibly binds to hemoglobin in red blood cells. Collecting a CBV map requires 10 min with continuous inhalation of C^{15}O.

Energy metabolism maps can be obtained in different ways: 10 min continuous inhalation of ^{15}O$_2$, coupled to additional CO and CO$_2$ inhalation studies in the same subject, allows the generation of cerebral oxygen consumption (CMRO$_2$) and extraction (OER) in addition to CBF and CBV maps. Glucose metabolism maps be obtained as well, using either ^{18}F-deoxyglucose (HUANG et al. 1980) or ^{11}C-glucose. The former is trapped after phosphorylation and can be used to map the cerebral metabolic rate of glucose (CMRGlu), independent of the nature of the final energy pathway (aerobic or anaerobic), while the latter will lead to maps of brain oxidative metabolism.

Other metabolisms, of lesser interest in the framework of the present chapter, can be investigated with PET such as amino acid transport and incorporation rate into proteins using ^{11}C-methionine, for example (MAZOYER et al. 1993), or even lipid metabolism using ^{11}C-palmitate.

38.2.3
Mapping Neurotransmission Parameters

A most exciting use of PET is the investigation of neurotransmission, since the human brain is thought to contain over 100 neurochemicals and more than 300 subtypes of receptors for these molecules. The brain concentrations of these elements are usually sub-nanomolar, which is still detectable by PET using adequate radiotracers. For several reasons, however, performing neurotransmission studies with PET is considerably more difficult than conducting hemodynamic or metabolic investigations.

The first difficulty is the choice and synthesis of an adequate tracer for the neurotransmission system of interest. Ideally, this tracer should passively cross the blood-brain barrier (BBB) and have the same properties as the natural neurotransmitter when interacting at the membrane neuroreceptor sites. It is, unfortunately, not always possible to label the natural neurotransmitter, or its labeled version may not cross the BBB, as is the case for dopamine. More often than not, one has then to turn either to a labeled precursor, confounding synthesis and receptor interaction steps in the same experiment, or to agonist and antagonist molecules that will only partly mimic the natural neurotransmission dynamics.

A second potential difficulty is that, during the time course of the PET experiment, the radioligand may enter in different metabolic pathways leading to the appearance in the blood and the tissue of radiolabeled metabolites that produce a signal that is hard to separate from that of the original ligand.

A third problem encountered in neurotransmission studies is that receptor-ligand interactions are essentially driven by nonlinear biochemical reactions. The rate at which a ligand binds to its receptor depends on the actual concentrations of both the free and bound ligand, while the rate at which the receptor-ligand pair dissociates linearly depends on its local concentration. Accordingly, rather sophisticated experimental protocols, some involving multiple injections of labeled and unlabeled ligands, and mathematical modeling must be used in order to obtain maps of receptor density (B_{max}) and affinity (K_d) (DELFORGE et al. 1989).

Nevertheless, PET radioligands have been and are currently being developed for the investigation of four major neurotransmission systems, namely, the monoaminergic, cholinergic, opiod and gabaergic/benzodiazepine systems. The dopaminergic system has been, by and large, the system that has received the most attention (BARON et al. 1991) (Fig. 38.1). Ligands have been developed for the presynaptic (^{11}C-cocaine; PEARLSON et al. 1993) and postsynaptic sites, including different receptor subtypes, e.g., ^{11}C-SCH23390 for D_1 (NORDSTRÖM et al. 1995) and ^{11}C-raclopride for D_2 and D_3 (FARDE et al. 1986). In addition, the metabolism of the neurotransmitter it-

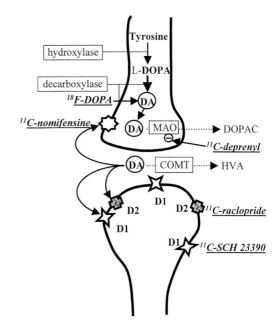

Fig. 38.1. A striatal dopaminergic synapse and its potential targets for positron emitter labeled ligands. The neurotransmitter (dopamine, DA) synthesis (from its precursor, the L-DOPA) or metabolism (by the monoamine oxydase, MAO) can be traced, as well as its pre- and postsynaptic receptor sites (only the D1 and D2 dopaminergic subtypes are represented in the figure)

self can be studied with ^{18}F-DOPA (MELEGA et al. 1996) serving as the neurotransmitter precursor. Similarly, competitive radiolabeled inactivators of monoamine oxidase A (^{11}C-deprenyl; FOWLER et al. 1996) can also be used, as well as ligands of the dopamine reuptake site (^{11}C-nomifensine; SALMON et al. 1990). Current tracers of interest for the PET investigation of the dopaminergic and other neurotransmission systems are presented in Table 38.1.

38.3
Synergistic Use of PET and FMRI

38.3.1
Technical Challenges

Combining PET and FMRI data raises a number of technical issues related both to the physical characteristics of each technique and to the biological nature of their respective signals. Although both methods provide true volumetric data, they differ in image resolution and characteristics. PET has an intrinsically lower resolution than FMRI, typically 6

Table 38.1. PET and SPECT radiotracers for neurotransmission studies

Radiotracer	Main target
^{11}C-SCH 23390	Dopamine D_1
^{11}C-raclopride	Dopamine D_2
^{11}C-FLB-457	Dopamine D_2
^{11}C-RTI 121 and 55	Dopamine re-uptake
^{18}F-fluorodopa	Dopaminergic neurone density
^{11}C-flumazenil	Central benzodiazepine
^{11}C-deprenyl	MAO-B activity
^{11}C-carfentanyl	m-opioid
^{11}C-diprenorphine	Nonselective opioid
^{18}F-altanserin	5-HT$_2$
^{18}F-setoperone	5-HT$_2$
^{11}C-methylspiperone	Cortical 5-HT$_2$, striatal D_2
^{11}C-MDL-100907	5-HT$_{2A}$
^{123}I-iodobenzamide	Dopamine D_2
^{123}I-epipride	Dopamine D_3
^{123}I-QNB	Muscarinic acetylcholine
^{123}I-CIT	Dopamine and 5-HT re-uptake

Adapted from GRASBY et al. 1996.

mm vs 3 mm, leading to larger partial volume effects for the former. Accordingly, one should not try to directly compare these signals but rather either acquire or interpolate FMRI data to that of PET when their combination is required. Ideally, a high resolution structural MR should also be acquired to serve as the common reference both for registration and to identify the structures that contribute to the PET signal. This may be especially important when gray nuclei or specific cortical areas are investigated, as their sizes are usually much smaller than twice the PET image resolution. Besides resolution, a second area of concern is that of image distortions. To a large extent, PET images are essentially free of geometric and homogeneity distortions, thanks to the attenuation and scatter correction applied to the raw data. There does exist, however, two phenomenon worth mentioning. First, due to the cylindrical geometry of most PET scanners, cross-talk between adjacent crystals increases as the radioactive source moves away from center, leading to a slight degradation of the transverse resolution in the radial direction (3–4 mm over 10 cm), or equivalently, to an elliptically shaped spatial autocorrelation. Although usually neglected, this phenomenon will have to be accounted for if accurate matching of FMRI activation and PET metabolic/neuroreceptor mapping is needed. The second and somewhat related issue has to do with the fact that upper and lower planes of the axial field of view are actually undersampled by the cylindrically shaped detector array (MURAYAMA and

NOHARA 1997). As a practical consequence, the actual efficient axial field of view (FOV) of current PET scanners is in fact limited to about 10 cm, meaning that subject positioning is critical when studying structures such as the supplementary area (SMA) or the cerebellum.

A second point to pay attention to is that of temporal resolution. Acquisition of PET data in the context of cognition may vary from 1 min (activation studies) up to 1 h (neurotransmission investigations), that is, one or two orders of magnitude larger than the time needed to collect FMRI data. Not taking into account this fundamental difference could have spurious effects on the interpretation of PET/FMRI joint experiments. Accordingly, one should restrict such experiments to cognitive tasks that can be sustained with reasonable stability over several minutes

38.3.2
Neurovascular Coupling

Although tremendous progress have recently been made regarding the understanding of the physiological bases of the FMRI BOLD signal (MALONEK and GRINVALD 1996), many questions remain unanswered that could benefit from a synergistic use of PET and FMRI.

A typical example of such studies has been recently published, dealing with the stability of the activation signal over long periods of time. Using a combined PET/FMRI experiment, differences in the stability of the BOLD and CBF signals in the visual cortex under stimulation were reported (BANDETTINI et al. 1997). Such studies clearly need to be extended to other parts of the cortex and to other types of stimuli, including more cognitive ones. In particular, it would be interesting to make full use of the PET potentialities by looking at CMRO$_2$ and CMRGlu in addition to CBF.

A second and somewhat overlooked, potential area of interest in combined PET/FMRI experiments is that of quantification. Since both methods rely on a difference paradigm, the amplitude of the signal conveys highly significant information in terms of neuronal activity. Since absolute measurements of CBF and CMRO$_2$ are, at this time, either difficult with or out of reach of FMRI, PET could provide critical information for the interpretation of FMRI data, thanks to its quantitative nature. One has, however, to acknowledge, that only long-term phenomenon (on the order of minutes) will fall under the scope of this approach.

38.3.3
Pharmacological Modulation of Local Hemodynamics and Metabolism

Apart from the two domains mentioned above, the question remains whether there will still be a use for PET activation studies 3 years from now. FMRI has clearly taken the lead in this area in all domains of cognition, including neurology, presurgical mapping, psychiatry and evaluation of developmental disorders. The fact that almost all PET units involved in cognitive neuroimaging are now equipped with state-of-the-art FMRI scanners provides the most obvious indicator that this field of research will, for years to come, be dominated by FMRI.

One field in which the quantitative nature of PET imaging is likely to be a strong argument in favor of its use is the investigation of interactions between pharmacological agents and local hemodynamics and/or energy metabolism. In fact, this approach has already been the subject of several reports, with studies focusing on the effects of drugs on flow/metabolism values either at rest (FIRESTONE et al. 1996; MEYER et al. 1996) or during activation studies (COULL et al. 1997; MATTAY et al. 1996). An example of such studies has been performed by our group, trying to look at brain structures involved in parkinsonian tremor (DUFFAU et al. 1996). The experimental protocol consisted of two different motor activation studies in the same session: one while the subject was trembling, the other 20 min after the subject was given a dopaminergic agonist that alleviated the tremor. In this way, modulation of cortical activation by restoring dopamine network integrity at the basal ganglia level was demonstrated. Several similar PET studies have been performed both in healthy individuals and in patients. These studies are particularly important for measuring the central effects of drugs and for unraveling the modulation of cortical networks by neurotransmission systems during cognitive activity.

38.3.4
Mapping Neurotransmitter Density and Occupancy

Quantitative mapping of neuroreceptor density will probably remain the exclusive domain of PET, since no other technique has the sensitivity to detect biological components at picomolar concentration. This approach has already been used to investigate several hypotheses regarding the perturbation of neurotransmission systems in psychiatric disorders,

the most typical example being the dopaminergic system and schizophrenia (SEDVALL et al. 1995). A number of sometimes conflicting results have been reported regarding the subtype (D_1–D_5) and the location (striatal or extrastriatal) of possible changes in dopaminergic receptor density in schizophrenia. Another example is depressive illness and the serotoninergic 5-HT_2 and 5-HT_{1A} system (ATTAR-LEVY et al. 1991). Studies of this kind are important for understanding the pathophysiology of psychiatric diseases and the design of therapeutic agents.

Measuring receptor occupancy is a closely related domain that will also remain exclusive to PET. Here, the binding potential (BP) of certain receptor is mapped under pharmacological intervention, providing a way to assess the dynamics of the relationship between the degree of receptor occupancy and the clinical efficacy of a drug. For example, it has been shown that a 65%–89% occupancy of striatal D_2 receptors is achieved 2 h after acute antipsychotic drug administration (FARDE et al. 1988), while extrapyramidal side effects appear only when occupancy is greater than 85%, defining a therapeutic window of occupancy of between 65% and 85% (FARDE et al. 1992). These and subsequent studies have demonstrated that PET will be an invaluable tool for pharmacological studies.

Finally, a very promising synergistic use of PET and FMRI in this domain could be the matching of hemodynamic and neuroreceptor maps. In this application, PET would provide the spatial distribution and interaction of various neurotransmitter systems, whereas FMRI would give the hemodynamic responses of cortical networks involved during the performance of cognitive activities. Such studies would help to unravel the relationships between cognition and neurotransmission. Preliminary reports of this sort, using autoradiography rather than PET, neuroreceptor mapping have recently been published (GEYER et al. 1996). Interestingly, the time may come at which such combined studies will be performed simultaneously using dedicated PET hardware that will fit inside a magnet (SHAO et al. 1997).

38.3.5
Measuring Endogenous Transmitter Release During Cognitive Activity

Because neurotransmission is one of the two major cellular events occurring during brain functioning (the other being ionic currents), there is considerable interest in trying to directly observe this phenomenon rather than more indirect events such as hemodynamic or metabolic responses. This is again a domain in which PET has unique potential because of its exquisite sensitivity and the availability of adequate radiolabeled tracers. The conceptual design of such studies is that, during cognitive activity or after pharmaceutical manipulation, synaptic activity generates endogenous neurotransmitter release which in turn increases receptor occupancy, a phenomenon that could be observed with PET (Fig. 38.2).

There are obviously tremendous difficulties and limitations in performing neuroreceptor activations, both from the technical point of view (choice of tracer, flow effects) and due to problems encountered in the biological interpretation of increases in receptor occupancy. Nevertheless, pioneering studies have already been performed showing, for example, that predosing subjects with drugs that release dopamine decreases the binding of ^{11}C-raclopride, a dopaminergic D$_2$ ligand (DEWEY et al. 1993). Similarly, behavioral manipulations may also modulate neurotransmitter release, as indicated by a study in which increased elimination of ^{11}C-diprenorphine, a tracer of central μ, δ, and κ opioid receptors, was observed in associative cortex during serial epileptic seizures (BARTENSEIN et al. 1993). This result was later shown to be not solely explainable by blood flow effects, but more likely also by the presence of endogenous opioids during seizures.

As for cognitive studies, there have been very few attempts to directly map neurotransmitter release during the performance of activation tasks. There are numerous technical difficulties to be overcome before achieving this goal (FRISTON et al. 1997; MORRIS et al. 1996). First, almost all neurotransmission PET tracers are labeled with either ^{11}C or ^{18}F, both isotopes having a somewhat long half-life for cognitive neuroimaging studies. Thus, in the best case, these studies will be limited to cognitive tasks that can be sustained for at least several minutes. Similarly, because of the long isotope half-life, a very limited number of scans can be performed in the same subject, even when using a split-dose experiment, and a minimum delay of at least a half-day will be required between two scans (control and activation). Finally, the expected activation signal in such studies will consist of a slight reduction in radiotracer uptake during the activated state, due to increased receptor occupancy by the released endogenous neurotransmitter. This signal is likely to be very weak and the practical feasibility of such studies in the cognitive neuroscience domain remains to be demonstrated.

References

Attar-Levy D, Blin J, Crouzel C, Martinot JL, Dao-Castallana MH, Mazoyer BM, Poirier MF, Feline A, Hantouche E, Fiorelli M, Pappata S, Syrota A (1991) Cortical 5-HT2 receptors studied with PET and 18F-labelled setoperone during depressive illness and antidepressant treatment with clomipramine. J Cereb Blood Flow Metab 11:S653(Abstract)

Bandettini PA, Kwong KK, Davis TL, Tootell RBH, Wong EC, Fox PT, Belliveau JW, Weisskoff RM, Rosen BR (1997) Characterization of cerebral blood oxygenation and flow changes during prolonged brain activation. Human Brain Mapping 5:93–109

Baron JC, Comar D, Farde L, Martinot J-L, Mazoyer B (1991) Brain dopaminergic systems: imaging with positron tomography. Kluwer Academic, Dordrecht

Bartensein PA, Duncan JS, Prevett MC, et al. (1993) Investigation of the opioid system in absence seizures with positron emission tomography. J Neurol Neurosurg Psych 56:1295–1302

Coull JT, Frith CD, Dolan RJ, Frackowiak RSJ, Grasby PM (1997) The neural correlates of the noradrenergic modulation of human attention, arousal and learning. Eur J Neurosci 9:589–598

Delforge J, Syrota A, Mazoyer BM (1989) Experimental design optimization: theory and application to estimation of receptor model parameters using dynamic positron emission tomography. Phys Med Biol 34:419–435

Dewey SL, Smith GS, Logan J (1993) Effects of central cholinergic blockade on striatal dopamine release measured

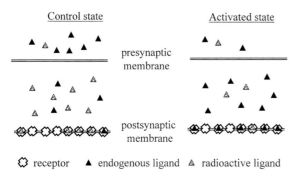

Fig. **38.2.** Principles of the measurement of endogenous neurotransmitter release during activation by positron emission tomography. During the control state (*left*), the endogenous neurotransmitter concentration in the synaptic cleft is small, which leaves free access for the radiolabeled ligand to the postsynaptic membrane receptors. During the activated state (*right*), endogenous neurotransmitter is released through the presynaptic membrane that binds to the postsynaptic sites, reducing the amount of receptor sites available for binding with the radiotracer and thus the local radioactive concentration

with positron emission tomography in normal human subjects. Proc Natl Acad Sci USA 90:11816–11820

Duffau H, Tzourio N, Caparros-Lefebvre D, Parker F, Mazoyer B (1996) Tremor and voluntary repetitive movement in Parkinson's disease: comparison before and after L-dopa with positron emission tomography. Exp Brain Res 107:453–462

Farde L, Hall H, Ehrin E, Sedvall G (1986) Quantitative analysis of D2 dopamine receptor binding in the living human brain by PET. Science 231:258–261

Farde L, Nordström AL, Wiesel FA, Pauli S, Halldin C, Sedvall G (1992) Positron emission tomographic analysis of central D_1 and D_2 dopamine receptor occupancy in patients treated with classical neuroleptics and clozapine relation to extrapyramidal side effects. Arch Gen Psychiatry 49:538–554

Farde L, Wiesel FA, Halldin C, Sedvall G (1988) Central D_2-dopamine receptor occupancy in schizophrenic patients treated with antipsychotic drugs. Arch Gen Psychiatry 45:71–76

Firestone LL, Gyulai F, Mintun M, Adler LJ, Urso K, Winter PM (1996) Human brain activity response to fentanyl imaged by positron emission tomography. Anesth Analg 82:1247–1251

Fowler JS, Volkow ND, Wang G-J, Pappas N, Logan J, MacGregor R, Alexoff D, Shea C, Schlyer D, Wolf AP, Warner D, Zezulkova I, Cliento R (1996) Inhibition of monoamine oxidase B in the brains of smokers. Nature 379:733–736

Friston KJ, Malizia AL, Wilson S, Cunningham VJ, Jones T, Nutt DJ (1997) Analysis of dynamic radioligand displacement for activation studies. J Cereb Blood Flow Metab 17:80–93

Geyer S, Ledberg A, Schleicher A, Kinomura S, Schormann T, Bürgel U, Klingberg T, Larsson J, Zilles K, Roland PE (1996) Two different areas within the primary motor cortex of man. Nature 382:805–807

Grasby P, Malizia P, Bench C (1996) Psychopharmacology – in vivo neurochemistry and pharmacology. Brit Med Bull 52:513–526

Herscovitch P, Markham J, Raichle ME (1983) Brain blood flow measured with intravenous H215O I theory and error analysis. J Nucl Med 24:782–789

Huang SC, Phelps ME, Hoffman EJ, Sideris K, Selin CJ, Kuhl DE (1980) Noninvasive determination of local cerebral metabolic rate of glucose in man. Am J Physiol 238:E69–E82

Malonek D, Grinvald A (1996) Interactions between electrical activity and cortical microcirculation revealed by imaging spectroscopy: implications for functional brain mapping. Science 272:551–554

Mattay VS, Berman KF, Ostrem JL, Esposito G, Van Horn JD, Bigelow LB, Weinberger DR (1996) Dextroamphetamine enhances "neural network-specific" physiological signals: a positron-emission tomography rCBF study. J Neurol Sci 16:4816–4822

Mazoyer B (1996) Human brain mapping: state of the art. In: Pavone P, Rossi P (eds) Functional MRI. Springer-Verlag, Rome, pp 66–69

Mazoyer B, Heiss D, Comar D (1993) PET studies of amino acid metabolism and protein synthesis. Kluwer Academic, Dordrecht

Mazoyer B, Trebossen R, Deutch R, Casey M, Blohm K (1991) Physical characteristics of the ECAT 953B/31: a new high resolution brain positron tomograph. IEEE Trans Med Imaging 10:499–504

Mazoyer BM, Huesman RH, Budinger TF, Knittel BL (1986) Dynamic PET data analysis. J Comput Assist Tomogr 10–4:645–653

Melega WP, Quintana J, Raleigh MJ, Stout DB, Yu D-C, Lin K-P, Huang S-C, Phelps ME (1996) 6-[^{18}F]Fluoro-L-DOPA-PET studies show partial reversibility of long-term effects of chronic amphetamine in monkeys. Synapse 22:63–69

Meyer JH, Kapur S, Wilson AA, DaSilva JN, Houle S, Brown GM (1996) Neuromodulation of frontal and temporal cortex by intravenous d-fenfluramine: an [^{15}O]H$_2$O PET study in humans. Neurosci Lett 207:25–28

Morris ED, Fisher RE, Rauch SL, Fischman AJ, Alpert NM (1996) PET imaging of neuromodulation designing experiments to detect endogenous transmitter release. In: Myers R, Cunningham V, Bailey D, Jones T (eds) Quantification of brain function using PET. Academic, San Diego, pp 425–433

Muehllehner G, Karp JS (1988) Advances in SPECT and PET. IEEE Trans Nucl Sci 35:639–643

Murayama H, Nohara N (1997) The local noise property in positron volume imaging and optimal conditions for the signal-to-noise ratio of the 3D reconstructed image. Phys Med Biol 42:231–249

Nordström A-L, Farde L, Nyberg S, Karlsson P, Halldin C, Sedvall G (1995) D_1, D_2, and 5-HT$_2$ receptor occupancy in relation to clozapine serum concentration: a PET study of schizophrenic patients. Am J Psychiatry 152:1444–1449

Pearlson GD, Jeffery PJ, Harris GJ, Ross CA, Fischman MW, Camargo EE (1993) Correlation of acute cocaine-induced changes in local cerebral blood flow with subjecticve effects. Am J Psychiatry 150:495–497

Salmon E, Brooks DJ, Leenders KL, Turton DR, Hume SP, Cremer JE, Jones T, Frackowiak RSJ (1990) A two-compartment description and kinetic procedure for measuring regional cerebral (^{11}C)nomifensine uptake using positron emission tomography. J Cereb Blood Flow Metab 10:307–316

Sedvall G, Pauli S, Karlsson P, Farde L, Nordström A-L, Nyberg S, Halldin C (1995) PET imaging of neuroreceptors in schizophrenia. European Neuro-Psychopharmacology Suppl :25–30

Shao Y, Cherry SR, Farahani K, Meadros K, Siegel S, Silverman RW, Marsden PK (1997) Simultaneous PET and MR imaging. Phys Med Biol 42:1965–1970

Turner R (1995) Functional mapping of the human brain with magnetic resonance imaging. The Neurosciences 7:179–194

Wagner, Jr. HN (1986) Quantitative imaging of neuroreceptors in the living human brain. Semin Nucl Med XVI:51–62

Clinical Applications

39 Functional MRI in Neurology

T.A. HAMMEKE

CONTENTS

39.1
Introduction

This book is testament to the rapid pace and excitement generated by functional magnetic resonance imaging (fMRI) as a tool for understanding normal and abnormal functions of the nervous system. Development of applications of fMRI for use in neurological patients for diagnostic and treatment purposes is in its infancy. Principle limitations to date include: (1) insufficient information about the nature of the signal and signal artifacts, particularly as they may relate to clinical applications, (2) inadequate understanding of normal cognitive operations to enable meaningful applications to neuropathological states, (3) less than whole-brain imaging capability in many centers, and (4) insufficient signal-to-noise ratio evoked by many experimental tasks to make them applicable in single case designs.

Despite these limitations, progress in application of the technology to neurological issues has occurred. This is perhaps most apparent in the realm of preoperative evaluations of patients with intrac-

T. A. HAMMEKE, PhD; Department of Neurology (Neuropsychology), Medical College of Wisconsin, 9200 West Wisconsin Avenue, Milwaukee, WI 53226, USA

table epilepsy, both in determining the lateralization of language and memory function and predicting seizure focus. Preliminary investigations have been carried out in studies of chronic pain and identification of boundaries of functional tissue with neoplasms and ischemia. Functional MRI holds promise for understanding the neurocognitive changes of Alzheimer's disease and predicting stroke and subsequent recovery. Progress in these areas will be briefly reviewed here.

39.2
Applications in Epilepsy

Brain surgery has proven to be an effective treatment for individuals with medically intractable epilepsy, particularly for those patients with a single seizure focus in one temporal lobe (ENGEL et al. 1993). However, successful epilepsy surgery hinges on accurate determination of the brain locus of seizure origin and of the risks of postoperative morbidity. Functional MRI can be used to address these issues in a number of ways. First, through determination of functionally viable brain tissue, fMRI may predict deficit in cognitive (e.g., language and memory), motor, and sensory perceptual functions that might arise from surgical intervention. Second, functional asymmetries or intrahemispheric anomalies in activation of memory circuits may facilitate the lateralization and localization of an ictal focus. Lastly, at least for a subset of the patients with intractable seizures, the technology may provide evidence for direct localization of the cerebral origin of seizures, either through signs of increased blood flow or blood oxygen level-dependent (BOLD) signal during the ictal period or signs of decreased flow or BOLD during the interictal period.

The current "gold standard" for determination of language and memory lateralization in the preoperative evaluation of epileptic patients is the Wada exam, also referred to as the intracarotid amobarbital test (IAT). In the context of an angiographic

decisions. Moreover, in our continuing investigations at the Medical College of Wisconsin, we have appreciated a significant discrepancy between fMRI and IAT lateralization indices in approximately one in ten patients. The reasons for these discrepant findings are only now being systematically investigated and will likely be multiple. Potential reasons for validity problems in each procedure are presented in Table 39.1. In some instances validity may be compromised because of inherent limitations of IAT. For example, during IAT a few patients become mildly sedated during the right hemisphere injection, which may have the effect of impairing their performance on language tasks, thereby suppressing the estimation of language capacities in the left hemisphere. In fMRI the adequacy of the patient's comprehension and compliance with task instructions may prove to be a critical factor in obtaining valid findings. In other cases, the discrepancies between IAT and fMRI may simply reflect differences in the tasks used between the two procedures. For example, there are infrequent cases of epilepsy in which the capacity for oral speech appears to reside in one hemisphere and language comprehension in the other (OJEMANN et al. 1989). When this occurs, it has been our impression that the fMRI results from the semantic decision task align more closely with the IAT estimate of comprehension capabilities than oral speech. Case B in Fig. 39.1 represents such a case in which oral speech capabilities appeared to reside in the left hemisphere and comprehension capacities in the right hemisphere as measured by IAT. It is possible that a word generation task used in fMRI in these patients might have produced a finding consistent with language asymmetries identified by measures of speech on IAT. Thus, clinical implementation of fMRI to determine lateralization of epilepsy patients must await further study of these validity issues and the refinements in methods that undoubtedly will occur.

39.2.2
Lateralization of Memory

The benefits of anterior temporal lobectomy in treatment of seizures must be weighed against the risks of decline in recent memory function. Another important function of the IAT test is to estimate this risk by determining which hemisphere, and specifically which temporal lobe, is capable of supporting explicit memory functions. Studies that systematically compare the memory assessment procedures

Table 39.1. Sources of procedural error

IAT (Wada test)	fMRI
Inadequate anesthetization	Field inhomogeneities in region of interest
Excessive anesthetization	
Abnormal vasculature	Movement artifacts
Vasospasm	Insensitive task or task contrasts
Task compliance	Task compliance
Intelligence	Intelligence
Motivation	Motivation
Emotional status	Emotional status

IAT, intracarotid amobarbital test.

in IAT with ones in fMRI have yet to be completed. To some extent these studies have awaited the development of tasks that can reliably activate mesial temporal regions thought to be critical to forming new explicit memories, i.e., the hippocampal formation and adjacent cortices (ZOLA 1997), and do so sufficiently well as to be detected in individual cases. Such tasks are now being refined and show promise for exploring memory lateralization capability in fMRI (e.g., BOOKHEIMER et al. 1996a, 1996b; STERN et al. 1996; PETERSSON et al. 1997). Cognitive procedures that simultaneously activate both mesial temporal lobes in neurologically normal individuals will be ideal.

Only preliminary studies of memory functions in epileptic patients are available at this time. BELLGOWAN et al. (1998) studied 28 patients with either left or right temporal lobe epilepsy performing the semantic decision test described above. Because patients were able to recognize a large number of animal names used during scanning, it was assumed that episodic encoding was occurring during the semantic decision task. While activation of language areas in the frontal and parietal lobes was similar in both groups, the right temporal lobe epilepsy group showed much stronger activation of left mesial temporal lobe including the hippocampus, parahippocampal gyrus, and collateral sulcus, than did patients with left temporal lobe epilepsy. Thus, in this study activation patterns in the mesial temporal lobe discriminated between those with left and right temporal lobe epilepsy on a group basis. Future investigations will be necessary before it is determined whether these results can be applied on an individual basis.

It is important to note that the IAT is designed to simulate memory function after resection of the an-

Case A: fMRI LI = +84; Wada LI = +100

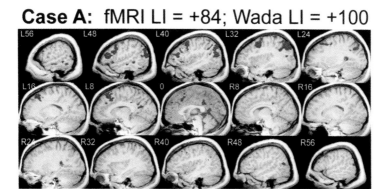

Case B: fMRI LI = - 81; Wada LI = -14

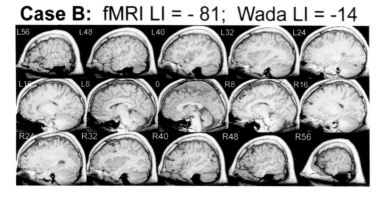

Fig. 39.1. Examples of brain activation images using a semantic decision-tone discrimination task contrast (see text for details) in two patients with intractable epilepsy. Functional MRI was completed at 1.5 Tesla on a General Electric (GE Medical Systems, Milwaukee, WI) scanner using a 3-axis local gradient and RF head coil designed for whole-brain echo-planar imaging. Areas of significant signal increase during the language task were identified by the cross-correlation method (BANDETTINI et al. 1993) using a correlation threshold of $r \geq 0.40$. Functional and high resolution anatomical images were then projected into stereotaxic space using MCW-AFNI software (Cox 1996). Sagittal images spaced at 8 mm and extending from 56 mm left to 56 mm right of midline are presented. Regions positively correlated with the language task are colored in *red*. Laterality indices (LI) from fMRI and Wada procedures are provided (see text for explanation of computation). Case A shows strong activation of association cortices in frontal, temporal, and parietal regions of the left hemisphere and illustrates the typical pattern of left hemisphere language dominance that was in close agreement with the Wada test. Case B shows relatively stronger activation of the right than left hemisphere by the language task in fMRI, implying a crossed dominance pattern, and shows less agreement with the Wada findings. This atypical activation pattern may be due to a separation of oral speech and language comprehension capacities between the hemispheres in this patient (see text for more detail)

terior temporal lobe and hippocampus in one or the other hemisphere. Since the procedure involves anesthesia of the hemisphere, it is presumed to be a direct test or prediction of amnesia following resection of a given temporal lobe. It will be an important step to determine whether results from activation studies in fMRI can be used to make the same prediction.

39.2.3
Identification of Boundaries of Functional Tissue

In the same way that fMRI might be used to predict deficits in language and memory that may occur fol-

lowing temporal lobectomy, prediction of functional deficits in other domains such as primary sensory and motor functions can also be made. Since activation of the primary sensory and motor areas yield robust BOLD signals, it is relatively easy to determine precise boundaries of functional tissue in these regions (PUCE 1995; ATLAS et al. 1996; LEE et al. 1996; MUELLER et al. 1996). A number of stimulus and response procedures are now available which enable study of the functional integrity of the retinotopic organization of the visual cortex (e.g., GRABOWSKI et al. 1995; DEYOE et al. 1996; ENGEL et al. 1997), tonotopic organization of auditory cortices (e.g., LANTOS et al. 1997; STRAINER et al. 1997; TALAVAGE et al. 1997; see also Chap. 32, this volume), and somatotopic organization in somatosensory and motor cortices (Puce et al. 1995; Rao et al. 1995; also see Chap. 31, this volume). The distributed systems for language (see Chap. 33, this volume) and working memory have been investigated in general. Still, the limitations here are the practicalities of completing multiple types of studies on an individual. Once more is known about task activation paradigms, it may be reasonable to design a set of activation procedures which can compress multiple functions into one or two activation runs, making the logistics more manageable. This again seems to be easily accomplished with stimulation of primary sensory and motor regions and is more difficult for activity in heteromodal cortices.

39.2.4
Identification of Seizure Focus

39.2.4.1
Through Direct Signal

The capability of both recording electrophysiological activity and BOLD signal has made it possible to more directly localize the focus of seizure onset or region of abnormal discharge (Ives et al. 1993; Huang-Hellinger et al. 1995; Lemieux et al. 1997). Several investigators now have been successful in using BOLD contrast for refining the estimate of or precisely localizing the origin of abnormal discharges (Jackson et al. 1994; Detre et al. 1995, 1996; Warach et al. 1994, 1996). These investigators have found evidence of increased perfusion during the intervals of abnormal electrical discharges. The initiation of a fMRI scan can be triggered by the first signs of abnormal discharges, then later compared with a scan without abnormal discharges (Warach et al. 1996). Bookheimer (1996) described a patient with reflex epilepsy in whom seizures occurred with eye closure, a circumstance of seizure control that is ideal for fMRI study. BOLD signal can also be used to identify the subcortical circuitry associated with the ictal events, thereby facilitating an understanding of the semiology of the seizure (Detre et al. 1996). This strategy of localizing the source and distribution of abnormal discharges is not limited to patients who have frank seizures in the MR scanner, but can be used to detect subclinical neuroelectrical events (Detre et al. 1995; Warach et al. 1996).

It remains to be seen how useful fMRI may be for routine use in intractable epilepsy. Abnormal electrical discharges would need to occur on a relatively frequent basis, either spontaneously or through elicitation from drugs or external stimulation, in order to make this practical. Ictal activity will need to be verified by EEG recordings that are acquired concurrent with fMRI, a feature that has been lacking in most studies to date. An additional interpretive problem of seizure origin arises when there are multiple areas of cortical activation (Witte et al. 1994), which will require further refinement of image processing methods to optimize temporal resolution of the signal. It will also be important to be able to discriminate movement artifacts from BOLD signal contrast (Hill et al. 1995). Patients who have secondary generalization from their partial seizures would likely be excluded from study due to movement artifacts.

39.2.4.2
Through Asymmetric Function

The IAT procedure has been shown to provide a fair estimate of lateralization of seizure focus (Loring et al. 1993; Perrine et al. 1995). Most informative has been the relative asymmetry in memory functions assessed during the IAT. Since fMRI may provide a similar estimation of the integrity of function in the mesial temporal lobes, it too could be used to estimate side of seizure focus. Indeed, in the Bellgowan et al. (1998) study described above, the asymmetry and distribution of activation in mesial temporal lobe structures by a language task discriminated groups of patients with a right vs left temporal seizure focus. While these results are encouraging, it is unclear whether such prediction can occur on an individual case basis and thus provide meaningful information to the preoperative assessment of intractable epilepsy.

39.3
Applications in Dementia

Understanding the neurological correlates of cognitive decline in degenerative neurological conditions may shed new light on neuropathological disease processes and treatment strategies. Functional neuroimaging that affords improved spatial resolution combined with repeatability can assist with this understanding. Of course this implies that we have a good foundation of knowledge about the distributed networks of cognitive function in healthy individuals and changes that occur with normal aging. A substantial foundation is emerging from the literature, including regional changes in resting metabolic rate with age, knowledge of the distributed networks for select cognitive operations, and changes associated with disease states. It is expected that fMRI will enable a significant acceleration of research and understanding of distributed cognitive networks and effects of disease processes on these.

At present most of our knowledge about functional neuroimaging of aging and dementia has been achieved with PET, and most studies have focused on changes in resting metabolism. LOESSNER et al. (1995) and MOELLER et al. (1996) provide information about the topography of resting cerebral metabolism in the elderly and identify distinct differences from younger individuals. The most consistent finding was decreased cortical metabolism with age, particularly in the frontal lobes, while little change was apparent in subcortical structures and the primary visual cortex. Several studies have found significant correlations between resting metabolic levels and age-related declines in memory functions (e.g., EUSTACHE et al. 1995). Other investigators have focused specifically on individuals with neurodegenerative conditions. For example, COLLETTE et al. (1997) correlated resting cerebral metabolism and performances on verbal and visuospatial span memory tests in patients with probable Alzheimer's disease. They found a positive correlation between task performance and metabolism rates in regions that have been identified as critical to the slave systems of working memory operations (e.g., SALMON et al. 1996), but a lack of correlation with prefrontal areas. The authors, citing research to support a disproportionate decline in the central executive capacities in Alzheimer's disease (BADDELEY et al. 1991), interpret the lack of correlation as evidence of a failure in these patients to engage executive resources to achieve optimal test performance. GONZALEZ et al. (1995) found good regional concordance between PET and fMRI estimates of blood flow volume in a group of patients with dementia, thereby enhancing the cross-generalization of findings from these two methodologies.

Since much of our understanding of networks of neuronal activity during cognitive operations has been generated in healthy young volunteers, it will be important to study how the topography of activation changes with age before functional neuroimaging studies of the elderly during activation paradigms can be properly interpreted. Similar to changes in resting metabolic rates in aging, there is reason to expect changes in regional activation profiles. For example, Grady and colleagues (GRADY et al. 1994, 1995; GRADY 1996) have completed a series of studies that confirm age-related changes in the distribution of functional activity during encoding and recognition of faces and locations. In general these studies found that during perceptual processing younger subjects showed greater activation than older subjects in prestriate areas, and older subjects showed greater activation of extrastriate and anterior cortices. While regional activation differences between young and old were also found on recognition memory task, the findings were less consistent. The authors interpret these findings as evidence of functional reorganization that occurs naturally with aging and may represent compensation that occurs when select abilities deteriorate. Still, functional activations in other domains may not show change with age. For example, TEMPEL and PERLMUTTER (1992) did not find significant correlation between age and regional activations induced by vibrotactile stimulation.

39.4
Applications in Stroke

MRI and perfusion-weighted imaging offer considerable potential for studying blood flow-related abnormalities and potential risks factors for stroke. This literature is considerable and will not be reviewed in any detail here. Two areas of clinical promise using BOLD contrast are nonetheless worth noting, i.e., use of fMRI to determine risk for stroke and to predict recovery of function after stroke.

Cerebral blood flow and volume depend largely on arterial reactivity to changes in partial pressure of arterial CO_2, with increasing levels of PCO_2 producing pronounced vasodilatation of cerebral arterioles and capillaries. Disturbance in this autoregulatory function is known to occur with age, but is particularly evident in the context of cerebral hemorrhage and ischemia (see MADDEN 1993 for review). Thus, cerebrovascular CO_2 reactivity (or that induced by administration of acetazolamide) has been viewed as a marker of vascular reserve capacity and, as such, a potential index of risk for stroke in those with ischemic disease (YAMAMOTO et al. 1980; TAKANO et al. 1988; GUR et al. 1996).

While PET offers a highly specific index of perfusion reserve capacity (LEVINE et al. 1988), BOLD fMRI offers a noninvasive and readily available technique for estimating cerebrovascular CO_2 reactivity (GRAHAM et al. 1994; ROSTRUP et al. 1994; BOOK et al. 1997). There is a growing body of literature using fMRI to study the effects of hypercapnia on BOLD in humans, but the procedure has not as yet been systematically applied to clinical populations.

Also of interest is a modest literature using functional neuroimaging to study motor recovery patterns in individuals with subcortical infarctions. Most of these studies have been accomplished using PET. Groups studies have shown that bilateral activation of motor cortices and recruitment of additional motor cortices have occurred in patients showing recovery of function (e.g., CHOLLET et al. 1991; WEILLER et al. 1992). PET studies have shown that there is considerable individual variability in functional reorganization that occurs to enable recovery of motor function (WEILLER et al. 1993; BOOKHEIMER et al. 1995). Still the factors that influence this variability have yet to be elucidated. FMRI offers improved resolution over PET technology for investigating the functional reorganization correlates of small subcortical infarcts and may improve prediction of outcome.

39.5
Applications in Chronic Pain

The study of nociception has proven to be scientifically challenging largely due to imprecise methods of measuring a subjective state. With the improved spatial resolution of fMRI, a new objective means of measuring pain in humans is available. Using electrical stimulation of the median nerve as the painful stimulus, DAVIS et al. (1995; 1997) identified a small region in the posterior portion of the anterior cingulate that is routinely activated during painful states and appears to be separate from an adjacent region activated by an attention demanding word-generation task. The magnitude of activation in the cingulate was correlated with the rated pain intensity ($r=0.49$, $p<0.0001$). KIRIAKOPOULOS et al. (1997) used fMRI to study the central effects of dorsal column stimulation on intractable spinal or neuralgic pain. After surgical placement of the spinal stimulators in each of three patients, the patients underwent fMRI study during states of activation and deactivation of the stimulators. Despite limited imaging parameters (one slice) and relatively insensitive signal detection procedures, the authors nonetheless found evidence of increased signal in the primary somatosensory cortex and cingulate at times of pain relief from spinal stimulation. Functional MRI has also been used to better understand the modulating effect of acupuncture on pain perception (WU et al. 1997). Studies of this character imply that fMRI may

provide an independent index of pain intensity and thereby facilitate differential diagnosis of psychiatric from chronic pain patients. Also, such studies may identify critical brain regions to be considered in psychosurgical treatment of intractable pain, and help determine optimal electrode placement for spinal stimulation.

39.6
Other Potential Applications

As a neuroimaging technique with mid-range spatial and temporal resolution, fMRI offers a methodology for improved measurement and understanding of a variety of neurological and neurobehavioral abnormalities. At it simplest, disorders affecting primary and secondary motor and sensory systems, where robust BOLD signals are typically available with system activation, lend themselves to convenient individual case investigation. One example of this is provided by DEYOE et al. (1997). These investigators use fMRI to study an art professor with visual field defects and dyschromotopsia following bilateral occipital strokes. Using a visual task with a flickering, black and white, checkered hemifield that rotated slowly about a central fixation point as well as one with checkered annulus that expanded outward from the fixation point (DEYOE et al. 1996), activation maps of the primary visual cortices were obtained and combined in a three-dimensional computer generated model of functional activity. This model showed good correspondence to tests of visual perimetry on the patient using retinotopic organizational patterns identified in neurologically normal individuals (DEYOE et al. 1996). Of interest is that, while activation maps showed relatively good correspondence to lesion localization based on standard MRI studies in that functional activity was generally not seen in regions of obvious infarct, functional activity was often seen in the edges of apparently damaged cortex. Also, there were small islands of tissue within damaged cortex that had distinct stimulus locked signal. Other investigators have utilized fMRI to better understand aberrations in neural activity associated with resting tremor (BUCHER et al. 1997) and ataxia (WESSEL and NITSCHKE 1997). BOLD signal contrast can be seen in spinal cord during hand movements (YOSHIZAWA et al. 1996), implying wider clinical applications than just investigation of brain functions.

The technology also may be exploited to study the integrity of neural connections in individual patients, even when they are unable or unwilling to comply with task activation procedures. Biswal et al. (1995) hypothesized that fluctuations in BOLD fMRI signal during the resting state have a physiologic origin. They first identified cerebral regions that were activated by bilateral finger tapping as target pixels. They then investigated the correlation of low frequency (<0.1 Hz) fluctuations occurring in these target pixels during the resting state with fluctuations occurring in all other regions in the brain. The low frequency fluctuations in the target pixels showed a high degree of correlation with all brain regions associated with motor function. They argued that such inter-regional correlations in the resting physiological state are a direct representation of functional connectivity of the brain. The absence of correlated activity between regions known to form a functional circuit might then be used to study disruption or degradation in neural connections caused by pathological processes, e.g., as in demyelinating disease.

39.7
Practical Issues in Neurological Patients

Several practical issues in using fMRI to investigate clinical populations are worth highlighting. First, body morphology imposes some practical limitation. For example, with regard to the General Electric Signa system that is used in many imaging centers, the table weight limit is 136 kg (300 lb.). The bore of the GE Signa 1.5 Tesla scanner is 55 cm ID and is further restricted by the gantry table, precluding patients of substantial girth from study. Other patients may fit into the magnet, but then have insufficient space around them in the bore for placement of peripheral devices needed for either the stimulus delivery or response recording necessary for the functional task. For example, it is not uncommon in our imaging work with epileptic patients to forego studies with visual stimuli due to insufficient space in the bore to enable view of a projection screen placed at the patient's feet.

It is useful to keep in mind that claustrophobic reactions are considerably higher in clinical populations than in normal volunteers. Also, sedating medications that are often used in standard MRI with anxious clinical patients will be contraindicated in many studies of functional activation. Compliance on motion restriction represents a substantially greater problem in clinical populations. Patients with resting movement disorders may pose a special challenge, both because of movement related

artifacts in the field of view (FOV), but also distortions in magnetic field created by movement immediately outside of the FOV (Yetkin et al. 1996). Extra time and effort is almost always necessary with patients relative to healthy volunteers.

Lastly, but hardly a trivial issue, is the matter of task compliance in clinical populations. It cannot be assumed that patients will easily understand and be adequately motivated to comply with activation tasks designed for them. In many neurological populations, impaired comprehension and reasoning capacities are common and motivational problems may be a core symptom of their disease. Reduced intelligence may affect activation parameters that are associated with task difficulty. Extra time for task training, reduced difficulty levels, and incentives for optimal performance may need to be incorporated into the study protocols. Methods to ensure adequate task performance for valid clinical interpretation of imaging data are mandatory.

39.8
Conclusions

It is difficult not to be excited about the use of fMRI in furthering our knowledge and treatment of neurological conditions. The exponential growth of functional neuroimaging studies has already accelerated our understanding of functional neuroanatomy. Still, it is useful to recognize that in order to make appropriate interpretations of any new investigational technology in studying pathological conditions, it is imperative that we understand the findings of that technology in neurologically healthy individuals. Even more stringent are standards of reliability and clinical validity that need to be met before replacing an established clinical procedure with one involving the new technology. In this regard, development of applications of fMRI in neurology remains in its infancy. Many clinical applications will await better understanding of cognitive functions in neurologically healthy individuals. Still, promising areas of potential application have already arisen in areas of preoperative evaluation of intractable epilepsy and chronic pain. There are exciting prospects in applications in stroke prediction, as well as studying connectivity in neural circuitry in neurological conditions. Future applications will be limited principally by one's creativity in designing activation and contrast tasks that are clinically revealing.

References

Alsop DC, Detre JA, D'Esposito M, Howard RS, Maldjian JA, Grossman M, Listerud J, Flamm ES, Judy KD, Atlas SW (1996) Functional activation during an auditory comprehension task in patients with temporal lobe lesions. Neuroimage 4:55–59

Atlas SW, Howard RS 2nd, Maldjian J, Alsop D, Detre JA, Listerud J, D'Esposito M, Judy KD, Zager E, Stecker M (1996) Functional magnetic resonance imaging of regional brain activity in patients with intracerebral gliomas: findings and implications for clinical management. Neurosurgery 38:329–338

Baddeley AD, Della Dalla S, Logie R, Spinnler H (1991) The decline of working memory in Alzheimer's disease. Brain 114:2521–2542

Bandettini PA, Jesmanowicz A, Wong EC, Hyde JS (1993) Processing strategies for time-course data sets in functional MRI of the human brain. Magn Reson Med 30:161–173

Bavelier D, Corina D, Jezzard P, Padmanabhan S, Clark VP, Karni A, Prinster A, Braun A, Lalwani A, Rauschecker JP, Turner R, Neville H (1997) Sentence reading: a functional MRI study at 4 Tesla. J Cogn Neurosci 9:664–686

Bellgowan PSF, Binder JR, Swanson SJ, Hammeke TA, Springer JA, Frost JA, Mueller WM, Morris GL (1998) Lateralization of seizure focus predicts activation of the left medial temporal lobe during semantic information encoding: an FMRI study. Neurology 51:479–484

Binder JR (1997) Neuroanatomy of language processing studied with functional MRI. Clin Neurosci 4:87–94

Binder JR, Rao SM, Hammeke TA, Frost JA, Bandettini PA, Jesmanowicz A, Hyde JS (1995) Lateralized human brain language systems demonstrated by task subtraction functional magnetic resonance imaging. Arch Neurol 52:593–601

Binder JR, Swanson SJ, Hammeke TA, Morris GL, Mueller WM, Fischer M, Benbadis S, Frost JA, Rao SM, Haughton VM (1996) Determination of language dominance using functional MRI: a comparison with the Wada test. Neurology 46:978–984

Binder JR, Frost JA, Hammeke TA, Cox RW, Rao SM, Prieto T (1997) Human brain language areas identified by functional magnetic resonance imaging. J Neurosci 17:353–362

Biswal B, Yetkin FZ, Haughton VM, Hyde JS (1995) Functional connectivity in the motor cortex of resting human brain using echo-planar MRI. Magn Reson Med 34:537–541

Book DS, Binder JR, Frost JA, Forster H, Bellgowan PS, Bandettini PA (1997) Assessment of cerebrovascular reserve with functional MRI. Neurol 48:A194–A195

Bookheimer SY (1996) Functional MRI applications in clinical epilepsy. Neuroimage 4:S139–146

Bookheimer S, Dapretto M, Cohen M, Wang J, Small G (1996) Functional MRI of the hippocampus during short term memory tasks: parametric responses to task difficulty and stimulus novelty. Neuroimage 3:531

Bucher SF, Seelos KC, Dodel RC, Reiser M, Oertel WH (1997) Activation mapping in essential tremor with functional magnetic resonance imaging. Ann Neurol 41:32–40

Chollet F, DiPiero V, Wise RJS, Brooks DJ, Dolan RJ, Frackowiak RSJ (1991) The functional anatomy of motor recovery after stroke in humans: a study with positron emission topography. Ann Neurol 29:63–71

Collette F, Salmon E, Van der Linden M, Degueldre C, Franck G (1997) Functional anatomy of verbal and visualspatial span tasks in Alzheimer's disease. Hum Brain Mapping 5:110–118

Courtney SM, Ungerleider LG (1997) What fMRI has taught us about human vision. Curr Opin Neurobiol 7:554–561

Cox RW (1996) AFNI: software for analysis and visualization of functional magnetic resonance neuroimages. Comput Biomed Res 29:162–173

Cuenod CA, Bookheimer SY, Hertz-Pannier L, Frank JA, Zeffiro TA, Theodore WH, Le Bihan D (1995) Functional MRI during word generation using conventional equipment: a potential tool for language localization in clinical environment. Neurology 45:1821–1827

Davis KD, Wood ML, Crawley AP, Mikulis DJ (1995) fMRI of human somatosensory and cingulate cortex during painful electrical nerve stimulation. Neuroreport 7:321–325

Davis KD, Taylor SJ, Crawley AP, Wood ML, Mikulis DJ (1997) Functional MRI of pain- and attention-related activations in the human cingulate cortex. J Neurophysiol 77:3370–3380

Desmond JE, Sum JM, Wagner AD, Demb JB, Shear PK, Glover GH, Gabrieli JD, Morrell MJ (1995) Functional MRI measurement of language lateralization in Wada-tested patients. Brain 118:1411–1419

Desmond JE, Gabrieli JD, Wagner AD, Ginier BL, Glover GH (1997) Lobular patterns of cerebellar activation in verbal working-memory and finger-tapping tasks as revealed by functional MRI. J Neurosci 17:9675–9685

Detre JA, Sirven JI, Alsop DC, O'Connor MJ, French JA (1995) Localization of subclinical ictal activity by functional magnetic resonance imaging: correlation with invasive monitoring. Ann Neurol 38:618–624

Detre JA, Alsop DC, Aguirre GK, Sperling MR (1996) Coupling of cortical and thalamic ictal activity in human partial epilepsy: demonstration by functional magnetic resonance imaging. Epilepsia 37:657–661

DeYoe EA, Carman GJ, Bandettini P, Glickman S, Wieser J, Cox R, Miller D, Neitz J (1996) Mapping striate and extrastriate visual areas in human cerebral cortex. Proc Natl Acad Sci U S A 93:2382–2386

DeYoe EA, Rosen AC, Williams K, Hammeke TA, Antuono P, Maas E (1997) Quantitative assessment of visual field defects and brain lesions with fMRI. Neuroimage 5:S312

Engel JJr, Van Ness PC, Rasmussen TB, Ojemann LM (1993) Outcome with respect to epileptic seizures. In: Engel J (ed) Surgical treatment of the epilepsies, 2nd edn. Raven, New York, pp 609–621

Engel SA, Glover GH, Wandell BA (1997) Retinotopic organization in human visual cortex and the spatial precision of functional MRI. Cereb Cortex 7:181–192

Eustache F, Rious P, Desgranges B, Marchal G, Petit-Taboue MC, Dary M, Lechevalier B, Baron JC (1995) Healthy aging, memory subsystems and regional cerebral oxygen consumption. Neuropsychologia 33:867–887

Gonzalez RG, Fischman AJ, Guimaraes AF, Carr CA, Stern CE, Halpern EF, Growdon JH, Rosen BR (1995) Functional MR in the evaluation of dementia: correlation of abnormal dynamic cerebral blood volume measurements with changes in cerebral metabolism on positron emission tomography with fludeoxyglucose F18. Am J Neuroradiol 16:1763–1770

Grabowski TJ, Damasio H, Frank RJ, Brown CK, Bolles Ponto LL, Watkins GL, Hichwa RD (1995) Neuroanatomical analysis of functional brain images: validation with retinotopic mapping. Hum Brain Mapping 2:134–148

Grady CL (1996) Age-related changes in cortical blood flow activation during perception and memory. Ann N Y Acad Sci 777:14–21

Grady CL (1998) Age-related changes in brain activity patterns during working memory. J Int Neuropsychol Soc 4:38

Grady CL, Maisog JM, Horwitz B, Ungerleider LG, Mentis MJ, Salerno JA, Pietrini P, Wagner E, Haxby JV (1994) Age-related changes in cortical blood flow activation during visual processing of faces and location. J Neurosci 14:1450–1462

Grady CL, McIntosh AR, Horwitz B, Maisog JM, Ungerleider LG, Mentis MJ, Pietrini P, Schapiro MB, Haxby JV (1995) Age-related reductions in human recognition memory due to impaired encoding. Science 269:218–221

Graham GD, Zhong J, Petroff AC, Constable RT, Prichard JW, Gore JC (1994) BOLD MRI monitoring of changes in cerebral perfusion induced by acetazolamide and hypercarbia in the rat. Magn Reson Med 31:557–560

Gur AY, Bova I, Bornstein NM (1996) Is impaired cerebral vasomotor reactivity a predictive factor of stroke? Stroke 27:2188–2190

Hertz-Pannier L, Gaillard WD, Mott SH, Cuenod CA, Bookheimer SY, Weinstein S, Conry J, Papero PH, Schiff SJ, Le Bihan D, Theodore WH (1997) Noninvasive assessment of language dominance in children and adolescents with functional MRI: a preliminary study. Neurology 48:1003–1012

Hill RA, Chiappa KH, Huang-Hellinger F, Jenkins BG (1995) EEG during MR imaging: differentiation of movement artifact from paroxysmal cortical activity. Neurology 45:1942–1943

Huang-Hellinger FR, Breiter HC, McCormack G, Cohen MS, Kwong KK, Sutton JP, Savoy RL, Weisskoff RM, Davis, TL, Baker JR, Belliveau JW, Rosen BR (1995) Simultaneous functional magnetic resonance imaging and electrophysiological recording. Hum Brain Mapping 3:13–23

Ives J, Warach L, Schmitt F, Edelman R, DL S (1993) Monitoring the patient's EEG during echo planar MRI. Electroencephalogr Clin Neurophysiol 87:417

Jackson GD, Connelly A, Cross JH, Gordon I, Gadian DG (1994) Functional magnetic resonance imaging of focal seizures. Neurology 44:850–856

Kiriakopoulos ET, Tasker RR, Nicosia S, Wood ML, Mikulis (1997) Functional magnetic resonance imaging: a potential tool for the evaluation of spinal cord stimulation: technical case report. Neurosurgery 41:501–504

Lantos G, Liu G, Shafer V, Knuth K, Vaughan H (1997) Tonotopic organization of primary auditory cortex: an fMRI study. Neuroimage 5:S174

Lee CC, Jack CR Jr, Riederer SJ (1996) Use of functional magnetic resonance imaging. Neurosurg Clin N Am 7:665–683

Lemieux L, Allen PJ, Franconi F, Symms MR, Fish DR (1997) Recording of EEG during fMRI experiments: patient safety. Magn Reson Med 38:943–952

Levine RL, Sunderland JJ, Lagreze HL, Nickles RJ, Rowe BR, Turski PA (1988) Cerebral perfusion reserve indexes determined by fluoromethane positron emission scanning. Stroke 19:19–27

Loessner A, Alavi A, Lewandrowski KU, Mosley D, Souder E, Gur RE (1995) Regional cerebral function determined by FDG-PET in healthy volunteers: normal patterns and changes with age. J Nucl Med 36:1141–1149

Loring DW, Meador KJ, Lee GP, King DW (1992) Amobarbital effects and lateralized brain function: The Wada test. Springer, Berlin Heidelberg New York

Loring DW, Murro AM, Meador KJ, Lee GP, Gratton CA, Nichols ME, Gallagher BB, King DW, Smith JR (1993) Wada memory testing and hippocampal volume measurements in the evaluation for temporal lobectomy. Neurology 43:1789–1793

Madden JA (1993) The effect of carbon dioxide on cerebral arteries. Pharmacol Ther 59:229–250

McCarthy G, Blamire AM, Rothman DL, Gruetter R, Schulman RG (1993) Echo-planar magnetic resonance imaging studies of frontal cortex activation during word generation in humans. Proc Natl Acad Sci USA 90:4952–4959

Moeller JR, Ishikawa T, Dhawan V, Spetsieris P, Mandel F, Alexander GE, Grady C, Pietrini P, Eidelberg D (1996) The metabolic topography of normal aging. J Cereb Blood Flow Metab 16:385–398

Mueller WM, Yetkin FZ, Hammeke TA, Morris GL 3rd, Swanson SJ, Reichert K, Cox R, Haughton VM (1996) Functional magnetic resonance imaging mapping of the motor cortex in patients with cerebral tumors. Neurosurgery 39:515–520

Ojemann G, Ofemann J, Lettich E, Berger M (1989) Cortical language localization in left, dominant hemisphere: an electrical stimulation mapping investigation in 117 patients. J Neurosurg 71:316–326

Perrine K, Westerveld M, Sass KJ, Devinsky O, Dogali M, Spencer DD, Luciano DJ, Nelson PK (1995) Wada memory disparities predict seizure laterality and postoperative seizure control. Epilepsia 36:851–856

Petersson KM, Elfgren C, Ingvar M. (1997) A dynamic role of the medial temporal lobe during retrieval of declarative memory in man. Neuroimage 6:1–11

Puce A (1995) Comparative assessment of sensorimotor function using functional magnetic resonance imaging and electrophysiological methods. J Clin Neurophysiol 12:450–459

Puce A, Constable RT, Luby ML, McCarthy G, Nobre AC, Spencer DD, Gore JC, Allison R (1995) Functional magnetic resonance imaging of sensory and motor cortex: comparison with electrophysiological localization. J Neurosurg 83:262–270

Rao SM, Binder JR, Hammeke TA, Bandettini PA, Bobholz JA, Frost JA, Myklebust BM, Jacobson RD, Hyde JS (1995) Somatotopic mapping of the human primary motor cortex with functional magnetic resonance imaging. Neurology 45:919–924

Rostrup E, Larsson HB, Toft PB, Garde K, Thomsen C, Ring P, Sondergaard L, Henriksen O (1994) Functional MRI of CO2 induced increase in cerebral perfusion. NMR in Biomedicine 7:29–34

Salmon E, Van der Linden M, Collette F, Delfiore F, Maguet P, Degueldre C, Luxen A, Franck G (1996) Regional brain activity during working memory tasks. Brain 119:1617–1625

Springer JA, Binder JR, Hammeke TA, Swanson SJ, Frost JA, Bellgowan PS, Brewer CC, Perry HM, Morris GL, Mueller

WM (1997). Variability of language lateralization in normal controls and epilepsy patients: an FMRI study. Neuroimage 5:S581

Stern CE, Corkin S, Gonzalez RG, Guimaraes AR, Baker JR, Jennings PJ, Carr CA, Sugiura RM, Vedantham V, Rosen BR, (1996) The hippocampal formation participates in novel picture encoding: evidence from functional magnetic resonance imaging. Proc Natl Acad Sci U S A 93:8660–8665

Strainer JC, Ulmer JL, Yetkin FZ, Haughton VM, Daniels DL, Millen SJ (1997) Functional MR of the primary auditory cortex: an analysis of pure tone activation and tone discrimination. Am J Neuroradiol 18:601–610

Takano T, Nagatsuka K, Ohnishi Y, Takamitsu Y, Matsuo H, Matsumoto M, Kimura K, Kamada T (1988) Vascular response to carbon dioxide in areas with and without diaschisis in patients with small, deep hemispheric infarction. Stroke 19:840-845

Talvage TM, Ledden PJ, Sereno MI, Rosen BR, Dale AM (1997) Multiple phase-encoded tonotopic maps in human auditory cortex. Neuroimage 5:S8

Tempel LW, Perlmutter JS (1992) Vibration-induced regional cerebral blood flow responses in normal aging. J Cereb Blood Flow Metab 12:554–561

Warach S, Levin JM, Schomer DL, Holman BL, Edelman RR (1994) Hyperperfusion of ictal seizure focus demonstrated by MR perfusion imaging. Am J Neuroradiol 15: 965–968

Warach S, Ives JR, Schlaug G, Patel MR, Darby DG, Thangaraj V, Edelman RR, Schomer DL (1996) EEG-triggered echoplanar functional MRI in epilepsy. Neurology 47:89–93

Weiller C, Chollet F, Friston KJ, Wise RJ, Frackowiak RS (1992) Functional reorganization of the brain in recovery from striatocapsular infarction in man. Ann Neurol 31:463-472

Weiller C, Ramsay SC, Wise RJ, Friston KJ, Frackowiak RS (1993) Individual patterns of functional reorganization in the human cerebral cortex after capsular infarction. Ann Neurol 33:181-189

Wessel K, Nitschke MF (1997) Cerebellar somatotopic representation and cerebro-cerebellar interconnections in ataxic patients. Prog Brain Res 114:577–588

Witte OW, Bruehl C, Schlaug G, Tuxhorn I, Lahl R, Villagran R, Seitz RJ (1994) Dynamic changes of focal hypometabolism in relation to epileptic activity. J Neurol Sci 124:188–197

Wu M-T, Xiong J, Yang P-C, Hsieh J-C, Tsai G, Rosen BR, Kwong KK (1997) Acupuncture modulating the limbic brain detected by functional MR imaging. Neuroimage 5:S15

Xiong JH, Rao S, Gao JH, Woldorff M, Fox PT (1998) Evaluation of hemispheric dominance for language using functional MRI: a comparison with positron emission tomography. Hum Brain Mapping 6:42-58

Yamamoto M, Meyer JS, Sakai F, Yamaguchi F (1980) Aging and cerebral vasodialator responses to hypercarbia. Arch Neurol 37:489–496

Yetkin FZ, Haughton VM, Cox RW, Hyde J, Birn RM, Wong EC, Prost R (1996) Effect of motion outside the field of view on functional MR. Am J Neuroradiol 17:1005–1009

Yoshizawa T, Nose T, Moore GJ, Sillerud LO (1996) Functional magnetic resonance imaging of motor activation in the human cervical spinal cord. Neuroimage 4:174–182

Zola S (1997) Amnesia:neuroanatomic and clinical aspects. In: Feinberg, Farah (eds) Behavioral neurology and neuropsychology. McGraw-Hill, New York, pp 447–462

40 Functional MRI in the Study of Emotion

R.J. Davidson, W. Irwin

40.1 Introduction

The purpose of this chapter is to present an overview of the use of functional magnetic resonance imaging (fMRI) to make inferences about the neural substrates of human affective processes. Emotion is a topic that lay dormant in the biobehavioral sciences for many decades. However, over the past 10 years, there has been an enormous increase in animal research that has provided a detailed foundation for understanding the neural circuitry of several basic emotional processes (e.g., LeDoux 1996). This corpus of literature has helped to make emotion a tractable problem in the neurosciences and has led to the development of affective neuroscience (Davidson and Sutton 1995). With recent advances

in functional brain imaging, the circuitry underlying emotion in the human brain can now be studied with unprecedented precision.

There is growing literature using positron emission tomography (PET) to look at the functional neuroanatomy of affective processes in both normal individuals and in patients with various mood and anxiety disorders (see, e.g., Drevets and Raichle 1995 for review). It is beyond the scope of this chapter to review the studies using PET. However, these studies have provided some basis for formulating hypotheses about circuitry to examine with fMRI. In the future, it will be particularly informative to combine studies of regional activation assessed using fMRI with PET studies of receptor and neurotransmitter function (see, e.g., Koepp et al. 1998). This combination promises to yield the most complete picture available yet of the functional neurochemistry and functional neuroanatomy of affective processes.

The next section of this chapter will consider some conceptual distinctions important to the study of emotion so that our review of the extant literature can then be considered in light of these distinctions. In addition, a number of crucial methodological issues will be noted at the central outset. These conceptual and methodological complexities are to the interpretation of extant data and have important implications for the design of future studies. Many of these issues have already been raised in the literature on psychophysiological correlates of emotion (e.g., Davidson et al. 1990), but unfortunately this body of research is rarely consulted by those in the neuroimaging community. The third section of the chapter will contain a review of extant studies using fMRI to make inferences about the neural circuitry associated with different aspects of affective processing. The last section will present a brief summary and conclusions.

R.J. Davidson, PhD; Laboratory for Affective Neuroscience, University of Wisconsin-Madison, 1202 West Johnson Street, Madison, WI 53706, USA
W. Irwin, BS; Laboratory for Affective Neuroscience, University of Wisconsin-Madison, 1202 West Johnson Street, Madison, WI 53706, USA

40.2
Conceptual and Methodological Complexities in fMRI Studies of Human Emotion

The issues addressed in this section are not unique to fMRI studies, but rather are pertinent to the application of a range of neuroimaging methods to the study of emotion. First we address certain properties of affective processes per se and consider their bearing on experimental strategies for neuroimaging research. Much has been written about the structure of affect (see EKMAN and DAVIDSON 1994 for review) and it is not our intention to provide a review of this complex issue. However, there are several distinctions that are important to highlight and the import of these distinctions for the experimental study of the neural substrates of affective processes will be described.

Affective processes can be conceptualized in both state and trait terms. Emotions are often considered phasic processes (e.g., EKMAN 1984) but there are also consistent differences in patterns of emotional reactivity and affective dispositions that have collectively been referred to as affective style (e.g., DAVIDSON 1992, 1998). Neuroimaging studies have been addressed to both state and trait properties of affect. For example, there are studies that measure regional brain activation during phasic emotional arousal elicited by using pictures (e.g., IRWIN et al. 1996), films (e.g., LANE et al. 1997) or other sensory stimuli (e.g., olfaction, e.g., SOBEL et al. 1998; sound, e.g., MADDOCK and BUONOCORE 1997). Another type of study is one in which two groups are compared that are assumed to differ in some dispositional emotional characteristic, e.g., depressed patients vs controls. These groups can be compared on both resting measures of regional brain activation (e.g., DREVETS et al. 1997) or on differences in reactivity to specific phasic affective stimuli (e.g., BREITER et al. 1996b). Of course, the adoption of one or the other experimental approach is most often dictated by the specific questions and interests of the investigators. However, critical to the interpretation of such studies as relevant to elucidating the underlying circuitry of emotion are several issues. It is essential to verify the presence of the intended emotional state or trait. It is insufficient to simply assume that the intended emotional state or trait is present given the particular independent variable chosen. For example, the presentation of emotional film clips or faces does not guarantee that the emotional state intended is actually elicited. Ideally the investigator can use con-

current or near-concurrent measures to objectively verify that the intended emotional state was actually produced by the manipulation of the independent variable. Thus, for example, in fear conditioning studies, investigators have used measures of skin conductance either during (e.g., BUCHEL et al. 1998) or after (e.g., LABAR et al. 1998a) the actual scanning session to confirm that conditioning in fact did occur. When clinical groups are being compared to normal control groups, it is imperative to examine the current emotional state of the participants since mood can be quite variable. Moreover, the manner in which psychiatric patients react to the demands of a neuroimaging study may differ considerably from normal controls. For example, we have found that depressed patients respond with more positive mood (compared with their own trait levels) while controls respond more negatively to a PET study (ABERCROMBIE et al. 1999).

One of the more convincing ways to demonstrate that the activations produced are emotion-related is to perform correlational analyses between regional activation measures and objective measures of emotional arousal. For example, LABAR et al. (1998a) demonstrated that the extent of amygdala activation during conditioned fear acquisition was strongly predicted by skin conductance changes during conditioning, the latter of which was collected 1–3 months following the scanning session. BREITER and colleagues (1997) examined correlations between each brain voxel and several self-report measures of response to cocaine. They reported a number of significant associations including a correlation between reports of craving and signal change in the nucleus accumbens. We have reported strong correlations between the magnitude of signal change in the amygdala in response to negative compared with neutral pictures and subjects' reports of dispositional negative affect (IRWIN et al. 1998a) and intensity of reactivity to negative stimuli (IRWIN et al. 1998b). These correlational analyses help to strengthen the interpretation that the activations that have been reported in these various studies are indeed emotion-related.

Another issue that may be important relates to whether the emotional changes produced by the investigator's choice of independent variable are discrete or more dimensional. If it is the intention of the investigator to elicit an increase in negative affect, then it is important that the stimuli used not be saturated with one specific discrete negative affect (e.g., disgust), but rather include a broad range of negative emotions. Inconsistencies in the literature may in part be due to the fact that different stimulus sets used to induce emotion may differ in the extent to which they weight one or another discrete emotion category. It is important to emphasize that we do not believe it is more appropriate to conceptualize emotion as either discrete or dimensional (see EKMAN and DAVIDSON 1994 for extensive discussion). Rather, it is apparent that both levels of analysis are appropriate for different questions. In the present context it is important to simply emphasize the importance of remaining sensitive to this issue in the choice of stimuli for fMRI studies of emotion.

An issue of crucial importance is to carefully distinguish between the perception and production of emotion. Unfortunately, this issue still gets confused in the literature. The presentation of facial expressions of emotion do not necessarily (nor even likely) elicit any emotion, yet some investigators write as if they are studying emotion when they examine activation in response to such stimuli. While it is perfectly reasonable to study the perception of facial expressions of emotion, it is imperative to carefully constrain conclusions based upon such studies to the perceptual domain. This issue has been of long-standing confusion in the psychophysiology, lesion and neuroimaging literatures (see DAVIDSON 1993).

Also of importance in fMRI studies of emotion is the nature of the control conditions used against which the effects of emotional stimuli are compared. It is clear that when using subtractive methodology, it is critical to control for as much of the stimulus content as possible to isolate the effects of emotion per se. There have been some PET studies that have compared the effects of self-generated emotional imagery to a resting control condition (e.g., PARDO et al. 1993). The problem with this design is that any effects observed might not be a function of the particular emotion (sadness in this case) that was aroused, but rather the cognitive processes involved in retrieving information from memory and voluntarily generating visual imagery. It is a good practice to include more than one emotion condition (e.g., both positive and negative) since any effects produced as a consequence of simply generating emotion per se should be common to the two emotions, while differences between conditions can be attributed to the specific nature of the emotional process elicited. It is also important when including more than one emotion condition that the emotions be matched on intensity or arousal (see DAVIDSON et al. 1990 for more detailed discussion). Arousal can be inferred in several different ways including self-report and skin conductance measures (e.g., LANG et

al. 1990). Differences in patterns of activation observed between two emotion conditions that are not matched on intensity or arousal can obviously be an artifact of failure to match appropriately.

A related issue that is of special importance in neuroimaging studies is the need to match stimuli across emotion and control conditions on physical properties such as color, the presence of faces, spatial frequency, etc. Some differences found between emotion conditions might conceivably be a function of physical differences between the stimuli that have nothing directly to do with emotion. For example, in our fMRI studies of emotion induced with pictures, we have found (IRWIN et al. 1997) that activation of secondary visual cortex by the negative pictures compared with the neutral pictures is in part a function of the color differences between these classes of stimuli. The negative pictures have a higher red-to-green ratio.

An issue of major importance in the analysis of imaging data, and one that has figured prominently in various studies of emotion, is laterality. Many investigators using both PET and fMRI have reported asymmetric changes associated with emotion (e.g., MORRIS et al. 1998). In most cases, claims about an activation being asymmetric were made on the basis of voxels in one hemisphere exceeding statistical threshold while homologous voxels in the opposite hemisphere did not. However, such an analytic strategy, while typical, is only testing for main effects of condition. Rarely has an investigator formally tested the Condition X Hemisphere or Group X Hemisphere interaction. This is likely largely a function of the fact that software is not commercially available to perform such analyses for the entire brain volume. Second, most investigators have not recognized the critical need to formally test this interaction prior to making claims about asymmetric effects. If this interaction is not significant, it is not legitimate to claim that an asymmetric finding was observed since the lack of a significant interaction means that the changes found in one hemisphere are not significantly different from those observed in the other, even if the effects are independently significant in one hemisphere. Moreover, it is possible for significant interactions to arise in the absence of any significant main effects. As will be seen below in the review of extant emotion studies using fMRI, very few investigators who have reported asymmetric effects have properly tested for the Condition X Hemisphere interaction.

40.3
Functional MRI Studies of Affective Processes in Review

To date, there is a paucity of published studies that have used fMRI to study affective processes compared to the number of studies of cognitive and sensory processes. As noted at the outset, the study of emotion with neuroimaging is plagued with complexities and complications that make such work challenging, particularly using fMRI. This review will cover all published studies that have used fMRI to make inferences about neural mechanisms underlying affective processes.

With the exception of a little-known report by the group at the University of Tübingen (GRODD et al. 1995), we published the first report which used fMRI to study normal affective processes (IRWIN et al. 1996). In that same month and year, BREITER et al. (1996b) published a report using fMRI to study obsessive-compulsive disordered patients. Since that time, many other studies have been published and the number likely to appear within the next several years will be several times that already in the literature, based upon the abstract presentations at several recent national and international meetings.

Table 40.1 summarizes the major methods and findings for all of the published studies using fMRI to study affective processes. The studies listed in Table 1 can be categorized into seven broad categories: studies of self-induced affect (2); studies of externally elicited affect using visual, auditory or olfactory stimuli (5); studies of the perception of facial expressions of emotion (3); studies of pain (2); studies of conditioned affect (2); studies of pharmacological manipulations of affect (1); and studies of affective disorders (3).

40.3.1
Studies of Affective Disorders

Three studies have examined affective disorders. In the first such report, BREITER et al. (1996b) examined the functional neuroanatomy underlying the activation of obsessive-compulsive symptoms in a group of clinically diagnosed patients. It is important to note that the affective challenges were individually tailored for each patient. For example, those patients with sanitary phobias were instructed to touch a towel putatively soaked in toilet water or a patient with a sexual assault obsession was presented with a picture of their victim relative. At first

pass, this may strike one as a noisy manipulation in that, by definition, different affective inputs (e.g., tactile vs visual) will activate different sensory systems. However, it could also be argued that to the extent that the various manipulations elicit a similar obsessional state across subjects, then the significant activations that emerge from group analyses will reflect the common underlying neural substrata. Table 40.1 lists all of the significant activation foci reported. Of note is activation in the orbitofrontal prefrontal cortex, consistent with the role of this cortical sector in obsessive/perseverative syndromes as derived from lesion and trauma studies (LEVIN et al. 1991), and activation of the amygdala which receives extensive projections from orbitofrontal cortex (AMARAL and PRICE 1984). No such activations were detected in control subjects exposed to the same stimuli as the patients.

We (KALIN et al. 1998) reported preliminary data from a study of control and clinically depressed patients exposed to affectively laden positive (e.g., puppy dogs), negative (e.g., mutilated face) and neutral (e.g., basket) complex visual stimuli. The protocol involved scanning subjects and patients on three separate occasions. During the first scanning session, all depressed patients were in an acute episode and off medication. After the first scanning session, patients were placed on Venlafaxine. All subjects were rescanned 2 and 6 weeks following the initial scan. In our preliminary data, we found that in response to the positive vs neutral stimuli, the controls showed a decrease in activation in secondary visual cortex (occipotemporal gyrus; Brodmann's area 19) at the second session compared with the first. For the depressed patients, no activation in response to positive vs neutral pictures was observed at session 1, while after 2 weeks of treatment, significant activation emerged in secondary visual cortex. This emergence of activation was concomitant with rather substantial decreases in self-reported depression severity from time 1 to time 2. This region of visual cortex has been reported to be activated in response to affectively relevant visual stimuli in both PET (e.g., FREDRIKSON et al. 1993; LANE et al. 1997) and fMRI (e.g., IRWIN et al. 1997; PHILLIPS et al. 1997) studies.

BIRBAUMER and colleagues (1998) reported bilateral amygdalar activation in a group of male social phobics in response to neutral facial expressions (compared to a resting baseline condition). Such a neural response appears to be consistent with social phobia being characterized as an irrational fear of social situations. The amygdalar activation in this patient group was comparable in magnitude to that elicited by an aversive odor (fermented yeast). This is in contrast to a control group who showed bilateral amygdalar activation in response to the odor, but showed no amygdalar activation in response to the facial expressions. Interestingly, subjects' affective ratings for the face stimuli were comparable for both patients and controls.

40.3.2
Studies of Conditioned Affective Responses

Two very recent reports examined the neural substrates of the conditioned emotional response (PAVLOV 1927). LABAR et al. (1998a) examined the acquisition and extinction of a classically conditioned response to a visual stimulus (colored square) paired with an electric shock delivered to the forearm. In wishing to extend what is known about the role of the amygdala in non-human animal studies of conditioning (e.g., LEDOUX 1996), they acquired data coronally from a limited region of the brain (22 mm) centered on the amygdala. Bilateral amygdalar activation was detected in both the early (i.e., first half of each trial) phases of acquisition and extinction. Due to technical difficulties, these investigators were unable to collect skin conductance responses (SCRs), the typical metric of conditioning, during scanning. However, a subset of the originally studied subjects were brought back to the laboratory and were presented with an identical conditioning protocol used during the scanning sessions. Analysis of the SCRs indicated typical conditioning and extinction. Interestingly, there was a significant positive correlation between the magnitude of SCR and the spatial extent of amygdalar activation that was measured 1–3 months earlier.

BUCHEL et al. (1998) reported an event-related study of classical conditioning in which neutral facial expressions were paired (or not) with an aversive loud tone on a 50% reinforcement schedule. They examined both the brain response and SCRs to the conditioned stimuli that were not paired with the tone. The complete set of activations reported is listed in Table 40.1. Importantly, these investigators performed interaction analyses that revealed that the amygdala response shows a rapid adaptation to the conditioned stimulus. This finding is consistent with that observed by LaBar and colleagues, as reviewed above. Amygdalar activation during aversive conditioning paradigms has been reported in abstract form by KNIGHT et al. (1996, 1997, 1998).

40.3.3
Studies of Perception of Facial Expressions of Emotion

Several studies have examined the neural response to presentation of the now classic Pictures of Facial Affect (EKMAN and FRIESEN 1976), a stimulus set comprised of several adults posing neutral and emotionally expressive facial expressions. In all of these studies, the hypotheses involve predictions about differential responses of various brain regions, notably the amygdala, to facial expressions of emotion compared to neutral faces. As noted in Sect. 40.2, there are important conceptual ambiguities associated with studies using facial expressions of emotion as stimuli. It is typically not clear in any given study whether the presentation of emotional faces actually elicits any emotion in the viewer. While changes in facial electromyography have been reported to the simple presentation of emotional faces (DIMBERG 1982), it is not clear whether these subtle changes in facial muscle tone are actually reflecting alterations in emotion or mood that are produced by the faces or rather are reflecting motor mimicry that may be recruited in the process of perceiving such faces. Without additional evidence to verify the presence of an emotional state, we believe it is prudent to assume that studies examining MR signal changes in response to facial expressions of emotion are revealing the circuitry associated with the perception of emotion rather than the production of emotion (see Sect. 40.2).

The first of these reports compared the response to happy and fearful facial expressions of emotion to that of neutral facial expressions. BREITER et al. (1996a) reported both bilateral amygdalar and fusiform gyrus (Brodmann's areas 19 and 37) in response to viewing both fear and happy facial expressions compared to neutral facial expressions. The amygdalar activation showed rapid habituation within run, while activation in fusiform gyrus did not. Despite the fact that subjects, post-scanning, reported more nonspecific arousal when viewing the emotional than the neutral facial expressions, there were no differences in heart rate when subjects were viewing the emotional compared to neutral facial expressions.

WHALEN and colleagues (1998) reported amygdalar activation in response to viewing fearful and happy facial expressions of emotion. The unique feature of this study is that the emotional facial expressions were presented masked with a neutral facial expression such that subjects were unaware of the

Table 40.1. Summary of methods and results for extant functional MRI studies of affective processes

Study	Subjects	Subject screening	Affect manipulation	Control condition	Manipulation check	Brain coverage	Brain regions	Behavioral indices
Davis et al. (1995)	5 males and 4 females; all right-handed	Healthy; screening for tolerance of electric stimulation	Electric shock to the right median nerve	Rest; non-painful (tingling pain) stimulation	Pain intensity ratings	1, 4 mm sagital slice in the left hemisphere, 3–4 mm lateral to the midline	Cingulate cortex activation in response to painful electrical stimulation, but not in response to tingling electrical stimulation	Subjects' pain ratings distinguished between painful and tingling electrical stimulation
Grodd et al. (1995)	12 subjects; all right-handed. Sex not reported	Healthy volunteers	View happy or sad facial expression and think affekt-congruent thoughts	View neutral facial expression with instructions to memorize names and resting with eyes open	Positive and Negative Affect Scales (PANAS) administered after each manipulation trial	3, 4 mm coronal slices, 2 mm gap	Left amygdala	Not reported
Breiter et al. (1996b)	10 obsessive-compulsive disordered (OCD) patients; 5 control subjects. Sex breakdown was not reported	Patients: DSM-III-R criteria for OCD without comorbidity of other axis I or II disorders. Controls: clinical screen for current and history of psychiatric disorders	Tactile presentation of subject-specific provocative stimuli (e.g., towel soaked in toilet water)	Tactile presentation of subject-specific innocuous stimuli (e.g., clean towel)	Pre- and post-scan ratings of anxiety and obsessionality	14, 7 mm contiguous coronal slices covering from the frontal pole past the thalamus	Patients: Bilateral anterior and posterior orbitofrontal, cingulate, temporal and insular cortices; bilateral superior, middle and inferior gyri; bilateral caudate; bilateral lenticulate; bilateral amygdala activation in response to provocative stimuli. Controls: no activations	Significant increases in anxiety and obsessionality during presentation of provocative stimuli
Breiter et al. (1996a)	Experiment 1: 10 males; experiment 2: 8 males; all right-handed	No history of psychiatric or neurological illness or treatment with medications	View happy and fearful facial expressions of emotion	View neutral facial expression	Post-scan ratings of the intensity of their feelings during scanning; pulse-oximetry (heart rate)	14–15, 8 mm contiguous coronal slices covering the whole brain	Bilateral amygdala and fusiform gyrus (Brod-mann's areas 19, 37) activations in response to both happy and fearful faces	Ratings of nonspecific arousal were higher for viewing happy and fearful faces; no changes in heart rate
Irwin et al. (1996)	3 females; all right-handed	Normal; no psychiatric conditions present or history of neurological disorders	Negatively valenced complex pictures (e.g., mutilated face)	Neutral complex pictures (e.g., book)	Post-scan ratings of stimuli valence	3, 5 mm contiguous coronal slices with the center slice "centered" on the amygdala	Bilateral amygdala activation in response to negative pictures compared to neutral pictures.	Subjects rated the negative stimuli significantly more negatively than the neutral stimuli

Study	Subjects	Subject screening	Affect manipulation	Control condition	Manipulation check	Brain coverage	Brain regions	Behavioral indices
BREITER et al. (1997)	Cocaine addicts: 13 males and 4 females; all right-handed	Selected using the Addiction Severity Index, Hamilton Anxiety Scale, and Hamilton Depression Scale	Cocaine infusion	Saline infusion	0–3 ratings of "rush", "high", "low" and "craving"; electrocardiogram; plasma urine levels	15, 8 mm contiguous axial slices covering the whole brain	Nucleus accumbens, subcallosal cortex, caudate, putamen, basal forebrain, anterior and posterior thalamus, lateral geniculate nucleus, insula, hippocampus, parahippocampal gyrus, anterior and posterior cingulate gyrus, lateral prefrontal, temporal, parietal, striate and extrastriate cortices, ventral tegmentum and pons activations in response to cocaine. Amygdala, temporal pole, medial frontal cortex deactivations in response to cocaine	Ratings of "rush" positively correlated with the left basal forebrain, ventral tegmentum, right anterior and posterior cingulate, caudate, right putamen, right insula, posterior thalamus, left posterior hippocampus; Ratings of "craving" positively correlated with the nucleus accumbens and right parahippocampal gyrus, and negatively with the left amygdala; Heart rate and urine plasma levels of cocaine increased following infusion of cocaine
DAVIS et al. (1997)	8 right-handed subjects. Sex breakdown not reported	Not reported	Electric shock to the right median nerve	Rest	Verbal (0–10) rating of the intensity of the pain	1, 4 mm sagittal slice in the left hemisphere 3–4 mm lateral to the midline	Anterior cingulate gyrus (posterior Brodmann's area 24)	Pain intensity ratings were positively correlated with percent signal change in anterior cingulate
PHILLIPS et al. (1997)	2 males and 5 females; all right-handed	No history of brain injury or of past or current psychiatric illness	View fear and disgust facial expressions of emotion with varying intensities. Concurrent sex discrimination and button press	View "slightly" happy facial expression of emotion with varying intensities. Concurrent sex discrimination and button press	None reported	14, 5 mm near-axial slices, 0.5 mm gap, covering the whole brain	75% fear vs. "neutral": left insula and left amygdala; 150% fear vs. "neutral": right putamen and right amygdala; 75% disgust vs. "neutral": right anterior-mid insula and right medial frontal cortex; 150% disgust vs. "neutral": left medial frontal cortex, left peristriate cortex, bilateral anterior insula posterior cingulate gyrus, right dorsolateral prefrontal cortex, right parastriate cortex, right thalamus, left inferior-posterior temporal cortex, left superior temporal cortex, right middle temporal cortex and right putamen	Sex discrimination performance averaged 96.6% correct

Table 40.1. Summary of methods and results for extant functional MRI studies of affective processes (Continued)

Study	Subjects	Subject screening	Affect manipulation	Control condition	Manipulation check	Brain coverage	Brain regions	Behavioral indices
MADDOCK and BUONORE (1997)	5 males and 5 females; all right-handed	Normal; no psychiatric conditions present	Listen to threat-related words and judge their pleasantness	Listen to neutral words	None reported	16, 6 mm coronal slices, 2 mm gap, covering from the middle occipital gyrus to the anterior tip of the cingulate gyrus	Posterior cingulate and retro-splenial cortex (Brodmann's areas 23, 29, 31); 8/10 left; 2/10 right	Memory for second (post scan) presentation of threat words was positively correlated with the number of significant voxels in the posterior cingulate
SCHNEIDER et al. (1997)	7 males and 5 females; all right-handed	Normal; no affective illness in themselves or first-degree relatives	View happy or sad facial expression and think affect-congruent thoughts	View neutral facial expression with instructions to memorize names and resting with eyes open	PANAS administered after each manipulation trial; emotion discrimination task	3, 4 mm coronal slices with the middle slice "centered" on the amygdala	Left amygdala and left cingulum (Brodmann's area 32, 33) more active during happy and sad manipulations compared to control conditions; analyses used ROIs drawn on structural MRIs	More negative affect reported during sad and less negative affect during happy induc-tion as indicated by the PANAS. The median perfor-mance on the emotion discrimi-nation task was 92.5%
STILLER et al. (1997)	20 right-handed subjects. Sex breakdown not reported	None reported	Auditory presentation of sad intoned adjectives for which subjects had to detect the phoneme /a/	Neutral intoned adjectives for which subjects had to detect the phoneme /a/	Detection of the phoneme was recorded by left-handed button pushes	5, 8 mm contiguous oblique axial slices	Group results: bilateral superior temporal gyrus, supratemporal plane (i.e., from caudal portion of the planum temporale), auditory cortex including medially the transi-tion zones to insular cortex, and anterior auditory association cortical activations for all phoneme detection tasks (i.e., no laterality) "Right responders": significantly greater right hemisphere activation for prosodic phoneme compared to neutral phoneme "Left responders": significantly greater left hemisphere acti-vation for prosodic phoneme compared to neutral phoneme	Phoneme detection performance averaged 99.8% correct
BIRBAUMER et al. (1998)	7 male social phobics; 5 male controls; handedness not reported	Social phobia was diagn-osed with the Social Phobia and Anxiety Inventory	View neutral faces; odorant (fermented yeast); neutral air puff	Rest	Subjects made online valence, arousal and intensity ratings of the stimuli	20, 3 mm coronal slices, 1 mm gap (slice locations not reported)	Bilateral amygdala in response to odors for phobics and controls; bilateral amygdala in response to faces for the phobics	Odors rated as more aversive than faces for both phobics and controls; faces rated similarly by phobics and controls

Study	Subjects	Screening	Task / stimuli	Control	Autonomic measure	Slices	Activations	Notes
al. (1998)	2 females; all right-handed		...cal condition-ing with 3 condi-tions: neutral facial expressions with ~100 dB tone (CS+, paired); neutral facial expression alone (CS+, unpaired); neutral facial expression (CS-)	...to the CS+, unpaired	...conductance response (SCR)	...mm axial slices covering the whole brain	bilateral anterior cingulate gyri; bilateral anterior insulae, medial parietal cortex; red nucleus; premotor cortex; supplementary motor area; bilateral amygdala activations in response to the CS+, unpaired	SCRs indicated acquired conditioned autonomic responses
LaBar et al. (1998b)	5 males and 5 females; all right-handed	No history of neurological impairment	Acquisition and extinction of aversive classical conditioning using a colored visual cue paired with shock (CS+)	Colored visual cue presented without shock	Post-scan skin conductance responses	3, 6 mm coronal slices, 2 mm gap centered on the amygdala	Early acquisition: rostral and caudal anterior cingulate, precentral gyrus, bilateral periamygdaloid cortex, striatum superior frontal gyrus. Late acquisition: Middle frontal gyrus, superior frontal gyrus, superior temporal gyrus, striatum, caudate anterior cingulate. Early extinction: Middle frontal gyrus, bilateral amygdala, precentral gyrus, superior frontal gyrus, head of caudate, superior temporal gyrus. Late extinction: Superior frontal gyrus	Post-scan measures of skin conductance correlated positively with spatial extent of amygdala activation
LANG et al. (1998)	12 males and 8 females; handedness not reported	None reported	Negatively (e.g., mutilated face), positively (e.g., kissing couple), and neutrally (e.g., book) valenced complex pictures	Colored checkerboard	None reported	4, 5 mm coronal slices, 1.5 mm gap, covering from 10 mm from the occipital pole to the anterior of the occipitoparietal fissure	Bilateral calcarine fissure (Brodmann's areas 17 and 18) activation in response to all pictures compared to the checker-board; right inferior and superior parietal lobules, bilateral occipital gyrus, right fusiform gyrus, and right superior temporal gyrus (Brodmann's area 19) acti-vations in response to positive and negative pictures; right fusiform gyrus, right parietal lobulus, and right Brodmann's area 18 activation in response only to negative pictures; right Brodmann's area 19, right lingual gyrus and left fusiform gyrus activa-tions in response only to positive pictures	None reported
SOBEL et al. (1998)	6 males and 7 females; all right-handed	One female was unilaterally anosmic	Odorants: decanoic acid and vanillin (concentrations not given)	Absence of odorant	On-line determi-nation of pres-ence or absence of odorant	8, 4 mm ob-lique slices, 2 mm gap (slice locations not reported)	Anterior and lateral orbitofrontal cortex, piriform cortex (also mention of peri-insular, superior temporal and "limbic system") activation in response to presence of odorant	Odor detection was between 89% and 100% correct
WHALEN et al. (1998)	8 males; all right-handed	None reported	View masked happy and fearful facial expressions of emotion	View masked neutral facial expressions	Post-scan inquiry about the aware-ness of seeing any facial expres-sions and ident-ification thereof	15, 8 mm contiguous axial slices covering the whole brain	Bilateral amygdala, substantia innominata and inferior prefrontal cortex activations in response to fearful faces compared to happy faces	Subjects did not report seeing any happy or fearful faces, and could only identify the neutral faces

CS+, conditioned stimuli; SCR, skin conductance responses 01, region of interest.

presence of the happy or fearful expressions. Differential amygdalar activation to the fearful and happy facial expressions was a product of signal increases in response to fearful faces and signal decreases in response to happy faces. Interesting, just dorsal to this activation, substantia innominata activation was present in response to both fearful and happy faces, with the fearful faces evoking a greater increase. This study further confirms, in humans, the unique roll the amygdala plays in the perception of faces which has been unambiguously demonstrated in non-human primates studies (ROLLS 1984), even when the subjects are unaware of the presence of the face.

Using fearful and disgust facial expressions of emotion, as well as neutral facial expressions, PHILLIPS et al. (1997) report, in addition to amygdala activation in response to fear faces (compared to neutral faces), an extended neural network of activation in response to disgust faces that did not include the amygdala. The network includes 12 foci of activation as listed in Table 40.1. Notable among those foci is activation in the anterior insular cortex, a region that is responsive to gustatory input as demonstrated in non-human primates (YAXLEY 1988).

40.3.4
Studies of Externally Elicited Affect

As mentioned above, a little-known study reported by GRODD et al. (1995) is the first known report to use fMRI to investigate the neural mechanisms of affective responses. In that study, the affect manipulation employed pictures of sad and happy facial expressions of emotion which served as cues for subjects to recall an affectively congruent experience in their life. Those conditions were compared to a condition in which subjects viewed neutral facial expressions and made identity judgements. GRODD et al. (1995) reported left amygdalar activation in response to the sad condition compared to the neutral condition. In a replication of that work, the same group, using the same manipulation, reported left amygdalar and left cingulum (Brodmann's areas 32 and 33) in response to both the happy and sad compared to the neutral conditions (SCHNEIDER et al. 1997).

In an initial study, we used affective and neutral pictures selected from the International Affective Picture System (IAPS; LANG et al. 1997). One of the virtues of this stimulus set is that it is known that the negative and positive high-arousal stimuli elicit reliable increases and decreases, respectively, in startle magnitude elicited by a background acoustic startle probe (LANG 1995; SUTTON et al. 1997). Thus, independent objective measures consistently verify that these stimuli reliably alter emotional state. In this study we compared the viewing of negatively valenced (e.g., mutilated face) to neutral (e.g., book) visual stimuli (IRWIN et al. 1996) and found that the former elicited significant bilateral activation in the amygdala compared with the latter. In this study we only imaged a limited region (15 mm) of brain and were, therefore, unable to examine activation in other brain regions. We have recently replicated the finding of bilateral amygdala activation in a different, larger sample with whole-brain imaging (IRWIN et al. 1997). LaBar et al. (1998b) have replicated our original amygdala activation finding using both negative and positive (e.g., erotica) compared to neutral stimuli.

As noted above, activation in striate and extrastriate visual cortices in response to affectively salient stimuli has been reported in both PET and fMRI studies. LANG et al. (1998), who have developed the IAPS, examined differences in activation in visual cortices as a function of differently valenced pictorial stimuli. They reported activation of the right fusiform gyrus and right inferior and superior parietal lobules in the negative and positive picture conditions compared to the neutral picture conditions. This pattern of activation in visual cortices using the same stimuli is exactly consistent with our own findings (IRWIN et al. 1997). Perhaps relevant to the finding of visual cortical activation in response to affectively salient stimuli are the known projections to effectively all sectors of visual cortices from the basal and accessory basal nuclei of the amygdala (AMARAL and PRICE 1984; AMARAL et al. 1992). However, the functional significance of these amygdalofugal projections is currently unknown (D. G. Amaral 1998, personal communication).

Two studies have reported unique patterns of activation in response to affectively ladden auditory stimuli. These stimuli, however, were unlikely to have elicited any emotion in the perceiver; thus, the findings should be understood as bearing on the perception of auditory emotional information rather than related to the circuitry of emotion generation. STILLER et al. (1997) used a phoneme detection paradigm to identify hemispheric lateralization of affective prosody processing. Group results did not reveal lateralized processing of affective compared to neutral prosody in primary auditory cortices (i.e., superior temporal gyrus, supratemporal plane, from the caudal portion of the planum temporale, auditory cortex including medially the transition zones to insular cortex, and anterior auditory association cortices). However, they were able to divide their subjects into right (n=7) and left (n=13) hemisphere responders revealing greater right and left lateralized activation, respectively, in response to the identification of affective prosody. STILLER et al. (1997) cite our electrophysiological work in their article (WHEELER et al. 1993) and suggest that their right vs left activators correspond to differences we have reported in stable asymmetric activation that predict individual differences in affective style.

MADDOCK and BUONOCORE (1997) compared patterns of activation in response to threat-related words compared to neutral words. They reported robust activation in the posterior cingulate and retrosplenial cortices (Brodmann's areas 23, 29 and 31) with a tallied asymmetry for a left (8/10) greater than right (2/10) bias. As a quasi-manipulation check, subjects were brought back to the laboratory and given a memory test for an additional presentation of the threat-related words. Interestingly, subjects' memory score for the threat-related words was positively correlated with the number of significant voxels in the posterior cingulate.

Finally, SOBEL et al. (1998) examined the neural responses to pure odorants (decanoic acid and vanillin). Consistent with what is known about the olfactory system from non-human studies, these odorants elicited activation in, primarily, the lateral and anterior orbitofrontal cortices. This activation was distinct from that elicited by the action of sniffing, per se, which elicited activation primarily in piriform and medial and posterior orbitofrontal cortices.

40.3.5
Studies of Pain

DAVIS et al. (1995) have published initial and follow-up (DAVIS et al. 1997) reports on neural responses to transcutaneous electrical stimulation to the median nerve, with specific focus on the anterior cingulate cortex (ACC; Brodmann's area 24). Given the role of the ACC in attentional processes, the activation patterns to electrical stimulation were contrasted with activation patterns elicited by an attention-demanding word generation task. Painful electrical stimulation, but not stimulation that evoked a tingling sensation, activated a focus in posterior ACC. The attention task elicited activation foci that were superior and anterior to the pain-elicited foci,

and of generally larger spatial extent. Of note was a positive correlation between the on-line ratings of subjective pain and the percent signal change in the ACC.

40.3.6
Studies of Pharmacological Manipulation of Affect

BREITER et al. (1997) have published an elaborate report of the neural responses to cocaine injection in cocaine addicts. The activation patterns to an intravenous injection of cocaine were compared to injections of saline solution, while on-line reports of "rush," "high," "low" and "craving" were obtained every minute. The complete list of activation foci is presented in Table 40.1, but it is noteworthy that there was robust activation in nucleus accumbens which is consistent with the large corpus of non-human animal data demonstrating the critical role of the mesoaccumbens dopaminergic pathway in addictive behaviors (KOOB 1992). Notably, activation in the area of the ventral tegmentum which is the primary source of dopamine for the nucleus accumbens was positively correlated with self-reported measures of euphoria (i.e., "rush" ratings). The robustness of these findings was demonstrated by re-testing a subset of the subjects 3.5–4 months later and finding similar patterns of activation for both experiments. Finally, in contrast to many of the studies reviewed above which reported amygdalar activation in response to a variety of affect manipulations, this study reported amygdalar deactivation in the group analyses and a heterogeneous response at the single-subject level.

40.4
Summary and Conclusions

While the use of fMRI in the study of human affective processes is just beginning, it is already apparent that this method for making inferences about regional brain activation will play an increasingly important role in our understanding of the neutral substrates of affective processes. At the outset of this chapter, we presented several conceptual and methodological issues especially pertinent to the use of neuroimaging in general and fMRI in particular to the study of affective processes. It is clear from our review of the extant literature that many of the methodological desiderata that we outlined are not systematically incorporated into the available studies. However, several general trends have emerged from the data reviewed. Most studies that have elicited negative emotion in subjects with any of the several methods that have been used in the laboratory have reported activation of the amygdala. While some investigators have reported asymmetric amygdalar effects (e.g., SCHNEIDER et al. 1997), most have not. This issue requires additional examination using proper procedures to formally test the interaction between Condition and Hemisphere.

Amygdalar activation has also been found in response to facial expressions of emotion, particularly to those displaying fear. The extent to which these effects might be due to the actual elicitation of emotion in the viewer or are simply associated with the perception of emotional significance of the stimuli requires further study with independent measures to objectively identify whether any emotion has been elicited in the viewer.

The study by BREITER et al. (1997) of the effects of cocaine on MR signal changes is particularly noteworthy since it is the first fMRI study of emotional changes produced by a pharmacological manipulation that were imaged with fMRI. They observed activation the classic dopaminergic accumbens circuit during of reported craving produced by cocaine. As noted in the Introduction, it is possible to combine fMRI studies of functional activation with PET studies of in vivo neurotransmission (e.g., KOEPP et al. 1998) in the same subjects to examine relations between activation and transmitter changes.

While at the time of this writing only three published reports had appeared using fMRI to study psychiatric patients, we are aware of many such efforts currently underway at institutions throughout the world. We believe that this technology will be increasingly important in understanding the circuitry underlying major mental illness, and the fact that it is non-invasive will allow longitudinal studies and repeated testing of the sort that is not possible with PET. We anticipate that the next 5 years will see explosive growth in the use of fMRI to study normal and abnormal affective processes.

Acknowledgments. Preparation of this chapter was supported in part by an NIMH Research Scientist Award (MH00875), a NARSAD Established Investigator Award, and an NIMH Behavioral Sciences Research Center Grant (P50-MH52354) to Richard J. Davidson and an NSF Predoctoral Fellowship to William Irwin.

References

Abercrombie HC, Davidson RJ, Larson CL, Henriques JB, Schaefer SM (1999) Differential affective responses to the PET scanning environment in depressed patients and controls (in preparation)

Amaral DG, Price JL (1984) Amygdalo-cortical projections in the monkey (Macaca fascicularis). J Comp Neurol 230:465–496

Amaral DG, Price JL, Pitkanen A, Carmichael ST (1992) Anatomical organization of the primate amygdaloid complex. In: Aggleton JP (ed) The amygdala: neurobiological aspects of emotion, memory, and mental dysfunction. Wiley-Liss, New York, p 1

Birbaumer N, Grodd W, Diedrich O et al (1998) fMRI reveals amygdala activation to human faces in social phobics. Neuroreport 9:1223–1226

Breiter HC, Etcoff NL, Whalen PJ et al (1996a) Response and habituation of the human amygdala during visual processing of facial expression. Neuron 17:875–887

Breiter HC, Rauch SL, Kwong KK et al (1996b) Functional magnetic resonance imaging of symptom provocation in obsessive-compulsive disorder. Arch Gen Psychiatry 53:595–606

Breiter HC, Gollub RL, Weisskoff RM et al (1997) Acute effects of cocaine on human brain activity and emotion. Neuron 19:591–611

Buchel C, Morris J, Dolan RJ, Friston KJ (1998) Brain systems mediating aversive conditioning: an event-related fMRI study. Neuron 20:947–957

Davidson RJ (1992) Emotion and affective style: Hemispheric substrates. Psychol Sci 3:39–43

Davidson RJ (1993) Cerebral asymmetry and emotion: conceptual and methodological conundrums. Cogn Emotion 7:115–138

Davidson RJ (1998) Affective style and affective disorders: perspectives from affective neuroscience. Cogn Emotion 12:307–330

Davidson RJ, Sutton SK (1995) Affective neuroscience: The emergence of a discipline. Curr Opin Neurobiol 5:217–224

Davidson RJ, Ekman P, Saron C, Senulis J, Friesen WV (1990) Approach/withdrawal and cerebral asymmetry: emotional expression and brain physiology, I. J Pers Soc Psychol 58:330–341

Davis KD, Wood ML, Crawley AP, Mikulis DJ (1995) fMRI of human somatosensory and cingulate cortex during painful electrical nerve stimulation. Neuroreport 7:321–325

Davis KD, Taylor SJ, Crawley AP, Wood ML, Mikulis DJ (1997) Functional MRI of pain- and attention-related activations in the human cingulate cortex. J Neurophysiol 77:3370–3380

Dimberg U (1982) Facial reactions fo facial expressions. Psychophysiology 19:643–647

Drevets WC, Raichle ME (1995) PET imaging studies of human emotional disorders. In: Gazzaniga MS (ed) The cognitive neurosciences. MIT, Cambridge, MA, pp 1153–1164

Drevets WC, Price JL, Simpson JR Jr, Todd RD, Reich T, Vannier M, Raichle M (1997) Subgenual prefrontal cortex abnormalities in mood disorders. Nature 386:824–827

Ekman P (1984) Expression and the nature of emotion. In: Scherer K, Ekman P (eds) Approaches to emotion. Erlbaum, Hillsdale, pp. 319–343

Ekman P, Davidson RJ (1994) The nature of emotion: fundamental questions. Oxford University, New York

Ekman P, Friesen WV (1976) Pictures of facial affect. Consulting Psychologist (in press), Palo Alto

Fredrikson M, Wik G, Greitz T, Erickson L, Stone-Elander S, Ericson K Sedvall G (1993) Regional cerebral blood flow during experimental phobic fear. Psychophysiology 30:126–130

Grodd W, Schneider F, Klose U, Nagele T (1995) Functional magnetic resonance imaging of psychological functions with experimentally induced emotion. Radiologe 35:283–289

Irwin W, Davidson RJ, Lowe MJ, Mock BJ, Sorenson JA, Turski PA (1996) Human amygdala activation detected with echo-planar functional magnetic resonance imaging. Neuroreport 7:1765–1769

Irwin W, Mock BJ, Sutton SK et al (1997) Positive and negative affective responses: neural circuitry revealed using functional magnetic resonance imaging. Soc Neurosci Abstr 23:1318

Irwin W, Davidson RJ, Kalin NH, Sorenson JA Turski PA (1998a) Relations between human amygdala activation and self-reported dispositional affect. J Cogn Neurosci [Suppl] S:109

Irwin W, Mock BJ, Sutton SK et al (1998b) Ratings of affective stimulus characteristics and measures of affective reactivity predict MR signal change in the human amygdala. Neuroimage 7:S908

Kalin NH, Davidson RJ, Irwin W et al (1998) Functional magnetic resonance imaging studies of emotional processing in normal and depressed patients: effects of venlafaxine. J Clin Psychiatry 58:32–39

Knight DC, Helmstetter FJ, Stein EA (1996) Functional imaging of brain regions involved in Pavlovian fear conditioning in humans. Soc Neurosci Abstr 22:1867

Knight DC, Smith CN, Stein EA, Helmstetter FJ (1997) Human fear conditioning. Soc Neurosci Abstr 23:209

Knight DC, Smith CN, Cheng DT, Stein EA, Helmstetter FJ (1998) Functional imaging of human conditional fear (abstract). Neuroimage 7:S53

Koepp MJ, Gunn RN, Lawrence AD et al (1998) Evidence for striatal dopamine release during a video game. Nature 393:266–268

Koob GF (1992) Neurobiological mechanisms of cocaine and opiate dependence. In: O'Brien CP, Faffe JH (eds) Addictive states. Raven, New York, p 171

LaBar KS, Gatenby JC, Gore JC, LeDoux JE, Phelps EA (1998a) Human amygdala activation during conditioned fear acquisition and extinction: a mixed-trail fMRI study. Neuron 20:937–945

LaBar KS, Gatenby JC, Gore JC, Phelps EA (1998b) Role of the amygdala in emotional picture evaluation as revealed by fMRI. J Cogn Neurosci [suppl]:S108

Lane RD, Reiman EM, Ahern GL, Schwartz GE, Davidson RJ (1997) Neuroanatomical correlates of happiness, sadness, and disgust. Am J Psychiatry 154:926–933

Lang PJ (1995) The emotion probe: studies of motivation and attention. Am Psychol 50:372–385

Lang PJ, Bradley MM, Cuthbert BN (1990) Emotion, attention and the startle reflex. Psychol Rev 97:377–398

Lang PJ, Bradley M, Cuthbert B (1997) International affective picture system (IAPS): technical manual and affective ratings. Center for Research in Psychophysiology, University of Florida, Gainesville, FL

Lang PJ, Bradley MM, Fitzsimmons JR, Cuthbert BN, Scott JD, Moulder B, Nangia V (1998) Emotional arousal and activation of the visual cortex: an fMRI analysis. Psychophysiology 35:199–210

LeDoux JE (1996) The emotional brain: the mysterious underpinnings of emotional lift. Simon and Schuster, New York

Levin HS, Goldstein FC, Williams DH, Eisenberg HM (1991) The contribution of frontal lobe lesions to the neurobehavioral outcome of closed head injury. In: Levin HS, Eisenberg HM, Benton AL (eds) Frontal lobe function and dysfunction. Oxford University, New York, p 318

Maddock RJ, Buonocore MH (1997) Activation of left posterior cingulate gyrus by the auditory presentation of threat-related words: an fMRI study. Psychiatry Res Neuroimaging Sect 75:1–14

Morris JS, Ohman A, Dolan RJ (1998) Modulation of amygdala activity by masking of aversively conditioned visual stimuli. Neuroimage 7:S52

Pardo JV, Pardo PJ, Raichle ME (1993) Neural correlates of self-induced dysphoria. Am J Psychiatry 150:713–719

Pavlov IP (1927) Conditioned reflexes. Oxford University, London

Phillips ML, Young AW, Senior C et al (1997) A specific neural substrate for perceiving facial expressions of disgust. Nature 389:495–498

Rolls ET (1984) Neurons in the cortex of the temporal lobe and in the amygdala of the monkey with responses selective for faces. Hum Neurobiol 3:209–222

Schneider F, Grodd W, Weiss U, Klose U, Mayer KR, Nägele T, Gur RC (1997) Functional MRI reveals left amygdala activation during emotion. Psychiatry Res Neuroimaging Sect 76:75–82

Sobel N, Prabhakaran V, Desmond JE, Glover GH, Goode RL, Sullivan EV, Gabrieli JDE (1998) Sniffing and smelling: separate subsystems in the human olfactory cortex. Nature 392:282–286

Stiller D, Gaschler-Markefski B, Baumgart F, Schindler F, Tempelmann C, Heinze HJ, Scheich H (1997) Lateralized processing of speech prosodies in the temporal cortex: a 3-T functional magnetic resoance imaging study. MAGMA 5:275–284

Sutton SK, Davidson RJ, Donzella B, Irwin W, Dottl DA (1997) Manipulating affective state using extended picture presentation. Psychophysiology 34:217–226

Whalen PJ, Rauch SL, Etcoff NL, McInerney SC, Lee MB, Jenike MA (1998) Masked presentations of emotional facial expressions modulate amygdala activiy without explicit knowledge. J Neurosci 18:411–418

Wheeler RE, Davidson RJ, Tomarken AJ (1993) Frontal brain asymmetry and emotional reactivity: a biological substrate of affective style. Psychophysiology 30:82–89

Yaxley S (1988) The responsiveness of neurons in the insular gustatory cortex of the macaque monkey is independent of hunger. Physiol Behav 42:223–229

41 Functional MRI in Psychiatry

J.H. Callicott and D.R. Weinberger

CONTENTS:

41.1
Introduction

No other technological advance of the latter twentieth century has contributed more to the in vivo study of mental illness than functional neuroimaging. Clearly, while vast amounts of "bottom-up" *in vitro* data are still needed to understand the complexities of mental illnesses like schizophrenia, such information will not be sufficient. The "top-down" *in vivo* vantage point provided by functional neuroimaging is necessary to navigate this complex terrain to reach clinically relevant interventions for mental illnesses. Furthermore, given the brain's complexity, one might anticipate that some key aspects of brain function might arise as emergent properties of this complexity – perhaps only appreciable from the top down (Goldman-Rakic 1996). For reasons related to subject tolerability, ease of repetition, and improved spatial and temporal resolution, functional magnetic resonance imaging – inclusive of both functional magnetic resonance imaging (fMRI) and proton magnetic resonance spectroscopy and spectroscopic imaging (^{1}H-MRS, ^{1}H-MRSI) – have shown particular promise in the study of mental illness.

Within only a few years of their introduction to psychiatric research, these techniques have reconfirmed the notion that there are identifiable, predictable functional abnormalities in patients with such disorders. At the same time, their ability to generate individual "brain maps" with the same ease previously available only for structural brain scans has reinvigorated discussions regarding the sensitivity and specificity of functional findings in mental illness. While these techniques have their own methodological vulnerabilities (e.g., sensitivity to subject movement), functional MRI provides unprecedented access to these potential sources of artifact (e.g., movement can be quantified during registration of image volumes). In this chapter, we will review recent findings in functional MRI (fMRI and MR spectroscopy) in psychiatry. In addition, we will present data from novel applications of individual brain mapping and discuss the unresolved methodological issues relevant to an informed appreciation of these data in psychiatry.

41.2
Historical Perspective

To place these newer techniques in historical perspective, their importance to psychiatry and psychology arises from a long-term quest to define the neurophysiological underpinnings of the so-called "functional illnesses", like schizophrenia and bipolar disorder, which were historically differentiated from "organic" illnesses, like stroke and epilepsy. Some might argue that this process began in earnest with the appreciation of gross anatomical structural abnormalities in schizophrenia made possible by computerized tomography (CT) in the late 1970s (Johnstone et al. 1976; Reider et al. 1979; Weinberger et al. 1979). Although earlier work had already demonstrated structural and functional abnormalities in these patients (Storey 1966; Vogel and Lange 1966; Ingvar and Franzen 1974), the

J.H. Callicott, MD; D.R. Weinberger, MD; Clinical Brain Disorders Branch, NIMH, NIH, Building 10, Room 4S237A, MSC 1379, 9000 Rockville Pike, Bethesda, MD 20892, USA

ease of use, the improvements in resolution, and the widespread availability of CT fostered an explosion of *in vivo* studies and thus helped swing psychiatry and psychology back towards the study of brain per se (KANDEL 1998). *In vivo* findings, such as increased ventricle to brain ratio (VBR) (ZIGUN and WEINBERGER 1992), coinciding with *in vitro* evidence of subtle cellular aberrations in post-mortem brain (BOGERTS 1993), intensified the search for their functional concomitants. However, then as now, a large gap remained between gross anatomical anomalies of individual brains and *in vivo* neuronal function. Furthermore, as these structural techniques were applied widely beyond schizophrenia, it became clear that anatomical pathology was neither a necessary nor a specific part of any particular mental illness (WEINBERGER 1995).

Throughout the 1980s, radiotracer studies using single photon emission tomography (SPECT) and positron emission tomography (PET) were developed to study *in vivo* brain function. For example, these techniques measured neuronal activity through glucose consumption and regional blood flow and estimated neuronal transmission via radiolabeled compounds specific to certain neurotransmitter receptors such as dopamine (LIDDLE 1995). Perhaps the greatest contribution of these efforts, even beyond the wealth of individual findings, was confirmation of the long-held notion that there were predictable functional abnormalities associated with mental illnesses, even in the absence of the more obvious pathology associated with organic illnesses. For example, patients with schizophrenia were found to have reduced prefrontal cortical activation (so-called hypofrontality), particularly when these patients were performing tasks that required working memory (WEINBERGER and BERMAN 1996). Ultimately, however, technical limitations may have contributed to the fact that, in spite of the numerous findings, this work failed to generate many clinical applications. The need for special facilities, the expense, the limitations in radiation exposure, the limited spatial and temporal resolution, and the need for complex algorithms to interpret these data diminished their clinical usefulness. Until recently, another limitation was that these methods utilized group-averaged data and could not reliably create functional maps for individual patients. However, both resolution approaching fMRI and single subject analyses are becoming feasible, at least for PET. While technical limitations can be addressed, the aforementioned lack of well-defined sensitivity or specificity of given functional abnormalities to specific psychiatric syndromes – the exception perhaps being the use of reduced brain metabolism as an adjunct to the diagnosis of Alzheimer's disease (SMALL 1996) – is more difficult to overcome. In fact, no pathognomonic functional lesions have yet been identified for the major mental illnesses. Given this historical perspective, it is important to remain mindful of the limitations relevant to the validity of functional MRI data and to the likelihood that these functional MRI techniques will generate significant clinical applications. Also, while the technical prowess of MRI is still growing, it is unlikely that the technical improvements alone will allow the identification of hitherto undiscovered lesions. Rather, it will be up to researchers and clinicians to refocus their attention on those questions functional neuroimaging can best address.

41.3
Functional MRI in Psychiatry

Functional MRI offers several advantages in comparison to nuclear medicine techniques for mental illness research, including low invasiveness, no radioactivity, widespread availability, and virtually unlimited study repetitions (LEVIN et al. 1995). These characteristics, plus the relative ease of creating individual brain maps, offer the unique potential to address a number of long-standing issues in psychiatry and psychology, including the distinction between state and trait characteristics, effects of medication, and reliability. Additionally, longitudinal studies and studies within novel populations, (e.g., children) may help address the historical dynamics of mental illness – including adaptation to, treatment of, and progression from brain pathology (WEINBERGER et al. 1996). Finally, the implementation of real-time fMRI will allow investigators to tailor examinations individually while a subject is still in the scanner, promising true interactive studies or physiological interviews (FRANK et al., in press).

fMRI studies of mental illness have included both dynamic contrast (BELLIVEAU et al. 1991) and blood oxygenation level-dependent (BOLD) (OGAWA et al. 1992; BANDETTINI et al. 1992) methods. The technical details of these approaches are covered in detail elsewhere in this volume. However, the fact that published fMRI studies have not been as numerous as ^{1}H-MRS or radionuclide based investigations in psychiatry speaks to the additional difficulty of applying these techniques to ill populations (WEIN-

BERGER et al. 1996). Ironically, one of the most significant contributions psychiatric fMRI investigations may make to the larger field of functional neuroimaging is an increased awareness of and
strategies for dealing with potential artifacts (e.g.,
susceptibility to motion) hidden within the data
(COHEN et al. 1995; FRISTON 1996; BULLMORE et al.
1996). The artifacts become especially prominent
when using these techniques outside of the usual
healthy, motivated control population (BREITER et
al. 1996; CALLICOTT et al. 1998). Unfortunately, it has
been increasingly apparent that failure to systematically control for artifact renders any such work difficult to interpret (Table 41.1). Furthermore, the additional level of stringency necessary to make popula-
tion-wide inferences across diagnostic groups may
mean that traditional solutions in fMRI (e.g., registration) for known and expected artifacts (e.g., subject motion) are inadequate without additional intervention in patient datasets (Fig. 41.1).

As an illustration, we studied a group of ten
matched schizophrenic patients and controls using
principles of echo shifting with a train of observa-

tions (PRESTO) 3-D fMRI (VANGELDEREN et al.
1995) and a variation of the n- back working
memory task (GEVINS et al. 1990). In addition to assessing prefrontal function, our version of the n-
back task incorporated a continual motor response
to generate a quality control signal in contralateral
sensorimotor cortex. Initially, we noted the predicted reduced prefrontal activation in patients.
However, we also found an apparent reduction in
sensorimotor cortex activation even though the patients made a similar number of responses as controls. Unfortunately, in spite of removing residual
subject motion using registration and assuring that
each subject had made appropriate motor responses,
we had failed to control for a systematic group difference in signal intensity variance most likely arising
from increased intrascan motion by a few of our patients. After matching for variance across the groups,
we eliminated the spurious finding within motor
cortex, yet retained and strengthened the hypothesized reduced activation within prefrontal cortex.

Similarly, work by RENSHAW and colleagues
(1994; COHEN et al. 1995) examining the occipital

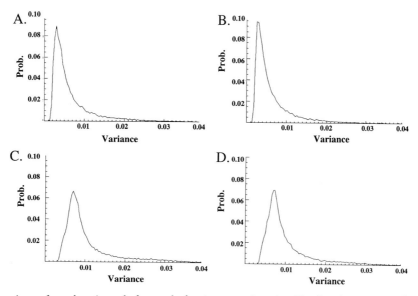

Fig. 41.1A–D. Comparison of voxel variance before and after image registration. Voxel variance across the whole brain is
displayed as a histogram (MATTAY et al. 1996). These histograms were obtained from two healthy male control subjects
matched for age and handedness (**A,B** subject 1; **C,D** subject 2) performing the n-back working memory task. Variance was
obtained following a simple subtraction of "on" and "off" working memory conditions (i.e., two back–no back). Whole brain
BOLD fMRI data were acquired on a standard 1.5 Tesla General Electric Signa scanner (Milwaukee, WI) using echo planar
imaging as described previously (effective whole brain TR=4 s, voxel dimensions 3.75 mm isotropic; MATTAY et al. 1996). The
y-axis represents the number of voxels possessing a given variance (expressed as probability). The *x-axis* represents increasing variance computed for each voxel as follows: [standard error of the mean difference (on-off)]/[average signal intensity].
Variance is presented both before (**A, C**) and after (**B, D**) image registration (windowed sinc algorithm (OSTUNI et al. 1997)).
No residual uncorrected motion was present for either subject following registration. While registration alters variance to
some degree in both subjects, registration, in spite of correcting for motion, does not remove the overall increased variance
for subject 2

Table 41.1. A structured approach to the evaluation of fMRI data

Parameter	Comments
Prevention of artifact	
Machine-related artifact: standardized assessment of machine stability	Signal drift, field characteristics, test-retest reliability
Subject-related artifact	Physiological variability: monitor physiological parameters (e.g., end-tidal CO2, pulse); use of "gated" pulse sequences
	Movement: prevention through head immobilization
Assessment of artifact (quality control)	
Standardized assessment of motion	Systematic correction for subject motion (e.g., realignment via registration, excitation history correction)
	Comparison across groups (or time) of motion correction parameters (translation, pitch, roll, yaw)
	Re-examination following analysis for residual artifact not corrected by registration (e.g., edge artifacts)
Examination of signal change time course in activated voxels	Correlation of time course with experimental paradigm
Comparison of activation in pathophysiologically neutral region	Internal activation standard
Examination of variance	Histogram of voxel-wise variance[a]
Evaluation of results	
Controlling across individuals and groups for differences in variance	
Use of stringently-defined threshold for activation	
Placing activation into context: cautious reification of activation in unexpected regions	

The information presented above is by no means exhaustive nor any individual step meant as necessary. Rather, it illustrates the notion that there are multiple aspects to vigilance regarding potential artifacts in fMRI. Adapted from CALLICOTT et al. (1998) with permission.

[a]See Fig. 41.1.

cortex of schizophrenic patients illustrates that the assumptions made by functional MRI methodologies (e.g., regarding the BOLD effect in fMRI or metabolite ratios in MR spectroscopy) are not always straightforward. As a result, these assumptions carry the attendant risks of error and over-simplification when applied to patient populations. In their initial study using echo planar imaging (RENSHAW et al. 1994), patients with schizophrenia were noted to have an exaggerated BOLD activation response to photic stimulation within primary visual cortex. In a follow-up study, COHEN et al. (1995) used dynamic susceptibility contrast MRI in schizophrenics and found significantly increased regional cerebral blood volume in the left occipital cortex and left caudate. Given the lack of compelling data to suggest clinically-relevant deficiencies in primary visual processing in schizophrenia, these findings raise a number of potentially troubling possibilities, includ-

ing fundamental anomalies in cerebral vasculature in schizophrenia, some alteration in the relationship between neuronal activity and the blood flow response introduced by illness, alterations in apparent blood flow or volume due to alterations in the ratio of gray to white matter (partial volume effects), medication effects, or perhaps some unanticipated artifact of experimental design (e.g., arising from the possibility that patients blink less because of medication effects). Using ^{15}O-$H_2$0 PET, TAYLOR et al. (1997) recently found increased activation (number of significant resels) within the occipital cortex of schizophrenic patients exposed to flashing lights at several frequencies, but did not find increased cerebral blood flow following acetazolamide challenge. The latter might have supported the hypothesis of a primary abnormality of cerebral vascular responsiveness. Further, TAYLOR et al. (1997) defined "increased activation" using spatial extent of activation (i.e., number of significant resels), while RENSHAW et al. (1994) used the magnitude of activation within a predetermined region surrounding a local maxima. Thus, the PET data are difficult to interpret as a simple replication of visual cortex abnormalities in schizophrenia. For example, TAYLOR et al. (1997) failed to find a significant difference in magnitude of activation within significantly activated resels. Whatever the ultimate significance of these data, they speak to the importance of attending to details of experimental design and interpretation. Another caveat is that many fMRI studies fail to cover the whole brain, raising similar issues of selective sampling that will be discussed below in regard to ^{1}H-MRS. This lack of whole brain coverage makes otherwise straightforward procedures, such as motion correction through registration and stereotactic normalization, much more difficult, though probably not insurmountable (MAAS et al. 1997).

Based in part on clinical observations of minor neurological anomalies in schizophrenia and in part on the central role that motor experiments (e.g., finger tapping) have played in the development of fMRI methodology, several groups have studied motor movement in schizophrenia. While two studies have found decreased magnitude of fMRI activation and diminished lateralization of the response (WENZ et al. 1994; SCHRODER et al. 1995), MATTAY and colleagues (1997) found similar alterations in laterality in complex, self-guided motor movements without an associated alteration in overall response. As an extension of earlier work that suggested alterations in activity within auditory association areas arising amidst manifest psychotic illness (CLEGHORN et al. 1990; SILBERSWEIG et al. 1995), DAVID et al. (1996) and WOODRUFF et al. (1997) have reported alterations in temporal cortex activation to external speech in patients with schizophrenia. In two schizophrenic patients with auditory hallucinations, DAVID and colleauges (1996) found reduced activation within auditory cortex to auditory stimuli concurrent with hallucinations – independent of medication status and not present in the visual cortex response to visual stimuli. In a subsequent study, WOODRUFF et al. (1997) replicated this reduction of auditory cortex response in the context of auditory hallucinations in a larger sample of such patients. In addition, both hallucinating and non-hallucinating schizophrenic patients had reduced left, but increased right, temporal cortical activation to word presentation. The findings were interpreted to mean that the auditory hallucinations competed with the auditory stimuli for the cortical physiological re-

sponse. In addition to the working memory task noted above (CALLICOTT et al. 1998), support for the association between prefrontal cortical dysfunction and schizophrenia was also reported by YURGELUN-TODD and colleagues (1996b), who used a verbal fluency paradigm. Using a surface coil placed over the left frontal and temporal cortices, they found that schizophrenic subjects underactivated the left prefrontal cortex while they overactivated the left superior temporal cortex during a word generation task.

Most of the studies mentioned above relied on rather traditional block designs in which subjects were asked to perform some motor or cognitive task. However, there have been several studies which have taken a more dynamic approach to mapping mental illness. BREITER and colleagues (1996) used symptom provocation in patients with obsessive-compulsive disorder to map activation within the limbic system (most notably in amygdala, orbitofrontal, and cingulate cortices). Several groups have also used either cocaine infusion (BREITER et al. 1997) or cocaine-associated cues (MAAS et al. 1998) to map activation in regions thought to be related to intoxication (e.g., nucleus accumbens, striatum, and prefrontal cortex) and those related to craving (e.g., prefrontal and cingulate cortices). PETERSON et al. (1998) studied patients with Tourette's disorder while they actively suppressed their tics. They found that activation within the basal ganglia and thalamus inversely correlated with tic severity – implying the potential importance of subcortical neuronal dysregulation in the pathogenesis of tics. Finally, BERTOLINO and colleagues (1997a) have used the dissociative anesthetic ketamine as a pharmacological model of cortical dysconnection. When given to healthy controls performing the n-back working memory task, ketamine seems to mimic the physiological capacity limitation seen in patients with schizophrenia given the same task. Such studies have been made more feasible with fMRI, given the need for repeated sessions inherent in such complex designs.

41.4
[1]H Magnetic Resonance Spectroscopy Studies in Psychiatry

Inhabiting a nebulous zone between structural MRI and blood-flow-based fMRI, ^{1}H-MRS has become a particularly intriguing imaging modality in psychiatry. While ^{1}H-MRS metabolites, especially N-acetylaspartate (NAA), were originally thought to reflect static brain phenomena, it now appears that these measures reflect dynamic processes (MURATA et al. 1993; CHARLES et al. 1994; DAGER et al. 1995) – albeit over a longer temporal scale than the blood flow changes in fMRI. In two recent cross-modality studies, BERTOLINO and colleagues have found that ^{1}H-MRSI-derived NAA measures are predictive of dynamic functional phenomena in schizophrenia, namely, subcortical dopamine release as measured with SPECT (BERTOLINO et al. 1997c) and activation within a larger cortical network subserving the Wisconsin Card Sorting Task as measured with ^{15}O-H$_2$0 PET (BERTOLINO et al. 1997b). For these reasons, ^{1}H-MRS is evolving into a truly functional neuroimaging methodology in psychiatric research. There are also several phosphorous 31 (P^{31}) MRS studies reported in psychiatry, which will not be addressed in this report.

Taking advantage of the fact that protons (^{1}H) resonate at slightly different frequencies depending on their particular chemical surroundings within certain molecules (so-called chemical-shift; OLDENDORF and OLDENDORF 1991), ^{1}H-MRS is able to identify several ubiquitous chemical moieties as small peaks separated from the dominant peak of H$_2$0. These peaks include (currently) n-acetyl aspartate containing compounds (NAA), choline-containing compounds (CHO), creatine- and phospho-creatine containing compounds (CRE), lactate, myoinositol (mI), and glutamate plus glutamine and γ-amino butyric acid (GABA) (Ross 1991; Ross and MICHAELIS 1994). Because creatine and phosphocreatine are metabolites involved in cellular energy production, the CRE signal may reflect relative neuronal and/or glial metabolism. Present mainly in membrane constituents like phosphocholine and glycerophosphocholine and found in higher concentrations within glial cells, CHO levels may reflect relative intensity of cell wall constituent turnover or astrocytic proliferation (URENJAK et al. 1993). Related to phophatidylinositol, the role of mI is less clear but, sharing characteristics of CHO and CRE, it may reflect turnover of internal neuronal cytoskeletal elements or cellular activity in the form of inositol second messenger systems (Ross and MICHAELIS 1994).

Of particular interest to neuroscientists, NAA is found only within neurons and has an easily identifiable peak in ^{1}H-MRS (TSAI and COYLE 1995). As such, relative reductions of NAA have been linked to neuronal dysfunction in several neurological and neuropsychiatric disorders (Ross and MICHAELIS

1994, for review). While ^{1}H-MRS is likely measuring at some distance from any inherent metabolic or physiological "lesion" present in mental illness, this distance may not be prohibitively large, as suggested by at least one postmortem study of the mesial temporal cortex in schizophrenia. In this study, TSAI et al. (1995) found alterations in the NAA-related enzyme N-acetyl-α-linked acidic dipeptidase (NAALADase), the NAA precursor N-acetyl-spartylglutamate (NAAG), aspartate and glutamate suggestive of alterations in excitatory neurotransmission (TSAI et al. 1995). As for ^{1}H-MRS metabolites in general, it remains unclear whether NAA concentrations are best viewed as state or trait markers, since details, e.g., the relative time course of their turnover, remain to be established (MILLER 1991). For example, dietary intake of choline may alter the CHO signal (STOLL et al. 1995). Nevertheless, by providing regionally localizable neurochemistry, ^{1}H-MRS has a unique place in the aforementioned resolution gap between functional neuroimaging and cell biology and may link top-down abnormalities such as cognitive function with intraneuronal processes.

Taking their lead from the wealth of structural neuroimaging abnormalities in patients with schizophrenia (particularly in prefrontal and mesial temporal cortices), MR spectroscopists initially focused on attempting to reconfirm the presence of regionally specific neuronal dysfunction. Initially, single voxel ^{1}H-MRS studies reported regional pathology in the frontal lobes and mesial temporal cortex in patients with schizophrenia (NASRALLAH et al. 1994; BUCKLEY et al. 1994; CHOE et al. 1994). These findings have been replicated by a number of centers (MAIER et al. 1995; RENSHAW et al. 1995; FUKUZAKO et al. 1995; YURGELUN-TODD et al. 1996a; DEICKEN et al. 1997a, 1998), although there have been exceptions (STANLEY et al. 1996). Single voxel studies have also found regional abnormalities in the anterior cingulate region (DEICKEN et al. 1997b) and basal ganglia (FUJIMOTO et al. 1996).

While regionally specific, these findings have been criticized for their limited spatial and spectral resolution. Voxel dimensions are often on the order of 5–10 cm, and thus often sample across a mixture of gray matter, white matter, and cerebrospinal fluid (CSF). Any regional abnormality in NAA, for example, might arise from abnormalities of gray or white matter and might also arise from partial volume effects. Further, concerns have arisen regarding the selective sampling implicit in single voxel studies. Uniform placement of these volumes of interest within and across diagnostic groups becomes critical and uncertainty arises regarding any regional pathology without simultaneously sampling an "unaffected" control region (e.g., the potential confound of global artifact). In addition, absolute quantitation of these metabolites remains an issue under investigation. Thus, metabolite concentrations have been determined by ratio to another metabolite (e.g., NAA/CRE) or to the larger H_2O peak in so-called water normalization. As in any ratio in which the numerator and denominator may change independently, these ratio measures introduce another level of uncertainty (i.e., decreased spectral resolution). Nonetheless, the fact that regional NAA reductions in schizophrenia have been replicated across laboratories with a variety of techniques likely indicates that regional NAA abnormalities are not simply artifactual. Improvements in resolution, both spatial and spectral, plus efforts to more fully characterize regions of interest using segmentation will likely be ongoing and will inform future replication efforts. Increased spectral resolution is possible using short echo time acquisitions, and small peaks for glutamate, glutamine, and GABA have been analyzed (Ross and Michaelis 1994). While the pattern of abnormalities in these metabolites is not as clear as for NAA (Stanley et al. 1996), probably in part because reliability has been poor, some studies seem to support a role for anomalous excitatory neurotransmission in schizophrenia (Choe et al. 1994, 1996; Bartha et al. 1997).

One potential solution for the problems of selective sampling mentioned above is provided by multiple voxel acquisitions. Combining a multislice ^{1}H-MRS technique with voxel segmentation, Lim et al. (1998) have attempted to differentiate the impact of reduced gray matter volume in the cortex of patients with schizophrenia on NAA measurements in hopes of assigning NAA reductions to either gray or white matter. In ten schizophrenic patients and nine healthy controls, they found gray matter volume deficits without associated NAA reductions coupled with normal white matter volume associated with reduced NAA – perhaps suggesting abnormal axonal connections. While this technique clearly covers more cortex than a single voxel, at this timeit is unable to regionally differentiate areas of cortex (e.g., dorsolateral prefrontal cortex from parietal cortex). Since there is evidence to suggest regionally specific pathology, such an approach might miss a regional NAA deficit particular to one, but not all, areas of cortex.

Using another multislice approach, the issue of regional pathology has also been addressed. Using ^{1}H-MRSI (Duyn et al. 1993) a ^{1}H-MRS technique with greater brain coverage and spatial resolution, Bertolino et al. (1996, 1998b) have found bilateral reductions in NAA measures in dorsolateral prefrontal cortex and mesial temporal cortex (inclusive of hippocampus, parahippocampal gyrus, and amygdala) in patients with schizophrenia. These findings have been expanded to include patients with childhood onset schizophrenia and neuroleptic-naïve subjects (Bertolino et al. 1998a, 1998c). Furthermore, as part of a large study of siblings of patients with schizophrenia, more than 100 subjects with schizophrenia have been studied and regional abnormalities have been found in prefrontal and mesial temporal cortex, but not in the anterior cingulate, prefrontal white matter, superior temporal gyrus, or basal ganglia/thalamus (Callicott et al., in press). Furthermore, while emphasis has been placed on NAA, the failure to find increased CHO, which might suggest gliosis or some other ongoing neurodegenerative process, appears consistent with prior neuropathological and neuroimaging studies that have posited a non-neurodegenerative etiology for schizophrenia (Weinberger 1995).

Studying a cohort of adult rhesus monkeys that included subjects with mesial temporal cortex ablations as neonates and subjects with similar ablations as adults, Bertolino and colleagues (1997d) have explored the hypothesis that developmental aberration of prefrontal-temporolimbic connectivity might lead to in vivo prefrontal NAA reductions using ^{1}H-MRSI. As hypothesized, the monkeys with neonatal disruption of temporal-prefrontal connectivity showed reduced prefrontal NAA, whereas adult-lesioned animals did not. These findings may add plausibility to the potential import of developmental aberrations in schizophrenia. In a larger sense, they demonstrate the potential power of an in vivo methodology that may be applied not only across diagnostic groups, but also across species. However, there are limitations to the ^{1}H-MRSI methodology, including all of the general criticisms regarding the proper interpretation of the metabolites measured, large voxel sizes and associated partial volume effects, the use of ratios, and variability in the data (Bertolino et al. 1996).

^{1}H MRS has been applied to other neuropsychiatric illnesses as well. In particular, Tupler et al. (1997) found elevations of CHO and mI in the cortex and basal ganglia of patients with social phobia. Reductions of NAA have also been reported in the anterior cingulate and right striatum of patients with obsessive-compulsive disorder (Ebert et al. 1997). In men-

tal retardation, reductions of NAA/CHO have been reported for the right parietal cortex (HASHIMOTO et al. 1995) and increased CHO has been found longitudinally in the prefrontal white matter of patients with Down's syndrome (MURATA et al. 1993), perhaps tracking ongoing neuronal degeneration. Several studies have reported NAA reductions in the frontal and parietal cortices of patient with Alzheimer's disease (TEDESCHI et al. 1996). In an intriguing use of ^{1}H-MRS as a truly functional MRI technique, DAGER and colleagues (1995) studied changes in the lactate (LAC) peak following hyperventilation in patients with panic disorder. As predicted by research indicating abnormal brain lactate in panic disorder, LAC was disproportionately increased in panic disorder patients in a subcortical voxel following hyperventilation. Finally, CHARLES et al. (1994) observed state-dependent changes in CHO in seven patients with major depression before and after treatment with nefazodone.

41.5
Novel Neurobiological Phenotypes

In addition to mapping the functional abnormalities associated with mental illness, one of the other major challenges facing researchers is the characterization of the genetic vulnerability to these illnesses. It now appears that such vulnerability likely arises from a number of genes, each of small effect interacting in a complex or epistatic fashion (KIDD 1997). Furthermore, due to their inherent imprecision, traditional phenotypes based on clinical diagnoses are likely contributing to the difficulty of this task (CROWE 1993). As suggested by earlier structural (WEINBERGER et al. 1981) and functional studies of phenotypic variability (WOLF et al. 1996), neuroimaging can generate quantifiable characteristics as alternatives to or supplements for traditional phenotypes in genetic linkage studies (HOLZMAN 1992). These so-called endo- or intermediate phenotypes depend on the assumption that they reflect some inherent and basic neurophysiological defect one or more steps closer to gene expression than complex behavioral phenomena like auditory hallucinations (EGAN and WEINBERGER 1997).

Given its ability to assess neurophysiology in individual subjects, functional MRI techniques are particularly attractive in this regard. Further, measures such as ^{1}H-MRS are relatively free of the behavioral confounds (like attention or poor test performance)

Table 41.2. Relative risk (λ_S) estimates of hippocampal NAA phenotype

Subjects	Left hippocampus	Right hippocampus	Bilateral hippocampus
Controls	17%	11%	8%
Patients	43%	41%	27%
Siblings	38%	40%	29%
Sibs of patients with phenotype	63%	46%	67%
Sibs of patients without phenotype	24%	35%	16%
Relative risk	3.8	4.3	8.8

The relative frequency of subjects within each diagnostic group (controls, patients with schizophrenia, and their non-psychotic, unaffected siblings) of the potential intermediate phenotype of reduced hippocampal N-acetylaspartate (NAA). Relative risk (λ_S) estimates were calculated as follows: λ_S=[(frequency of NAA phenotype in sibs of schizophrenic patients with phenotype)/(frequency of phenotype in healthy controls)].
Adapted from CALLICOTT et al. (in press) with permission.

that often bedevil other neuropsychological probes. Hopefully, whatever susceptibility loci are ultimately associated with the expression of these intermediate phenotypes will also represent loci underlying vulnerability to schizophrenia (HOLZMAN 1992; FARAONE et al. 1995). So far, three such studies, using P50 inhibition (FREEDMAN et al. 1997), increased ventricle-to-brain ratio (VBR) (SHIHABUDDIN et al. 1996), and eye-tracking dysfunction (ETD) (AROLT et al. 1996), have reported linkages to chromosomes 15, 5, and 6, respectively.

Recently, we have described a potential functional neuroimaging phenotype obtained using ^{1}H-MRSI in a large cohort of patients with schizophrenia and their siblings (CALLICOTT et al., 1998). Given the increased frequency of reduced NAA measures in the prefrontal cortex and hippocampal area of patients with schizophrenia, we sought the relative frequency of these abnormalities in schizophrenic patients, their unaffected, non-psychotic relatives, and a healthy control population (see Table 41.2).

We assumed that a heritable trait would be over-represented in the siblings of patients with low NAA as a consequence of the fact that siblings share on average 50% of their genes. In this regard, reduced hippocampal NAA appeared familial ($\lambda_{S=}3.8$–8.8). However, while NAA is a quantitative measure (as in height), it is unclear if it represents a quantitative or qualitative trait (analagous to dwarfism). As a matter of fact, direct intra-class correlation between a given patient and his or her sibling was low – counter to the notion of reduced NAA as a quantitative trait. Nonetheless, the generation of intermediate phenotypes using functional MRI techniques remains a particularly novel and potentially significant contribution to psychiatric neuroscience.

41.6
Conclusions

Many aspects of fMRI and ^{1}H-MRS/^{1}H-MRSI outlined above make them ideally suited to the study of the so-called functional neuropsychiatric illness. Because scanning sessions are not limited by radiation exposure, functional MRI techniques also generate larger amounts of data, potentially permitting more powerful single subject analyses. Thus, researchers may be in a better position than ever to accurately assess neurophysiological differences across groups. Furthermore, it is likely that within a few years much of this work can be done interactively in real time. Individual brain mapping may help address the long-standing diagnostic inconsistencies that have plagued the top-down approach to mental illness research. There is hope that functional MRI methodologies might characterize mental illness based on quantifiable neurophysiology. Ultimately, these neurophysiological parameters might be more meaningful, since these abnormalities likely reside one or more steps closer to neuronal function than more complex clinical phenomena like sadness or psychosis. Related to this theme of neurophysiological traits, the characterization of novel functional phenotypes is a particularly exciting new application for functional neuroimaging. However, the ultimate worth of these contributions will rest on our ability to appreciate both the strengths and weaknesses of this promising technology.

References

Arolt V, Lencer R, Nolte A, et al. (1996) Eye tracking dysfunction is a putative phenotypic susceptibility marker of schizophrenia and maps to a locus on chromosome 6p in families with multiple occurence of the disease. Am J Med Genet 67:564–579

Bandettini PA, Wong EC, Hinks RS, Tikofsky RS, Hyde JS (1992) Time course EPI of human brain function during task activation. Magn Reson Med 25:390–397

Bartha R, Williamson PC, Drost DJ, et al. (1997) Measurement of glutamate and glutamine in the medial prefrontal cortex of never-treated schizophrenic patients and healthy controls by proton magnetic resonance spectroscopy. Arch Gen Psychiatry 54:959–965

Belliveau JW, Kennedy DN, McKinstry RC, et al. (1991) Functional mapping of the human visual cortex by magnetic resonance imaging. Science 254:716–719

Bertolino A, Nawroz S, Mattay V, et al. (1996) Regionally specific pattern of neurochemical pathology in schizophrenia as assessed by multislice proton magnetic resonance spectroscopic imaging. Am J Psychiatry 153:1554–1563

Bertolino A, Adler C, Callicott J, et al. (1997a) Effects of ketamine on working memory circuitry as studied by whole brain fMRI. Biol Psychiatry 41:64 S

Bertolino A, Esposito G, Callicott JH, et al. (1997b) 1H-Magnetic spectroscopic imaging correlates with rCBF activation during working memory in patients with schizophrenia. Neuroimage 5:S281

Bertolino A, Knable MB, Callicott JH, et al. (1997c) Prefrontal cortical regulation of subcortical dopamine in patients with schizophrenia: a 1H-magnetic spectroscopic imaging and IBZM-SPECT study. In: Proceedings of th 27th annual meeting of the Society for Neuroscience, 25–30 Oct 1997. Society for Neuroscience, Washington DC

Bertolino A, Saunders R, Mattay V, Bachevalier J, Frank J, Weinberger D (1997d) Altered development of prefrontal neurons in rhesus monkeys with neonatal mesial temporo-limbic lesions: a proton magnetic resonance spectroscopic imaging study. Cereb Cortex 7:740–748

Bertolino A, Callicott J, Ellman I, et al. (1998a) Regionally specific neuronal pathology in untreated patients with schizophrenia: a proton magnetic resonance spectroscopic imaging study. Biol Psychiatry 43:641–648

Bertolino A, Callicott JH, Nawroz S, et al. (1998b) Reproducibility of proton magnetic resonance spectroscopic imaging in patients with schizophrenia. Neuropsychopharmacology 18:1–8

Bertolino A, Kumra S, Callicott JH, et al. (1998c) A common pattern of cortical pathology in childhood onset and adult onset schizophrenia as identified by proton magnetic resonance spectroscopic imaging. Am J Psychiatry 155:1376-1383

Bogerts BH (1993) The neuropathology of schizophrenia. Schizophr Bull 19:68–75

Breiter HC, Rauch SL, Kwong KK, et al. (1996) Functional magnetic resonance imaging of symptom provocation in obsessive-compulsive disorder. Arch Gen Psychiatry 53:595–606

Breiter HC, Gollub RL, Weisskoff RM, et al. (1997) Acute effects of cocaine on human brain activity and emotion. Neuron 19:591–611

Buckley PF, Moore C, Long H, et al. (1994) 1H-magnetic resonance spectroscopy of the left temporal and frontal lobes in schizophrenia: clinical, neurodevelopmental, cognitive correlates. Biol Psychiatry 36:792–800

Bullmore E, Brammer M, Williams SC, et al. (1996) Statistical methods of estimation and inference for functional MR image analysis. Mag Reson Med 35:261–277

Callicott J, Ramsey N, Tallent K, et al. (1998) fMRI brain mapping in psychiatry: methodological issues illustrated in a study of working memory in schizophrenia. Neuropsychopharmacology 18:186–196

Callicott JH, Egan MF, Bertolino A, et al. (1998) Proton magnetic resonance spectroscopic imaging abnormalities in unaffected siblings of patients with schizophrenia: identification of a possible intermediate neurobiological phenotype. Biol Psychiatry 44:941–950

Charles HC, Lazeyras F, Krishnan KRR, Boyko OB, Payne M, Moore D (1994) Brain choline in depression: in vivo detection of potential pharmacodynamic effects of antidepressant therapy using hydrogen localized spectroscopy. Prog Neuropsychopharmacol Biol Psychiatry 18:1121–1127

Choe BY, Kim KT, Suh TS, et al. (1994) 1H magnetic resonance spectroscopy characterization of neuronal dysfunction in drug-naive, chronic schizophrenia. Acad Radiol 1:211–216

Choe BY, Suh TS, Shinn KS, Lee CW, Lee C, Paik IH (1996) Observation of metabolic changes in chronic schizophrenia after neuroleptic treatment by in vivo hydrogen magnetic resonance spectroscopy. Invest Radiol 31:345–352

Cleghorn JM, Garnett ES, Nahmias C, et al. (1990) Regional brain metabolism during auditory hallucinations in chronic schizophrenia. Br J Psychiatry 157:562–570

Cohen BM, Yurgelun-Todd D, English CD, Renshaw PF (1995) Abnormalities of regional distribution of cerebral vasculature in schizophrenia detected by dynamic susceptibility contrast MRI. Am J Psychiatry 152:1801–1803

Crowe RR (1993) Candidate genes in psychiatry: an epidemiological perspective. Am J Med Genet 48:74–77

Dager SR, Strauss WL, Marro KI, Richards TL, Metzger GD, Artru AA (1995) Proton magnetic resonance spectroscopy investigation of hyperventilation in subjects with panic disorder and comparison subjects. Am J Psychiatry 152:666–672

David AS, Woodruff PWR, Howard R, et al. (1996) Auditory hallucinations inhibit exogenous activation of auditory association cortex. Neuroreport 7:932–936

Deicken RF, Zhou L, Corwin F, Vinogradov S, Weiner MW (1997a) Decreased frontal lobe N-acetylaspartate in schizophrenia. Am J Psychiatry 154:688–690

Deicken RF, Zhou L, Schuff N, Weiner MW (1997b) Proton magnetic resonance spectroscopy of the anterior cingulate region in schizophrenia. Schizophr Res 27:65–71

Deicken RF, Zhou L, Schuff N, Fein G, Weiner MW (1998) Hippocampal neuronal dysfunction in schizophrenia as measured by proton magnetic resonance spectroscopy. Biol Psychiatry 43:483–488

Duyn J, Gillen J, Sobering G, Van ZP, Moonen C (1993) Multisection proton MR spectroscopic imaging of the brain. Radiology 188:277–282

Ebert D, Speck O, Konig A, Berger M, Hennig J, Hohagen F (1997) 1H-magnetic resonance spectroscopy in obsessive-compulsive disorder: evidence for neuronal loss in the cingulate gyrus and the right striatum. Psychiatry Res 74:173–176

Egan MF, Weinberger DR (1997) Neurobiology of schizophrenia. Curr Opin Neurobiol 7:701–707

Faraone SV, Kremen WS, Lyons MJ, Pepple JR, Seidman LJ, Tsuang MT (1995) Diagnostic accuracy and linkage analysis: how useful are schizophrenia spectrum phenotypes? Am J Psychiatry 152:1286–1290

Frank J, Ostuni J, Yang Y, et al. A technical solution for an interactive fMRI examination: application to a physiological interview and the study of cerebral physiology. Radiology (in press)

Freedman R, Coon H, Myles-Worsley M, et al. (1997) Linkage of a neurophysiological deficit in schizophrenia to a chromosome 15 locus. Proc Natl Acad Sci USA 94:587–592

Friston KJ, Williams S, Howard R, et al. (1996) Movement-related effects in fMRI time series. Magn Reson Med 35:346–355

Fujimoto T, Nakano T, Takano T, Takeuchi K, Yamada K, Fukuzako T, Akimoto H (1996) Proton magnetic resonance spectroscopy of basal ganglia in schizophrenia. Biol Psychiatry 40:14–18

Fukuzako H, Kouzou T, Hokazono Y, et al. (1995) Proton magnetic resonance spectroscopy of the left medial temporal and frontal lobes in chronic schizophrenia: preliminary report. Psychiatr Res 61:193–200

Gevins AS, Bressler S, Cutillo B, Illes J, Miller J, Stern J, et al. (1990) Effects of prolonged mental work on functional brain topography. Electroencephalogr Clin Neurophysiol 76:339–350

Goldman-Rakic PS (1996) The prefrontal landscape: implications of functional architecture for understanding human mentation and the central executive. Philos Trans R Soc Lond B Biol Sci 351:1445–1453

Hashimoto T, Tayama M, Miyazaki M, et al. (1995) Reduced N-acetylaspartate in the brain observed on in vivo proton magnetic resonance spectroscopy in patients with mental retardation. Pediatr Neurol 13:205–208

Holzman PS (1992) Behavioural markers of schizophrenia useful for genetic studies. J Psychiatr Res 26:427–445

Ingvar D, Franzen G (1974) Distribution of cerebral activity in chronic schizophrenia. Lancet 2:1484–1486

Johnstone EC, Crow TJ, Frith CD, Husband J, Kreel L (1976) Cerebral ventricular size and cognitive impairment in chronic schizophrenia. Lancet 2:924–926

Kandel EK (1998) A new intellectual framework for psychiatry. Am J Psychiatry 155:457–469

Kidd KK (1997) Can we find genes for schizophrenia? Am J Med Genet 74:104–111

Levin J, Ross M, Renshaw P (1995) Clinical applications of functional MRI in neuropsychiatry. J Neuropsychiatry 7:511–522

Liddle P (1995) Brain imaging. In: Hirsch S, Weinberger DR (eds) Schizophrenia. Blackwood, London, pp 425–439

Lim KO, Adalsteinsson E, Spielman D, Sullivan EV, Rosenbloom MJ, Pfefferbaum A (1998) Proton magnetic resonance spectroscopic imaging of cortical gray and white matter in schizophrenia. Arch Gen Psychiatry 55:346–352

Maas LC, Frederick BD, Renshaw PF (1997) Decoupled automated rotational and translational registration for functional MRI time series data: the DART registration algorithm. Magn Reson Med 37:131–139

Maas LC, Lukas SE, Kaufman MJ, et al. (1998) Functional magnetic resonance imaging of human brain activation during cue-induced cocaine craving. Am J Psychiatry 155:124–126

Maier M, Ron M, Barker G, Tofts P, et al. (1995) Proton magnetic resonance spectroscopy: an in-vivo method of estimating hippocampal neuronal depletion in schizophrenia. Psychol Med 25:1201–1209

Mattay VS, Frank JA, Santha AKS, et al. (1996) Whole brain functional mapping with isotropic MR imaging. Radiology 201:399–404

Mattay VS, Callicott JH, Bertolino A, Santha A, Tallent K, Frank J, Weinberger DR (1997) Sensorimotor cortex lateralization is anomalous in patients with schizophrenia: a whole brain fMRI study. Neuroimage 5:S23

Miller B (1991) A review of chemical issues in 1H NMR spectroscopy: n-acetyl-l-aspartate, creatine and choline. NMR Biomed 4:47–52

Murata T, Koshino Y, Omori M, et al. (1993) In vivo proton magnetic resonance spectroscopy study on premature aging in adult Down's syndrome. Biol Psychiatry 34:290–297

Nasrallah HA, Skinner TE, Schmalbrock P, Robitaille PM (1994) Proton magnetic resonance spectroscopy (1H MRS) of the hippocampal formation in schizophrenia: a pilot study. Br J Psychiatry 165:481–485

Ogawa S, Tank DW, Menon R, et al. (1992) Intrinsic signal changes accompanying sensory stimulation: functional brain mapping with magnetic resonance imaging. Proc Natl Acad Sci USA 89:5951–5955

Oldendorf W, Oldendorf W (1991) MRI primer. Raven, New York

Ostuni J, Santha A, Mattay V, Weinberger D, Levin R, Frank J (1997) Analysis of interpolation effects in the reslicing of functional MR images. J Comput Assist Tomogr 21:803–810

Peterson BS, Skudlarski P, Anderson AW, et al. (1998) A functional magnetic resonance imaging study of tic suppression in Tourette syndrome. Arch Gen Psychiatry 55:326–333

Reider RO, Donnelly EF, Herdt JR, Waldman IN (1979) Sulcul prominence in young schizophrenic patients: CT scan findings associated with impairment on neuropsychological tests. Psychiatry Res 1:1–8

Renshaw PF, Yurgelun-Todd DA, Cohen BM (1994) Greater hemodynamic response to photic stimulation in schizophrenic patients: an echo planar MRI study. Am J Psychiatry 151:1493–1495

Renshaw P, Yurgelun-Todd D, Tohen M, Gruber S, Cohen B (1995) Temporal lobe proton magnetic resonance spectroscopy of patients with first-episode psychosis. Am J Psychiatry 152:444–446

Ross BD (1991) Biochemical considerations in 1H spectroscopy. Glutamate and glutamine; myo-inositol and related metabolites. NRM Biomed 4:59–63

Ross BD, Michaelis T (1994) Clinical applications of magnetic resonance spectroscopy. Magn Reson Med 10:191–247

Schroder J, Wenz F, Schad LR, Baudenistel K, Knopp MV (1995) Sensorimotor cortex and supplementary motor area changes in schizophrenia: a study with functional magnetic resonance imaging. Br J Psychiatry 167:197–201

Shihabuddin L, Silverman JM, Buchsbaum MS, et al. (1996) Ventricular enlargement associated with linkage marker for schizophrenia-related disorders in one pedigree. Mol Psychiatry 1:215–222

Silbersweig DA, Stern E, Frith C, et al. (1995) A functional neuroanatomy of hallucinations in schizophrenia. Nature 378:176–179

Small GW (1996) Neuroimaging and genetic assessment for early diagnosis of Alzheimer's disease. J Clin Psychiatry 57:9–13

Stanley JA, Williamson PC, Drost DJ, Rylett RJ, Carr TJ, Malla A, Thompson RT (1996) An in vivo proton magnetic resonance spectroscopy study of schizophrenia patients. Schizophr Bull 22:597–609

Stoll AL, Renshaw PF, Micheli ED, Wurtman R, Pillay SS, Cohen BM (1995) Choline ingestion increases the resonance of choline-containing compounds in human brain: an in vivo proton magnetic resonance spectroscopy study. Biol Psychiatry 37:170–174

Storey PB (1966) Lumbar air encephalography in chronic schizophrenia: a controlled experiment. Br J Psychiatry 112:135–144

Taylor SF, Tandon R, Koeppe RA (1997) PET study of greater visual activation in schizophrenia. Am J Psychiatry 154:1296–1298

Tedeschi G, Bertolino A, Lundbom N, et al. (1996) Cortical and subcortical chemical pathology in Alzheimer's disease as assessed by multislice proton magnetic resonance spectroscopic imaging. Neurology 47:696–704

Tsai C, Coyle JT (1995) N-acetylaspartate in neuropsychiatric disorders. Prog Neurobiol 46:531–540

Tsai G, Passani LA, Slusher BS, Carter R, Baer L, Kleinman JE, Coyle JT (1995) Abnormal excitatory neurotransmitter metabolism in schizophrenic brain. Arch Gen Psychiatry 52:829–836

Tupler LA, Davidson JRT, Smith RD, Lazeyras F, Charles HC, Krishnan KRK (1997) A repeat proton magnetic resonance spectroscopy study in social phobia. Biol Psychiatry 42:419–424

Urenjak J, Williams S, Gadian D, Noble M (1993) Proton nuclear magnetic resonance spectroscopy unambiguously identifies different neural cell types. J Neurosci 13:981–989

VanGelderen P, Ramsey NF, Liu G, Duyn JH, Frank JA, Weinberger DR, Moonen CTW (1995) Three-dimensional functional magnetic resonance imaging of human brain on a clinical 1.5-T scanner. Proc Natl Acad Sci USA 92:6906–6910

Vogel T, Lange HJ (1966) Pneumoencephalographic and psychopathological pictures in endogenous psychoses. (Statisitical study on the material published by G Huber in 1957). Arch Psychiatr Nervenkr 208:371–384

Weinberger DR (1995) Schizophrenia as a neurodevelopmental disorder: a review of the concept. In: Hirsch SR, Weinberger DR (eds) Schizophrenia. Blackwood, London, pp 293–323

Weinberger DR, Berman KF (1996) Prefrontal function in schizophrenia: confounds and controversies. Philos Trans R Soc Med 351:1495–1503

Weinberger DR, Torrey EF, Neophytides AN, Wyatt RJ (1979) Lateral cerebral ventricular enlargement in chronic schizophrenia. Arch Gen Psychiatry 36:735–739

Weinberger DR, DeLisi LE, Neophytides AN, Wyatt RJ (1981) Familial aspects of CT scan abnormalities in chronic schizophrenic patients. Psychiatry Res 4:65–71

Weinberger DR, Mattay V, Callicott J, et al. (1996) fMRI applications in schizophrenia research. Neuroimage 4:S118–S126

Wenz F, Schad LR, Knopp MV, Baudendistel KT, Flomer F, Schroder J, Van Kaik G (1994) Functional magnetic resonance imaging at 1.5 T:activation pattern in schizophrenic patients receiving neuroleptic medication. Magn Reson Med 12:975–982

Wolf S, Jones D, Knable M, et al. (1996) Tourette syndrome: prediction of phenotypic variation in monozygotic twins by caudate nucleus D2 receptor binding. Science 273:1225–1227

Woodruff PWR, Wright IC, Bullmore ET, et al. (1997) Auditory hallucinations and the temporal cortical response to speech in schizophrenia: a functional magnetic resonance imaging study. Am J Psychiatry 154:1676–1682

Yurgelun-Todd D, Renshaw P, Gruber S, Waternaux C, Cohen B (1996a) Proton magnetic resonance spectroscopy of patients with first-episode psychosis. Schizophrenia Res 152:444–446

Yurgelun-Todd DA, Waternaux CM, Cohen BM, Gruber SA, English CD, Renshaw PR (1996b) Functional magnetic resonance imaging of schizophrenic patients and comparison subjects during word production. Am J Psychiatry 153:200–205

Zigun JR, Weinberger DR (1992) In vivo studies of brain morphology in schizophrenia. In: Lindenmayer J, Kay SR (eds) New biological vistas on schizophrenia. Brunner/Mazel, New York, pp 57–81

42 Functional MRI in Pediatrics

K.M. Thomas and B.J. Casey

CONTENTS

42.1
The Potential of fMRI for Pediatrics

For decades, scientists and clinicians who work with children have been interested in understanding the brain mechanisms of developmental change, from the development of basic motor and sensory functions, to the onset and maturation of cognitive capabilities such as language. To date, very little is known regarding the neural bases of cognition in normally developing children, and the neural correlates of developmental disorders are less well understood. Certain developmental psychiatric disorders (e.g., attention deficit hyperactivity disorder, obsessive compulsive disorder, childhood depression) have shown abnormal brain metabolism in adult brain imaging studies. Despite the clinical significance of these findings, most childhood onset disorders have been studied in adulthood, long after the appearance of the psychiatric symptoms. In order to address the

neural circuits underlying such disorders, developmentalists require a means of assessing in vivo the physiological progression of the disorder. Noninvasive functional magnetic resonance imaging (fMRI) techniques provide a preferred means of addressing such developmental issues.

Until recently, studies of functional brain development have been limited to relatively indirect techniques such as scalp-recorded electroencephalography and event-related brain potentials, which provide excellent information regarding the timing of sensory and cognitive events (DONCHIN 1984), but are insufficient for localizing the neural circuits which maintain these functions. Although other brain imaging techniques have been available and actively used with normal adult and patient populations, e.g., positron emission tomography (PET), computerized tomography (CT), and single photon emission computed tomography (SPECT), these techniques frequently require exposure to radiation. While these techniques may be used with pediatric patient populations when medically warranted, the ethics of exposing children to unnecessary radiation for the advancement of research are still under debate. With the development of the blood oxygenation level-dependent (BOLD) contrast (KWONG et al. 1992; OGAWA et al. 1990; TURNER et al. 1991), the field of magnetic resonance imaging (MRI) has been opened to developmental research. This technique capitalizes on the fact that hemoglobin becomes strongly paramagnetic in its deoxygenated state and can therefore be used as a naturally occurring contrast agent, with highly oxygenated brain regions producing a larger MR signal than less oxygenated areas. This method eliminates the need for exogenous contrast agents, including radioactive isotopes, and should hallmark the end of studies exposing children to unnecessary radiation.

The significance of studying these blood oxygenation changes in a developmental context becomes more apparent when we consider aspects of brain development in general. Clearly the brain continues to develop after birth and well into childhood.

K.M. THOMAS, PhD; B.J. CASEY, PhD; Western Psychiatric Institute and Clinic, Room E-735, Univ. of Pittsburgh, 3811 O'Hara Street, Pittsburgh, PA 15213, USA

HUTTENLOCHER (1990, 1997) has demonstrated that pruning and reorganization of some cortical regions are relatively protracted. While synaptic density reaches adult levels by approximately 5 months in visual cortex, prefrontal cortex still shows 10% greater synaptic density at 7 years than later in adulthood. Similarly, PET studies of glucose metabolism suggest that maturation of local metabolic rates in prefrontal cortex closely parallel the time course of this overproduction and subsequent pruning of synapses (CHUGANI et al. 1987). The higher metabolic rates observed in the developing brain may reflect the processes needed to maintain membrane potentials over a larger surface area or, alternatively, the higher glucose metabolism may be due to increased energy expenditure during the height of the myelination process (CHUGANI et al. 1987; KENNEDY and SOKOLOFF 1957). A logical conclusion from these findings is that cognitive processes such as memory, inhibition, and language, which rely heavily on the prefrontal, temporal, and association cortices, may function in a physiologically different manner in children than in adults. Whether this difference is qualitative or quantitative is yet to be determined.

Several research laboratories have demonstrated the utility of using structural MRI techniques for examining developmental issues, especially questions surrounding abnormal development or developmental psychiatric disorders. For example, GIEDD et al.(1996) have used morphometric measures to examine normative brain development across childhood. In addition, these authors have demonstrated that particular clinical groups show abnormal or reduced volume of particular brain structures, implicating specific brain regions in the pathology of the disorder (e.g., CASTELLANOS et al. 1996; GIEDD et al. 1994). Using these morphometric data as a building block, the next step for developmentalists is to address the brain state changes that are occurring during the onset of symptoms of these disorders.

42.2
Review of the Pediatric fMRI Literature

Although the technology for noninvasive fMRI has been available for over 5 years, the foray into developmental research has been surprisingly slow. This delay may be due to the hesitancy of developmentalists to leap into a relatively new and expensive research arena. Currently, the published fMRI literature contains very few pediatric contributions;

however, this situation should improve in the near future as a number of laboratories around the world are actively engaged in pediatric research.

A major criticism of the developmental neuroimaging literature to date has been the use of pediatric patient populations to study normal behavior. For example, although CHUGANI et al. (1987) have provided invaluable data concerning the development of various aspects of brain metabolism with PET, the children included in that study all had a history of neurologic events. Much of the work reviewed in this chapter relies on neuroimaging data from clinical populations to address normal development, although a small number of studies have examined brain activity in healthy children. These currently reported pediatric fMRI endeavors are reviewed in the following sections covering studies of the development of sensorimotor systems, language, functional reorganization, and frontal lobe functions, including memory and inhibition (Table 42.1).

42.2.1
Studies of Sensorimotor Systems

If functional MRI is to be used with the very young child, then basic sensorimotor paradigms must be developed. For example, fMRI may be useful in describing the normal functional development of sensory and motor systems and corresponding changes in brain plasticity with age and experience. Although several neuroimaging studies have examined developing sensorimotor systems, interpretations of these data are limited by the use of sedation, since most fail to include unsedated children or sedated adults as comparison groups.

42.2.1.1
Visual Studies

At least three fMRI studies of visual stimulation with infants have been completed to date. In general, these studies show decreases and/or a lack of change in the MR signal in the visual cortex of infants. For example, BORN et al. (1996) scanned sedated infants between 6 weeks and 36 months of age and observed an overall deactivation of occipital cortex during passive visual stimulation. A follow-up study (BORN et al. 1997) including premature and full-term newborns showed similar decreases in MR signal intensity in visual cortex for all but one infant, who showed no activity. Infants under 6 weeks of age were not sedated, but data from 11 of these 13 new-

Table 42.1. Summary of pediatric fMRI literature

Behavioral tasks	Age of participants	Citation	Comments
Sensorimotor studies			
Passive visual stimulation	6 weeks–36 months (*n*=7) Healthy adults (*n*=3)	Born et al. (1996)[a]	Infants were sedated patients; adults were unsedated
Passive visual stimulation	28 weeks gestation– 36 months (*n*=30)	Born et al. (1997)	Infants over 6 weeks were sedated
Passive visual stimulation	4 days–8 years (n=7) Healthy adults (*n*=10)	Joeri et al. (1996a)	Children were sedated; adults were unsedated
Undescribed motor, speech, and visual tasks	22 months–18 years (*n*=25)	Kiriakopoulos et al. (1996)	Children were neurosurgery patients
Unilateral and bilateral hand and finger movement	8 years–14 years (*n*=7)	Popp et al. (1996)	Children were unsedated; 6 healthy, 1 with parietal tumor
Language studies			
Verbal fluency and language tasks	9-year old (*n*=1)	Benson et al. (1996)[a]	Child was unsedated; child had epilepsy and learning disability
Spelling and rhyming tasks	Children and adults[b]	Dapretto et al. (1996)	Some participants were dyslexic
Phoneme deletion and discrimination	13 years–19 years (*n*=20)	Frost et al. (1997)	Children were dyslexics (*n*=10) and age-matched controls (*n*=10)
Undescribed lateralization task	9 years–18 years[c] Healthy adults[c]	Hertz-Pannier et al. (1995)	Some children were epileptic patients
Word generation	8 years–18 years (*n*=11)	Hertz-Pannier et al. (1997)[a]	Patients with partial epilepsy
Passive listening task	15-month old (*n*=1)	Hirsch et al. (1997)	Child was a sedated patient
Word generation and object naming	6 years–16 years (*n*=20)	Logan et al. (1998)	Participants were presurgical patients
Living/nonliving word decisions	8 years–12 years (*n*=6)	Vaidya et al. (1998)	Healthy volunteers
Cortical reorganization studies			
Sentence comprehension, verb generation, and mental rotation	11 years–12 years (*n*=2) Healthy adults (*n*=4)	MacWhinney et al. (1998)	Children had left hemisphere lesions prior to 1 year of age
Hierarchical spatial analysis of shape forms	10 years–15 years (*n*=7)	Moses et al. (1997)	Five healthy volunteers, 1 child left lesion, 1 child right lesion
Memory and inhibition studies			
Nonspatial working memory	9 years–11 years (*n*=6)	Casey et al. (1995)[a]	Healthy volunteers
Spatial working memory	8 years–10 years (*n*=6)	Casey et al. (1997a)	Healthy volunteers
Spatial working memory	8 years–10 years (*n*=6)	Orendi et al. (1997)	Healthy volunteers
Spatial working memory	8 years–12 years (*n*=7)	Truwit et al. (1996)	Healthy volunteers
Go/no-go paradigm	7 years–12 years (*n*=9) Adults (*n*=9)	Casey et al. (1997b)[a]	Healthy volunteers
Go/no-go paradigm	6 years–9 years (*n*=10)	Casey et al. (1998)	Children had perinatal IVH
Go/no-go paradigm	Children (*n*=10)[d]	Vaidya et al. (1997)	Children had ADD; each tested both on and off medication

ADD, attention deficit disorder; IVH, intraventricular hemorrhage.
[a]Refereed journal article, not a conference abstract.
[b]Age range and sample sizes unavailable.
[c]Unknown sample size.
[d]Age range unavailable.

borns were excluded due to excessive motion artifact. Finally, Joeri et al. (1996a) scanned seven sedated children between the ages of 4 days and 8
years and ten unsedated adults. They observed no
visual cortex activity for the two neonates, while
older infants showed a deactivation of occipital cortex, and the 8-year-old child and unsedated adults
showed activation of the occipital cortex.

The findings from these three studies were taken
primarily from data of sedated children compared to
unsedated adults. Thus, the results may reflect the effect of sedation rather than brain maturation. In fact,
Joeri et al. (1996b) reported that adults sedated with
phenobarbitol showed cortical deactivation in the
same areas that were activated during unsedated
passive visual stimulation. Such comparisons are
critical for our interpretations of pediatric data,
given the large number of studies employing sedation methods with infants.

42.2.1.2
Motor Studies

At least one study of motor cortex has been completed in children 8–12 years of age without sedation. Popp et al. (1996) assessed patterns of brain
activity in children during unilateral and bilateral
finger wiggling and hand opening and closing. Like
many pediatric fMRI studies, the main goal of this
research was to assess the feasibility of fMRI techniques with children. Initial data showed 2%–6%
increases in signal intensity, primarily in the contralateral sensorimotor area for unilateral tasks, and
bilaterally for the bilateral tasks. Activation was often observed in the supplementary motor area as
well, similar to reported adult findings during
simple motor movements.

42.2.2
Studies of Language

A prevalent area of research in developmental psychology has been the study of language development
(e.g., Locke, 1993, for review). How is it that children
learn their native languages so naturally and without formal instruction? What are the brain mechanisms underlying this complex development? A
number of investigators have begun to use fMRI to
study language use in children. However, these studies primarily have investigated language function in
children with epilepsy, dyslexia, or early left hemisphere lesions.

A number of studies have examined the functional mapping of language in children prior to neurosurgery for epilepsy. According to these studies,
functional MRI provides a noninvasive alternative to
the common intra-carotid amobarbital test for
hemispheric language dominance used with epilepsy patients undergoing temporal lobectomy for
seizure control. Hertz-Pannier et al. (1997) reported that fMRI scanning during word generation
tasks produced lateralized activation in language areas of epileptic children and showed 100% compatibility with amobarbital test results. Kiriakopoulos
et al. (1996) have reported success in localizing
speech, motor, sensory, and visual cortices in alert 2-
18 year old neurosurgery patients that was 94% reproducible and correlated 100% with intraoperative
electrocortical stimulation, electrocorticography,
and magnetic source imaging. Similar findings have
been observed for speech, motor, sensation, and visual cortices in children by Logan and coworkers
(Logan et al. 1998; Benson et al. 1996). However, results from such studies emphasize the importance of
behavioral paradigm development, since it was reported that verb and word generation tasks were
more effective in producing lateralized language activity than a simple object naming task (Logan et al.
1998).

Diffuse and anatomically disparate areas of brain
activation in children relative to adults has been reported using both active and passive language tasks.
Hertz-Pannier et al. (1995) compared language-related brain activity in adults and children. Results
showed distinct lateralized frontal regions of activation for adults during word generation as compared
to rest. However, children and adolescents produced
more varied patterns of frontal activation, ranging
from the adult pattern to a very diffuse and poorly
lateralized pattern. It should be noted that the most
diffuse and least lateralized patterns in the Hertz-
Pannier et al. (1995) study occurred in two children
who were epileptic. A similar finding of diffuse and
anatomically disparate areas of activation has been
reported using a passive language task with a sedated 15-month-old (Hirsch et al. 1997). With the
mother's voice as a stimulus, these authors observed
activation in Heschl's gyrus, superior temporal gyrus, inferior and middle frontal gyri, cingulate gyrus,
thalamus and putamen. The interpretations from
these studies with regard to normal language development are limited due to the reliance on pediatric
patients in their samples.

At least two pediatric fMRI studies of dyslexia
have been described to date. Dapretto et al. (1996)

reported that children and adolescents with dyslexia show restricted activation of brain regions during various language tasks when compared to normal adults. Data presented for an individual child (age 13) demonstrated similar activation in the left inferior frontal cortex during spelling and rhyming when compared to a normal adult, but lacked activation of the left superior temporal lobe and angular gyrus. Instead, the dyslexic child demonstrated more posteriorly located activity in the right hemisphere. FROST et al. (1997) demonstrated that dyslexic adolescents (ages 13–19) failed to activate the supramarginal gyrus during a phoneme discrimination task and showed significantly less activity than age-matched controls in the inferior frontal gyrus and supramarginal gyrus during a phoneme deletion task. These data lend support to the notion that fMRI can provide clues about the locus of functional abnormalities in the brains of children with developmental disorders, but underscore the importance of examining normative development.

At least one normative study of language development was reported recently in an abstract by VAIDYA et al. (1998). They evaluated frontal activity during semantic processing in 8–12 year old boys. These authors report activation of left superior, middle, and inferior frontal cortices during living/nonliving word judgments as compared to uppercase/lowercase judgments, as well as left cingulate gyrus and temporal pole activity. Such normative work will be critical for understanding the biological substrates of language development.

42.2.3
Studies of Reorganization of Verbal and Spatial Abilities

The reorganization of the brain following early lateralized lesions has been a topic of much interest. Is it the case that an early left hemisphere lesion results in the reorganization of hemisphere-specialized functions (e.g., language) to the contralateral side? MACWHINNEY et al. (1998) reported preliminary 3 T fMRI data examining this question with regard to language. They scanned two school-age children with lesions to the left hemisphere prior to 1 year of age. These children demonstrated difficulties in behavioral tests of sentence comprehension although intelligence and spoken vocabulary were normal. The child with the largest lesion demonstrated regions of activation in the undamaged hemisphere which were homologous to the regions activated in

healthy adults for sentence comprehension, verb generation, and mental rotation of alphanumeric characters (e.g., superior temporal, inferior temporal, and parietal cortices, respectively). However, the other child showed activation which was uncorrelated with adult activity for sentence comprehension and mental rotation, activating for example, bilateral inferior temporal and occipital regions for sentence comprehension rather than superior temporal and prefrontal cortices. These results may have implications for the plasticity of function following early brain lesions, specifically, the relation between lesion size and location, and subsequent cortical reorganization.

This question of functional reorganization is also being addressed in other cognitive domains. For example, MOSES et al. (1997) reported preliminary findings from a study of spatial analytic processing. Normally developing children demonstrated similar but more variable patterns of inferior temporal-occipital cortex activation during spatial analysis of hierarchical stimuli than observed in adult participants, including patterns of right lateralization for global-level processing, and left lateralized activity for local-level processing. In contrast, children with unilateral parietal-superior temporal cortex lesions demonstrated activity in the contralateral hemisphere for both global and local processing. Again, a large scale study of this hemispheric lateralization may provide insights into the plasticity of brain function following injury.

42.2.4
Studies of Memory and Inhibition

Given the prolonged physiological development of the prefrontal cortex, tasks thought to tap this region are ideal for investigating development. Two cognitive processes which have been attributed to the frontal lobe are memory and inhibition (FUSTER 1989). A number of normative pediatric fMRI studies have examined brain activity in children during memory and response inhibition tasks. In fact, the first published pediatric fMRI study examined prefrontal cortex activation in children performing a nonspatial working memory task (CASEY et al. 1995). The results replicated an earlier adult fMRI study showing inferior and middle frontal gyrus activity using the same paradigm (COHEN et al. 1994). Several groups (CASEY et al. 1997a; ORENDI et al. 1997; TRUWIT et al. 1996) have also examined brain activity during a spatial working memory task. One

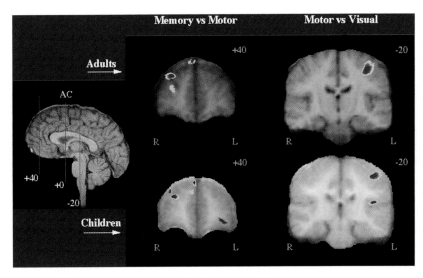

Fig. 42.1. The mid-sagittal image on the *left* identifies the location of the pictured slices relative to the anterior commissure. Slices indicate activation for adults (*top row*) and children (*bottom row*) during the memory and motor tasks of the n-back spatial working memory paradigm respectively. These results are based on a pooled analysis across each age-group

goal of this research was to equate task difficulty across age groups. The results suggest that children show similar patterns of predominantly right dorso-lateral prefrontal activation when compared to adults, although individual studies differed in the exact Brodmann's areas activated. Children may activate a slightly more anterior and superior region of prefrontal cortex (area 9 rather than 46) during working memory as compared to adults (Fig. 42.1).

Given the prevalence of inhibitory problems in the general pediatric population and related symptomatology in various developmental disorders (e.g., attention deficit hyperactivity disorder, obsessive compulsive disorder, Tourette syndrome), the neural substrate of inhibitory control has received much attention. At least one fMRI study using a go/no-go paradigm with healthy children has been published to date (CASEY et al. 1997b). Activity in the orbital frontal cortex and anterior cingulate gyrus in children and adults correlated with behavioral performance on this response inhibition task. In this investigation, the general location of activation in prefrontal cortex did not differ for children as compared to adults, but overall volume of prefrontal activation was greater for children than adults.

Two recent abstracts have been published assessing inhibitory processing in clinical pediatric populations. VAIDYA et al. (1997) applied a go/no-go task identical to that used by CASEY et al. (1997b) to probe the circuitry underlying attention and impulsivity problems inherent in attention deficit disorder (ADD), and the effects of methylphenidate (Ritalin) on the function of this circuitry. Children performed the behavioral task with fewer errors and showed greater activation of the anterior frontal brain regions during the response inhibition condition when they were on Ritalin than when they were off medication. The authors interpret these results to suggest that Ritalin enhances frontal cortex mechanisms of inhibitory function in children with ADD. Unlike the previous studies with pediatric patients, conclusions from such work are more convincing since the same children were tested in both medicated and unmedicated states.

Our laboratory has also addressed inhibition in a clinical population. Building on our model of inhibitory mechanisms of attention and our previous pediatric fMRI study using the go/no-go paradigm (CASEY et al. 1997b), we examined children with perinatal histories of intraventricular hemorrhage (IVH) (CASEY et al. 1998). This study tests our theory regarding the role of fronto-striatal circuitry in inhibition by examining children known to have early damage to this circuitry. IVH can damage neural tissue in the lateral ventricles and nearby structures (e.g., caudate nucleus), and is a frequent consequence of premature birth. In contrast to our previous study, preliminary results indicate that, while children with IVH reliably activate orbitofrontal cortex, this activity is not correlated with false alarm rate. These results suggest that early damage to the striatum may be sufficient to disrupt the normal mechanisms underlying behavioral inhibition. This research will not be complete until the appropriate comparison group has been tested (i.e., children born prematurely without IVH).

42.3
Issues in Working with a Developmental Population

These preliminary studies of pediatric populations indicate the feasibility of using fMRI techniques with children, but also raise a number of issues regarding interpretation of results and methodological problems common to pediatric research in this field. As in behavioral research, statistical and practical issues arise when working with any special population, including the ability to detect a difference between groups (power and effect size), differences in between-groups variance, interpretation of observed differences, and methodological issues (e.g., motion). In the case of fMRI research, artifact minimization becomes extremely relevant with developmental populations and may require some practical modifications in the standard fMRI methods and procedures. The following sections address these issues.

42.3.1
Behavioral Paradigm Development

A simplistic but necessary step in pediatric research is the design of age appropriate tasks. Not only must these tasks be easy to explain, and relatively easy to complete, but they must also engage a child's attention for long enough to collect fMRI data. Although many of the behavioral tasks used with adults are exciting and should be applied to pediatric settings, most will require minor, if not substantial, adaptations for use with children. In addition, adult behavioral tasks should not be applied indiscriminately to pediatric groups, but rather should be theoretically motivated to examine development.

In addition to choosing an age appropriate behavioral task, investigators need to train children on the task outside of the scanner to ensure a high rate of performance. We have observed that children (and adults) do not usually perform as well in the scanner as they do outside of the scanner, perhaps due to anxiety, the unusual posture for completing tasks, or the excessive noise produced by the machine. Once the subject has entered the scanner, the investigator must have some means of assessing task performance. For example, tasks can be designed to include auditory feedback in the control room regarding behavioral responding by the participant. Without this feedback, the investigator may be blind to any performance problems until the scan is complete.

Current techniques for motion minimization and behavioral response with pediatric populations severely limit the age groups which can be tested as well as the paradigms which can be applied. The majority of behavioral tasks used in pediatric fMRI involve either passive stimulation of a sensory system or require some form of motor response. Given the limited motor coordination of some patient populations and age groups, such paradigms will not be practical. A future direction for pediatric fMRI research will most likely include monitoring of alternative behavioral responses, including voice response and eye movements.

42.3.2
Scanner Acclimation and/or Desensitization

Most children feel uncomfortable in unfamiliar environments. This discomfort may manifest as shyness with investigators, disinterest in preliminary explanations or task instructions, crying and other symptoms of anxiety, or refusal to participate. An important step in preventing and alleviating this distress is to create an environment that is child friendly. This step includes not only the physical scanner environment, but also the flexibility and demeanor of the investigators.

While the physical appearance of the scanner may be beyond the investigator's control, small concessions, such as allowing young children to bring blankets or stuffed toys into the magnet, can provide a big boost not only in the child's comfort with the scanner, but also in the child's confidence toward the investigators. In addition, allowing the child to have a parent stay in the room with him/her and/or giving the child something to do during times when functional data are not being collected can improve the child's impressions of the experience, as well as assist with motion minimization and subject attrition. The use of fabric or painted facades to make the scanner appear more like a child's playroom or bedroom may prove effective in alleviating anxiety. Novelty facades such as castle, dinosaur or cartoon motifs may be appropriate, and can easily be velcroed to the outside of the scanner.

A child friendly environment also requires providing the child with sufficient and developmentally appropriate information so that she/he knows what to expect during the scanning session. For example, a simple explanation of the importance of remaining still might be achieved by explaining to the child that the pictures of her brain will be blurry if she moves.

A more clear understanding of what we are trying to achieve proves to be a better motivator for child compliance than obedience to authority.

42.3.2.1
Simulator

A simulation of a scanner is one of the most valuable tools that investigators can use when working with children. Although it has been noted that young children do not seem to experience the feelings of claustrophobia that sometimes plague adult subjects, many children do show fear of the unknown or hospital-like environment. Children who show no discomfort or anxiety in anticipation of the scan may feel extreme distress upon actually seeing and entering the magnet.

Several groups of investigators (e.g., CASEY et al. 1995; ORENDI et al. 1996) have reported that a simulator which reproduces the look, feel, and sounds of the scanner can significantly reduce subjects' self-reported anxiety and can provide a realistic measure of how the child might perform during the scan. In addition to assessing the child's anxiety, this setting can provide an opportunity to give children feedback about their head and body motion before they enter the scanner (SLIFER et al. 1993). This simulation also allows the child an opportunity to ask further questions about the session without jeopardizing the results of the scan (Fig. 42.2).

In our research with 5- to 10-year-old children, we have implemented a practice of providing the child with a pre-simulator experience. Many of our participants seem intimidated by the medical environment, even in the simulator setting. In order to put these children more at ease, we first explain the study in the context of a large play tunnel, similar to those found at school playgrounds and fast-food restaurants. In this setting, we allow the child to lie down in the tunnel, hear recordings of the scanner sounds while wearing ear plugs, and use a mirror to see out of the tunnel. Children treat this experience like a game or an unusual adventure and subsequently appear more comfortable moving on to the simulator and later to the actual scan environment.

42.3.3
Motion Minimization

As with structural MRI, fMRI data are quite sensitive to motion artifact. Slight movements of the head, face, throat, hands or other body parts can significantly affect measurements. This problem is more prevalent when working with certain patient populations and proves to be a concern when working with children.

Although most children are unaccustomed to lying perfectly still for long periods of time, several of the methods used to minimize or prevent motion in adult participants are also effective with children. Less intrusive methods include a head clamp consisting of padded plastic clamps that press on either side of the head (TRUWIT et al. 1996), a pillow clamp consisting of a large pillow wrapped around the back of the head and foam padding (CASEY et al. 1997b), or some combination of these methods. Measures such as a bite bar or form fitting chemical foam which have been used with adults are more successful at restricting movement, but may be more unappealing to children and may increase attrition rates. A combination of a flexible chin strap or strap across the forehead with a head or pillow clamp may be more appealing.

In addition to physical restraints, children often require specific instructions and periodic reminders regarding acceptable and unacceptable behaviors. Humming, singing, and talking to oneself are common behaviors in young children. Our group has had success in movement reduction by allowing children to watch their favorite videotape between functional scans. We have observed that children move less when they have a task or some form of entertainment. Child tendencies toward movement and self-entertainment also imply that scanning sessions must be as short as possible. Although most children are amiable participants, 1–2 h is more than enough to try a child's patience.

Technological advances are needed in motion minimization methods. Methods to give a child im-

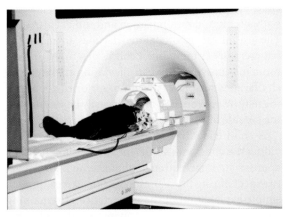

Fig. 42.2. Acclimation of a 5-year-old child to the MR scanner environment

mediate feedback regarding body motion could prove useful in training children to remain motionless during scanning. For example, a system of operant training could be imposed such that a visual display remains on only as long as the child maintains head position. This effect can be accomplished through a mechanical potentiometer apparatus or infrared detectors of head position. Systems like these are already in place at Johns Hopkins University and Children's Hospital of Philadelphia (SLIFER et al. 1993; J.C. Haselgrove, personal communication).

Regardless of the type of motion minimization techniques which are used, all motion cannot be removed completely. Therefore, off-line 3D motion correction algorithms have proven quite useful in pediatric studies (e.g., WOODS et al. 1992). Pediatric data from multiple laboratories (e.g., CASEY et al. 1995, 1997, 1998; HERTZ-PANNIER et al. 1995; TRUWIT et al. 1996; VAIDYA et al. 1997, 1998) indicate that medical sedation is not necessary. Sedation of normally developing children is an ethically tenuous position. Sedation is acceptable primarily in very young children undergoing scans for clinical purposes. Given the appropriate environment, and age appropriate expectations, children are generally willing and able to remain still in the scanner environment.

42.3.4
Assessment of Group Differences

42.3.4.1
Power or Effect Size

One issue that arises when trying to interpret differences between age groups (e.g., children and adults), or between normal volunteers and clinical populations, is that of statistical power, or effect size. Using the standard 1.5 Tesla clinical scanner, reliable differences may reflect a change of only 1%–2% in the magnitude of the MR signal (KWONG et al. 1992). One concern in pediatric or clinical fMRI is the feasibility of detecting group differences when the expected effect sizes for signal intensity are quite small. This issue of power becomes more evident when variance due to movement artifact, unreliable measures of cognition, or other sources are added to the equation. In our study of prefrontal activation in children (CASEY et al. 1997b), we evaluated statistical power in a comparison of volume of activation between children and adults. Effect size was on the order of 1.3 standard deviations, with children showing more activation than adults. With a significance criterion of 0.05 and a sample size of 10, the estimated power of our effect was calculated to be 0.78. Although power was sufficient in this instance, investigators should be aware that pediatric research may require larger sample sizes in some cases to achieve sufficient statistical power.

42.3.4.2
Variance Between Groups

Between-group variance may be a factor when comparing different age groups. Given the continued physiological brain changes during early childhood, it is possible that variance in the MR signal may change with development. Significant differences between children and adults in synaptic density, blood oxygenation, and metabolism may increase biological noise in the MR signal. In order to assess such effects in our study of prefrontal cortex function, we generated MR signal variance maps for each group across each condition (CASEY et al. 1997b). Results suggested that children did not differ from adults in the variance of the MR signal ($t_{142}=0.68$, $p<0.52$), with average variances of 168 (SD=111) and 147 (SD=136) for children and adults, respectively.

Overall brain size also can vary throughout early childhood but, more importantly, the location of specific anatomical landmarks and functional gyri can vary significantly across individuals, especially in later developing regions (e.g., prefrontal cortex). This problem is especially noticeable in studies of clinical populations. The difference in brain size complicates comparisons of brain regions across age groups. For example, standard adult atlases may be inadequate when studying children. Similarly, previous research has indicated that patient groups can demonstrate overall volume differences for specific brain regions (e.g., CASTELLANOS et al. 1996). Any subsequent group differences in functional brain activation must take morphometric group differences into account. A smaller region of activation may reflect only a smaller structure rather than a differential use of that brain region.

42.3.5
Interpreting Differences

Once motion artifact and other sources of variance have been rejected as possible factors for group differences, challenges still arise in interpreting the observed differences. Do group differences in the magnitude and volume of MR signal represent maturational changes in the neural circuitry underlying the cognitive process (i.e., brain development), differences in the cognitive strategies used (i.e., cognitive development), or do these differences simply reflect physiological states, such as anxiety? The easiest of these to assess is physiological anxiety. Pulse rate and blood pressure can easily be monitored before and after scans, assuring that physiologic measures are within normal resting levels for the child's age. In addition, some investigators employ a self-rating system to elicit information concerning subjective feelings of anxiety, such as a 1–10 scale or a happy face/sad face rating. However, we have found the number system confusing for young children.

Behavioral performance plays an important role in the interpretation of developmental differences. Behavioral data are essential for evaluating whether the participant was performing the desired task. Correlations between behavioral performance and the volume or magnitude of the MR signal can provide additional information regarding the relationship between the behavior and the observed activity. Likewise, behavioral performance data aid in determining whether group differences in MR measurements may be attributable to maturation alone, or whether behavioral measures correlate with age, suggesting a functional development such as a change in cognitive strategy or efficiency.

The importance of equating task difficulty across groups is evident in a study by Braver et al. (1997). They showed that the MR signal in prefrontal cortex increased monotonically as memory load increased, suggesting that changes in blood flow can be due to the cognitive demands of the task. Logically, if children find a particular working memory task more difficult than adults, we would expect to find greater signal intensity changes in children than in adults on the identical task. Behavioral paradigms may be designed to control for possible group differences in task difficulty. For example, the studies of spatial working memory discussed previously (Orendi et al. 1996; Truwitt et al. 1996; Casey et al. 1997a) tested all participants at a memory load of 1, 2, or 3, whichever elicited 70%–90% accuracy. For some individuals, this performance was achieved in a 2-back paradigm, while others required the 1-back or 3-back paradigms to produce this level of accuracy.

42.4
Conclusions

Clearly, the number of preliminary reports and completed fMRI studies with children strengthens the claim that fMRI is a feasible and preferred method for developmental neuroimaging. Other methods for brain imaging have drawbacks, such as exposure to harmful radiation, which make them inappropriate for use with children. Although many scientists have begun to study development using fMRI, the field lacks a substantive body of literature tracing normative development. At the very least, studies of pediatric patients need to include a normal control group matched in age.

References

Benson RR, Logan WJ, Cosgrove GR, et al. (1996) Functional MRI localization of language in a 9-year-old child. Can J Neurol Sci 23: 213–219

Born P, Rostrup E, Leth H, Peitersen B, Lou HC (1996) Change of visually induced cortical activation patterns during development. Lancet 347: 543

Born P, Rostrup E, Larsson HBW, Leth H, Miranda M, Peitersen B, Lou HC (1997) Infant visual cortex function evaluated by fMRI. Neuroimage 5(4): S171 (Abstract)

Braver TS, Cohen JD, Nystrom LE, Jonides J, Smith EE, Noll DC (1997) A parametric study of prefrontal cortex involvement in human working memory. Neuroimage 5: 49–62

Casey BJ, Thomas KM, Welsh TF, Eccard CH, Livnat R, Pierri JN (1998) An fMRI study of response inhibition in children with striatal lesions. Abstracts of the 4th International Conference on Functional Mapping of the Human Brain (Abstract)

Casey BJ, Cohen JD, King SW, et al. (1997a) A developmental functional MRI study of cortical activation during a spatial working memory task. Neuroimage 23: S69 (Abstract)

Casey BJ, Trainor RJ, Orendi JL, et al. (1997b) A developmental functional MRI study of prefrontal activation during performance of a go-no-go task. J Cog Neurol 9(6): 835–847

Casey BJ, Cohen JD, Jezzard P, et al. (1995) Activation of prefrontal cortex in children during a nonspatial working memory task with functional MRI. Neuroimage 2:221–229

Castellanos FX, Giedd JN, Hamburger SD, Marsh WL, Rapoport JL (1996) Brain morphometry in Tourette's syndrome: The influence of comorbid attention deficit/hyperactivity disorder. Neurology 47(6): 1581–1583

Chugani HT, Phelps ME, Mazziotta JC (1987) Positron emission tomography study of human brain functional development. Ann Neurol 22: 487–497

Cohen JD, Forman SD, Braver TS, Casey BJ, Servan-Schreiber D, Noll DC (1994) Activation of prefrontal cortex in a nonspatial working memory task with functional MRI. Hum Brain Map 1: 293–304

Dapretto M, Bookheimer SY, Cohen MS, Wang J (1996) fMRI of language in dyslexic and normally developing children. Neuroimage 3(3): S434 (Abstract)

Donchin E (1984) Cognitive psychophysiology. Lawrence Erlbaum, New Jersey

Frost JA, Binder JR, Newby RF, Hammeke TA, Bellgowan PSF, Springer JA, Cox RW (1997) Phonological processing in developmental dyslexia: An fMRI study. Neuroimage 5: S568 (Abstract)

Fuster JM (1989) The prefrontal cortex: Anatomy, physiology and neuropsychology of the frontal lobe. Raven, New York

Giedd JN, Snell JW, Lange N, et al. (1996) Quantitative magnetic resonance imaging of human brain development: Ages 4–18. Cereb Cortex 6: 551–60

Giedd JN, Castellanos FX, Casey BJ, Kozuch P, King AC, Hamburger SD, Rapoport JL (1994) Quantitative morphology of the corpus callosum in attention deficit hyperactivity disorder. Am J Psychiatry 151: 665–669

Hertz-Pannier L, Gaillard WD, Mott SH, et al. (1997) Noninvasive assessment of language dominance in children and adolescents with functional MRI: A preliminary study. Neurology 48: 1003–1012

Hertz-Pannier L, Gaillard WD, Mott S, Weinstein S, Conry J, Theodore WH, Le Bihan D (1995) Functional MRI of language tasks: Frontal diffuse activation patterns in children. Hum Brain Map Supp 1: 231 (Abstract)

Hirsch J, Kim KHS, Souweidane MM, McDowell R, Ruge MI, Correa DD, Krol G (1997) fMRI reveals a developing language system in a 15-month old sedated infant. Abst Soc Neurosci 23: 2227

Huttenlocher PR (1997) Regional differences in synaptogenesis in human cerebral cortex. J. Comp Neurol 387: 167–178.

Huttenlocher PR (1990) Morphometric study of human cerebral cortex development. Neuropsychologia 28: 517–527

Joeri P, Loenneker T, Huisman D, Ekatodramis D, Rumpel H, Martin E (1996a) fMRI of the visual cortex in infants and children. Neuroimage 3: S279 (Abstract)

Joeri P, Huisman T, Loenneker T, Ekatodramis D, Rumpel H, Martin E (1996b) Reproducibility of fMRI and effects of pentobarbital sedation on cortical activation during visual stimulation. Neuroimage 3: S280 (Abstract)

Kennedy C, Sokoloff L (1957) An adaptation of the nitrous oxide method to the study of the cerebral circulation in children: Normal values for cerebral blood flow and cerebral metabolic rate in childhood. J Clin Invest 36: 1130–1137

Kiriakopoulos ET, Wood ML, Mikulis DJ (1996) fMRI in pediatric neurosurgical patients. Neuroimage 3: S490 (Abstract)

Kwong KK, Belliveau JW, Chesler DA, et al. (1992) Dynamic magnetic resonance imaging of human brain activity during primary sensory motor stimulation. Proc Nat Acad Sci USA 89: 5675

Locke JL (1993) The child's path to spoken language. Harvard University, Cambridge, MA

Logan WJ (1998) Functional MRI language localization in children. Abst Cogn Neurosci Soc, p. 127

MacWhinney B, Booth JR, Thulborn KR, et al. (1998) Functional reorganization of activation patterns in children with brain lesions: Whole brain fMRI imaging during three different cognitive tasks. Abstracts of the Annual Meeting of the American Association for the Advancement of Science (Abstract)

Moses P, Martinez A, Roe K, et al. (1997) Functional MR imaging of children's spatial analysis of hierarchical forms. Neuroimage 5: S97 (Abstract)

Ogawa S, Lee TS, Nayak AS, Glynn P (1990) Oxygenation-sensitive contrast in magnetic resonance image of rodent brain at high magnetic fields. Mag Res Med 26: 68–78

Orendi JL, Irwin W, Ward RT, et al. (1997) A fMRI study of cortical activity in children and adults during a spatial working memory task. Neuroimage 5: S603 (Abstract)

Popp CA, Trudeau JD, Durden D et al. (1996) Functional MR imaging in children. Neuroimage 3: S594 (Abstract)

Slifer KJ, Cataldo MF, Cataldo MD, Llorente AM, Gerson AC (1993) Behavior analysis of motion control for pediatric neuroimaging, J Appl Beh Anal 26: 469–470

Truwit CL, Le TH, Hu X, et al. (1996) Functional MR imaging of working memory task activation in children: Preliminary findings. Neuroimage 3: S564 (Abstract)

Turner R, Le Bihan D, Moonen CTW, Despres D, Frank J (1991) Echo-planar time course MRI of cat brain oxygenation changes. Mag Res Med 22: 159–166

Vaidya CJ, Gabrieli JDE, Desmond JE, Glover GH (1998) fMRI of semantic processing in children. Abst Cogn Neurosci Soc, p. 127

Vaidya CJ, Gabrieli JDE, Rypma B, et al. (1997) fMRI of frontal lobe function in children with attention deficit disorder on and off Ritalin. Abst Soc Neurosci 23: 859

Woods RP, Cherry SR, Mazziotta JC (1992) Rapid automated algorithm for aligning and reslicing PET images. J Comp Assist Tomog 16: 620–633

43 Functional MRI in Pharmacology

E.A. Stein, R. Risinger, A.S. Bloom

CONTENTS

E.A. Stein, PhD; R. Risinger, MD; Department of Psychiatry, Medical College of Wisconsin, 8701 W. Watertown Plank Road, Milwaukee, WI 53226, USA
A.S. Bloom, PhD; Department of Pharmacology, Medical College of Wisconsin, 8701 W. Watertown Plank Road, Milwaukee, WI 53226, USA

43.1 Introduction

There is great potential for the use of fMRI in pharmacological research. Currently, the use of pharmacological agents in fMRI experiments has, for the most part, been rather limited. This situation is likely to change in the next several years as more investigators become comfortable with, and cognizant of, the applications and limitations of pharmacology in fMRI. The intrinsic advantages of an imaging method with rapid, noninvasive and massively repeatable measures over lengthy periods lends naturally to studies of CNS drug effects. While other techniques (e.g. flicker fusion, evoked potentials) are able to establish that a given drug compound has CNS activity, they offer no information as to the pathways or neuroanatomical localization of drug effect. Currently, predicting a drug's CNS effect is based primarily upon regional CNS receptor binding and extrapolation from animal models of behavior. Since there has been ample demonstration of mismatches between receptor localization and functional sites of drug action (Herkenham 1987), fMRI fills a gap by directly examining changes in the functioning nervous system.

Neuropharmacological studies can be divided into two principal categories: those that have as their goal to understand the sites and mechanisms of action of a drug (e.g., where does nicotine act in the brain) and those experiments that employ a drug as a tool or probe to better understand the functioning of various brain systems (e.g., the effect of nicotinic activation on working memory). This chapter will review aspects of each approach. Because of the multicausal nature of the fMRI signal, issues of experimental design, data analysis and specific control procedures require special attention over and above the issues in standard, non-pharmacological fMRI experiments.

43.1.1
Advantages of fMRI vs Other Imaging Techniques in Neuropharmacology

Due to its unique properties, fMRI presents numerous advantages over other imaging procedures in the use of drugs to study brain physiology. Conversely, as an indirect marker of neuronal activity, fMRI presents unique challenges for the scientist wishing to combine the use of drugs in their experiments. In addition to knowledge of the drug's mechanisms of action, the physiological and biophysical transduction mechanisms underlying the generation of the functional MR signal must be considered and specific control procedures included in order to make appropriate data interpretations. Data analysis issues also need to be tailored when combining fMRI with pharmacology.

Briefly, positron emission tomography (PET) possesses two main advantages and two disadvantages to the application of pharmacological studies. Perhaps its main strength is its ability to directly address questions regarding the localization of neurotransmitter receptors since one can radiolabel compounds that will specifically bind to receptor subtypes. In addition, with the ability to sample arterial blood tracer concentration, PET can be used to quantify changes in drug-induced metabolic activity using standard physiological measures of blood flow (ml/100 g per min) or glucose metabolism (µmoles/ 100 g per min). In contrast, the relatively poor temporal and spatial resolution limitation of PET, the limited number of times isotopes can be administered to a subject, and great expense restrict the types of experiments and experimental designs available.

Functional MRI, in contrast, has as its main advantages, excellent temporal and spatial resolution and, as no radiotracers are used, the ability to develop within-subjects, longitudinal design protocols. Thus, the interaction of cognitive, sensory or motor tasks with pharmacological manipulation of the CNS becomes more tractable. In addition to its inability to directly observe receptor localization, its main disadvantage is the nature of the complex transduction processes that gives rise to the functional MR signal and the need to control for factors other than drug actions on neurons as the origin of the signal. Each of these issues will be discussed below.

43.1.2
Types of Pharmacological Studies That Can Be Performed Using fMRI

With adequate control procedures (see below), fMRI can be used to answer many of the questions addressed in pharmacological research, specifically, questions of where a particular drug acts within the brain, when its onset of action begins, its magnitude of effect and duration of action. Dose-response issues are also directly addressable. Issues of tolerance (the decreasing action of a drug with repeated administration) and sensitization (an enhanced drug effect following repeated administration) can also be directly studied. Because of the ability to repeatedly study the same individual over many days, weeks or months, experiments can be designed to follow the effects of chronic drug administration on brain function (for example, in the case of a slowly developing therapeutic effect with agents such as antidepressants) or the effects of withdrawal from chronic drug use, as in the case of cigarette smoking cessation.

43.2
Specific Design Issues

Using pharmacological agents in fMRI studies presents numerous unique procedural issues that must be confronted including those of subject safety, experimental design, data collection, analysis and interpretation. Some of these are particular to pharmacological studies; others become exacerbated when using drugs and therefore require greater attention than in non-drug experiments. Perhaps the most obvious source of drug-induced error is head movement. While this problem is certainly not restricted to drug studies, various drugs may exacerbate the problem, notably the administration of stimulants such as nicotine and cocaine. Vigilant quality control examination of time series data sets as well as both active head restraint (e.g., bite bar, restrictive padding) and post-processing image realignment software (Woods et al. 1992) are necessary first-step solutions.

43.2.1
Safety Issues

Experiments performed in an MRI environment are logistically and environmentally complicated. The need to restrict metal from the magnet vicinity and the restricted physical space available to the investigator limits emergency medical treatment possible within the magnet. As such, several procedural steps should be routinely performed to minimize safety concerns. First, all subjects should be carefully screened prior to acceptance into the study, beginning in general with extensive medical histories taken both on the telephone and in person. Careful inclusion/exclusion criteria review and enforcement can obviate many later problems. Depending upon the drug to be administered, a physical exam that includes appropriate urine and blood tests should be performed. Second, key research medical personnel should be ACLS trained and regularly certified. Third, personnel should practice emergency procedures on a regular basis including rapid removal of the subject from the scanner (often requiring the removal of multiple monitoring and projection equipment), followed by life support and code procedure reviews. Perhaps most important, however, is the administration of the drug to the subject prior to scanning in a controlled environment. Our group routinely administers all doses of the drug to be studied to each subject in a hospital bed in the General Clinical Research Center in the presence of a physician, research nurse and crash cart. In the event of an adverse response, appropriate medical treatment can be administered rapidly within the confines of the hospital. Equally important, both the subject and physician get experience with that individual's drug response. For the subject, this leads to less subsequent anxiety in the scanner, while the physician can be better prepared for any adverse effects and can use this opportunity to tailor drug doses when necessary.

43.2.2
Physiological Monitoring

Because drugs always act upon both desired and nontargeted physiological systems and because fMRI is, by definition, an indirect measure of brain activity, it is critical that careful monitoring of relevant physiological systems be performed during scanning. Such "on-line" monitoring of drug action should be performed for several reasons: to insure subject safety (see below), as a possible way to parse data based upon an objective measure of drug effect, and for proper fMRI data interpretation, since observed signal changes may be due not to neuronal activation, but secondary to peripheral, autonomic effects. Arterial blood pressure, heart rate, respiration and end tidal CO_2 should be routinely monitored in pharmacological experiments. If signs of behavioral anxiety are sought, galvanic skin resistance (GSR) and skin temperature are also easily monitored. Finally, several research centers are now also obtaining electroencephalograms during scanning (LEMIEUX et al. 1997). Needless to say, all instruments placed within the scanning room and attached to a subject must be fully MR compatible and care taken that no wire loops be formed that can induce current flow to the subject.

43.2.3
Route of Administration

The goal of most fMRI pharmacology experiments is to determine the effects of a drug on the CNS and/or the effects of the drug upon specific CNS processes. As such, coordinating the scan session with the period when the drug is inducing its maximal or steady state effect is generally desirable. Thus, knowledge of the drug's pharmacodynamics and pharmacokinetics are critical in experimental design. Choice of route of drug administration will depend upon these and other experimental design issues. Specifically, if comparisons are to be made between or across several drug states within subjects, oral administration is generally preferred. For example, a comparison of several medications on task-induced activation in a population of individuals with schizophrenia will probably be performed only after multiple dosings are given to achieve steady state drug levels. However, if the acute time course of the drug (especially a very lipophilic one) is to be studied, it is likely that the IV route will be necessary. Other means to rapidly obtain peak blood levels, e.g. inhalation and insufflation, are less compatible within the fMRI setting due to the difficulty in maintaining head stability. When delivering drugs via the IV route, the injection volume, temperature and, most importantly, the rate of drug administration should be tightly controlled. Various commercial syringe pumps are available and should be used whenever possible to assure constant drug delivery parameters.

43.2.4
Behavioral Ratings

Most drugs used in fMRI experiments will likely cause specific behavioral as well as physiological effects. The magnitude of the effects seen will be dependent upon multiple factors including the route of administration (see above), the dose and rate of administration, the subject's level of tolerance and previous experience with the drug (e.g., cigarette smoking) and, to some extent, the individual's personality and reactivity to the drug's effect (GORDON and GLANTZ 1996). All or some of these factors might alter the neuropharmacological response to the drug and thus the fMRI signal. As such, one means to post-hoc parse data is to group subjects based upon their behavioral and/or physiological responses, rather than the drug dose. Likert scale questionnaires, consisting of a series of questions projected onto a screen visible from within the scanner, may be administered to subjects immediately after each scan session. Questions can be tailored to the drug being studied and may include such constructs as subject "liking," "high," "craving," etc., and can be answered with a joy stick manipulandum.

43.3
Control Procedures

Since the fMRI signal is an indirect measure of neuronal activity, one must always be cognizant of, and control for, other sources of drug-induced signal changes. It is critical to eliminate the possibility that the drug being examined is not altering blood flow (or oxygenation) by acting either directly or indirectly upon the cerebral vasculature independent of neuronal activation. These procedures can be divided into MR controls, physiological controls and behavioral controls and should be carried out in a recursive fashion in parallel with drug administration protocols.

43.3.1
Magnetic Resonance Controls

To help determine drug mechanisms of action and to separate out possible drug-induced vascular or autonomic effects from specific neuronal effects, the use of specialized pulse sequences is recommended to produce fMR signals that are weighted towards blood flow (e.g., FAIR, QUIPPS), oxygenation (e.g., BOLD), small vessel (gradient echo) or large vessel (spin echo) effects (BIRN et al. 1998). Controls for pulsatile motion, flow velocity and blood volume also may be necessary. While complete fMRI transduction mechanisms are still being determined (BANDETTINI and WONG 1995, 1998), the coherence of data from multiple pulse sequences sensitive to different dependent variables adds to the confidence that fMRI data are the result of drug-induced neuronal activation.

43.3.2
Physiological Controls

Drug-induced changes in respiration may alter pCO_2 levels which may, in turn, induce vasodilatation independent of neuronal activity. Such a sequence of events would produce changes in MR signal that do not reflect changes in neuronal activity. Likewise, increases in blood pressure could alter pulsatile motion (notably around sinuses) and blood flow, even transiently, to alter the MR signal (BANDETTINI and WONG 1995). In an attempt to reconcile these issues, we give all subjects (both drug and non-drug control subjects) a brief, 4 min exposure to CO_2 (generally 5%–7%) during the same scan session that the drug is to be given. It is generally accepted that CO_2 will increase flow without appreciably altering neuronal metabolism (MRAOVITCH and SERCOMBE 1996). The resultant MR signal increase should be homogeneously expressed in the brain, temporally linked to the CO_2 inhalation, and rapidly reversed after breathing normal air resumes. In contrast, drug-induced neuronal activation should be manifest with a longer onset and offset latency dependent upon the drug's lipophilicity and metabolism, should be heterogeneously localized and reflect the known chemical neuroanatomy of the brain. Two questions can be addressed in this control procedure: (1) If CO_2 is given in the absence and presence of some task performance (e.g. finger tapping), that individual's capacity to vasodilate to a vascular challenge as well as the "ceiling" response during task-induced activation can be determined. (2) If the procedure is later repeated after the subject has been given the drug, a measure of the capacity of the drug to alter both the tonic resting vascular tone and the physiological transduction processes leading to task-induced vasodilatation can be calculated.

43.3.3
Behavioral Controls

Well controlled animal neuropharmacological studies have suggested that the effect of a drug on neurochemical systems is modified, to a greater or lesser extent, by the behavioral state of the animal (STEWART et al. 1984). For example, the dopamine release pattern in the nucleus accumbens of rats following cocaine administration is dependent upon whether the animal self-administers the drug or whether it is passively delivered by the experimenter (KIYATKIN and STEIN 1995). In humans, drug administration may alter the psychological state of the subject to modulate a number of cognitive neuronal systems (e.g., anxiety) that may, in turn, modulate the effect of the drug. For this reason, all subjects receiving drug in fMRI experiments should be experienced with the effects of the drug prior to scanning. In the case of addictive (e.g., nicotine) and controlled substances (e.g., cocaine, marijuana), all subjects should be experienced drug users, meet the criteria for drug dependence (AMERICAN PSYCHIATRIC ASSOCIATION 1994), and have used the drug by the route of administration relevant to the study. Use of a mock scanner to train subjects in the performance of tasks while recumbent also serves to assure that subject state is relatively normal during the actual scanning experience. Drug pre-exposure within the mock scanner can also be used to establish conditioned place-specific drug effects.

43.4
Analysis of fMRI Signals from Pharmacological Experiments

Traditionally, fMRI studies have examined signal changes occurring between an active and resting state using alternating repetitive presentations of sensory stimuli or cognitive or motor tasks interspersed with either a no stimulus or alternative task period. The most common method to identify regions of brain activation using this presentation format is based upon a cross-correlation statistic calculated against an alternating on/off input function that exactly matches the temporal pattern of each stimulus or task (BANDETTINI et al. 1993) However, the fMRI response to non-alternating events such as a pharmacological challenge has not been widely addressed. What does seem evident is that the use of cross-correlation analysis is inappropriate for most acute drug studies since drug injections and their response input functions tend to be of relatively long duration and thus do not permit rapidly alternating periods of activation and rest. The power of cross-correlation analysis increases with the number of on/off reversals in a data set and requires several epochs for adequate statistical sensitivity (BANDETTINI et al. 1993).

With that in mind, we have developed alternative strategies for the determination of brain activation that results from the administration of pharmacological agents. A drug's pharmacokinetics or the time-related changes in drug concentration within the bloodstream or other compartments of the body are measurable, predictable and known for most commonly used drugs. Similarly, the time course of a drug's physiological actions, such as change in heart rate, can be measured and quantified. As such, an input function based upon the single dose pharmacokinetics and/or pharmacological time course of each drug studied can be used for signal detection.

Several assumptions must be made to merge pharmacokinetics with fMRI signal processing. First, the concentration of a drug in the brain is directly proportional to its concentration in the circulation. This is usually true after an acute administration of lipophilic, short-acting drugs such as nicotine and cocaine. These drugs are ideal prototypes for this type of analysis, since, when administered by the IV route, they have a rapid onset and a relatively short duration of action (HARDMAN et al. 1996). The total time of drug action in a single dose experiment should be within the range of a single fMRI run, generally between 10 and 20 min. With longer acting drugs, such as the cannabinoids and methylphenidate, several sequential imaging runs may need to be concatenated if this method is to be applied.

With IV administration, the pharmacokinetics of these drugs are characterized by a rapid distribution phase during which they distribute throughout the body, including the brain, proportional to the organ's blood flow. Thus brain concentration of drug is thought to reflect blood drug concentration during this early distribution phase. An elimination phase follows during which the drug first leaves the brain by redistribution and/or metabolism and is ultimately metabolized and excreted from the body. For most drugs, the elimination follows first order kinetics characterized by an exponential decline in circulating blood concentrations of the drug. This may not be the case for highly lipophilic drugs such as nicotine. Second, it is hypothesized that brain activity, as reflected by changes in fMRI BOLD signal, is directly and proportionately driven by a drug's concentration at its receptor in the brain. Finally, it is assumed that the drug is acting upon neuronal elements and not indirectly via actions on the cerebral vasculature or upon peripheral cardiovascular variables (see above).

We have developed two signal detection and extraction procedures for the fMRI analysis of drug effects. The first procedure is based upon a binary decision making model in which the waveform in any given voxel must meet all of a set of criteria based upon that drug's pharmacokinetics to be considered activated (BLOOM et al., submitted). The second procedure is based upon a nonlinear fitting of each voxel's fMRI signal waveform to a generalized pharmacokinetic equation with constraints based upon a drug's characteristic pharmacokinetics. Activation decisions are then based upon goodness of fit using an F-test statistic against the null hypothesis of a straight line (WARD et al. 1998).

In the binary decision making model, active voxels are detected using six criteria including time to peak effect, magnitude and statistical significance of peak vs baseline effect, slope of the rising phase of the response curve, time to decline back to 50% of peak and baseline period. The acceptable range for each parameter is determined from both the known pharmacokinetics of each drug and the observed physiological and behavioral effects (Fig. 43.1, Table 43.1). In order to be considered active, a voxel has to meet all criteria. Statistical significance can be determined based upon a probability function derived from a beta distribution of each individuals responses after a saline injection (BLOOM et al., submitted).

An alternative model for the determination of drug-induced changes in fMRI signal is the application of a nonlinear curve fitting method. This method detects an arbitrary signal waveform, in which the user specifies the signal as a function of certain parameters. A nonlinear optimization algorithm is used to find the least squares estimate of these parameters.

A simple model that is commonly used to describe drug levels in a compartment as a function of time, absorption and elimination rate constants (and hypothetically the relative concentration in the brain), is given by the difference of two exponentials:

$$Y_i = k[e^{-\alpha_1(t_1-t_0)} - e^{-\alpha_2(t_1-t_0)}] \qquad (43.1)$$

where Y1 is the response at time t_i, and the model parameters k, t_0, a_1, and a_2 are unknown (and so

Waveform Analysis Protocol

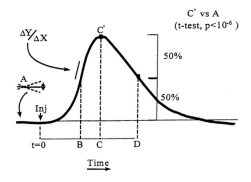

Fig. 43.1. An idealized drug response fMRI waveform based upon our pharmacokinetic binary decision making model. The model requires the input of a limited range of values to define relevant waveform parameters. Specific parameters are defined from both the known pharmacokinetics of the drug and empirically modified following visual inspection of specific waveform characteristics of the data. As an example, the waveform analysis parameters used for IV nicotine are shown in Table 43.1

Table 43.1. Waveform analysis parameters used for IV nicotine[a]

Parameter	Acceptable range
Time to peak response (t=0 to C)	1–8 min after start of injection
Peak response (C)	≥0.5% over baseline
Time for response to decline to 50% of peak (t=0 to D)	4–12 min after injection
Slope of rising phase of response ($\Delta Y/\Delta X$) at time B	0.5–5.0
t test of peak height vs baseline	$p \leq 10^{-6}$
Baseline stability	Range of ≤11% of mean range for all voxels in brain[a]

[a]See Fig. 43.1.

must be estimated). If it is assumed that the above signal is measured in the presence of noise, including a constant offset plus linear trend, then those terms must be added to the model as well. Therefore, the full model would be:

$$Y_i = \gamma_0 + \gamma_1 t_1 + k[e^{-\alpha_1(t_1-t_0)} - e^{-\alpha_2(t_1-t_0)}] + \varepsilon_i \qquad (43.2)$$

where

Y_i= measured time series data (i=1,...,n)
γ_0= constant offset term
γ_1= coefficient of linear trend
k= multiplicative constant
t_0= time delay to drug response
α_1= elimination rate constant
α_2= absorption rate constant
ε_i= Gaussian noise, i.i.d. $N(o, \sigma^2)$

and $u(t)$ is the unit step function: 0, for t≥0, and 1, for t+0. Thus, the full model has six unknown parameters: g_0, g_1, k, t_0, a_1, and a_2.

A constrained, nonlinear optimization to find constants for the least squares estimate for each of the parameters is performed individually for each voxel in the data set. Determining whether the time series for a particular voxel corresponds to a given signal waveform can be expressed in terms of a statistical hypothesis test. The null hypothesis is: H_0: time series is "noise". The alternative hypothesis is: H_a: time series is "signal+noise." Using the above drug response model, the hypothesis can be expressed as:

$$H_0: Y_i = \beta_0 + \beta_1 t_i + \varepsilon_i \qquad (43.3)$$

$$H_a: Y_i = \gamma_0 + \gamma_1 t_i + k[e^{-\alpha_1(t_i-t_0)} - e^{-\alpha_2(t_i-t_0)}]u(t_i - t_0) + \varepsilon_i \qquad (43.4)$$

A test of the null hypothesis is made by first determining the parameters which yield the least squares fit for the noise model (also called the reduced model) and the parameters which yield the least squares fit for the signal+noise model (also called the full model). One can reject the null hypothesis if the error sum of squares from fitting the full model [SSE(F)] is much less than the error sum of squares from fitting the reduced model [SSE(R)]. However, if SSE(F) is only slightly smaller than SSE(R), than we do not have reason to reject the null hypothesis. Consider the test statistic F^{**}:

$$F^{**} = \frac{MS(\text{Regression})}{MS(\text{Error})} = \frac{\dfrac{SSE(R) - SSE(F)}{df_R - df_F}}{\dfrac{SSE(F)}{df_F}} \qquad (43.5)$$

where df_R is the number of degrees of freedom for the reduced model, and df_F is the number of degrees of freedom for the full model.

By the above reasoning, a large value for F^{**} indicates that the described signal is present, whereas a small value for F^{**} suggests that only noise is present. For large sample size n, the statistic F^{**} has an approximate F(df_R–df_F, df_F distribution) under the null hypothesis. The F^{**} statistic for each voxel is calculated and used to determine activation under this model.

Functional images are generated by applying criteria for either the binary decision model or the nonlinear curve fitting method to each voxel and overlaying the activate d voxels upon high resolution 3D Spoiled GRASS (gradient recalled at steady state) images. Nearest neighbor pixel analysis can be applied to preclude isolated pixel recognition. Transformation of each subject's data into stereotaxic space and averaging across subjects allows the production of mean activation maps that can be displayed using AFNI (Cox 1996) or other 3D display programs. A cluster analysis is typically used to distinguish regions of interest with a volume of tissue minimum (i.e. 150 µl) based upon acceptable false positive rates. Clusters below this size can be ignored. For example, in the case of IV nicotine (see below), less than 3% of the voxels in the brain met the criteria for nicotine activation after saline injection, and in the mean activation maps, no clusters of 150 µl or greater were formed. This indicates a very low probability of a false positive using this method of waveform analysis.

43.5
Specific fMRI Pharmacological Research Examples

43.5.1
Effects of IV Cocaine

In a study of the acute effects of cocaine-induced changes in fMRI signal, BREITER et al. (1997) administered 0.6 mg/kg cocaine IV in cocaine-dependent subjects. Whole brain fMRI were acquired for 5 min before and 13 min after infusion while subjects rated the "rush" "high" "low" and "craving". Regions of activation and deactivation were identified using nonparametric Kolmogorov-Smirnov statistical maps comparing pre and post-drug periods. Cocaine infusion was associated with robust increases in nucleus accumbens/subcallosal cortex, insula, cingulate gyrus and parahippocampal gyrus in at least eight of ten subjects. Decreases in BOLD signal following cocaine infusion were found in temporal pole and medial frontal cortex and were similarly consistent across a majority of subjects. Several subjects underwent repeat studies and showed good replication of the regional activation pattern following cocaine and saline infusions. Multiple correlation of signal time series in these regions with averaged subjective ratings suggested that subjective euphoria correlated with short duration, focal BOLD signal increases in putative brain reward pathways (ventral tegmentum, nucleus accumbens) as well as basal forebrain, caudate, insula, cingulate and prefrontal cortex.

43.5.2
Dose-Response Effects of IV Cocaine

Taking a somewhat different approach, we (STEIN et al. 1995) are performing a dose-response study, administering IV saline and three doses of cocaine (10, 20 and 40 mg/70 kg) every 30 min in an ascending order. Eight subjects have been tested to date. During the drug run-up, transient, dose-dependent increases in mean arterial blood pressure (MAP) and heart rate were seen following cocaine administration. Subjects generally reported minimal to no subjective effects following the low dose, slight to mild sensations after the medium dose, and a definite rush and high after the 40 mg dose. Preliminary fMRI analysis using the waveform analysis program described above revealed cerebral activation in several brain regions including the dorsolateral, inferior and medial frontal gyri, insular and cingulate gyri. (Fig. 43.2)

43.5.3
Dose-Response Effects of IV Nicotine

After alcohol, nicotine is the second most commonly psychoactive substance abused by humans (JAFFE 1990). However the sites and mechanisms underlying its dependence-producing properties in the human brain are not well understood. As such, we administered IV saline and three doses of nicotine (0.75, 1.5 and 2.25 mg) in a population of dependent smokers while acquiring BOLD fMRI (STEIN et al. 1998). Subjects generally reported positive subjective effects after nicotine injection. Plasma nicotine levels peaked at 2 min after administration and decreased to about two thirds of peak at 15 min.

Drug-induced changes in fMRI signal were extracted using the binary decision algorithm described above. Representative, single time course fMRI data from one subject are shown in Fig. 43.3 and a composite map of the 2.25 mg dose from all subjects is displayed in Fig. 43.4. Activation was seen in several brain areas including insula, cingulate, frontal lobe (orbital, dorsolateral and medial) and portions of the temporal and visual cortex. A number of limbic subcortical regions were also activated including the nucleus accumbens, amygdala, hypothalamus and limbic thalamus. Comparable with measured plasma nicotine levels, the average peak fMRI signal intensity increased above pre-drug baseline levels between 2.5 and 3 min after nicotine injection, and returned back to 50% of baseline at 4.6 min after the peak. These data suggest that nicotine produces a regionally selective increase in brain ac-

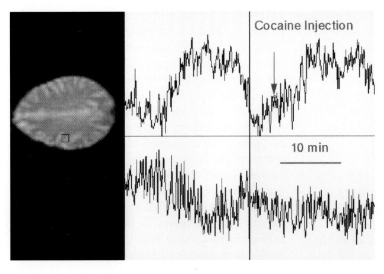

Fig. 43.2. Functional MRI waveforms recorded from a region of the left parietal lobe following a single 20 mg injection of cocaine in one subject. The *red arrow* indicates time of injection. Note the time course of pixel activation and the distinct patterns seen in adjacent pixels (the total displayed area is 11.25 mm² as depicted in the *box* on the accompanying first shot echo-planar image)

Fig. 43.3. Single subject fMRI waveforms recorded following a single 1.5 mg iv injection of nicotine. Illustrated superimposed upon the T1-weighted, fast spin echo anatomic image is a map of all nicotine activated voxels (*white boxes*) from that brain slice. The *box* outlined in the anterior cingulate denotes the 2×2 voxel region of interest corresponding to the time course data shown on the right

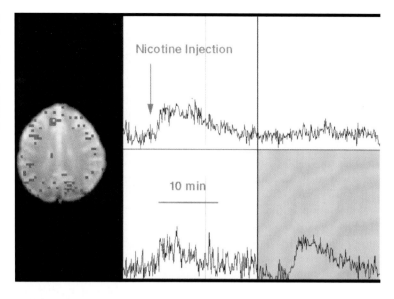

Fig. 43.4. Grouped fMRI activation data from all subjects given 2.25 mg nicotine superimposed upon a single anatomical data set placed into stereotaxic coordinates. Orthogonal views are linked by the *blue cross-hairs*. Note the statistically significant activation in the anterior cingulate, dorsolateral frontal, insular and posterior orbital gyri

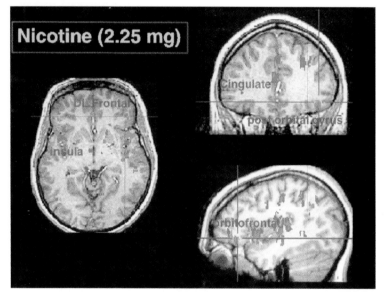

tivity that is temporally consistent with the observed behavioral actions of the drug. Data from this and the above cocaine experiments demonstrate the effectiveness of fMRI and the described waveform recognition algorithm in studying drug effects in the human brain.

43.5.4
Cognitive Task-Induced Brain Activation During Nicotine Withdrawal

Chronic use of nicotine products such as cigarettes produces physiological and/or psychological dependence. Smoking cessation is associated with a withdrawal syndrome consisting of alterations in mood along with an impairment of attention and cognitive performance. To better understand the biological substrates of nicotine dependence, we have examined the time course of nicotine withdrawal effects on brain activation induced by cognitive tasks using fMRI. Smokers performed three cognitive tasks: (1) a delayed match to sample-DMTS-working memory (JONIDES et al. 1993), (2) a visuospatial working memory (VSWM) (COHEN et al. 1993) and (3) a concept formation (CF) task (RAO et al. 1997) while undergoing whole brain fMRI scanning. Scanning was performed prior to smoking cessation and at 1 day, 1 week and 3 weeks of abstinence. An age matched nonsmoking control group was also studied using the same experimental schedule.

There was a significant decrease ($p<0.01$) in performance (73% vs 93% accuracy) on the CF task between the two groups. While there were no significant differences in the performance on the two spatial working memory tasks between the groups, the cognitive demands of these tasks appear to be less than for the CF task. Activation by the VSWM and CF tasks was very consistent over time in the nonsmoking control group. The VSWM task produced bilateral activation in the dorsolateral prefrontal cortex (DLF), primary motor, premotor and supplemental motor areas (SMA). Posterior parietal and occipital lobes were also strongly activated. Preliminary data analyses in smokers suggest a decrease in brain activation, even prior to nicotine withdrawal (day 0). Activation of the left DLF was minimal and decreases were seen in other areas. As nicotine withdrawal progressed, activation in left DLF did not increase, while posterior parietal activation increased.

The CF taskinduced bilateral activation in DLF, motor, premotor and SMA areas, superior frontal gyrus, posterior parietal and occipital lobes in the control group. Activation also occurred in thalamus and left insular cortex. Again, activation was very stable over repeated sessions. In agreement with the VSWM task, the total extent of activation in smokers was decreased when compared to controls prior to nicotine withdrawal (day 0). DLF activation was still decreased during withdrawal as was posterior parietal and occipital lobe activation (Fig 43.5).

These data suggest that chronic nicotine use and smoking cessation produce major changes in brain activation induced by the performance of two cogni-

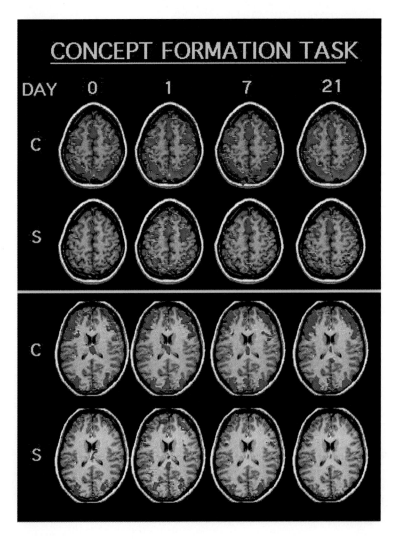

Fig. 43.5. Grouped fMRI activation data from both control (*c*) subjects and smokers (*s*) taken after performing the concept formation task and illustrated at two axial levels. Data are superimposed upon a single subjects grouped anatomical data set placed into stereotaxic coordinates and were acquired on four separate occasions: during a baseline period while smokers were still using cigarettes (day 0), and following 17 and 21 days of withdrawal. Control subjects were scanned at comparable intervals. Note the intragroup activation reproducibility in the control subjects over the four scan sessions. Also note the similar activation pattern, but reduced areas of activation, in the smoker group both at baseline and during withdrawal. Data were derived from a 2way 3-D ANOVA of group x days (subjects nested) and threshold at p ≤ 0.01

tive tasks when compared to nonsmoking controls. Effects of the CF tasks were more profound and persistent than on the VSWM task. Nicotine use is known to effect activation in brain regions associated with memory, attention and choice behavior, suggesting cholinergic involvement in these processes. These data suggest that chronic nicotine intake produces long lasting changes in these regions. Finally, this study demonstrates the feasibility of using fMRI to study the effects of chronic drug use and cessation of drug use over extended periods of time.

43.6
Use of fMRI in Drug Discovery

Currently, modern imaging methods play a limited role in the pharmaceutical discovery process. However, the utility of fMRI suggests that its role will increase in the near term, since the capability of within-subject repeated measures over a short time offers unique advantages – both in terms of individually adjusting doses to achieve specific pharmacological effects and in monitoring long term neurocognitive effects. Importantly, the insights gained from fMRI pharmacological studies may be obtainable with populations of individuals much smaller than traditionally used in drug discovery. Below are presented some ways in which fMRI may impact drug discovery.

43.6.1
Determining the Site of Drug Activity

Where a potential pharmacological agent acts in the human nervous system can be readily determined by the use of fMRI as demonstrated above with nicotine and cocaine. Such localization of action is important to both better characterize the desired actions of a new drug as well as anticipate potential undesirable, cognitive-behavioral side effects. Given appropriate biophysical controls, design and analysis consideration (see above), fMRI may prove to be useful in establishing a minimal dose capable of inducing regional CNS changes – a dose that is potentially far different from that predicted from CNS kinetic studies. As brain mapping advances our understanding of the modular cognitive systems involved in a given behavior, knowledge of regional activity changes with drug challenge will enable a more precise determination (and potential prediction) of the cognitive effects of a drug based upon the overlap of pharmacologically activated brain regions with imputed cognitive functional regions. Thus determining regional activity changes associated with a drug may enable a more precise assessment of its cognitive-behavioral effects.

Inter-individual variability plagues all neuroimaging techniques, and fMRI is no exception. The ability, however, to perform repeated measures within the same individual offers unique advantages to other types of pharmacological studies. FMRI's spatial and temporal resolution can be exploited for the purpose of better characterizing individual drug response variability. Individual differences in time of onset, extent or degree of change in regional activations can be characterized. Pharmacological studies can be designed as single individual trials correlating onset of behavioral changes (e.g., tremor, nausea, etc.) with regional activation (e.g., basal ganglia or brainstem activation) within each subject.

43.6.2
Relative Drug Effects, Comparative Agonist-Antagonist Studies

Comparing regional fMRI activation patterns between two agents with similar in vitro binding or behavioral pharmacological profiles may predict novel clinical effects for the new compound. Conversely, dose-ranging of antagonist effects can be tested in agonist-reversal paradigms to determine doses required to achieve a given regional neuronal effect (e.g., a partial agonist-antagonist anticipated to be useful in blocking drug withdrawal). Similarly, since receptor down-regulation and other neural adaptations to chronic drug administration can occur rapidly (over minutes to hours), characterizing the time-course of the fMRI neural response may be useful to more directly relate drug plasma concentration to desired neurobehavioral effect(s).

Hypothesized differences in neuronal activation patterns between drugs with similar receptor binding profiles have proven difficult to demonstrate given the limitations of radionuclide-based neuroimaging techniques (Nyberg et al. 1996; Volkow et al. 1996). Of note is the current plethora of novel antipsychotic compounds available clinically and at various stages of development. Development of these compounds followed the clinical success of clozapine, a drug with a broad receptor binding profile. The new generation of antipsychotic drugs is distinguishable by subtle variations in receptor specificity across a range of receptors. Aside from unwanted side-effects, differentiating these drugs in terms of clinical efficacy has proven difficult. By merging modern cognitive neuroscience with fMRI, unique insight into the neuropharmacological modulation of cognition by these and other agents may provide not only better matching of drug to patient, but also additional new knowledge of the neurochemical anatomy of human cognition.

43.6.3
Regional Differences in Drug Tolerance/Sensitization and Withdrawal

An area of pharmaceutical development that can be difficult to document is the potential for, and extent of, drug tolerance. Simply defined, tolerance is the requirement for higher doses of drug to be administered over time in order to achieve the same pharmacological effect. fMRI may help characterize the time course and localization of neuronal changes that occur during the development of tolerance by examining changes during long term, repeated drug administration. For example, alterations in regional signal change localization may correlate with the development of tolerance to drug-induced side effects. Similarly, the degree or extent of neural activation in prefrontal cortex after cessation of drug treatment may correlate with cognitive impairments during withdrawal.

43.6.4
Real-Time Neuropharmacological Effects

Drugs under consideration for clinical development are frequently radiolabeled with positron emitters to determine CNS kinetics (i.e., binding, uptake and half-life). Although these studies yield regional binding density and speak to the process of drug delivery, they do not produce a functional profile of drug action. The exception to this is dopamine reuptake studies, which presumably yield information on the relative ability of agents to alter synaptic transmitter reuptake. However, PET imaging lacks the spatial and temporal sensitivity to determine time course of these changes anywhere but basal ganglia. Since dosimetry guidelines limits the total number of acquisition sessions, PET does not allow a complete sampling of the full time course of effects within an individual. This is important since acute receptor occupancy does not necessarily predict al-

tered biological function (e.g., psychotropic agents are generally behaviorally effective only after semichronic intake, whereas receptors become bound virtually immediately). Given the multiplicity of positive and negative feedback circuits for any neural system, altering activity in one area may effect neural function many synapses away. The net effect of these countermining processes may be differentially affected by both drug concentration and secondary effects over time. fMRI may thus afford unique insight into both functional alteration and time course of drug effects that may be useful in drug development.

43.6.5
Clinical Utility

As knowledge of the functional neuroanatomical substrates of normal CNS processes and disease states progresses, the need to monitor and individualize therapeutic interventions will grow. In addition to the long term monitoring of drug-induced pathological processes (e.g., the development of neuroleptic-induced motor dysfunction), if core symptoms of an illness or representative pathways can be captured utilizing a standardized paradigm, clinicians may be able to rapidly assess if a given agent will be effective for an individual, thus saving days, weeks or months of morbidity. Rapidly selecting agents, a range of doses, or combinations of agents with desired effects, based upon direct measurement of CNS activity (rather than a more diffuse behavioral end point), may enable a more rapid relief of suffering and more certainty of therapeutic effect. In the case of medications that possess a narrow therapeutic window, dose ranging studies to prevent undesirable effects are similarly possible, e.g., selecting the dose range over which cognition (task performance) improves while not altering neural activity in remote brain regions.

fMRI may also prove useful for monitoring CNS changes following chronic drug administration. After patients are stabilized on a psychotropic regimen, the function of specific regions may be observed using standard neuropsychiatric tests. For example, after years of treatment with typical antipsychotics, the development of movement disorder symptoms is common and felt to be due to the chronic effects of drug on basal ganglia (BARRIO et al. 1997; ELKASHEF et al. 1994). Monitoring basal ganglia activity in response to a standard task may help to identify subjects prone to develop or actually developing parkinsonian or other movement disorder symptoms.

43.7
Summary

Functional MRI, as a still emerging tool, has been applied to a wide range of questions in sensory, motor control and cognitive psychology. This chapter has presented evidence that it may also be useful in helping to understand the sites and mechanisms of action of pharmacological agents within the human CNS. However, in so doing, a new set of problems and concerns surrounding the technique arises because of the unique transduction mechanisms (both physiological and biophysical) that exist to produce the fMRI signal from the underlying neuronal activity. Experimental design and control issues become paramount in designing fMRI pharmacology protocols and in signal interpretation. With these caveats, the use of pharmacological agents with fMRI is likely to greatly increase in the near term as new questions about both brain physiology and neuropharmacological mechanisms become addressable for the first time.

Acknowledgements. Supported by USPHS grants DA09465 (EAS) and GCRC 5M01 RR00058

References

American Psychiatric Association (1994) DSM-IV. Diagnostic and statistical manual of mental disorders, 4th edn. American Psychiatric Association, Washington DC

Bandettini PA, Wong EC (1995) The effects of biophysical and physiological parameters on brain activation-induced DR2* and DR2 changes: simulations using a deterministic diffusion model. Int J Imaging Syst Technol 6:133-152

Bandettini PA, Wong EC (1998) Echo planar magnetic resonance imaging of human brain activation. In: Schmitt F, Stehling MK, Turner R (eds) Echo-planar imaging. Springer, Berlin Heidelberg New York

Bandettini PA, Jesmanowicz A, Wong EC, Hyde JS (1993) Processing strategies for time-course data sets in functional MRI of the human brain. Magn Reson Med 30:161-173

Barrio JR, Huang SC, Phelps ME (1997) Biological imaging and the molecular basis of dopaminergic diseases. Biochem Pharmacol 54:341-348

Birn RM, Donahue KM, Bandettini PA (1998) Magnetic resonance imaging: principles, pulse sequences and functional imaging. In: Hendee WH (ed) Biomedical uses of radiation. Wiley-VCH, Weinheim Germany

Bloom AS, Hoffmann RG, Fuller SA et al An activation detection algorithm for drug-induced changes in functional MRI signal using a pharmacokinetic model (submitted)

Breiter HC, Gollub RL, Weisskoff RM et al (1997) Acute effects of cocaine on human brain activity and emotion. Neuron 19:591-611

Cohen JD, Forman S, Casey BJ, Servan-Schreiber D, Noll DC, Lewis DA (1993) Activation of dorsolateral prefrontal cortex in humans during a working memory task using functional MRI. Neurosci Abstr 19:1285

Cox RW (1996) AFNI: software for analysis and visualization of functional magnetic resonance neuroimages. Comput Biomed Res 29:162-173

Elkashef AM, Buchanan RW, Gellad F, Munson RC, Breier A (1994) Basal ganglia pathology in schizophrenia and tardive dyskinesia: an MRI quantitative study. Am J Psychiatry 151:752-725

Gordon HW, Glantz MD (eds) (1996) Individual differences in the biobehavioral etiology of drug abuse. National Institutes on Drug Abuse. NIH Publication no 96-4034 (NIDA research monograph, vol 159)

Hardman JG, Limbird LE, Molinoff PB, Ruddon RW, Gilman AG (eds) (1996) The pharmacological basis of therapeutics, 9th edn. McGraw-Hill, New York

Herkenham M (1987) Mismatches between neurotransmitter and receptor localizations in brain: observations and implications. Neuroscience 23:1-28

Jaffe J (1990) Tobacco smoking and nicotine dependence. In: Wonnacott S, Russell MAH, Stolerman IP (eds) Nicotine psychopharmacology: molecular, cellular and behavioral aspects. Oxford University Press, Oxford

Jonides J, Smith EE, Koeppe RA, Awh E, Minoshima S, Mintun MA (1993) Spatial working memory in humans as revealed by PET. Nature 363:623-625

Kiyatkin EA, Stein EA (1995) Fluctuations in nucleus accumbens dopamine during cocaine self-administration behavior: an in vivo electrochemical study. Neuroscience 64:599-617

Lemieux L, Allen PJ, Franconi F, Symms MR, Fish DR (1997) Recording of EEG during fMRI experiments: patient safety. Magn Reson Med 38:943-952

Mraovitch S, Sercombe R (1996) Neurophysiological basis of cerebral blood flow control: an introduction. Libbey, London

Nyberg S, Nakashima Y, Nordstrom AL, Halldin C, Farde L (1996) Positron emission tomography of in-vivo binding characteristics of atypical antipsychotic drugs. Review of D2 and 5-HT2 receptor occupancy studies and clinical response. Br J Psychiatry [Suppl] 29:40-44

Rao SM, Bobholz JA, Hammeke TA et al (1997) Functional MRI evidence for subcortical participation in conceptual reasoning skills. Neuroreport 8:1987-1993

Stein EA, Pankiewicz J, Harsch HH et al (1995) Cocaine- induced alterations of brain activity in humans: An fMRI study. Neurosci Abstr 21:1956

Stein EA, Pankiewicz J, Harsch HH et al (1998) Nicotine-induced limbic cortical activation in the human brain: a functional MRI study. American J. Psychiatry 155:1009-1015

Stewart J, deWit H, Eikelboom R (1984) Role of unconditioned and conditioned drug effects in the self-administration of opiates and stimulants. Psychol Rev 91:251-268

Volkow ND, Fowler JS, Gatley SJ, Logan J, Wang GJ, Ding YS, Dewey S (1996) PET evaluation of the dopamine system of the human brain. J Nucl Medi 37:1242-1256

Ward BD, Garavan H, Ross TJ, Bloom AS, Cox RW, Stein EA (1998) Nonlinear regression for FMRI time series analysis. Neuroimage 7, S767

Woods RP, Cherry SR, Mazziota JC (1992) Rapid automated algorithm for aligning and reslicing PET images. J Comput Assist Tomogr 16:620–633

44 The Role of Functional MRI in Planning Perirolandic Surgery

C.R. Jack, Jr., C.C. Lee, H.A. Ward, S.J. Riederer

CONTENTS

44.1
Introduction

The goal of neurosurgical resection of brain pathology is complete removal of the abnormality. This is only feasible, however, when the proposed margin of the surgical resection does not violate functionally eloquent cortical areas. Mapping of cortical function for the purpose of surgical planning is generally considered in the context of neuro-oncologic or resective epilepsy procedures. Traditional invasive methods for localizing functionally eloquent cortical areas include intraoperative cortical stimulation in the awake patient, implantation of subdural grids with extraoperative stimulation mapping, or operative sensory evoked potential recording (Berger et al. 1990; Gregorie and Goldring 1984; Ojemann et al. 1993; Skirboll et al. 1996; Woolsey et al.

C.R. Jack, Jr., MD; C.C. Lee, PhD; H.A. Ward, B.A.; S.J. Riederer, PhD; Department of Diagnostic Radiology and MR Research Laboratory, 200 First Street SW, Mayo Clinic and Foundation, Rochester, MN 55905, USA

1979). While accurate, a major disadvantage of these approaches is that a surgical procedure itself is required before any functional information can be obtained. As a result, important patient management decisions must be made without complete knowledge of the anatomic relationship between the lesion borders and functionally eloquent cortex. Conversely, with functional magnetic resonance imaging (fMRI) functional information is acquired preoperatively, and as a result, knowledge of the precise anatomic relationship between functionally eloquent tissue and a proposed surgical target can be incorporated into preoperative clinical decision making and surgical planning.

44.2
Functional Neuroanatomy of the Perirolandic Region

The term perirolandic refers to that region of the brain which encompasses the central sulcus. Primary motor function is located in Brodman's area 4 – the pre-central gyrus (Fig. 44.1). Primary somatosensory function is located in Brodman's areas 3, 2, and 1 – the post-central gyrus. These two gyri are separated by the central sulcus. Classically, the anterior bank of the central sulcus contains motor neurons, while the posterior bank of the central sulcus contains sensory neurons (Blume 1993). More detailed electrophysiologic recording studies, however, reveal that anatomic demarcation of motor from sensory function is often not rigorously defined by the central sulcus (Cedzich et al. 1996; Lehman 1994; Riddle and Purves 1995; Uematsu et al. 1992a,b). The pre- and post-central gyri are functionally organized according to a somatopic homunculus (Penfield and Rasmussen 1950; Fig. 44.2). While considerable inter-individual variation exists in the exact proportions of the motor and sensory homunculi, in general, the lower extremity is located on the medial surface and the vertex of the hemi-

...

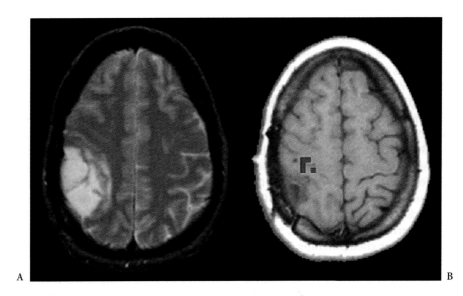

A   B

Fig. 44.5A,B. Risk-benefit assessment – tumor surgery. This 40-year-old woman experienced a single convulsive seizure, and an imaging study revealed a tumor near the central sulcus region which by imaging criteria was most likely a medium to low grade glioma. The patient wished to have the tumor excised as completely as possible, but was neurologically intact and unwilling to accept any surgically induced functional deficit. **A** T2-weighted image illustrating the tumor. **B** fMRI activation map superimposed on a T1-weighted anatomic image. Activation pixels are located in the central sulcus. The tumor therefore abutted the posterior margin of the post-central gyrus. The patient elected to proceed with the surgery only after this preoperative fMRI study demonstrated that the sensorimotor functional area was at the periphery, and not inside the margins of gross visible tumor. Results of the fMRI study were validated with intraoperative cortical stimulation mapping

Finally, with regard to planning the surgical procedure itself, if a proposed surgical resection is felt preoperatively to place the primary motor area at risk, then an invasive operative mapping procedure is generally done. This is either accomplished with cortical stimulation mapping in the awake patient, or operative sensory evoked potential recording. If on the other hand, the position of the tumor is a sufficient distance from the primary sensorimotor area, then operative functional mapping is not necessary. fMRI can help in selecting appropriate candidates for intraoperative functional mapping because the precise functional-anatomic relationship of interest can be ascertained extraoperatively.

44.4
The Role of fMRI in Perirolandic Epilepsy Surgery

Epilepsy surgery differs from tumor surgery in several ways (JACK 1993, 1995). First, epilepsy is not a life threatening condition, and this must be factored into the therapeutic decision making process when

assessing the risk benefit ratio of different therapeutic options. While in tumor surgery the potential benefit to the patient may be prolongation of life, in epilepsy surgery the potential benefit to the patient is an improvement in the quality of life that results from eliminating or reducing seizure frequency. In this sense epilepsy surgery may be viewed as an elective rather than a necessary procedure, and patients may be less willing to accept the risk of surgical morbidity when undergoing epilepsy surgery than when undergoing resection of a malignant brain tumor. Epilepsy surgery also differs from tumor surgery in that epilepsy is fundamentally an electrophysiologic not a histologic abnormality. While perirolandic epilepsy is often associated with a focal structure lesion, this need not be the case. The objective in epilepsy surgery is to resect the epileptogenic zone, which is defined as that area of cortex whose resection is both necessary and sufficient to eliminate the seizure disorder.

As is the case with tumor surgery, several important management decisions must be made for a patient with a medically intractable seizure disorder with the site of onset in or near the primary sensorimotor area. These are:

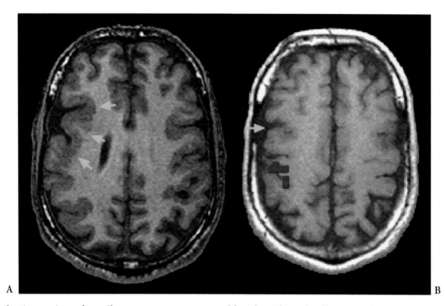

Fig. 44.6A,B. Selecting patients for epilepsy surgery. A 27-year-old male with medically intractable epilepsy. Ictal EEG recordings revealed that a right frontal cortical dysplasia (*arrows* in **A**) was the site of seizure onset. Partial resection of cortical dysplasia typically does not result in seizure relief. Therefore, the patient would be a surgical candidate only if the functional sensorimotor area was separated from the anatomic margins of the cortical dysplasia thus allowing complete resection. **B** An fMRI study was performed to determine the relationship between the cortical dysplasia and the functional sensorimotor hand area. The fMRI study revealed that the most inferior extent of the functional hand area was separate from the posterosuperior margin of the cortical dysplasia (*arrow*). The patient elected to proceed with resective surgery. After the immediate postoperative period, the patient has had no further seizures and suffered no surgical morbidity. Results of the fMRI findings were confirmed by intraoperative evoked potential recording

1. Is the patient a surgical candidate?
2. If so, which surgical procedure will produce the best outcome?
3. Does the patient require invasive EEG mapping?
4. Should intraoperative functional mapping be performed?

fMRI can play a useful clinical role in appropriately selecting patients for resective perirolandic epilepsy surgery if a structural epileptogenic lesion such as an area of cortical dysplasia or one of the biologically indolent tumors commonly associated with epilepsy is present. As with tumor surgery, a critical piece of information which determines the ultimate safety of any resective procedure is the anatomic relationship between proposed surgical target and the functional sensorimotor area. fMRI is uniquely capable of providing this information preoperatively and hence influencing this important patient management decision. If an fMRI study demonstrates that the primary sensorimotor area is located at a "safe" distance from the lesion, then the probability of a seizure free outcome with no surgical morbidity is fairly good. In such a scenario the results of the fMRI study may well influence the patient to pursue surgery (Fig. 44.6). However, if an

fMRI study demonstrates that the epileptogenic lesion directly involves the primary sensorimotor area, then the likelihood of surgical morbidity is substantially greater. In this scenario the potential benefit of seizure relief would be overshadowed by the risk of a contralateral hemiparesis and the patient might decide to forego surgery entirely and live with his/her seizure disorder.

With regard to selecting the appropriate surgical procedure several options exist for surgical treatment of patients with intractable focal seizure disorders due to epileptogenic lesions in or near the primary sensorimotor area. The most common type of surgery by far is focal cortical resection. Several variants of focal cortical resection exist. The area or volume of tissue which is resected can be limited to the lesion itself and this is commonly referred to as a lesionectomy. The lesion plus a variable amount of surrounding "normal" cortical tissue may be resected. This is sometimes referred to as a "lesionectomy plus." If an epileptogenic lesion does not involve the primary sensorimotor area, then it may be resected in its entirety. If on the other hand, the epileptogenic lesion does involve the primary sensorimotor area, then a cortical resection of this tissue is generally precluded. An al-

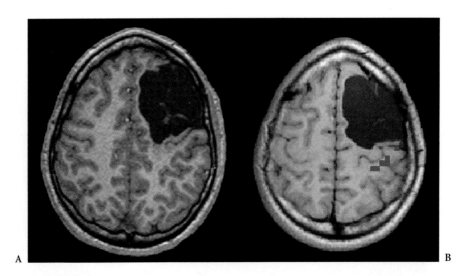

A   B

Fig. 44.7. fMRI used to guide placement of subdural EEG recording strips. An 18-year-old male with a life-long medically intractable seizure disorder likely due to a perinatal hemorrhage. The patient had a spastic right hemiparesis, but had retained some right-hand function. Due to the perceived proximity of the left frontal encephalomalacic cyst (**A**) to the anatomic central sulcus, and the fact that the injury occurred in the perinatal period, the possibility of functional cortical reorganization was raised. Scalp EEG recordings revealed the site of seizure onset to be near the posterior margin of the encephalomalacic cyst. An fMRI study was performed (**B**) to clarify the relationship between the epileptogenic zone and the functional sensorimotor area. The fMRI study (**B**) revealed that the functional sensorimotor area was located along the posterior margin of the encephalomalacic cyst. A series of subdural strips were implanted and these extraoperative recordings revealed that the epileptogenic zone of cortex was located adjacent to, but clearly demarcated from, the functional hand area. A resection of the epileptogenic zone was carried out and the patient has been seizure free postoperatively

ternative procedure in this case is a subpial transection. Subpial transection involves making a series of cross-hatched cuts through the full thickness of the cortex. This has been proposed as a way stop the spread of seizures out of the epileptogenic zone without inducing significant surgical morbidity. fMRI can help guide the selection among these various surgical options. For example, if an epileptogenic lesion is demonstrated to be some distance from the functional sensorimotor area, a lesionectomy, or lesionectomy plus may be pursued without fear of surgical morbidity (Fig. 44.6). However, if the fMRI study were to demonstrate direct involvement of the primary sensorimotor area by an epileptogenic lesion then the most prudent surgical option might be a subpial transection.

Many, but not all, patients with perirolandic focal onset seizure disorders who are being evaluated as surgical candidates undergo some form of prolonged invasive cortical mapping. This is accomplished by surgically placing either a grid or several recording strips on the surface of the brain and then recording the patient's spontaneous seizures over the ensuing few days. This enables the epileptologist to map out on the surface of the brain the precise extent of the epileptogenic zone, and with the same implanted grid functional cortical stimulation mapping can be performed extraoperatively. fMRI may play a useful clinical role in helping to determine whether invasive EEG monitoring with or without extraoperative stimulation mapping is necessary. If it can be demonstrated on a preoperative fMRI study that the functional sensorimotor area is a safe distance from an epileptogenic lesion, then the surgeon and epileptologist may forgo invasive EEG monitoring. Conversely, if the suspected epileptogenic zone is close to the functional sensorimotor area, then grid implantation with EEG recording and extraoperative function stimulation mapping would be prudent (Fig. 44.7). This is not a trivial issue. Invasive EEG monitoring carries with it the risks of subdural hemorrhage or infection. Also, invasive EEG monitoring can be quite expensive, with costs ranging from $20,000–$50,000 for the surgical implantation and removal, and the EEG monitoring.

Finally, for every epilepsy patient who is operated on in the primary sensorimotor area, the decision must be made whether or not to perform intraoperative functional cortical mapping. Performing cortical stimulation mapping in the awake patient intraoperatively is a fairly straightforward procedure which can be accomplished quickly and provides the surgeon with an accurate intraoperative "road map." For this reason, it is highly doubtful that fMRI will replace direct cortical stimulation mapping in the operating room. However, if it can be demonstrated on a preoperative fMRI study that the surgical target is sufficiently distant from the functional sensorimotor area, then the surgeon may elect not to perform intraoperative cortical stimulation mapping, thus saving the time and expense associated with this procedure.

44.5
Is Functional Mapping of the Central Sulcus Necessary?

The central sulcus separates the pre-central gyrus from the post-central gyrus. Brodman's area 4 (primary motor) occupies the anterior bank of the central sulcus while Brodman's areas 3, 2, and 1 (primary sensory) occupy the posterior bank of the central sulcus (Fig. 44.1). Anatomic criteria based on cross-sectional imaging studies are quite accurate in identifying the central sulcus in normal individuals. On axial MR images several highly reliable criteria can be used to locate the superior portion of the central sulcus where hand function typically resides (BERGER et al. 1990; IWASAKI et al. 1991; RUMEAU et al. 1994; SOBEL et al. 1993; YOUSRY et al. 1997). These are:

1. The paracentral lobule caps the medial extent of the central sulcus.
2. The medullary branching pattern in axial sections through the vertex of the brain is characteristic with the post-central gyrus forming the first medullary branch anterior to the superior parietal lobule.
3. A distinct "knuckle" is present in the superior portion of the central sulcus which represents its superior genu.

Similar criteria have been developed for identifying the inferior portion of the central sulcus on sagittal images. Given the fact that anatomic criteria can be used to locate the central sulcus one might reasonably ask is presurgical sensorimotor functional mapping necessary? The most straightforward answer to this question is that it is necessary only in those circumstances in which normal structural-functional relationships are either not discernible or are suspect on clinical grounds. For example, the normal anatomic landmarks used to identify the central sulcus can be obliterated in patients in whom

tumor and associated mass effect distort normal cortical anatomy in the perirolandic region (Fig. 44.4). A second situation in which normal cortical topographic landmarks may fail to locate the functional sensorimotor area is in cases of functional cortical reorganization. This issue is particularly pertinent in epilepsy patients because both intractable epilepsy and cortical functional reorganization often share a common etiology: (a) destructive brain lesions, such as infarction, infection, or trauma, which occur in utero or in early childhood, or (b) malformations of cortical development. fMRI can be quite useful in presurgical evaluation of these patients (Fig. 44.7). Even if the normal anatomy of the central sulcus appears to be intact in patients with developmental anomalies or early life destructive lesions, one cannot know with certainty whether functional reorganization of sensorimotor function has occurred simply by inspecting anatomic images. In these situations clinicians are justifiably less trustful of the fidelity of classical anatomic landmarks as indicators of the location of sensorimotor function.

Which portions of the sensorimotor functional complex must be mapped? While one might presume that none of the sensorimotor areas can be safely violated during a surgical procedure, neurosurgical experience accumulated over several decades has shown this is not true (OLIVIER 1996; ZENTER et al. 1996). Cortical resections involving functionally eloquent areas of the premotor cortex and supplementary motor area (area 6) may result in transient postoperative clumsiness of the involved extremity. However, this typically resolves with no long term morbidity (OLIVIER 1996; ZENTER et al. 1996). It is also the experience of most experienced neurosurgeons that resections involving the inferior portion of the homunculus of the primary motor area– the face and tongue area– can be performed with little or no long term morbidity (Fig. 44.2). This is likely due to the presence of bilateral hemispheric representation of motor function in this portion of the homunculus (TAYLOR and JONES 1997). On the other hand, if the primary motor area of the upper extremity or lower extremity is violated surgically, a disabling contralateral hemiparesis will result. Thus the pressing need in clinical fMRI is to provide reliable localization of the position of the upper or lower extremity homunculi in the primary motor cortex.

Can functionally eloquent tissue exist within an infiltrative brain tumor? If the answer to this question were no, then one could legitimately question the value of functional mapping in patients who have tumors which have infiltrated the perirolandic region, with the understanding that no functionally eloquent tissue would exist within the body of the tumor itself. However, intraoperative surgical mapping studies have definitely shown that functional eloquent tissue can reside within the body of an infiltrative primary neoplasm (OJEMANN et al. 1996; SKIRBOLL et al. 1996). Therefore, functional mapping is necessary even if it is clear that the central sulcus region is infiltrated by tumor.

44.6
Challenges to
Clinical Implementation of fMRI

44.6.1
Anatomic/Functional Specificity of fMRI

Blood oxygen level-dependent contrast (BOLD) is the most widely used method in fMRI, and most clinical studies are performed with this technique (BANDETTINI et al. 1992; KWONG et al. 1992; OGAWA et al. 1992). BOLD fMRI contrast is derived from the local hemodynamic changes which accompany task activation. The point source of the activation signal is located in the vascular bed and in surrounding perivascular tissues. Optimal functional-anatomic specificity would occur when the fMRI contrast point source was located in the microcirculation (capillary bed) which perfuses only those neurons involved in a given mental task. Because the proportion of hemoglobin molecules which have exchanged O_2 for CO_2 increases as a bolus of blood traverses the capillary bed, BOLD contrast is maximum at the distal capillary and venous level. A concern with BOLD imaging has been that the point source of fMRI contrast may be located predominantly in macroscopic draining veins rather than in the microcirculation. If the bolus of oxyhemoglobin produced by mental activation must move downstream in the venous drainage system away from the activated neurons in order to be detected, then there is loss of spatial resolution with BOLD fMRI and concomitant loss of functional-anatomic specificity. Conversely, if the point source of the BOLD activation signal is located in the pial venules immediately adjacent to the group of activated neurons, functional-anatomic specificity would be preserved. Both modeling and in vivo studies have demonstrated that the echo type and field strength influence location of the point source of the BOLD signal (OGAWA et al. 1993; WEISSKOFF et al. 1993). High

field strength (i.e., 3 or 4 T) weights the point source of the activation signal toward the microcirculation. Spin echo pulse sequences also improve the anatomic specificity by weighting contrast toward the capillary side of the circulation; however, the sensitivity of spin echo to the BOLD phenomenon is substantially less than that of gradient recalled pulse sequences. Several authors have raised the concern that gradient recalled fMRI exams at field strengths <3 T image predominantly large draining cortical veins (DUYN et al. 1994; HAACKE et al. 1994; KIM et al. 1994; LAI et al. 1993; MENON et al. 1992, 1995; SEGEBARTH et al. 1994; YOUSRY et al. 1996). And, several of these 1.5 T studies have clearly shown predominant localization of the fMRI signal in large draining cortical veins. However, pulse sequence parameters in these studies have also emphasized inflow effects – single slice, large flip angle, short TR gradient echo sequences (DUYN et al. 1994; HAACKE et al. 1994; KIM et al. 1996; LAI et al. 1993; SEGEBARTH et al. 1994; YOUSRY et al. 1996). GAO et al. (1996) have shown that fMRI images weighted toward the microcirculation may be obtained at 1.5 T *if* the pulse sequence is designed to minimize inflow contrast – multi-slice, long TR, echo planar images. In addition, several publications with carefully done correlation analysis between preoperative fMRI and intraoperative cortical mapping have shown good correspondence between the two (ATLAS et al. 1996; COSGROVE and BUCHBINDER 1996; JACK et al. 1994; MALDJIAN et al. 1996; MORIOKA et al. 1995; PUCE 1995; PUCE et al. 1995; PUJOL et al. 1996; YETKIN et al. 1995, 1997; YOUSRY et al. 1995). It seems reasonable to assume at this point therefore that functional-anatomic specificity which is adequate for presurgical mapping is possible at field strengths in the 1.0–2.0 T range if care is taken to employ imaging parameters that minimize inflow effects.

44.6.2
Difficulties with fMRI Interpretation

As mentioned in Sect. 44.5, the critical piece of information that a surgeon needs from a sensorimotor fMRI study is the location of the primary motor cortical area, particularly in the upper or lower extremity portion of the motor homunculus. However, other associated sensorimotor areas often are activated during commonly used sensorimotor activation paradigms such as finger to thumb tapping or palm brushing (BOECKER et al. 1994; RAO et al. 1993, 1995). Such tasks may activate the pre-motor or supplementary motor cortex or the primary sensory cortical areas, which if violated during an operative procedure does not result in significant morbidity. A difficulty for presurgical sensorimotor mapping with fMRI is its inability at this point to distinguish between activation that represents surgically "expendable" and surgically "nonexpendable" cortical areas.

A related issue is the specificity of the fMRI for the central sulcus. Anatomically three parallel sulci exist in the perirolandic region – the pre-central sulcus, the central sulcus, and post-central sulcus (Fig. 44.1). In our experience both palm brushing and finger tapping activation paradigms may produce activation in two adjacent perirolandic sulci. When this occurs uncertainty may exist as to how to interpret the fMRI results to indicate which is *the* central sulcus. In a study on normal volunteers, we have concluded that in this situation, activation typically is located in the central and post-central sulci, and is rarely seen in the pre-central sulcus with simple finger to thumb tapping or palm brushing tasks (LEE et al. 1996c, 1998b).

44.6.3
Peritumoral fMRI Activation

Challenges to the validity of fMRI mapping of brain tumors have arisen on two fronts. First, the ability of the brain to locally autoregulate its blood supply must be intact in order for the BOLD response to occur. It is conceivable that mass effect from tumor and peritumoral vasogenic edema could produce mechanical arteriolar compression which in turn would eliminate or dampen the vascular response expected during functional brain activation. In our experience, however, and also that of several centers who have published on the subject, a BOLD response has been seen in the sensory motor cortex of patients in whom this area of the brain is involved by considerable peritumoral mass effect (Fig. 44.4). A second challenge that has been raised with regard to the validity of fMRI mapping in brain tumors is the possibility that metabolic changes seen in some brain tumors, for example changes in tissue pH, may eliminate or diminish the physiologic vascular response on which BOLD contrast is dependent. Both this and the issue of mechanical arteriolar compression merit further study.

44.6.4
Motion

In fMRI motion artifacts can originate from: (1) thoraco-abdominal excursion during respiration, (2) cardiac driven pulsatility of the brain, overlying vessels, and cerebral spinal fluid, and (3) bulk head motion. Motion occurring during an fMRI time series can be conceptually divided into two categories; intra-image motion and inter-image motion. Intra-image motion refers to view-to-view motion and this results in image blurring and ghosting. Navigator echoes (EHMAN and FELMLEE 1989) have been employed to reduce motion related view-to-view fluctuations in phase during fMRI studies using non-EPI acquisition sequences (HU and KIM 1994; NOLL et al. 1993). However, for fMRI studies performed with single shot EPI acquisition in which all data for an image are collected in under 100 ms, intra-image (view-to-view) motion is rarely a problem. Inter-image motion is defined as that occurring between acquisition of successive images in an fMRI time series. It can not be rectified simply by fast scanning. Algorithms used to extract functional activity from an fMRI time series are based on the assumption that signal intensity fluctuations in each voxel are dependent only on the physiologic changes induced by the functional activation task itself. Image-to-image bulk head motion invalidates this assumption.

The effect of inter-image bulk head motion during fMRI examinations is particularly problematic in clinical examinations in which incorrect results may lead to errors in clinical management. Inter-image motion can result in activation maps which are false negative, i.e., physiologic changes driven by the activation task go undetected because of motion artifacts. Stimulus correlated inter-image head motion may lead to false positive, i.e. spurious or artifactual, "activation" areas which appear where none exist physiologically. The result may be an fMRI examination which is uninterpretable due to either the absence of any clear cut physiologic activation, misleading due to the presence of artifactual activation, or both.

Solutions for inter-image motion and fMRI have been proposed. One solution is simply to discard individual fMRI runs that were degraded by motion. Not only is this inefficient, but it leads to the scientifically undesirable practice of repeating fMRI runs until some preconceived idea of the "correct" result is achieved. Head fixation would seem to be a logical solution. Foam padding and straps provide some level of head fixation; thermoplastic masks or vacuum head holders provide an intermediate level of head fixation; and, dental molded bite bars provide highly rigid head fixation. While it is acceptable to hold the head rigidly in place with a custom molded bite bar while imaging normal volunteers, this is unacceptable from a safety standpoint when imaging patients with brain lesions who are at risk for seizures, the typical patient group in whom functional brain mapping would be performed for preoperative planning. One of our patients in fact did experience a generalized tonic-clonic seizure during an fMRI study (LEE et al. 1997b). Therefore, from the perspective of patient safety, the only feasible types of head restraint in the clinical setting would be minimal or intermediate restraint systems which may lessen but do not eliminate bulk head motion.

Voxel-based (FRISTON et al. 1994, 1996; HAJNAL et al. 1994; JIANG et al. 1995) or Fourier-based (EDDY et al. 1996; MAAS et al. 1997) retrospective image registration methods have been advocated to correct for inter-image head motion in fMRI time series. Retrospective approaches, however, are fundamentally limited by the inability to recapture information lost due to through-plane motion, that is, motion in which the anatomic section of interest moves in and out of the fixed planes of excitation over the course of the time series. Inter-image through-plane motion will corrupt the spin excitation history in individual voxels. Moreover, retrospective approaches necessitate interpolation and/or modeling, which are at best educated guesses and could blur and reduce the amplitude of the already small (3%–5%) fMRI signal at 1.5 T. The interpolation techniques required for subvoxel registration methods also change the variance of the statistical intensity distribution in corrected images (WU et al. 1996). This defeats the statistical assumption of stationary variance that is a basic requirement for most fMRI analysis protocols. These limitations have motivated our group to pursue prospective motion detection and correction in real-time as a means to reduce motion related artifacts and thereby improve the reliability of fMRI (LEE et al. 1996, 1997, 1998).

44.6.5
Ease of Use

fMRI is logistically more complex than standard anatomic MR imaging. Additional requirements for fMRI which are not present for standard anatomic MR imaging are: (a) During the fMRI time series the patient must execute a proscribed series of mental or physical tasks. (b) Some means of communicating to the patient what to do and when to do it in the time series is needed. (c) The activation task must be coordinated with the execution of the imaging pulse sequence. (d) The fMRI data must be subjected to a statistical analysis algorithm which generally involves multiple steps before a activation map is generated. (e) The activation map must be superimposed on a anatomic imaging template. These additional requirements for fMRI have served as a logistic impediment to its dissemination into general clinical practice. However, as manufacturers begin to provide automated or semi-automated software for fMRI data analysis, superimposition of fMRI data on anatomic images, and archiving of these hybrid functional/anatomic images into the digital database of hospital PACS systems, these "ease of use" impediments to clinical dissemination of fMRI should gradually disappear.

44.7
Conclusions

Many patients in whom surgery is being considered in or near the perirolandic region are candidates for a fMRI sensorimotor mapping procedure. It is unlikely that fMRI will completely replace invasive direct surgical cortical mapping of the sensorimotor area, because the latter procedure is relatively straightforward and provides the surgeon with an accurate intraoperative functional road map. However, fMRI has a fundamental advantage over invasive surgical mapping in that the relevant functional mapping information can be acquired preoperatively. fMRI is therefore uniquely positioned to provide critical information preoperatively that is useful in selection of patients for surgery, selection among various surgical options, and for surgical planning. A single fMRI study will often provide information that is helpful at each step of the clinical decision making tree. As the items raised in the preceding Sect. 44.6 are addressed, presurgical sensorimotor mapping with fMRI should find an increasing role in the management of tumor and epilepsy patients with lesions in or near the perirolandic region.

References

Atlas SW, Howard RS, Maldjian J, et al. (1996) Functional magnetic resonance imaging of regional brain activity in patients with intracerebral gliomas: findings and implications for clinical management. Neurosurgery 38:329–338

Bandettini PA, Wong EC, Hinks RS, et al. (1992) Time course EPI of human brain function during task activation. Magn Reson Med 25:390–397

Berger MS, Cohen WA, Ojemann GA (1990) Correlation of motor cortex brain mapping data with magnetic resonance imaging. J Neurosurg 72:383–387

Blume WT (1993) Motor cortex: anatomy, physiology, and epileptogenesis. In: Wyllie E (ed) The treatment of epilepsy: principles and practice. Lea and Febiger, Philadelphia, p. 16–25

Boecker H, Kleinschmidt A, Requardt M, et al. (1994) Functional cooperativity of human cortical motor areas during self-paced simple finger movements a high-resolution MRI study. Brain 117:1231–1239

Carpentar MB (1985) Core text of neuroanatomy, vol. 3. Williams and Wilkins, Baltimore

Cedzich C, Taniguchi M, Schafer S, et al. (1996) Somatosensory evoked potential phase reversal and direct motor cortex stimulation during surgery in and around the central region. Neurosurgery 38:962–970

Cosgrove GR, Buchbinder BR (1996) Functional magnetic resonance imaging for intracranial navigation. Neurosurg Clin North Am 7:313–322

Duyn JH, Moonen CTW, van Yperen GH, et al. (1994) Inflow versus deoxyhemoglobin effects in BOLD functional MRI using gradient echoes at 1.5 T. NMR Biomed 7:83–88

Eddy W, Fitzgerald M, Noll D (1996) Improved image registration by using Fourier interpolation. Magn Reson Med 36:923–931

Ehman RL, Felmlee JP (1989) Adaptive technique for high-definition MR imaging of moving structures. Radiology 173:255–263

Friston KJ, Jezzard P, Turner R (1994) Analysis of functional MRI time-series. Hum Brain Mapping 1:153–171

Friston KJ, Williams S, Howard R, et al. (1996) Movement-related effects in fMRI time-series. Mag Reson Med 35:346–355

Gao JH, Miller I, Lai S et al. (1996) Quantitative assessment of blood inflow effects in functional MRI signals. MRM 36:314–319

Gregorie EM, Goldring S (1984) Localization of function in the excision of lesions from the sensorimotor region. J Neurosurg 61:1047–1058

Haacke EM, Hopkins A, Lai S, et al. (1994) 2D and 3D High resolution gradient echo functional imaging of the brain: venous contributions to signal in motor cortex studies. NMR Biomed 7:54–62

Hajnal JV, Myers R, Oatride A, et al. (1994) Artifacts due to stimulus correlated motion in functional imaging of the brain. Magn Reson Med 31:283–291

Hu X, Kim SG (1994) Reduction of signal fluctuation in functional MRI using navigator echoes. Magn Reson Med 31:495–503

Iwasaki S, Nakagawa H, Fukusumi A, et al. (1991) Identification of pre-and postcentral gyri on CT and MR images on the basis of the medullary pattern of cerebral white matter. Radiology 179:207–213

Jack CR Jr (1993) Epilepsy: surgery and imaging (state-of-the-art). Radiology 189:635

Jack CR (1995) Magnetic resonance imaging. In: Latchow RE, Jack CR (eds) Neuroimaging and anatomy. Neuroimaging Clinics of North America 5:597–622

Jack CR Jr, Twomey CK, Zinsmeister AR, et al. (1994) Sensory motor cortex: correlation of presurgical mapping with functional MR imaging and invasive cortical mapping. Radiology 190:85–92

Jiang A, Kennedy DN, Baker JR et al. (1995) Motion detection and correction in functional MR imaging. Hum Brain Mapping 3:224–235

Kim JH, Shin T, Kim JS, et al. (1996) MR imaging of cerebral activation performed with a gradient echo technique at 1.5 T: source of activation signals. AJR 167:1277–1281

Kim SG, Hendrich K, Hu X, et al. (1994) Potential pitfalls of functional MRI using conventional gradient-recalled echo techniques. NMR Biomed 7:69–74

Kwong KK, Belliveau JW, Chesler DA et al. (1992) Dynamic magnetic resonance imaging of human brain activity during primary sensory stimulation. Proc Natl Acad Sci USA 89:5675–5679

Lai S, Hopkins AL, Haacke EM, et al. (1993) Identification of vascular structures as a major source of signal contrast in high resolution 2D and 3D functional activation imaging of the motor cortex at 1.5 T: preliminary results. Magn Reson Med 30:387–392

Lee CC, Jack CRJ, Grimm RC, et al. (1996a) Real-time approach to correct for rotational head motion in functional MR imaging. Radiology 201:258 (Abstracts RSNA Meeting 1996)

Lee CC, Jack CRJ, Grimm RC et al. (1996b) Real-time adaptive motion correction in functional MRI. Magn Reson Med 36:436–444

Lee CC, Riederer SJ, Jack CRJ (1996c) The specificity of sensorimotor mapping using functional MRI. Epilepsia 37:206 (Abstract, suppl. 5)

Lee CC, Jack CR, Grimm RC, et al. (1997a) A prospective approach to correct for through-plane rotational head motion in fMRI. ISMRM annual meeting, platform presentation. Vancouver, B.C., April 12–18, 1997

Lee CC, Jack CRJ, Sharbrough FW, et al. (1997b) Presurgical functial mapping with fMRI: experience to date with 34 patients. ISMRM annual meeting, platform presentation. Vancouver, B.C., April 12–18, 1997

Lee CC, Grimm RC, Manduca A, et al. (1998a) A prospective approach to correct for inter-image head rotation in fMRI. Magn Reson Med 39:234–243

Lee CC, Riederer SJ, Jack CR (1998b) Mapping of the central sulcus with functional MRI: active vs passive activation tasks. AJNR 19:847–852

Lehman RM (1994) Motor and sensory cortex in humans: topographic study with chronic subdural stimulation. Neurosurgery 35:1188–1189

Maas LC, Frederick BD, Renshaw PF (1997) Decoupled automated rotational and translational registration for functional MRI time series data: the DART registration algorithm. Magn Reson Med 37:131–139

Maldjian J, Atlas S, Howard RS, et al. (1996) Functional magnetic resonance imaging of regional brain activity in patients with intracerebral arteriovenous malformations before surgical or endovascular therapy. J Neurosurg 84:477–483

Menon RS, Ogawa S, Kim S-G, et al. (1992) Functional brain mapping using magnetic resonance imaging: signal changes accompanying visual stimulation. Invest Radiol 27:S47–S53

Menon RS, Ogawa S, Hu X, et al. (1995) BOLD based functional MRI at 4 Tesla includes a capillary bed contribution: echo-planar imaging correlates with previous optical imaging usign intrinsic signals. Magn Reson Med 33:453–459

Morioka T, Yamamoto T, Mizushima A, et al. (1995) Comparison of magnetoencephalography, functinal MRI, and motor evoked potentials in the localization of the sensory-motor cortex. Neurol Res 17:361–367

Noll DC, Schneider W, Cohen JD (1993) Artifacts in functional MRI using conventional scanning. Proc Soc Magn Reson Med 1:1407

Ogawa S, Tank D, Menon R, et al. (1992) Intrinsic signal changes accompanying sensory stimulation: functional brain mapping with magnetic resonance imaging. Proc Natl Acad Sci USA 89:5951–5955

Ogawa S, Menon RS, Tank DW, et al. (1993) Functional brain mapping by blood oxygenation level-dependent contrast magnetic resonance imaging. Biophys J 64:803

Ojemann GA, Sutherling WW, Lesser RP et al. (1993) Cortical stimulation. In: Engel JJ (ed) Surgical treatment of the epilepsies. Raven, New York, p. 399–414

Ojemann JG, Miller JW, Silbergeld DL (1996) Preserved function in brain invaded by tumor. Neurosurgery 39:253–259

Olivier A (1996) Surgical strategies for patients with supplementary sensorimotor area epilepsy. Adv Neurol 70:429–443

Penfield W, Rasmussen T (1950) The cerebral cortex of man. MacMillan, New York, p. 57

Puce A (1995) Comparative assessment of sensorimotor function usign functional magnetic resonance imaging and electrophysiological methods. J Clin Neurophysiol 12:450–459

Puce A, Constable RT, Luby ML, et al. (1995) Functional magnetic resonance imaging of sensory and motor cortex: comparison with electrophysiological localization. J Neurosurg 83:262–270

Pujol J, Conesa G, Deus J, et al. (1996) Presurgical identificant of the primary sensorimotor cortex by functional magnetic resonance imaging. J Neurosurg 84:7–13

Rao SM, Binder JR, Bandettini PA, et al. (1993) Functional magnetic resonance imaging of complex human movements. Neurology 43:2311–2318

Rao SM, Binder JR, Hammeke TA, et al. (1995) Somatotopic mapping of the human primary motor cortex with functional magnetic resonance imaging. Neurology 45:919–924

Riddle DR, Purves D (1995) Individual variation and lateral asymmetry of the rat primary somatosensory cortex. J Neurosci 15:4184–4195

Roland PE (1993) Brain activation. Wiley-Liss, New York

Rumeau C, Tzourio N, Murayama N, et al. (1994) Location of hand function in the sensorimotor cortex: MR and functional correlation. AJNR 15:567–572

Segebarth C, Belle V, Delon C, et al. (1994) Functional MRI of the human brain: predominance of signals from extracerebral veins. Neuroreport 5:813–816

Skirboll SS, Ojemann GA, Berger MS, et al. (1996) Functional cortex and subcortical white matter located within gliomas. Neurosurgery 38:678–685

Sobel DF, Gallen CC, Schwartz BJ, et al. (1993) Locating the central sulcus: comparison of MR anatomic and magnetoencephalographic functional methods. AJNR 14:915–925

Taylor L, Jones L (1997) Effects of lesions invading the post-central gyrus on somatosensory thresholds on the face. Neuropsycholgia 35:953–961

Uematsu S, Lesser R, Fisher RS, et al. (1992a) Motor and sensory cortex in humans: topography studied with chronic subdural stimulation. Neurosurgery 31:59–72

Uematsu S, Lesser RP, Gordon B (1992b) Localization of sensorimotor cortex: the influence of Sherrington and Cushing on the modern concept. Neurosurgery 30:904–913

Weisskoff RM, Boxerman JL, Zvo CS, et al. (1993) Endogenous susceptibility contrast: principles of relationship between blood oxygenation and MR signal change. Functional MRI of the brain workshop, p. 103–110

Woolsey CN, Erickson TC, Gilson WE (1979) Localization in somatic sensory and motor areas of human cerebral cortex as determined by direct recording of evoked potentials and electrical stimulation. J Neurosurg 51:476–506

Wu DH, Duerk JL, Lewin JS, et al. (1996) Inadequacy of motion correction algorithms in functional MRI: role of susceptibility induced artifacts. J Magn Reson Imaging 7:365–370

Yetkin FZ, Papke RA, Mark LP, et al. (1995) Location of the sensorimotor cortex: functional and conventional MR compared. AJNR 16:2109–2113

Yetkin FZ, Mueller WM, Morris GL, et al. (1997) Functional MR activation correlated with intraoperative cortical mapping. AJNR 18:1311–1315

Yousry T, Schmid UD, Jassoy A, et al. (1995) Topography of the cortical motor hand area: prospective study with functional MR imaging and direct motor mapping at surgery. Radiology 195:23–29

Yousry TA, Schmid UD, Schmitdt D, et al. (1996) The central sulcal vein: a landmark for identification of the central sulcus using functional magnetic resonance imaging. J Neurosurg 85:608–617

Yousry TA, Schmid UD, Alkadhi H (1997) Localization of the motor hand area to a knob on the precentral gyrus. A new landmark. Brain 120:141–157

Zenter J, Hufnagel A, Pechstein U, et al. (1996) Functional results after resective procedures involving the supplementary motor area. J Neurosurg 85:542549

45 Functional Neuroimaging in Developmental Dyslexia

G.F. Eden and T.A. Zeffiro

CONTENTS

45.1 Introduction

In this century, the transition from an agrarian and industrial to a service-based economy has lead to a steady increase in the requirement for literacy in the general population. This growing need for better reading skills has resulted in identification of reading problems. A principal cause of reading disability in younger individuals is developmental dyslexia, defined as a failure to acquire reading that cannot be explained by deficient intellectual ability, educational opportunities or socioeconomic factors. This learning disorder is characterized by a wide range of reading-related perceptual and cognitive deficits and can result in serious difficulties for affected school age children. Although many individuals show substantial improvement in reading skills with time, the many behavioral deficits characteristic of dyslexia, such as poor spelling, often persist into adult life. In response to the increasing number of individuals identified with dyslexia, a growing effort has been directed towards gaining a better understanding of this developmental learning disorder.

Although the first clinical descriptions of developmental dyslexia were made over 100 years ago (MORGAN 1896; HINSHELWOOD 1895), little is yet known about the pathophysiology of this disorder. It is known that dyslexia is heritable (OLSON et al. 1989) and there is some evidence that it occurs in significantly more males than females (however, see SHAYWITZ et al. 1990 for an alternative view). Explanations concerning the mechanism of developmental dyslexia have changed numerous times in this century and today accounts of the cause(s) of this disorder remain controversial. Teachers, clinicians, and scientists have all tried to characterize and identify the roots of developmental dyslexia in an attempt to develop new approaches to its remediation. One strategy has been to first identify the individual cognitive components of normal reading and then chart their growth during reading development. From this perspective, dyslexia could represent a failure to elaborate one or more of these components at a critical period in the development of reading. Indeed, skills that are lacking in dyslexics are related to the ability to apply sound-letter correspondence rules (BRADLEY and BRYANT 1978). However, it has also been demonstrated with a variety of behavioral approaches that these individuals are also impaired in multiple perceptual abilities (LOVEGROVE 1993; TALLAL et al. 1993). These results suggest that the pathophysiology of dyslexia is more complex than originally thought, extending beyond the classically defined language areas of the brain. Results from recent functional neuroimaging investigations have provided new information concerning cortical localization of reading processes, adding to knowledge gained from previous studies on focal cerebral lesions. It is likely that functional neuroimaging, by revealing more about the neural systems involved in

G. F. EDEN, D.Phil.; Georgetown Institute for Cognitive and Computational Sciences, Georgetown University Medical Center, 3870 Reservoir Road, Washington, DC 20007, USA
T.A. ZEFFIRO, MD, PhD; Sensor Systems, Inc., 103a Carpenter Drive, Sterling, VA 20164-4423, USA

reading, will continue to provide important new information concerning the neurobiological basis of developmental dyslexia.

45.2
Models of Reading

Models of the neural organization of reading have been developed from studies of the development of reading skills and their failure following cerebral injury. The behavioral consequences of focal brain injury provided the first clues concerning neuroanatomical localization of reading processes. When reading skills are lost following cerebral insult, the resulting clinical syndrome is referred to as acquired dyslexia. The specific nature of the resulting reading disturbance is dependent upon the cortical locus of the insult. From studies of acquired dyslexia, a number of biologically based reading models have been constructed (for review see MESULAM 1985; FRIEDMAN et al. 1993). In these cases, specific behavioral consequences have been observed following damage to different perisylvian areas in the left hemisphere. For example, phonological acquired dyslexics who exhibit impairments in the ability to sound out new words have lesions including the angular and supramarginal gyri. Damage to Broca's area (the left posterior inferior frontal gyrus) has been associated with speech production abnormalities. Patients with Wernicke's aphasia (lesion in the left posterior superior temporal gyrus) have difficulty comprehending both auditory and written material. DEJERINE (1892) first suggested that the angular gyrus was the visual word form area after having observed a lesion involving the angular gyrus in a patient with acquired illiteracy. The locations of these areas are depicted in Fig. 45.1.

Patients with focal cerebral lesions sometimes manifest reading impairments specific to a particular word type. These observations have resulted in accounts of reading that involve three major elements: (1) an orthographic processing system that analyzes information concerning letter identification, (2) a phonological system that encodes the phonemic constituents of text, and (3) a lexical/semantic system that extracts word meaning. Demonstration that a dissociation in the ability of acquired dyslexics to read irregular words and pseudowords has given rise to a model of reading. This posits the existence of "dual-routes" to access word meaning (COLTHEART et al. 1993). Irregular words are those that do not follow the

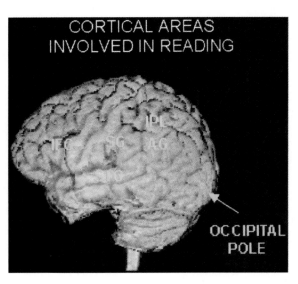

Fig. 45.1. Location of areas involved in reading: *AG*, angular gyrus; *IFG*, inferior frontal gyrus; *IPL*, inferior parietal lobule; *SG*, supramarginal gyrus; *STG*, superior temporal gyrus. Occipital pole includes areas V1 and V2

regular rules of spelling (e.g., yacht). Pseudowords are non-words that conform to rules and therefore can be read out, but do not have any meaning (e.g. wril). Based on the computational processes engaged in reading, namely orthographic, phonologic and semantic/lexical processing, the dual-route theory states that these components are integrated into direct and indirect mechanisms for word identification. The direct or orthographic route allows straight mapping of orthographic units onto their corresponding semantic/lexical representations. The indirect or phonological route requires orthographic information to be converted into its corresponding sound, and these phonological representations are in turn mapped onto the semantic/lexical system. Irregular words are thereby identified by the orthographic, or direct route; the phonological route would be inappropriate, because irregular words do not conform to the sound-correspondence rules. Regular words, whether real or pseudowords, are encoded via the indirect or phonological route. Beginning readers rely more heavily on the indirect route, as they sound out each new word, but become more reliant on the direct route with increased experience. Accomplished readers access the indirect route whenever a new word has to be decoded.

The structure/function relationships identified in focal cerebral injury studies have provided the primary evidence upon which investigators have proposed schemes to explain the reading failure in the developmental type of dyslexia. One obvious problem with this general strategy is that very few acquired dyslexics exhibit the same constellation of reading problems displayed by the more heterogeneous group of developmental dyslexics. Also, comparing behavioral profiles of patients who were once accomplished readers, then suddenly lost these skills, with those of children who have been unable to overcome even the initial hurdles of reading must be interpreted cautiously. The neural circuitry of beginning readers might be quite different from those of accomplished readers. Neuroanatomical abnormalities have been observed in developmental dyslexia (GALABURDA et al. 1985, 1994; LIVINGSTONE et al. 1991), and it is likely that these abnormalities may have been present prior to the first attempts to read.

Based on behavioral analysis of focal brain injury, the precise neuronal mechanisms underlying normal reading have not been fully identified. Consequently, an effort has begun to systematically study the functional organization of language using functional neuroimaging. With the advent of these noninvasive techniques to probe the regional functional specialization of reading, there is now a rapid increase in the ability to explore the effects of development, instruction and gender on reading and language. These findings are providing new information allowing construction of more biologically based models of reading and the mechanisms of its developmental failure.

45.3
Functional Neuroimaging Investigations of Reading

Functional neuroimaging offers powerful and novel methods to better delineate the regional functional specialization of reading in the intact brain. Positron emission tomography (PET) studies focusing on the cortical organization of visual word form processing have agreed, in part, with the original models of Dejerine and others. Some neuroimaging studies have attempted to identify the neuroanatomical substrates for reading by attempting to selectively activate one of two routes predicted from the dual-route reading model described above. Identification of spatially separated pathways (direct and indirect) was supported by evidence obtained in studies of the Japanese language. In these experiments it was found that selective impairment in recognizing Kana, the phonologically coded Japanese writing system, resulted after damage to the left angular/su-

pramarginal region. In the same individuals, the orthographically coded writing system, Kanji, remained intact. In addition, damage to the left posterior inferior temporal region interferes with reading Kanji. Functional neuroimaging studies have mostly confirmed this finding (KAWAMURA et al. 1987; SAKURAI et al. 1992).

Additional evidence supporting functional segregation of the direct and the indirect pathways in the dual-route model for word processing comes from a PET study comparing object naming to reading (BOOKHEIMER et al. 1995). Visual information presented as a simple line drawing, such as a picture of a boat, is assumed to be mapped onto the semantic/lexical representation of this word ("boat") via the direct route. That is, naming the object does not require the phonological and indirect sounding-out mechanisms that are used when reading the word "boat." Although reading a high-frequency word like "boat" poses less of a phonological challenge than decoding a non-word (pseudoword), as described above, oral reading of this word should invoke the phonological pathways when compared to reading silently or picture naming. The results of this comparison did indeed demonstrate that object naming aloud (engaging the direct route) selectively activated more frontal cortical regions (superior frontal gyrus). This area has been associated with lexical retrieval or semantic association. By contrast, areas specifically involved in the indirect, phonological pathway (sounding of words when reading) included the anterior superior temporal and supramarginal gyri. The areas involved in object naming, both silent and aloud, are depicted in Fig. 45.2a.

Another study using PET recently addressed the issue of the existence of direct and indirect routes for reading by using written stimuli (RUMSEY et al. 1997a; RUMSEY and EDEN 1997). In this study, it was not possible to identify two routes differentiating orthographic and phonological word reading, using irregular words and pseudowords. The study did reveal that activation location could be more strongly predicted by the covert vs overt nature of the response. Pronunciation tasks activated the superior temporal gyrus bilaterally but decision-making tasks (i.e., no pronunciation) preferentially activated the left inferior frontal cortex. These findings confirm an earlier investigation of overt and covert responses (PRICE et al. 1994), as well as the differences observed comparing reading aloud to reading silently (BOOKHEIMER et al. 1995). These studies all agree in finding that oral word pronunciation engages a superior temporal/inferior parietal route. Si-

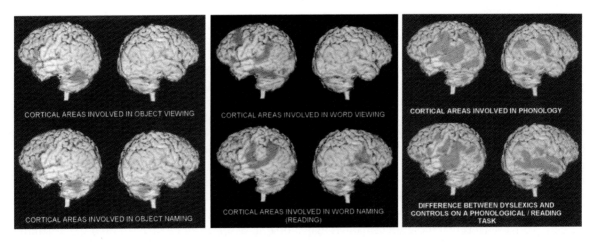

Fig. 45.2a–c. Composite of studies identifying the cortical areas involved during (**a**) viewing of objects, naming of objects, and (**b**) viewing of words and naming of words (i.e., reading aloud). (**c**) Composite of studies identifying the cortical areas subserving phonological processing and identifying differences between dyslexics and non-dyslexics during phonological processing. *Purple* identifies those areas in which dyslexics show less activations than controls. (From BOOKHEIMER et al. 1995; PRICE et al. 1994; PAULESU et al. 1996; RUMSEY and EDEN 1997; SHAYWITZ et al. 1998)

lent reading is less likely to utilize these temporoparietal areas and may more strongly utilize inferior temporal/extrastriate visual and inferior frontal cortical areas. The findings from these studies are depicted in Fig. 45.2b.

In summary, some functional neuroimaging studies have provided support for the dual-route model, while others have not. The differences may be explained by task variation among the experimental approaches. In contrast, the studies cited all provide evidence to support involvement of the superior temporal/inferior parietal areas of the left hemisphere during reading aloud, a task requiring considerable phonological processing. This is consistent with the early lesion data, as damage to the angular gyrus resulted in the loss of reading skills. Other evidence that attributes phonological processing to the anterior temporal lobe and semantic processing to the posterior temporal regions is based on tasks that do not elicit pronunciation (PUGH et al. 1996). It is likely that these differences will be resolved as experimental tasks become more comparable. Concerning dyslexia, the identification of the areas involved in phonological processing, even more than reading itself, is important, because a deficit in phonological awareness is strongly correlated with developmental dyslexia.

45.4
Behavioral Investigations of Language in Dyslexia

Although poor reading is the most prominent clinical manifestation, dyslexia is characterized by a wide range of perceptual and cognitive deficits. In addition to reading difficulties (decoding and recognition of single words), individuals with developmental dyslexia exhibit impairments in the ability to process phonological features of written or spoken language. It has long been clear that the ability to isolate and manipulate the constituent sounds of words is related to reading outcome (BRUCE 1964). Moreover, individuals with dyslexia exhibit deficits in numerous measures of phonological awareness (LIEBERMAN et al. 1985; LINDAMOOD et al. 1992; OLSON et al. 1992; STANOVICH 1988; WAGNER and TORGESEN 1987; BRADLEY and BRYANT 1978). There is also mounting evidence that dyslexics exhibit abnormalities in visual (LOVEGROVE 1993) and auditory (TALLAL et al. 1993) processing. These perceptual abnormalities may interfere with some aspects of the reading process.

We shall first discuss the deficits considered under the global category of phonological processing, as these abnormalities are invoked in most current explanations of the reading difficulties in dyslexia. The term "phonological awareness" refers to abilities pertaining to the manipulation and segmentation of the constituent sounds of words. Phonological awareness was first described by BRUCE (1964), who asked children to repeat the words after they had removed a particular sound. LIEBERMAN et al. (1985) devised a similar task, in which mono- and poly-syllabic words were read to children, who in turn tapped out the number of phonemes and syllables of particular words. It was discovered that tasks such as segmentation and phoneme blending accurately predict reading ability. Following these observations, a large body of evidence has shown that certain phonological abilities can predict reading acquisition.

In addition to these phonological tasks, two other measures have proven particularly useful in predicting reading ability. These are: (1) rapid automatized naming (RAN), a measure of phonological recoding (DENCKLA and RUDEL 1976; BOWERS and WOLF 1993), and (2) phonological coding in working memory (HULME and ROODENRYS 1995; JORM 1983; TORGESEN et al. 1990). Although both these tasks differ from the direct phonological manipulations described above, there is much evidence that deficits in these skills are cardinal characteristics of dyslexia. There have been numerous investigations into the precise relationship between performance on these tasks and reading at different age levels (WOLF and OBREGON 1992; BOWERS and WOLF 1993). For example, kindergarten children who later become reading disabled are slower at naming letters, numbers, colors and objects during RAN. Children with both poor RAN and phonological deficits are poorer readers than are those with either deficit alone (WOLF and GOODGLASS 1986). Compensated dyslexics perform better on rapid RAN tasks than those dyslexics who remain impaired at reading tasks. Moreover, these "improved readers" retain deficits in phonological manipulation tasks (FELTON et al. 1990).

Other behavioral abnormalities attributable to the phonological domain involve verbal working memory. It has been suggested that phonological recoding in working memory is an essential component of learning to read (BADDELEY 1992; HULME and ROODENRYS 1995). This is because efficient phonetic recoding depends on the accurate and efficient temporary storage of letter-sound representation while the blending of these sounds into words occurs simultaneously. A significant portion of reading disabled children (15%–35%) show deficits in short term memory (also referred to as working memory) in tasks requiring the recall of random digits, words or letters. For example, listening to and repeating a string of numbers (digit span) or words can be difficult for dyslexics. Most of the behavioral deficits described are consistent with the presence of a core phonological deficit in developmental dyslexia.

In summary, there are a number or reading-related tasks in which dyslexics experience difficulty. Skill in phonological awareness (e.g., segmentation), phonological recoding (e.g., RAN) and phonological coding in working memory (e.g., word lists) all strongly correlate with reading ability. Although often considered as components of phonological awareness, it is possible that each of these measures may involve subtly different cognitive components of the reading process.

45.5
Functional Neuroimaging Investigations of Phonological Processing in Dyslexia

Both PET and functional magnetic resonance imaging (fMRI) studies have provided new information about the cortical areas involved in reading, object naming and verbal working memory. Even so, very few studies have been conducted using the exact behavioral measures that have been so useful in identifying dyslexia. Despite abundant evidence supporting the relationship between phonological awareness and reading ability, the mechanisms underlying the sounding out or decoding of words in the brain are only just beginning to emerge from a controversial body of literature. The results from functional neuroimaging studies investigating phonological tasks in normal subjects are summarized in Fig. 45.2c. These experiments have been designed to identify the mechanisms specifically involved in phonological processing, as opposed to reading in the more general sense. The tasks utilized require the subject to make a decision about whether two visually presented letters rhyme (RUMSEY et al. 1997b; PAULESU et al. 1996; SHAYWITZ et al. 1998). These studies have revealed bilateral activation along the entire anterior-posterior axis of the brain. Spatial overlap of task-related activity has been observed in the left inferior parietal lobule, the superior temporal gyrus and the inferior frontal gyrus (for a thorough review see POEPPEL 1996). In at least one study, the right-hemisphere homologues of these areas were found to be activated, a result that would not have necessarily been predicted from the effects of focal cerebral damage.

Early investigations identified left hemisphere dysfunction in individuals with dyslexia. These findings were based on anatomical (GALABURDA and KEMPER 1978; GALABURDA et al. 1985), electrophysiological (DUFFY et al. 1980), and cerebral blood flow

(Xenon-133) abnormalities (FLOWERS et al. 1991). More recently, functional neuroimaging studies (PET and fMRI) have provided new information concerning the neural systems related to phonological processing that are abnormal in dyslexia. RUMSEY et al. (1992) demonstrated that controls exhibited regional cerebral blood flow (rCBF) increases in the left temporoparietal, left middle temporal, left posterior frontal, right middle temporal and right parietal regions while performing a phonological detection task. By contrast, dyslexics showed significantly less task-related signal increase than controls in these temporoparietal areas. A more recent study also finds comparatively lower task-related activation in bilateral posterior temporal and inferior parietal cortex in the dyslexics (RUMSEY et al. 1997a). These studies have clearly demonstrated functional differences in dyslexics in temporoparietal cortex.

However, other studies have identified dysfunction in other brain regions. In a PET study (PAULESU et al. 1996), dyslexics exhibited normal task-related activity in frontal cortex (Broca's area) during rhyme judgment and in the superior temporal gyrus (Wernicke's area) during a working memory task. However, the controls activated both of these areas, as well as the insula, during both tasks. The absence of activation in the insula linking the two other sites led the authors to suggest that dyslexia is a "disconnection syndrome." It is important to note that the pattern of task-related activity observed during rhyming was consistent with RUMSEY et al. (1997a), as the dyslexics again failed to activate the temporoparietal area during the rhyming task. However, the two studies differ with respect to the activity observed in the insula, as it was found to be normal in the dyslexics by RUMSEY and therefore failed to provide support for the disconnection account of dyslexia. More recently, a fMRI study has identified increased task-related activity in the inferior frontal gyrus in dyslexics compared to controls during a rhyme judgment task (SHAYWITZ et al. 1998). Less activation in the superior temporal gyrus and angular gyrus observed in the dyslexics in this same study is consistent with earlier studies described above. While the increased activity seen in frontal cortex may represent compensatory mechanisms, this explanation requires further exploration.

As mentioned previously, phonological processing abnormalities also involve verbal working memory (short-term memory). Difficulty remembering sequences of verbal information over brief periods is one of the clinical hallmarks of dyslexia.

PAULESU et al. (1996) also examined verbal short-term memory in dyslexia using functional neuroimaging. In addition to their description of impaired task-related activation of temporoparietal areas during a phonological task, in the same study they also identified decreased activity in frontal cortex during a working memory task. These results suggest that there is a neurobiological basis for the behavioral working memory deficit, with a presumptive localization to lateral inferior frontal cortex. Working memory has become an area of intense interest in functional neuroimaging and the cortical areas identified appear to show spatial overlap with those implicated in phonological processing. Presently, it is unclear whether verbal working memory is localized to Broca's or Wernicke's area (or both) and whether its organization is altered in dyslexia.

In summary, functional neuroimaging studies utilizing phonological tasks are congruent regarding findings of altered activity in the temporoparietal area in dyslexia. However, controversy persists regarding involvement of the insula and frontal cortex. The differences among studies may well reflect different approaches to subject selection and subtle cognitive differences associated with the phonological processing tasks employed in these different studies.

45.6
Behavioral Investigations of the Visual System in Dyslexia

Obviously, the visual system plays an extensive role in many aspects of reading. As we read, visual information is processed during short fixations and integrated between saccades to extract the written word form that is then linguistically encoded. An early explanation for the type of hesitant reading observed in dyslexia made reference to malfunction of the visual apparatus, somewhere between the primary input and the visual integration processors. This theory was proposed by Samuel Orton early in this century (ORTON 1925). He attributed the confused visual impression reported by individuals with dyslexia to a miscommunication of visual information between the two hemispheres. While this theory has fallen into disfavor, a more convincing visual deficit hypothesis of dyslexia has been put forward in the framework of two visual pathways, the magno-cellular and parvocellular systems (LOVEGROVE et al.

1980). A number of studies have demonstrated that parallel pathways can be identified in the primate visual system (UNGERLEIDER and MISHKIN 1982). These pathways can be identified anatomically (best observed at the level of the lateral geniculate nucleus or LGN), physiologically (based on single-unit properties) and psychophysically. The magnocellular (transient) and parvocellular (sustained) systems have been described in detail concerning their respective response properties. Neurons in the magnocellular system respond preferentially to lower spatial frequency, lower contrast and higher temporal frequency. These cells exhibit a rapid and brief response. At the level of the LGN the cells are large and myelinated, supporting rapid information processing. In a series of behavioral studies differences were identified in dyslexics compared to controls in visual tasks specifically designed to involve the magnocellular visual pathway (for review see LOVEGROVE 1993). For example, the contrast sensitivity of normal and reading disabled children was observed to be different, with the largest effects observed at low stimulus contrast, a situation designed to selectively stimulate the magnocellular system. When this experiment was repeated in the presence of uniform field flicker, causing diminished magnocellular sensitivity, the differences between controls and dyslexics decreased. Further, it has been demonstrated that the duration of visual persistence (perception of a visual stimulus after it has been physically removed) increases as spatial frequency increases. This increase was less in reading disabled children than in controls. That is, at low spatial frequencies, when the magnocellular system is expected to be predominantly involved, reading disabled children exhibited longer visual persistence (SLAGHUIS and LOVEGROVE 1985).

The magnocellular deficit theory is supported by physiological and anatomical studies as well. Electrophysiological recordings have revealed physiological differences in dyslexics' visual-evoked potential onset latencies during viewing of stimuli believed to preferentially engage the magnocellular or transient system (LIVINGSTONE et al. 1991). Whole-scalp neuromagnetic recordings (MEG) have shown that the signal elicited by apparent motion stimuli results in longer latencies in dyslexics (VANNI et al. 1997). Anatomical studies of postmortem tissue has provided further evidence for neuroanatomical abnormalities in the magnocellular system of dyslexics at the level of the LGN (LIVINGSTONE et al. 1991). It is also known that the magnocellular system is involved in the processing of global form, movement,

and temporal resolution. Numerous studies have observed differences in dyslexics during rapid visual temporal processing (EDEN et al. 1995), visual motion processing (CORNELISSEN et al. 1995; EDEN et al. 1996; DEMB et al. 1997), and eye movement control (EDEN et al. 1994; RAYNER 1990; STARK et al. 1990; FOWLER et al. 1990). To relate these findings to the reading difficulties experienced by dyslexics, it has been hypothesized that a magnocellular (transient) deficit may result in insufficient suppression of the sustained system (parvocellular) during saccades. In reading this could lead to superimposition of visual information that should have been separated by each eye movement, thereby leading to visual confusion (LOVEGROVE 1993). Although visual difficulties are reported by dyslexics (CORNELISSEN et al. 1991; EDEN et al. 1994), these perceptual problems are unlikely to explain the entire constellation of problems experienced by dyslexic individuals (such as phonological processing abnormalities and visual confusion).

45.7
Functional Neuroimaging Investigations of the Visual System in Dyslexia

In contrast with language studies, human visual processing experiments have benefited from a more detailed understanding of the anatomy and physiology of the visual system gained from experiments with non-human primates. From these studies, schemes for regional functional specialization of the visual cortical pathways have been described (UNGERLEIDER and MISHKIN 1982; LIVINGSTONE and HUBEL 1988; MAUNSELL and NEWSOME 1987; VAN ESSEN and MAUNSELL 1983; ZEKI 1973; ZEKI and SHIPP 1988). More recently, functional neuroimaging experiments utilizing PET and fMRI have identified a specific motion-sensitive area, the MT/V5 complex, dominated by input from the transient system or magnocellular stream. Because the visual behavioral abnormalities known to be present in dyslexia are expected to be associated with transient or magnocellular processing, this area of extrastriate cortex has been studied in dyslexics using fMRI (reviewed by EDEN and ZEFFIRO 1998). If dyslexics have a magnocellular deficit, then they should also have poorer visual motion discrimination due to aberrant motion processing. In the first functional imaging study investigating the visual deficit hypothesis, presentation of moving stimuli to dyslexics

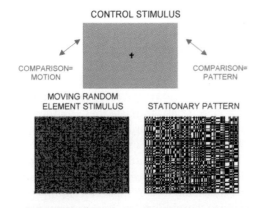

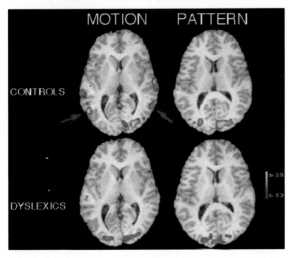

Fig. 45.3. Stimuli used to elicit visual motion processing and pattern processing (*top*); the motion stimulus moved alternating directions, while the pattern stimulus remained stationary. Task-related signal change revealed differences between the group of dyslexics and controls during motion processing (area MT/V5), but not pattern processing. (From EDEN et al. 1996)

failed to produce the same task-related functional activation in the MT/V5 complex as in controls (Fig. 45.3). This deficit was confined to the motion processing system, as presentation of stationary patterns resulted in equivalent task-related activation in both groups (EDEN et al. 1996). This finding was confirmed in a subsequent study in which it was also possible to demonstrate a direct relationship between the amplitude of fMRI signal change in the MT/V5 complex and reading skill (DEMB et al. 1997). In neuroimaging studies of dyslexia, the cortical and subcortical components of the visual motion pathway outside area MT/V5 have not yet been thoroughly investigated. The MT/V5 complex provides a strong input to the inferior parietal cortex and cerebellum, areas involved in visual motion processing.

Of note is the fact that both of these regions exhibit abnormal linguistic task-related activity in functional brain imaging studies of dyslexia.

Both of these studies found that the presentation of moving stimuli to dyslexics failed to produce the same task-related functional activation in the MT/V5 complex as that observed in controls. This deficit was confined to the motion processing system, as presentation of stationary patterns resulted in equivalent activation in both groups in other extrastriate areas. The results demonstrate the feasibility of using fMRI as a tool to detect and localize abnormal neuronal processing in dyslexia using tasks that do not involve language processing or reading. It has also been possible to demonstrate a direct correlation between the amount of signal change in the area MT/V5 and reading levels (DEMB et al. 1997, 1998). An individual mildly affected with dyslexia would be predicted to show weaker signals in this extrastriate area. Very low or absent signals would be expected in the case of severe dyslexia.

45.8
Summary

Although dyslexia has been viewed by some as primarily a perceptual deficit, others have argued that the deficit occurs at a cognitive level involving language processing. Here we have reviewed experimental results supporting the existence of both perceptual and cognitive deficits in this disorder. The results discussed suggest that there is congruence among these studies with respect to abnormal processing in the superior temporal gyrus and inferior parietal lobule. Combining the experimental results from neuroimaging studies of reading and reading-related processing with those demonstrating a magnocellular visual system deficit, the superior temporal and inferior parietal areas emerge as likely candidates for the principal locus of cerebral dysfunction in dyslexia. Visual input to the temporoparietal area is predominantly provided by the magnocellular system. This system originates in the magnocellular layers of the LGN and projects to the MT/V5 complex and parietal cortex (UNGERLEIDER and MISHKIN 1982; LIVINGSTONE and HUBEL 1988; MAUNSELL and NEWSOME 1987; VAN ESSEN and MAUNSELL 1983). Functional neuroimaging studies have demonstrated responses in visual motion processing in the MT/V5 complex and inferior parietal cortex of the human visual system (CORBETTA et al.

1990; Watson et al. 1993; Tootell et al. 1995). In addition, PET studies examining reading-related processes have regularly identified activity in the superior temporal gyrus and inferior parietal lobules.

In addition to poor reading, dyslexia is characterized by poor phonological awareness, poor phonological recoding, verbal working memory deficits and a subtle but significant rapid visual processing deficit. The functional neuroimaging data to date are not sufficient to provide information on the neuronal processes engaged during all phonological tasks that have been examined in the behavioral studies of dyslexia. For example, there are no existing neuroimaging studies exploring task-related activity during rapid automatized naming. Future work in this area may explore the spatial colocalization of processes underlying these perceptual and cognitive tasks.

The various neuroimaging studies of dyslexia have yielded somewhat inconsistent findings. Better agreement among experimental results may result from closer attention to details of: (1) subject selection, (2) task selection, and (3) stimulus presentation rate and duration. These experimental conditions are likely to play an important role in defining the nature of deficits observed in dyslexics.

With respect to the first point, the definition and selection of dyslexic individuals in general is a controversial issue (Stanovich 1994). In the functional neuroimaging studies considered here, different approaches to subject selection were utilized. Selection of the dyslexics in the study by Paulesu and colleagues (1996) was based on the presence of poor phonological skills, not on an absolute reading deficit as the other studies discussed. Although it is interesting to identify the "network" that is expressed during phonological processing in a group of individuals who are unskillful at this task, it is not clear how this then generalizes to other poor readers.

Second, the choice of task continues to confound comparison of results from different groups. For example, it could be that some of the tests utilized to measure phonological processing make different demands on working memory, a skill impaired in many dyslexics. There is a also need for studies that employ tasks that are the same as those commonly employed to assess reading or reading-related functions. These tasks usually require subjects to verbalize responses, which has been rarely used in studies to date, mainly because of concerns of introducing motion artifacts. From the above described studies comparing covert and overt reading, such limita-

tions may bring about unexpected results in the neural circuitry under investigation and could alone account for any differences in study outcome. With fMRI in particular, overt responses have been largely avoided because of the resulting artifacts introduced by head and jaw movements caused during articulation of responses. Improvement of head stabilization devices will promote studies employing vocalization of responses. Another way to circumvent this problem in the case of fMRI is to alternate data acquisition with task execution. With this approach, the jaw movement occurs in a period different from the data acquisition interval. Because of the delay of the hemodynamic response, the signal is captured in the delayed acquisition period (Eden et al. 1999). A further advantage of this "behavior interleaved gradient" (BIG) technique is that the acoustic noise associated with the gradients is also excluded from the task period, thereby providing a quieter environment in which to perform language studies. Further developments in data acquisition techniques will improve the signal derived from language neuroimaging studies and reduce inter and intra-subject reliability. Ideally, this will lead to data on dyslexics' phonological skills derived from single subjects, information that is noticeably absent at this time. This is an important issue, given the phenotypic heterogeneity of this group and the attempts to subgroup these individuals (Lyon 1996).

Third, in early PET experiments it was apparent that the regional CBF response in primary visual cortex was strongly influenced by the rate of stimulus presentation, with an 8 Hz reversing checkerboard stimulus producing the maximal activation. A serious hurdle in any comparison of a clinical and control group is the difficulty in matching speed of presentation in the two groups so as to avoid rate-related modulation of task-related activity (Price et al. 1992). Speed of presentation is largely determined by reaction time, which usually tend to be much longer in dyslexics. Often during these tests, accuracy is also significantly lower in the dyslexics. The resulting activation maps are difficult to interpret when reaction time and accuracy skills are not carefully matched. When presenting stimuli that are processed equally in accuracy, there is most likely to be a reaction time difference between the two groups. In order for the two groups to respond within the same time, it is likely that different difficulty levels will have to be used in each group. Alternatively, parametric study designs may be used to assess modulation of the areas of interest with respect to variation of presentation rate or task difficulty.

45.9
Conclusion

Functional neuroimaging has provided many novel insights into the pathophysiology of developmental dyslexia. Studies examining phonological skill in dyslexics have found altered activation in the superior temporal gyrus and inferior parietal lobule in individuals with dyslexia. It appears that these posterior areas are involved in the phonological manipulations related to reading. They also play a role in word pronunciation, which also makes demands on phonological skills. Visual perceptual processing deficits have been identified with functional neuroimaging in a subdivision of the visual system localized near those identified during linguistic studies of dyslexia. Future neuroimaging studies may elucidate the exact relationship between these perceptual and cognitive information processing deficits in dyslexia.

References

Baddeley A (1992) Working memory. Science 255:556–559

Bookheimer SY, Zeffiro TA, Blaxton T, Gaillard W, Theodore W (1995) Regional cerebral blood flow during object naming and word reading. Hum Brain Map 3:93–106

Bowers P, Wolf M (1993) Theoretical links among naming speed, precise timing mechanisms, and orthographic skill in dyslexia. Read Wri 5:69–86

Bradley L, Bryant P (1978) Difficulties in auditory organisation as a possible cause of reading backwardness. Nature 271:746–747

Bruce DJ (1964) The analysis of word sounds. Br J Educ Psychol 34:158–170

Coltheart M, Curtis B, Atkins P, Haller M (1993) Models of reading aloud: dual-route and parallel-distributed-processing approaches. Psychol Rev 100:589–608

Corbetta M, Miezin FM, Dobmeyer S, Shulman GL, Petersen SE (1990) Attentional modulation of neural processing of shape, color, and velocity in humans. Science 248:1556–1559

Cornelissen P, Bradley L, Fowler S, Stein J (1991) What children see affects how they read. Dev Med Child Neurol 33:755–762

Cornelissen P, Richardson A, Mason A, Fowler S, Stein J (1995) Contrast sensitivity and coherent motion detection measured at photopic luminance levels in dyslexic controls. Vision Res 35:1483–1494

Dejerine J (1892) Contribution à l'étude anatomo-pathologique et clinique des differentes varietes de cecite verbale. Mem Soc Biol 4:61–90

Demb JB, Boynton GM, Heeger DJ (1997) Brain activity in visual cortex predicts individual differences in reading performance. Proc Natl Acad Sci USA 94:13363–13366

Demb JB, Boynton GM, Heeger DJ (1998) FMR imaging of early visual pathways in dyslexia. J Neurosci (in press)

Denckla MB, Rudel RG (1976) Rapid "automized" naming (RAN): dyslexia differentiated from other learning disabilities. Neuropsychologia 14:471–479

Duffy FH, Denckla MB, Bartels PH, Sandini G (1980) Dyslexia: regional differences in brain electrical activity by topographic mapping. Ann Neurol 7:412–420

Eden GF, Zeffiro TA (1998) Neural systems affected in developmental dyslexia revealed by functional neuroimaging. Neuron (in press)

Eden GF, Stein JF, Wood HM, Wood FB (1994) Differences in eye movements and reading problems in dyslexic and normal children. Vision Res 34:1345–1358

Eden GF, Stein JF, Wood MH, Wood FB (1995) Temporal and spatial processing in reading disabled and normal children. Cortex 31:451–468

Eden GF, VanMeter JW, Rumsey JM, Maisog JM, Woods RP, Zeffiro TA (1996) Abnormal processing of visual motion in dyslexia revealed by functional brain imaging. Nature 382:66–69

Eden GF, Joseph JE, Brown HE, Brown CP, Zeffiro TA (1999) Utilizing the hemodynamic delay and dispersion to detect fMRI signal change without auditory interference: the behavior interleaved gradients technique. J Magn Reson Med 41:13–20

Felton RH, Naylor CE, Wood FB (1990) Neuropsychological profile of adult dyslexics. Brain Lang 39:485–497

Flowers DL, Wood FB, Naylor CE (1991) Regional cerebral blood flow correlates of language processes in reading disability. Arch Neurol 48:637–643

Fowler MS, Riddell PM, Stein JF (1990) Vergence eye movement control and spatial discrimination in normal and dyslexic children. In: Pavlidis, GT (ed)_Perspectives on dyslexia. Wiley, Chichester, pp 253–273

Friedman RF, Ween JE, Albert ML (1993) Alexia. In: Heilman KM, Valenstein E (eds)Clinical neuropsychology. Oxford University, New York, pp 37–62

Galaburda AM, Kemper TL (1978) Cytoarchitectonic abnormalities in developmental dyslexia: a case study. Ann Neurol 6:94–100

Galaburda AM, Sherman G, Rosen GD, Aboitiz F, Geschwind N (1985) Developmental dyslexia: Four consecutive cases with cortical anomalies. Ann Neurol 18:222–233

Galaburda AM, Menard MT, Rosen GD (1994) Evidence for aberrant auditory anatomy in developmental dyslexia. Proc Natl Acad Sci USA 91:8010–8013

Hinshelwood J (1895) Word blindness and visual memory. Lancet 2:1564–1570

Hulme C, Roodenrys S (1995) Practitioner review: verbal working memory development and its disorders. J Child Psychol Psychiatry 36:373–398

Jorm AF (1983) Specific reading retardation and working memory: a review. Br J Psychol 74:311–342

Kawamura M, Hirayama K, Hasegawa K, Takahashi N, Yamaura A (1987) Alexia with agraphia of kanji (Japanese morphograms). J Neurol Neurosurg Psychiatry 50:1125–1129

Lieberman P, Meskill RH, Chatillon M, Schupack H (1985) Phonetic speech perception deficits in dyslexia. J Speech Hear Res 28:480–486

Lindamood PC, Bell N, Lindamood P (1992) Issues in phonological awareness assessment. Ann Dyslexia 42:242–259

Livingstone M, Hubel D (1988) Segregation of form, colour, movement and depth: anatomy, physiology, and perception. Science 240:740–749

Livingstone MS, Rosen GD, Drislane FW, Galaburda AM (1991) Physiological and anatomical evidence for a magnocellular defect in developmental dyslexia. Proc Natl Acad Sci USA 88:7943–7947

Lovegrove W (1993) Weakness in transient visual system: a causal factor in dyslexia? Ann NY Acad Sci 14:57–69

Lovegrove WJ, Heddle M, Slaghuis W (1980) Reading disability: spatial frequency specific deficits in visual information store. Neuropsychologia 18:111–115

Lyon GR (1996) Learning disabilities. In: Mash E, Berkley R (eds) Child psychopathology. Guilford, New York, pp 390–435

Maunsell JHR, Newsome WT (1987) Visual processing in monkey extrastriate cortex. Annu Rev Neurosci 10:363–401

Mesulam M-M (1985) Attention, confusional states, and neglect. In: Mesulam M-M (ed) Principles of behavioral neurology. Davis, Philadelphia, pp 125–168

Morgan WP (1896) A case of congenital word blindness. Br Med J 7:1378

Olson R, Wise B, Conners F, Rack J, Fulker D (1989) Specific deficits in component reading and language skills: genetic and environmental influences. J Learn Disabil 22:339–348

Olson R, Forsberg H, Wise B, Rack J (1992) Measurement or word recognition, orthographic, and phonological skills. Measurement of learning disabilities conference. NIH, Bethesda

Orton ST (1925) "Word-blindness" in school children. Arch Neurol Psychiatry 14:581–615

Paulesu E, Frith C, Snowling M, Gallagher A, Morton J, Frackowiak RSJ, Frith C (1996) Is developmental dyslexia a disconnection syndrome? Evidence from PET scanning. Brain 119:143–157

Poeppel D (1996) A critical review of PET studies of phonological processing. Brain Lang 55:317–351

Price C, Wise R, Ramsay S, Friston K, Howard D, Patterson K, Frackowiak R (1992) Regional response differences within the human auditory cortex when listening to words. Neurosci Lett 146:179–182

Price CJ, Wise RJS, Watson JDG, Patterson K, Howard D, Frackowiak RSJ (1994) Brain activity during reading: the effects of exposure duration and task. Brain 117:1255–1269

Pugh KR, Shaywitz BA, Shaywitz SE, et al. (1996) Cerebral organization of component processes in reading. Brain 119:1221–1238

Rayner K (1990) Eye movements and dyslexia. In: Stein JF (ed) Vision and visual dyslexia. Macmillan, London

Rumsey JM, Eden GF (1997) Functional neuroimaging of developmental dyslexia: regional cerebral blood flow in dyslexic men. In: Specific reading disability: a view of the spectrum. Timonium, York, pp 35–62

Rumsey JM, Andreason P, Zametkin AJ, et al. (1992) Failure to activate the left temporoparietal cortex in dyslexia. Arch Neurol 49:527–534

Rumsey JM, Horwitz B, Donohue BC, Nace K, Maisoy JM, Andreason P (1997a) Phonologic and orthographic compents of word recognition: a PET-rCBF study. Brain 120:739–759

Rumsey JM, Nace K, Donohue BC, Wise D, Maisog JM, Andreason P (1997b) A PET study of impaired word recognition and phonological processing in dyslexic men. Arch Neurol 54:562–573

Sakurai Y, Momose T, Iwata M, Watanabe T, Ishikawa T, Takeda K, Kanazawa I (1992) Kanji word reading process analysed by PET. Neuroreport 3:445–448

Shaywitz SE, Shaywitz BA, Fletcher JM, Escobar MD (1990) Prevalence of reading disability in boys and girls. JAMA 264:998–1002

Shaywitz SE, Shaywitz BA, Pugh KR, et al. (1998) Functional disruption in the organization of the brain for reading in dyslexia. Proc Natl Acad Sci USA 95:2636–2641

Slaghuis WL, Lovegrove WJ (1985) Spatial-frequency-dependent visible persistence and specific reading disability. Brain Cogn 4:219–240

Stanovich KE (1988) Explaining the differences between the dyslexic and the garden-variety poor reader: the phonological-core variable-difference model. J Learn Disabil 21:590–612

Stanovich KE (1994) Annotation: does dyslexia exist? J Child Psychol Psychiatry 35:579–595

Stark LW, Giveen SC, Terdiman JF (1990) Specific dyslexia and eye movements. In: Stein JF (ed) Vision and visual dyslexia. Macmillan, London

Tallal P, Miller S, Fitch RH (1993) Neurobiological basis of speech: a case for the preminence of temporal processing. In: Tallal P, Galaburda AM, Llinas RK, von Euler C (eds) Temporal information processing in the nervous system: special reference to dyslexia and dysphasia. New York Academy of Sciences, New York, pp 27–47

Tootell RB, Reppas JB, Kwong KK, et al. (1995) Functional analysis of human MT and related visual cortical areas using magnetic resonance imaging. J Neurosci 15:3215–3230

Torgesen JK, Wagner RK, Simmons K, Laughon P (1990) Identifying phonological coding problems in disabled readers: naming, counting, or span measures? Learn Dis Q 13:236–243

Ungerleider LG, Mishkin M (1982) Two cortical visual systems. In: Ingle DJ, Goodale MA, Memsfield RJW (eds) Analysis of visual behavior. MIT, Cambridge, pp 549–586

Van Essen D, Maunsell JHR (1983) Hierarchical organization and functional streams in the visual cortex. Trends Neurosci 9:370–75

Vanni S, Uusitalo MA, Kiesila P, Hari R (1997) Visual motion activates V5 in dyslexics. 8:1939–1942

Wagner RK, Torgesen JK (1987) The nature of phonological processing and its causal role in the acquisition of reading skills. Psychol Bull 101:192–212

Watson JDG, Myers R, Frackowiak RSJ, et al. (1993) Area V5 of the human brain: evidence from a combined study using positron emission tomography and magnetic resonance imaging. Cereb Cortex 3:79–94

Wolf M, Goodglass H (1986) Dyslexia, dysnomia, and lexical retrieval: a longitudinal investigation. Brain Lang 28:154–168

Wolf M, Obregon M (1992) Early naming deficits, developmental dyslexia, and a specific deficit hypothesis. Brain Lang 42:219–247

Zeki SM (1973) Colour coding in rhesus monkey prestriate cortex. Brain Res 53:422–27

Zeki SM, Shipp S (1988) The functional logic of cortical connections. Nature 335:311–317

Subject Index

List of Contributors

GEOFFREY K. AGUIRRE, MD
Department of Neurology
Hospital of the University of Pennsylvania
3400 Spruce Street
Philadelphia, PA 19104-4283
USA

DAVID C. ALSOP, MD
Departments of Neurology and Radiology
University of Pennsylvania School of Medicine
3400 Spruce Street
Philadelphia. PA 19104-4283
USA

HANNU J. ARONEN, MD, PhD
Department of Clinical Radiology
Kuopio University Hospital
FIN-70100 Kuopio
Finland
and
Department of Radiology
Helsinki University Central Hospital
P.O.Box 380
FIN-00029 Hyks
Finland

JOHN ASHBURNER, MD
The Wellcome Department of Cognitive Neurology
Institute of Neurology
12 Queen Square
London WC1N 3BG
UK

PETER A. BANDETTINI, PhD
Assistant Professor
Biophysics Research Institute
Medical College of Wisconsin
8701 W. Watertown Plank Rd.
Milwaukee, WI 53226
USA

VALÉRIE BELLE, PhD
INSERM U438 (RMN Bioclinique)
Université Joseph Fourier
Laboratoire de Neurobiophysique
Centre Hospitalier Universitaire
Pavillon B, BP 217
F-38043 Grenoble Cedex 9
France

KAREN F. BERMAN, MD
Clinical Brain Disorders Branch
National Institute of Mental Health
Building 10; Room B1D-125
National Institutes of Health
9000 Rockville Pike
Bethesda, MD 20892
USA

JEFF R. BINDER, PhD
Department of Neurology
Medical College of Wisconsin
9200 W.Wisconsin Ave.
Milwaukee, WI 53226
USA

BHARAT B. BISWAL, PhD
Biophysics Research Institute
Medical College of Wisconsin
8701 W. Watertown Plank Rd.
Milwaukee, WI 53226
USA

ALAN S. BLOOM, PhD
Professor of Pharmacology
Department of Pharmacology
Medical College of Wisconsin
8701 W. Watertown Plank Rd.
Milwaukee, WI 53226
USA

TODD S. BRAVER, PhD
Department of Psychology
Washington University
Campus Box 1125
One Brookings Drive
St. Louis, MO 63130
USA

RANDY L. BUCKNER, PhD
Department of Psychology
Washington University
Campus Box 1125
One Brookings Drive
St. Louis, MO 63130
USA

KHALAF BUSHARA, MD
Clinical Associate
Human Motor Control Section
National Institute of Neurological Disorders and Stroke
National Institutes of Health
Building 10, Room 5N226
10 Center Dr. MSC 1428
Bethesda, MA 20892-1428
USA

RICHARD B. BUXTON, PhD
Associate Professor, Department of Radiology
University of California at San Diego
200 West Arbor Drive
San Diego, CA 92103-8756
USA

JOSEPH H. CALLICOTT, MD
Clinical Brain Disorders Branch
National Institute of Mental Health, NIH
Building 10; Room 4S237A, MSC 1379
9000 Rockville Pike
Bethesda, MD 20892
USA

B.J. CASEY, PhD
Assistant Professor of Psychiatry & Psychology
Western Psychiatric Institute and Clinic, Room E-735
University of Pittsburgh Health System
3811 O'Hara Street
Pittsburgh, PA 15213
USA

WEI CHEN, PhD
Center for Magnetic Resonance Research
Department of Radiology
University of Minnesota, School of Medicine
3021 6th Street SE
Minneapolis, MN 55455
USA

ERIC R. COHEN, BS
Department of Radiology
Center for Magnetic Resonance Research
University of Minnesota Medical School
385 East River Road
Minneapolis, MN 55455
USA

MARK S. COHEN, PhD
Associate Professor
Ahmanson-Lovelake Brain Mapping Center, Room 215A
604 Charles E Young Drive South
Los Angeles, CA 90095-7085
USA

RICHARD J. DAVIDSON, PhD
Laboratory for Affective Neuroscience
University of Wisconsin-Madison
1202 West Johnson Street
Madison, WI 53706
USA

MICHEL DÉCORPS, PhD
INSERM U438 (RMN Bioclinique)
Université Joseph Fourier
Laboratoire de Neurobiophysique
Centre Hospitalier Universitaire
Pavillon B, BP 217
F-38043 Grenoble Cedex 9
France

CHANTAL DELON-MARTIN, PhD
INSERM U438 (RMN Bioclinique)
Université Joseph Fourier
Laboratoire de Neurobiophysique
Centre Hospitalier Universitaire
Pavillon B, BP 217
F-38043 Grenoble Cedex 9
France

MARK D'ESPOSITO, MD
Department of Neurology
Hospital of the University of Pennsylvania
3400 Spruce Street
Philadelphia, PA 19104-4283
USA

JOHN A. DETRE, MD
Departments of Neurology and Radiology
University of Pennsylvania School of Medicine
3400 Spruce Street
Philadelphia, PA 19104-4283
USA

JEFF H. DUYN, PhD
Laboratory of Diagnostic Radiology Research
Clinical Center
Building 10 Room B1N256
National Institutes of Health
9000 Rockville Pike
Bethesda MD 20892
USA

GUINEVERE F. EDEN, PhD
Assistant Professor
Georgetown Institute for Cognitive and Computational
Sciences
Georgetown University Medical Center
3870 Reservoir Road
Washington DC 20007
USA

JOSEPH A. FRANK, MD
Laboratory of Diagnostic Radiology, Clinical Center
National Institutes of Health
9000 Rockville Pike
Bethesda, MD 20892
USA

LAWRENCE R. FRANK, PhD
VA Medical Center
9114/MRI, 3350 La Jolla
San Diego, CA 92161
USA

KARL J. FRISTON, MD
The Wellcome Department of Cognitive Neurology
Institute of Neurology
12 Queen Square
London WC1N 3BG
UK

JOSEPH S. GATI, MSC
The Laboratory for Functional Magnetic Resonance
John P. Robarts Research Institute
P.O. Box 5015, 100 Perth Drive
London, Ontario
Canada N6A 5K8

GARY H. GLOVER, PhD
Department of Radiology
Stanford University School of Medicine
Lucas MR Center, MC 5488
Corner of Welch Road and Pasteur Drive
Stanford, CA 94305-5488
USA

RANDY GOLLUB, PhD
Department of Psychiatry
Massachusetts General Hospital
Psychiatric Neuroloimaging
Room 9109, Building 149
13th Street
Charleston, MA 02129
USA

BRAD GOODYEAR, MS
Laboratory for Functional Magnetic Resonance Research
University of Western Ontario
London, Ontario N6A 5K8
Canada

E. MARK HAACKE, PhD
Mallinckrodt Institute of Radiology
Washington University
St. Louis, MO 63110
USA

MARK HALLETT, MD
Clinical Director NINDS
Human Motor Control Section
National Institute of Neurological Disorders and Stroke
National Institutes Of Health
Building 10, Room 5N226, 10 Center Dr MSC 1428
Bethesda, MA 20892-1428
USA

THOMAS A. HAMMEKE, PhD
Department of Neurology (Neuropsychology)
Medical College of Wisconsin
9200 W.Wisconsin Avenue
Milwaukee, WI 53226
USA

MICHAEL P. HARMS
Speech and Hearing Sciences Program
Harvard-Massachusetts Institute of Technology
Division of Health Sciences and Technology
NMR-Center, Massachusetts General Hospital
149 Thirteenth St.
Charlestown, MA 02129
USA

JÜRGEN HENNIG, PhD
Professor
Uniklinik Freiburg, Radiologische Klinik
Abteilung Kernspintomographie
Hugstetterstrasse 55
D-79106 Freiburg
Germany

MANABU HONDA, MD, PhD
Research Associate
Department of Brain Pathophysiology
Kyoto University
School of Medicine
54 Shogoin
Sakyo, Kyoto 606-8507
Japan

XIAOPING HU, PhD
Associate Professor, Department of Radiology
Center for Magnetic Resonance Research
385 East River Road
Minneapolis, MN 55455
USA

WEI HUANG, PhD
Department of Radiology
State University of New York
Stony Brook, NY 11794
USA

JAMES S. HYDE, PhD
Biophysics Research Institute
Medical College of Wisconsin
8701 Watertown Plank Rd.
Milwaukee, WI 53226
USA

RISTO J. ILMONIEMI
BioMag Laboratory
Medical Engineering Centre
Helsinki University Central Hospital
P.O. Box 508
FIN-00029 HYKS
Finland

WILLIAM IRWIN, BS
Laboratory for Affective Neuroscience
University of Wisconsin-Madison
1202 West Johnson Street
Madison, WI 53706
USA

KENJI ISHII, MD
Visiting Scientist
Human Motor Control Section
National Institute of Neurological Disorders and Stroke
National Institutes of Health
Building 10, Room 5N226
10 Center Drive
MSC 1428
Bethesda, MA 20892-1428
USA

CLIFFORD R. JACK JR., MD
Department of Diagnostic Radiology and MR Research
Laboratory
Mayo Clinic and Foundation
200 First St SW,
Rochester, MN 55905
USA

C. JANZ, MD
Professor
Uniklinik Freiburg, Radiologische Klinik
Abteilung Kernspintomographie
Hugstetterstrasse 55
D-79106 Freiburg
Germany

PETER JEZZARD, PhD
Head of MR Physics
FMRIB Centre
Department of Clinical Neurology
John Radcliffe Hospital
University of Oxford
Headington, Oxford OX3 9DU
United Kingdom

ANDREAS KASTRUP, MD
Department of Radiology
Lucas MRS Center
Stanford University School of Medicine
1201 Welch Road
Stanford, CA 94305-5488
USA

RICHARD P. KENNAN, PhD
Professor, Department of Diagnostic Radiology
and Department of Biomedical Engineering
Yale University School of Medicine
333 Cedar Street, Fitkin B.
New Haven, CT 06510
USA

SEONG-GI KIM, PhD
CMRR (Center for Magnetic Resonance Research)
University of Minnesota Medical School
2021 Sixth Street S.E.
Minneapolis, MN 55455
USA

WOLFGANG KUSCHINSKY, MD
Professor
Department of Physiology
University of Heidelberg
Im Neuenheimer Feld 326
D-69120 Heidelberg
Germany

SONG LAI, MD
Department of Diagnostic
Imaging and Therapeutics
University of Connecticut
School of Medicine
263 Farmington Avenue
Farmington, CT 06030-2017
USA

L. LAMALLE, PhD
INSERM U438 (RMN Bioclinique)
Université Joseph Fourier
Laboratorie de Neurobiophysique
Center Hospitalier Universitaire
Pavillon B, BP 217
F-38043 Grenoble Cedex 9
France

NICHOLAS LANGE, MD
Associate Professor, Department of Psychiatry
Faculty of Medicine, Harvard University and
Chief Biostatistician, Brain Imaging Center, McLean Hospital
115 Mill Street
Belmont, MA 02178
USA

TUONG HUU LE, MD, PhD
Department of Radiology
Center for Magnetic Resonance Research
University of Minnesota Medical School
385 East River Road
Minneapolis, MN 55455
USA

CHRISTINE C. LEE, PhD
Department of Diagnostic Radiology and MR Research
Laboratory
Mayo Clinic and Foundation
200 First St SW,
Rochester, MN 55905
USA

SANG PIL LEE, MS
CMRR (Center for Magnetic Resonance Research)
University of Minnesota Medical School
2021 Sixth Street S.E.
Minneapolis, MN 55455
USA

TIE QIANG LI, PhD
Department of Radiology
Lucas MRS Center
Stanford University School of Medicine
1201 Welch Road
Stanford, CA 94305-5488
USA

PIERRE J. MAGISTRETTI, MD, PhD
Professor
Institute of Physiology and Department of Neurology
Université de Lausanne
7, Rue du Bugnon
CH-1005 Lausanne
Switzerland

RAPHAEL MASSARELLI, PhD
INSERM U438 (RMN Bioclinique)
Université Joseph Fourier
Laboratoire de Neurobiophysique
Centre Hospitalier Universitaire
Pavillon B, BP 217
F-38043 Grenoble Cedex 9
France

Venkata S. Mattay, MD
Clinical Brain Disorders Branch
National Institute of Mental Health
Building 10; Room B1D-125
National Institutes of Health
9000 Rockville Pike
Bethesda, MD 20892
USA

Bernard Mazoyer, PhD, MD
Professor of Radiology and Medical Imaging
Groupe d'Imagerie Neurofonctionnelle
UPRES EA 2127 Université de Caen, LRC-CEA n 13V
GIP Cyceron, BP 5229
F-14074 Caen
France

Alan C. McLaughlin, PhD
Clinical Brain Disorders Branch
National Institute of Mental Health
Building 10; Room B1D-125
National Institutes of Health
9000 Rockville Pike
Bethesda, MD 20892
USA

Jennifer R. Melcher, PhD
Assistant Professor of Otology and Laryngology
Harvard Medical School
Eaton-Peabody Laboratory
Massachusetts Eye and Ear Infirmary
243 Charles Street
Boston, MA 02114
USA

Ravi S. Menon, PhD
The Laboratory for Functional Magnetic Resonance
John P. Robarts Research Institute
P.O. Box 5015
100 Perth Drive
London, Ontario
Canada N6A 5K8

Chrit Moonen, PhD
Résonance Magnétique des Systèmes Biologiques
UMR 5536 CNRS/Université Victor Segalen Bordeaux 2
146 rue Léo-Saignat, Case 93
F-33076 Bordeaux Cedex
France

Michael E. Moseley, PhD
Associate Professor
Department of Radiology
Lucas MRS Center
Stanford University School of Medicine
1201 Welch Road
Stanford, CA 94305-5488
USA

Douglas C. Noll, PhD
MR Research Center
Department of Radiology
B-804 PUH
University of Pittsburgh Medical Center
200 Lothrop Street
Pittsburgh, PA 15213
USA

Seiji Ogawa, PhD
Biological Computation Research
Bell Laboratories / Lucent Technologies
700 Mountain Avenue
Murray Hill, NJ 07974
USA

Ildikó Pályka, PhD
Department of Chemistry
Brookhaven National Laboratory
State University of New York
Building 555
Stony Brook, NY 11973
USA

Clifford S. Patlak, PhD
Department of Surgery
State University of New York
Stony Brook, NY 11794
USA

Luc Pellerin, PhD
Institute of Physiology
Université de Lausanne
7, Rue du Bugnon
CH-1005 Lausanne
Switzerland

Scott J. Peltier, PhD
MR Research Center
Department of Radiology
B-804 PUH
University of Pittsburgh Medical Center
200 Lothrop Street
Pittsburgh, PA 15213
USA

Nick F. Ramsey, PhD
Assistent Professor, Department Psychiatry
University Hospital of Utrecht
Room A.01.126
Heidelberglaan 100
3584 CX, Utrecht
The Netherlands

Michael E. Ravicz, MS
Eaton-Peabody Laboratory
Massachusetts Eye and Ear Infirmary
Boston, MA 02114
USA

Stephen J. Riederer, PhD
Department of Diagnostic Radiology and MR Research
Laboratory
Mayo Clinic and Foundation
200 First St SW,
Rochester, MN 55905
USA

Robert Risinger, MD
Assistant Professor, Department of Psychiatry
Medical College of Wisconsin
8701 W. Watertown Plank Rd.
Milwaukee, WI 53226
USA

MEDICAL RADIOLOGY
Diagnostic Imaging and Radiation Oncology

Titles in the series already published

MEDICAL RADIOLOGY
Diagnostic Imaging and Radiation Oncology

Titles in the series already published